Medical Immunology
Seventh Edition

Medical Immunology
Seventh Edition

Edited by
Dr. Gabriel Virella
Medical University of South Carolina
Charleston, South Carolina, U.S.A.

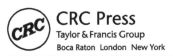

CRC Press
Taylor & Francis Group
Boca Raton London New York

CRC Press is an imprint of the
Taylor & Francis Group, an **informa** business

CRC Press
Taylor & Francis Group
6000 Broken Sound Parkway NW, Suite 300
Boca Raton, FL 33487-2742

First issued in paperback 2021

© 2020 by Taylor & Francis Group, LLC
CRC Press is an imprint of Taylor & Francis Group, an Informa business

No claim to original U.S. Government works

Printed on acid-free paper

ISBN-13: 978-0-367-22488-2 (hbk)
ISBN-13: 978-1-03-208777-1 (pbk)

Library of Congress Cataloging-in-Publication Data

Names: Virella, Gabriel, 1943- editor.
Title: Medical immunology / [edited by] Gabriel Virella.
Other titles: Medical immunology (Virella)
Description: 7th edition. | Boca Raton : Taylor & Francis, 2020. | Includes bibliographical references and index.
Identifiers: LCCN 2019018768| ISBN 9780367224882 (hardback : alk. paper) | ISBN 9780429278990 (ebook)
Subjects: | MESH: Immune System Phenomena | Immune System Diseases
Classification: LCC RC582 | NLM QW 504 | DDC 616.07/9--dc23
LC record available at https://lccn.loc.gov/2019018768

Visit the Taylor & Francis Web site at
http://www.taylorandfrancis.com

and the CRC Press Web site at
http://www.crcpress.com

This book is dedicated to my wife, Maria Lopes-Virella, my daughters, Isabel and Sara, and grandchildren, Daniel, Logan, Kelsey, Haley, and Samantha. Their love and friendship have been essential for me to keep active and willing to take on a task as demanding as preparing a seventh edition of Medical Immunology *33 years after the first edition.*

Contents

Preface

Thirty-three years ago, in 1986, the first edition of *Introduction to Medical Immunology* was published. I could not have imagined then that 33 years later I would be editing the seventh edition of *Medical Immunology*. This is a classic text in a traditional format, ideal for presenting clinically relevant and updated content from the overwhelming flow of information in the literature. Purposely, we emphasize knowledge for which there is a clear clinical application (or at the very least a clear experimental proof of concept). I believe that this approach is best suited for a general introductory book that provides a good balance between basic and clinical science.

This new edition of *Medical Immunology* has been thoroughly revised and reorganized following the described general guidelines.

The scientific basis of immunology is clearly conveyed in a general and succinct overview, including coverage of important emerging topics in terms that should be accessible to nonimmunologists, with emphasis on the application to medicine. The book should stimulate readers to seek more information and further develop their own education. Lists of recommended readings are included in each chapter.

The book starts with basic immunology followed by diagnostic immunology. We give special attention to diagnostic immunology because this area has fertile applications and has been the basis for important new knowledge. The last 15 chapters of this book are dedicated to clinical immunology, and the chapters have been thoroughly revised and updated. The final section on immunodeficiency diseases reflects the extraordinary significance of immunodeficiency diseases in clinical immunology. The study of primary immune deficiencies gives the best perspective about the intimate works of the human immune system, and secondary immunodeficiencies (including those caused iatrogenically as well as HIV induced) are encountered in virtually all fields of medicine.

The result is a concise book that conveys our collective intrinsic fascination with a discipline that seeks understanding of fundamental biological knowledge, with the goal of applying that knowledge to the diagnosis and treatment of human diseases.

Gabriel Virella, MD, PhD

Acknowledgments

I wish to acknowledge the efforts of all contributors to this book. Without their dedication and professionalism, this new edition of *Medical Immunology* would not have been possible. Also, the students at our medical school who continue to seek my guidance in the complex and ever-expanding field of immunology are responsible for my continuing interest in providing a concise introductory book for those wishing to open the door to a fundamental area of medical knowledge.

Editor

Gabriel Virella obtained his MD and PhD degrees at the University of Lisbon, Portugal, in 1967 and 1974. He completed postdoctoral studies in immunology at the Department of Experimental Pathology, University of Birmingham, England (1968–1969) and at the National Institute for Medical Research, Mill Hill, London, England (1969–1970). From 1970 to 1975, he was a researcher at the Gulbenkian Institute of Science, Oeiras, Portugal. He moved to the Medical University of South Carolina (MUSC) in 1975, where he is an emeritus professor of Immunology and Microbiology. He has published 260 articles in topics related primarily to immunology, with particular emphasis on the involvement of autoimmune phenomena in the pathogenesis of atherosclerosis. He has described original techniques for the isolation and characterization of antigen-antibody complexes, immunoassays for tetanus and diphtheria antibodies, and for the assay of modified LDL and corresponding antibodies. In 1989 he was corecipient with Drs. Christoph Gisinger and Maria F. Lopes-Virella of the Squibb Award of the Austrian Society of Internal Medicine for the work entitled "Metabolic Effects of Lipoprotein Immune Complexes in Macrophages." He co-edited the first edition of *Introduction to Medical Immunology* in 1986 and became the single editor of the third edition in 1993. The fourth edition (1999) was translated into Italian. He has now edited the seventh edition of *Medical Immunology*. In addition, he published *NMS Microbiology and Infectious Diseases*, third edition (1997), and *NMS Q&A: Microbiology, Immunology, and Infectious Diseases* (1999). He was section editor of *Clinical Immunology* from 1989 to 2003. During his tenure at the Medical University of South Carolina, he received numerous teaching awards from the students, the Health Sciences Foundation Teaching Excellence Award, MUSC in 1996 and 2006, Governor's Distinguished Professor Award in 1996 and 2006, the National AΩA Robert J. Glaser Distinguished Teacher Award in 2003, and was cited as Master Teacher by the Board of Trustees of the Medical University of South Carolina in 2007.

Contributors

Carl Atkinson PhD
Departments of Microbiology and
Immunology, and Surgery
Medical University of South Carolina
Charleston, South Carolina

José C. Crispín MD PhD
Department of Immunology and
Rheumatology
Instituto Nacional de Ciencias Médicas y
Nutrición Salvador Zubirán
Mexico City, Mexico

Stephen Elmore MD
Department of Rheumatology and Clinical
Immunology
Medical University of South Carolina
Charleston, South Carolina

Albert F. Finn, Jr. MD
Department of Medicine
Medical University of South Carolina
Charleston, South Carolina

Armand Glassman MD
Department of Microbiology and
Immunology
Medical University of South Carolina
Charleston, South Carolina

Ajay Grover PhD
Hematology/Flow Cytometry
Covance Inc.
Indianapolis, Indiana

Jane C. Kilkenny MD
Department of Surgery
Medical University of South Carolina
Charleston, South Carolina

Ellen Klohe PhD D(ABHI)
HLA Laboratory
Inland Northwest Blood Center
Spokane, Washington

Virginia Litwin PhD
Immunology
Caprion Biosciences Inc.
Montreal, Canada

Damien Montamat-Sicotte PhD
ImmuneCarta
Caprion Biosciences Inc.
Montreal, Canada

Joseph Murphy PhD
ImmunePCS LLC
Boston, Massachusetts

Satish N. Nadig MD PhD FACS
Departments of Surgery,
Pediatrics-Critical Care, and
Microbiology and Immunology
Medical University of
South Carolina
Charleston, South Carolina

Janardan P. Pandey PhD
Department of Microbiology and
Immunology
Medical University of South Carolina
Charleston, South Carolina

Richard M. Silver MD
Department of Rheumatology and Clinical
Immunology
Medical University of South Carolina
Charleston, South Carolina

John W. Sleasman MD
Division of Allergy, Immunology,
and Pulmonary Medicine
Department of Pediatrics
Duke University School of Medicine
Durham, North Carolina

Scott Sugden PhD
ImmuneCarta
Caprion Biosciences Inc.
Montreal, Canada

George C. Tsokos MD
Department of Medicine
Beth Israel Deaconess Medical Center
Harvard Medical School
Boston, Massachusetts

Juan Carlos Varela MD PhD
Blood and Marrow Transplant Program
Florida Hospital Cancer Institute
Orlando, Florida

Gabriel Virella MD PhD
Department of Microbiology and
Immunology
Medical University of South Carolina
Charleston, South Carolina

Karen K. Yam PhD
ImmuneCarta
Caprion Biosciences Inc.
Montreal, Canada

Bader Yassine Diab PhD
ImmuneCarta
Caprion Biosciences Inc.
Montreal, Canada

Introduction

GABRIEL VIRELLA

HISTORICAL OVERVIEW

The fundamental observation that led to the development of immunology as a scientific discipline was that an individual might become resistant for life to a certain disease after having contracted it only once. The term *immunity*, derived from the Latin "immunis" (exempt), was adopted to designate this naturally acquired protection against diseases such as measles or smallpox.

The emergence of immunology as a discipline was closely tied to the development of microbiology. The work of Pasteur, Koch, Metchnikoff, and of many other pioneers of the golden age of microbiology resulted in the rapid identification of new infectious agents. This was closely followed by the discovery that infectious diseases could be prevented by exposure to killed or attenuated organisms, or to compounds extracted from the infectious agents. The impact of immunization against infectious diseases such as tetanus, mumps, diphtheria, poliomyelitis, and smallpox, to name just a few examples, can be grasped when we reflect on the fact that these diseases, which were significant causes of mortality and morbidity, are now either extinct or very rarely seen. Indeed, it is fair to state that the impact of vaccination and sanitation on the welfare and life expectancy of humans has had no parallel in any other developments of medical science.

In the second part of this century, immunology started to transcend its early boundaries and became a more general biomedical discipline. Today, the study of immunological defense mechanisms is still an important area of research, but immunologists are involved in a much wider array of problems, such as self and non-self discrimination, control of cell and tissue differentiation, transplantation, immunomodulation of autoimmune diseases, cancer immunotherapy, etc. The focus of interest has shifted toward the basic understanding of how the immune system works in the hope that this insight will allow novel approaches to its manipulation.

GENERAL CONCEPTS

Specific and nonspecific defenses

The protection of our organism against infectious agents involves many different mechanisms, some nonspecific (i.e., generically applicable to many different pathogenic organisms) and others specific (i.e., their protective effect is directed to one single organism).

Nonspecific defenses, which as a rule are innate (i.e., all normal individuals are born with them), include the following:

- Mechanical barriers such as the integrity of the epidermis and mucosal membranes
- Physicochemical barriers, such as the acidity of the stomach fluid
- Antibacterial substances (e.g., lysozyme, defensins) present in external secretions
- Normal intestinal transit and normal flow of bronchial secretions and urine, which eliminate infectious agents from the respective systems
- Nonimmune mechanisms for ingestion of bacteria and particulate matter by a variety of cells, but particularly well developed in **granulocytes**

Specific defenses, as a rule, are induced during the life of the individual as part of the complex sequence of events designated as the immune response. The immune response has two unique characteristics:

- **Specificity for the eliciting antigen**, for example, immunization with inactivated poliovirus only protects against poliomyelitis, not against viral influenza. The specificity of the immune response is due to the existence of exquisitely discriminative antigen receptors on lymphocytes. Only a single or a very limited number of similar structures (epitopes) can be accommodated by the receptors of any given lymphocyte. When those receptors are occupied, an activating signal is delivered to the lymphocytes. Therefore, only those lymphocytes with specific

receptors for the antigen in question will be activated. A significant caveat, however, is that epitopes may be unexpectedly shared by microbial organisms and human tissues, and this may result in the emergence of antibodies reacting with totally unrelated entities. One classical example is antibodies elicited by intestinal bacteria that react with the AB antigens of human red cells, as discussed in detail in Chapter 14.

- **Memory**, meaning that repeated exposure to a given antigen elicits progressively more intense specific responses. Most immunizations involve repeated administration of the immunizing compound, with the goal of establishing a long-lasting, protective response. The increase in the magnitude and duration of the immune response with repeated exposure to the same antigen is due to the proliferation of antigen-specific lymphocytes after each exposure. The numbers of responding cells will remain increased even after the immune response subsides. Therefore, whenever the organism is exposed again to that particular antigen, there is an expanded population of specific lymphocytes available for activation, and as a consequence, the time needed to mount a response is shorter and the magnitude of the response is higher. This immunological memory is more effectively induced by protein antigens.

Stages of immune response

To better understand how the immune response is generated, it is useful to consider it as divided into

Table 1.1 Simplified overview of the three main stages of the immune response

Stage of the immune response	Induction	Amplification	Effector
Cells/molecules involved	Antigen-presenting cells; lymphocytes	Antigen-presenting cells; helper T lymphocytes	Antibodies (+ complement or cytotoxic cells); cytotoxic T lymphocytes; macrophages
Mechanisms	Processing and/or presentation of antigen; recognition by specific receptors on lymphocytes	Release of cytokines; signals mediated by interaction between membrane molecules	Complement-mediated lysis; phagocytosis; cytotoxicity
Consequences	Activation of T and B lymphocytes	Proliferation and differentiation of T and B lymphocytes	Elimination of non-self; neutralization of toxins and viruses

separate sequential stages (Table 1.1). The first stage (**induction**) involves a small lymphocyte population with specific receptors able to recognize an antigen or antigen fragments generated by specialized cells known as antigen-presenting cells (APCs). The second stage (amplification) is mediated by activated APCs and by specialized T cell subpopulations (T-helper cells, defined later) that enhance each other's proliferation and differentiation. This is followed by the production of effector molecules (antibodies) or by the differentiation of effector cells (cells that directly or indirectly mediate the elimination of undesirable elements). The final outcome, therefore, is the elimination of the organism or compound that triggered the reaction by means of activated immune cells or by defensive reactions triggered by mediators released by the immune system.

CELLS OF IMMUNE SYSTEM

Lymphocytes and lymphocyte subpopulations

The peripheral blood contains two large populations of cells: the red cells, whose main physiological role is to carry oxygen to tissues, and the white blood cells, which have as their main physiological role the elimination of potentially harmful organisms or compounds. Among the white blood cells, lymphocytes are particularly important because of their central role in the adaptive immune response. Several subpopulations of lymphocytes have been defined:

- **B lymphocytes**, which are the precursors of antibody-producing cells, known as plasma cells.
- **T lymphocytes**, which can be divided into several subpopulations:
  - **Helper T lymphocytes (Th)**, which play a significant amplification role in the immune response. Two functionally distinct subpopulations of T-helper lymphocytes emerging from a precursor population (Th0) have been defined. In broad strokes, the Th1 population assists the differentiation of cytotoxic cells and also activates macrophages. Activated macrophages, in turn, play a role as effectors of the immune response. The Th2 lymphocytes, in turn, are mainly involved in the amplification of B-lymphocyte responses.

    The amplifying effects of helper T lymphocytes are mediated in part by soluble

mediators—(cytokines)—and in part by signals delivered as a consequence of cell-cell interactions.

- **Cytotoxic T lymphocytes**, which are the main immunologic effector mechanism involved in the elimination of non-self or infected cells.
- **Immunoregulatory T lymphocytes**, which have the ability to downregulate the immune response through the release of cytokines such as interleukin-10 (IL-10) and through the expression of membrane molecules, such as CTLA-4, whose interaction with the corresponding receptors delivers a downregulatory signal.

Antigen-presenting cells (APC)

Antigen-presenting cells (APCs), such as the dendritic cells and the macrophages and macrophage-related cells, play a significant role in the induction stages of the immune response by trapping and presenting both native antigens and antigen fragments in a most favorable way for recognition by lymphocytes. In addition, these cells deliver activating signals to lymphocytes engaged in antigen recognition, both in the form of soluble mediators (interleukins such as IL-1, IL-12, and IL-18) and in the form of signals delivered by cell-cell contact.

The monocytes and macrophages also play significant roles as effectors of the immune response. One of their main functions is to eliminate antigens that have elicited an immune response. Antigens coated by antibodies and complement are ingested and digested after recognition by receptors for antibodies and complement on the membrane of monocytes and macrophages. However, if the antigen is located on the surface of a cell, antibody induces the attachment of cytotoxic cells that cause the death of the antibody-coated cell (**antibody-dependent cellular cytotoxicity [ADCC]**).

Natural killer (NK) cells

Natural killer (NK) cells play a dual role in the elimination of infected and malignant cells. These cells are unique in that they have two different mechanisms of recognition: they can identify malignant or viral-infected cells by their decreased expression of histocompatibility antigens, and they can recognize antibody-coated cells and mediate ADCC.

ANTIGENS AND ANTIBODIES

Antigens are usually exogenous substances (cells, proteins, and polysaccharides) that are recognized by receptors on lymphocytes, thereby eliciting the immune response. The receptor molecules located on the membrane of lymphocytes interact with small portions of those foreign cells or proteins, designated as antigenic determinants or epitopes. An adult human being has the capability to recognize millions of different antigens, and consequently produce antibodies, proteins that appear in circulation after infection or immunization and that have the ability to react specifically with epitopes of the antigen introduced in the organism. Because antibodies are soluble and are present in virtually all body fluids ("humors"), the term *humoral immunity* was introduced to designate the immune responses in which antibodies play the principal role as effector mechanism. Antibodies are also generically designated as immunoglobulins. This term derives from the fact that antibody molecules structurally belong to the family of proteins known as globulins (globular proteins) and from their involvement in immunity.

Antigen-antibody reactions, complement, and opsonization

The knowledge that the serum of an immunized animal contained protein molecules able to bind specifically to the antigen led to exhaustive investigations of the characteristics and consequences of the antigen-antibody reactions. At a morphological level, two types of reactions were defined:

- If the antigen is soluble, the reaction with specific antibody under appropriate conditions results in precipitation of aggregates.
- If the antigen is expressed on a cell membrane, cells carrying the antigen will be cross-linked by antibody and form visible clumps (agglutination).

Functionally, antigen-antibody reactions can be classified by their biological consequences:

- Viruses and soluble toxins released by bacteria lose their infectivity or pathogenic properties after reaction with the corresponding antibodies (neutralization).
- Antibodies complexed with antigens can activate the complement system. Nine major proteins or components that are sequentially activated constitute this system. Some of the complement components are able to promote ingestion of microorganisms by phagocytic cells, while others are inserted into cytoplasmic membranes and cause their disruption, leading to lysis of the offending microbial cell.
- Antibodies can cause the destruction of microorganisms by promoting their ingestion by phagocytic cells or their destruction by cells mediating ADCC. Phagocytosis is particularly important for the elimination of bacteria and involves the binding of antibodies and complement components to the outer surface of the infectious agent (opsonization) and recognition of the bound antibody and/or complement components as a signal for ingestion by the phagocytic cell.
- Antigen-antibody reactions are the basis of certain pathological conditions, such as allergic reactions. Allergic reactions have a very rapid onset, in a matter of minutes, and are also known as immediate hypersensitivity reactions.

LYMPHOCYTES AND CELL-MEDIATED IMMUNITY

Lymphocytes play a significant role as effector cells in three main types of situations, all of them considered as expression of cell-mediated immunity, i.e., immune reactions in which T lymphocytes are the predominant effector cells.

Immune elimination of intracellular infectious agents

Viruses, and some bacteria, parasites, and fungi have developed strategies that allow them to survive inside phagocytic cells or cells of other types. Infected cells are generally not amenable to destruction by phagocytosis or complement-mediated lysis. The study of how the immune system recognizes and eliminates infected cells resulted in the definition of the biological role of the histocompatibility antigens (human leukocyte antigens [HLAs]) that had been described as responsible for graft rejection (see the next section). Those membrane molecules have a peptide-binding pouch that needs to be occupied, with peptides derived either from endogenous or from exogenous proteins. The immune system does not recognize self peptides associated with self HLA molecules. In the case of infected cells, peptides split from microbial proteins synthesized by the infected cell as part of the microbial replication cycle become associated with HLA molecules. The HLA-peptide complexes are presented to the immune system and activate specific cytotoxic T lymphocytes as well as specific Th1 lymphocytes. Both cytotoxic T cells and Th1 lymphocytes can mediate killing of the infected cells against which they became sensitized. Cytotoxic T cells kill the infected cells directly, stopping the replication of the intracellular organism, while activated Th1 cells release cytokines, such as interferon-γ, which activate macrophages and increase their ability to destroy the intracellular infectious agents.

Transplant (graft) rejection

As stated in the previous section, the immune system does not respond (i.e., is tolerant) to self antigens, including antigens of the major histocompatibility complex (MHC), which includes the HLA molecules. However, transplantation of tissues among genetically different individuals of the same species or across species is followed by rejection of the grafted organs or tissues. The rejection reaction can be triggered by the presentation of peptides generated from non-self MHC molecules or, also possibly, for the direct recognition of non-self MHC molecules by the recipient's T cell.

Delayed hypersensitivity

While the elimination of intracellular infectious agents can be considered as the main physiological role of cell-mediated immunity and graft rejection is an unexpected and undesirable consequence of a medical procedure, other lymphocyte-mediated immune reactions can be considered as pathological conditions arising spontaneously in genetically predisposed individuals. The most common examples are skin reactions induced by direct skin contact or by intradermal injection of antigenic substances. These reactions express themselves 24–48 hours after exposure to an antigen to which the patient had been previously sensitized, and because of this timing factor received the designation of delayed hypersensitivity reactions.

SELF VERSUS NON-SELF KEEP NON-SELF DISCRIMINATION

The immune response is triggered by the interaction of an antigenic determinant with specific receptors on lymphocytes. It is calculated that there are several millions of different receptors in lymphocytes—10^{15} to 10^{18} on T cells and 10^{11} on B cells—sufficient to respond to a wide diversity of epitopes presented by microbial agents and potentially noxious exogenous compounds. At the same time, the immune system has the capacity to generate lymphocytes with receptors able to interact with epitopes expressed by self antigens. During embryonic differentiation and adult life, the organism uses a variety of mechanisms to ensure that potentially autoreactive lymphocytes are eliminated or turned off. This lack of response is known as tolerance to self.

When the immune system is exposed to exogenous compounds, it tends to develop a vigorous immune response. The discrimination between self and non-self is based the fact that the immune system has the ability to recognize a wide variety of structural differences on exogenous compounds. For example, infectious agents have marked differences in their chemical structure, easily recognizable by the immune system. Cells, proteins, and polysaccharides from animals of different species have differences in chemical constitution that, as a rule, are directly related to the degree of phylogenetic divergence between species. Those also elicit potent immune responses. Finally, many polysaccharides and proteins from individuals of any given species show antigenic heterogeneity, reflecting the genetic diversity of individuals within a species. Those differences are usually minor (relative to differences between species) but can still be recognized by the immune system. Transfusion reactions, graft rejection, and hypersensitivity reactions to exogenous human proteins are clinical expressions of the recognition of this type of differences between individuals.

GENERAL OVERVIEW

One of the most difficult intellectual exercises in immunology is to try to understand the global organization and control of the immune system. Its extreme complexity and the wide array of regulatory circuits involved in fine-tuning the immune response pose a formidable obstacle to our understanding. A diagrammatic depiction of the main elements and steps involved in the adaptive immune response is reproduced in Figure 1.1.

If we use as an example the activation of the immune system by an infectious agent that has managed to overcome the innate anti-infectious defenses, the first step in the induction of an immune response is the uptake of the infectious agent by a cell capable of degrading it and presenting fragments to cells involved in the adaptive immune response. A variety of cells can function as APCs, mainly tissue macrophages and dendritic cells. Those cells adsorb and ingest the infectious agent that is then broken down into small antigenic subunits. These subunits become intracellularly associated with histocompatibility antigens of the MHC-II family, and the resulting complex is transported to the cytoplasmic membrane, allowing stimulation of helper T lymphocytes. The interaction between surface proteins expressed by APCs and T lymphocytes, as well as signals delivered by cytokines released by the APCs, act as costimulants of the helper T cells. B cells can recognize epitopes in free or cell-associated antigens that do not need to be associated with an MHC molecule. It is well established that the activation of an immune response takes place in a lymphoid organ (lymph

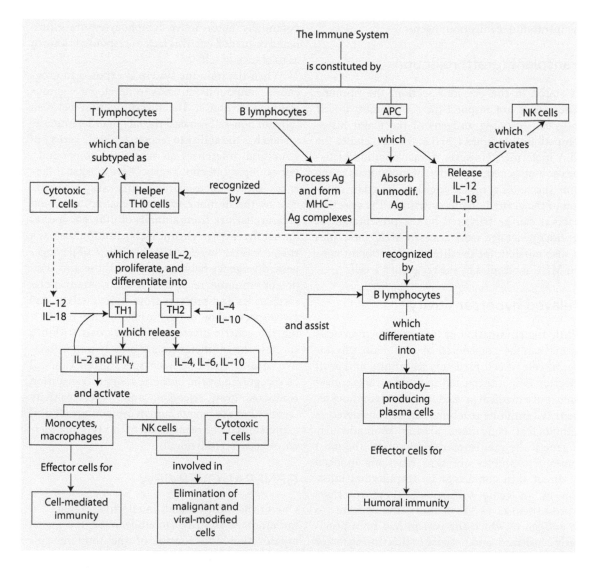

Figure 1.1 The major elements involved in the adaptive immune response.

node, peri-intestinal lymphoid tissues, spleen). All cellular elements necessary for the inductive and effector stages of an immune response are present on the lymphoid tissues, where there is ample opportunity for interactions and cooperation between those different cells.

Once stimulated to proliferate and differentiate, helper T cells become able to assist the differentiation of effector cells. However, not all helper T cells seem to assist all types of effector cells that require their help. In broad strokes, activated Th1 helper lymphocytes secrete cytokines that act on a variety of cells, including macrophages (further increasing their level of activation and enhancing their ability to eliminate infectious agents that may be surviving intracellularly), and cytotoxic T cells, which are very efficient in the elimination of virus-infected cells. In contrast, activated Th2 helper lymphocytes secrete a different set of cytokines that will assist the proliferation and differentiation of antigen-stimulated B lymphocytes which, in turn, will differentiate into plasma cells. The plasma cells are engaged in the synthesis of large amounts of antibody.

As stated earlier, antibodies are the main effector molecules of the humoral immune response. As specific antibodies bind to a microorganism, a complex series of proteins, the complement system, is activated, and the microorganisms will either be ingested and destroyed by phagocytic cells or be killed by complement-mediated lysis or by leukocytes able to mediate ADCC.

Once the microorganism is removed, negative feedback mechanisms become predominant, turning off the immune response. The downregulation of the immune response appears to result from the combination of several factors, such as the elimination of the positive stimulus that the microorganism represented, and the activation of lymphocytes with immunoregulatory activity that secrete cytokines that deliver inactivating signals to other lymphocytes.

At the end of the immune response, a residual population of long-lived lymphocytes specific for the offending antigen will remain. This is the population of memory cells that is responsible for protection after natural exposure or immunization. It is also the same generic cell subpopulation that may cause accelerated graft rejections in recipients of multiple grafts. As discussed in greater detail in the next section, the same immune system that protects us can be responsible for a variety of pathological conditions.

IMMUNOLOGY AND MEDICINE

Immunological concepts have found ample applications in medicine, in areas related to diagnosis, treatment, prevention, and pathogenesis.

The exquisite specificity of the antigen-antibody reaction has been extensively applied to the development of diagnostic assays for a variety of substances. Such applications received a strong boost when experiments with malignant plasma cell lines and normal antibody-producing cells resulted serendipitously in the discovery of the technique of hybridoma production, the basis for the production of monoclonal antibodies, which have had an enormous impact in the fields of diagnosis and immunotherapy.

Immunotherapy has been applied to a variety of diseases, ranging from neoplasias and autoimmune diseases to atherosclerosis. Efforts to stimulate the immune system of patients with malignancies have also met with some success. A major area of interest has been the induction of tolerance to grafts, but the excellent results obtained in studies with animal models have not been replicated in humans. In transplantation, the main clinical successes have been obtained in the prevention and treatment of graft rejection with monoclonal antibodies directed against the T cells involved in graft rejection.

The study of children with deficient development of their immune system (immunodeficiency diseases) has provided the best tools for the study of the immune system in humans, while at the same time giving us ample opportunity to devise corrective therapies. The acquired immunodeficiency syndrome (AIDS) underscored the delicate balance that is maintained between the immune system and infectious agents in the healthy individual and has stimulated a considerable amount of basic research into the regulation of the immune system.

The importance of maintaining self tolerance in adult life is obvious when we consider the consequences of the loss of tolerance. Several diseases, some affecting single organs, others of a systemic nature, have been classified as autoimmune diseases. In those diseases, the immune system reacts against cells and tissues, and this reactivity can either be the primary insult leading to the disease or may represent a factor contributing to the evolution and increasing severity of the disease.

Considerable effort has been dedicated to the study of conditions that could reconstitute the state of tolerance in these patients, but so far without clinical translation. The use of monoclonal antibodies or soluble receptors able to curtain the inflammatory reaction has been successfully applied to a variety of autoimmune and hypersensitivity diseases, such as asthma.

In the following chapters of this book, we illustrate the productive interaction that has always existed in immunology between basic concepts and clinical applications. In fact, no other biological discipline illustrates better the importance of the interplay between basic and clinical scientists; this is the main reason for the prominence of immunology as a biomedical discipline.

2

Leukocytes and lymphoid tissues: The framework of the immune system

GABRIEL VIRELLA

INTRODUCTION

The fully developed immune system of humans and most mammalians is constituted by a variety of cells and tissues whose different functions are remarkably well integrated. Among the cells, the lymphocytes play the key roles in the control and regulation of immune responses as well as in the recognition of infected or heterologous cells, which the lymphocytes can recognize as undesirable and promptly eliminate. Among the tissues, the thymus is the site of differentiation for T lymphocytes, and as such, is directly involved in critical steps in the differentiation of the immune system.

CELLS OF IMMUNE SYSTEM

Lymphocytes

The lymphocytes (Figure 2.1a) occupy a very special place among the leukocytes that participate in one way or another in immune reactions due to their ability to recognize non-self antigenic determinants and be consequentially activated. Lymphocytes differentiate from stem cells in the fetal liver, bone marrow, and thymus and are found in the peripheral blood and in all lymphoid tissues. They exist as two main functional classes.

B lymphocytes or **B cells** are so designated because the bursa of Fabricius, a lymphoid organ located close to the caudal end of the gut in birds, plays a key role in their differentiation in birds. Removal of this organ, at or shortly before hatching, is associated with lack of differentiation, maturation of B lymphocytes, and the inability to produce antibodies. A mammalian counterpart to the avian bursa has not yet been found. Some investigators believe that the bone marrow is the most likely organ for B-lymphocyte differentiation, while others propose that the peri-intestinal lymphoid tissues play this role.

B lymphocytes carry immunoglobulins on their cell membrane, which function as antigen receptors. As a consequence of that interaction, B cells are activated and undergo blastogenic transformation. After several rounds of division, they differentiate into antibody-producing cells (plasma cells). Activated B lymphocytes may also play the role of antigen-presenting cells, more commonly played by cells of monocytic/macrophagic lineage (see Chapters 3 and 4).

T lymphocytes or **T cells** are so designated because the thymus plays a key role in their differentiation. The functions of the T lymphocytes include the regulation of immune responses, and various effector functions (cytotoxicity and

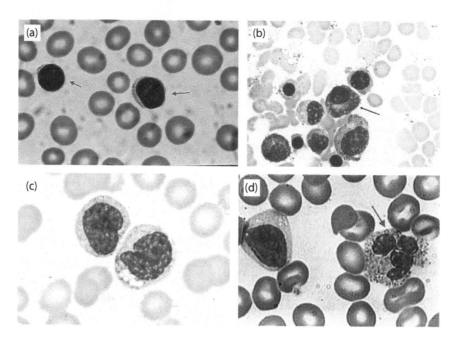

Figure 2.1 Morphology of the main types of human leukocytes: (a) lymphocyte, (b) plasma cell, (c) monocyte, (d) granulocyte. (Reproduced with permission from Reich PR. *Manual of Hematology.* Upjohn, Kalamazoo, MI, 1976.)

lymphokine production being the main ones) that are the basis of cell-mediated immunity (CMI). T lymphocytes also carry antigen-recognition units on their membranes, known as T-cell receptors (TCRs). TCRs and immunoglobulin molecules are structurally unrelated.

Several subpopulations of T lymphocytes with separate functions have been identified:

- **Helper T lymphocytes** are involved in the induction and regulation of immune responses.
- **Cytotoxic T lymphocytes** are involved in the elimination of infected cells.
- **Regulatory T cells (T_{reg})** have regulatory functions, and it appears that there are several subpopulations of regulatory T lymphocytes with the capacity to suppress immune responses.

Membrane markers have been used to define T-lymphocyte subpopulations, although it seems obvious that the phenotype can only be correlated with a predominant function, not to the exclusion of others. For example, it is possible to differentiate cells with predominant helper function from those with predominant cytotoxic function, but it is well known that phenotypically helper T lymphocytes can also behave as cytotoxic effector cells.

T lymphocytes have a longer life span than B lymphocytes. Long-lasting lymphocytes are particularly important because of their involvement in immunological memory.

T-lymphocyte activation requires the interaction of the T-cell receptor with an antigen-derived polypeptide and additional costimulatory signals from auxiliary cells. When properly stimulated, a small, resting T lymphocyte rapidly undergoes blastogenic transformation into a large lymphocyte (13–15 μm). This large lymphocyte (lymphoblast) then divides several times to produce an expanded population of medium (9–12 μm) and small lymphocytes (5–8 μm) with the same antigenic specificity. Activated and differentiated T lymphocytes are morphologically indistinguishable from a small, resting lymphocyte.

Plasma cells are morphologically characterized by their eccentric nuclei with clumped chromatin and a large cytoplasm with abundant rough endoplasmic reticulum (Figure 2.1b). Plasma cells produce and secrete large amounts of immunoglobulins but do not express membrane immunoglobulins. Plasma cells divide very poorly, if at all. Plasma cells are usually found in the bone marrow and in the perimucosal lymphoid tissues.

Natural killer (NK) cells morphologically are described as large granular lymphocytes. These cells do not carry antigen receptors of any kind but can recognize antibody molecules bound to target cells and destroy those cells using the same general mechanisms involved in T-lymphocyte cytotoxicity (antibody-dependent cellular cytotoxicity). They also have a recognition mechanism that allows them to destroy tumor cells and viral-infected cells.

Antigen-presenting cells: Monocytes, macrophages, and dendritic cells

Monocytes and macrophages are closely related. The monocyte (Figure 2.1c) is considered a leukocyte in transit through the blood which, when "fixed" in a tissue, will become a macrophage. Monocytes and macrophages, as well as granulocytes (see later in chapter), are able to ingest particulate matter (microorganisms, cells, inert particles) and for this reason are said to have phagocytic functions. The phagocytic activity is greater in macrophages (particularly after activation by soluble mediators released during immune responses) than in monocytes.

Macrophages and monocytes play an important role in the inductive stages of the immune response by processing complex antigens and presenting antigen-derived oligopeptides associated with class II major histocompatibility complex (MHC-II) on the cell membrane. In this form, the oligopeptides are recognized by helper T lymphocytes, as discussed in detail in Chapters 3 and 4. For this reason, these cells are antigen-presenting cells (APCs). The most specialized and efficient APCs are the dendritic cells, which are also heterogenous, including at least two populations, one of myeloid origin and the other of lymphoid origin. Some dendritic cells tend to be present in tissues such as the kidney, brain (microglia), capillary walls, and mucosae. In the resting state they seem very inefficient as APCs, but after activation by microbial substances or other stimuli, they migrate to the lymphoid tissues where they differentiate into efficient APCs, able to stimulate naive T cells. The **Langerhans cells** of the epidermis are of myeloid origin and are the prototype for migrating dendritic cells. When they reach the lymph nodes, Langerhans cells assume the morphological characteristics of dendritic cells (Figure 2.2) and interact with T lymphocytes and B lymphocytes, as described in Chapter 4.

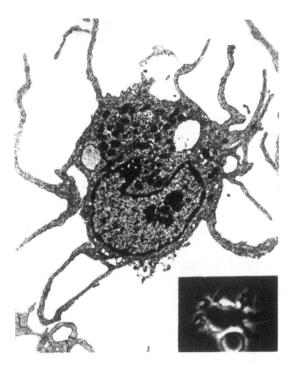

Figure 2.2 Electron microphotograph of a follicular dendritic cell isolated from a rat lymph node (×5000). The inset illustrates the *in vitro* interaction between a dendritic cell and a lymphocyte as seen in phase contrast microscopy (×300). (Reproduced with permission from Klinkert WEF. et al. *Proc Natl Acad Sci USA,* 1980;77:5414.)

A defining property of all APCs is the expression of a special class of histocompatibility antigens, designated as class-II MHC antigens (see Chapter 3). The expression of MHC-II molecules is essential for the interaction with helper T lymphocytes. APCs also release cytokines that assist the proliferation of antigen-stimulated lymphocytes, including interleukins-1, -6, and -12.

Another type of cell involved in the inductive stages of the immune response is the follicular dendritic cell, present in the spleen and lymph nodes, particularly in follicles and germinal centers. This cell, apparently of monocytic lineage, is not phagocytic and does not express MHC-II molecules on the membrane but appears particularly suited to carry out the antigen-presenting function in relation to B lymphocytes. Follicular dendritic cells concentrate unprocessed antigen on microvesicles of the membrane and keep it there for relatively long periods of time, a factor that may be crucial for a sustained B-cell response. The follicular dendritic cells form a network in the germinal centers, known as the antigen-retaining reticulum.

Granulocytes

Granulocytes are a collection of white blood cells with segmented or lobulated nuclei and granules in their cytoplasm, which are visible with special stains. Because of their segmented nuclei, which assume variable sizes and shapes, these cells are generically designated as polymorphonuclear (PMN) leukocytes (Figure 2.1d). Different subpopulations of granulocytes (neutrophils, eosinophils, and basophils) can be distinguished by differential staining of the cytoplasmic granules, reflecting their different chemical constitution.

Neutrophils are the largest subpopulation of white blood cells and have two types of cytoplasmic granules containing compounds with bactericidal activity. Their biological importance derives from their phagocytic activity. As most other phagocytic cells, they ingest with greatest efficiency microorganisms and particulate matter coated by antibody and complement (see Chapter 9). However, nonimmunological mechanisms have also been shown to lead to phagocytosis by neutrophils, perhaps reflecting phylogenetically more primitive mechanisms of recognition.

Neutrophils are attracted by chemotactic factors to areas of inflammation. Those factors may be released by microbes (particularly bacteria) or may be generated during complement activation as a consequence of an antigen-antibody reaction. The attraction of neutrophils is especially intense in bacterial infections. Great numbers of neutrophils may die trying to eliminate the invading bacteria. Dead PMN leukocytes and their debris become the primary component of pus, characteristic of many bacterial infections. Bacterial infections associated with the formation of pus are designated as purulent.

Eosinophils are PMN leukocytes with granules that stain orange-red with cytological stains containing eosin. These cells are found in high concentrations in allergic reactions and during parasitic infections, and their roles in both areas are discussed in later chapters.

Basophils have granules that stain metachromatically due to their contents of histamine and heparin. The tissue-fixed **mast cells** are similar to basophils, even though they appear to evolve from different precursor cells. Both basophils and mast cells play a key pathogenic role in allergic reactions.

LYMPHOID ORGANS AND TISSUES

The immune system is organized on several special tissues, collectively designated as lymphoid or immune tissues. These tissues, as shown in Figure 2.3, are distributed throughout the entire body. Those tissues where the lymphoid cells develop, bone marrow and thymus, are known as primary lymphoid tissues, while the tissues and organs where lymphocytes recognize antigens and differentiate into effector cells–lymph nodes, spleen, and mucosal-associated lymphoid tissue (MALT), are known as secondary lymphoid tissues. The most ubiquitous of the secondary lymphoid organs are the lymph nodes that are located in groups along major blood vessels and loose connective tissues and the spleen (white pulp). The MALTs include the gut-associated lymphoid tissues (GALTs), tonsils, Peyer's patches, and appendix, as well as aggregates of lymphoid tissue in the submucosal spaces of the respiratory and genitourinary tracts. The distribution of T and B lymphocytes within human lymphoid tissues is not homogeneous. As shown in Table 2.1,

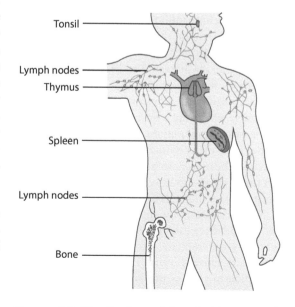

Figure 2.3 Distribution of lymphoid tissues in humans. Those tissues include the lymph nodes, spleen, bone marrow, thymus, mucosal-associated lymphoid tissues, Peyer's patches, and tonsils.

Table 2.1 Distribution of T and B lymphocytes in humans

Immune tissue	Lymphocyte distribution (%)[a]	
	T lymphocyte	B lymphocyte
Peripheral blood	80	10[b]
Thoracic duct	90	10
Lymph node	75	25
Spleen	50	50
Thymus	100	<5
Bone marrow	<25	>75
Peyer's patch	10–20	70

[a] Approximate values.
[b] The remaining 10% would correspond to non-T, non-B lymphocytes.

T lymphocytes predominate in the lymph, peripheral blood, and, above all, the thymus. B lymphocytes predominate in the bone marrow and MALT.

Lymph nodes

The lymph nodes are extremely numerous and disseminated all over the body. They measure 1–25 mm in diameter and play a very important and dynamic role in the initial or inductive states of the immune response.

ANATOMICAL ORGANIZATION

A connective tissue capsule circumscribes the lymph nodes. Afferent lymphatics draining peripheral interstitial spaces enter the capsule of the node and open into the subcapsular sinus. The lymph node also receives blood from the systemic circulation through the hilar arteriole. Two main regions can be distinguished in a lymph node: the cortex and the medulla. The cortex and the deep cortex (also known as paracortical area) are densely populated by lymphocytes, in constant traffic between the lymphatic and systemic circulation. In the cortex, at low magnification, one can distinguish roughly spherical areas containing densely packed lymphocytes, termed *follicles* or *nodules* (Figure 2.4).

T and B lymphocytes occupy different areas in the cortex. B lymphocytes predominate in the follicles (hence, the follicles are designated as T-independent areas), which also contain macrophages, follicular dendritic cells, and some T lymphocytes. The follicles can assume two different morphologies:

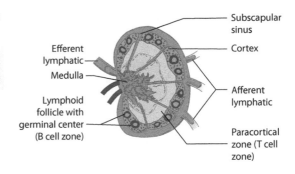

Figure 2.4 Lymph node structure. B lymphocytes are predominantly located on the lymphoid follicles and medullary cords (B-dependent areas), while T lymphocytes are mostly found in the paracortical area (T-dependent area). The germinal centers on the follicles are zones of intense cell proliferation.

- **Primary follicles** are densely packed with small naive B lymphocytes.
- **Secondary follicles** are larger, less dense follicles found in lymph nodes draining an area in which an infection has taken place. The secondary follicles contain a dark, packed mantle, where naive B cells predominate, and clear germinal centers where B lymphocytes are actively dividing as a result of antigenic stimulation.

Nonstimulated B cells enter the germinal center by the mantle area of the basal dark zone. In the light zone, B cells interact with antigens retained by the follicular dendritic cells, and start to proliferate. The proliferation of B cells in germinal centers is associated with phenotypic changes and with somatic mutations affecting the genes coding for the variable regions of the immunoglobulin molecule (see Chapters 5 and 7). The proliferation and differentiation of B cells continues on the apical light zone, where they eventually differentiate into plasma cells and memory B cells. In humans, both plasmablasts and memory B cells leave the lymph node through the medullary cords. Memory B cells enter recirculation patterns that are described later in this chapter. Plasmablasts "home" to the bone marrow where they fully differentiate into plasma cells.

In the deep cortex or paracortical area, which is not as densely populated as the follicles, T lymphocytes are the predominant cell population, and for this reason, the paracortical area is designated as T dependent. MHC-II expressing dendritic cells are also present in this area, where they present antigen to T lymphocytes.

The medulla, less densely populated, is organized into medullary cords draining into the hilar efferent lymphatic vessels. Plasmablasts can be easily identified in the medullary cords.

PHYSIOLOGICAL ROLE

The lymph nodes can be compared to a network of filtration and communication stations where antigens are trapped and messages are interchanged between the different cells involved in the immune response. This complex system of interactions is made possible by the dual circulation in the lymph nodes. Lymph nodes receive both lymph and arterial blood flow. The afferent lymph, with its cellular elements, percolates from the subcapsular sinus to the efferent lymphatics via cortical and medullary sinuses, and the cellular elements of the lymph have ample opportunity to migrate into the lymphocyte-rich cortical structures during their transit through the nodes. The artery that penetrates through the hilus brings peripheral blood lymphocytes into the lymph node; these lymphocytes can leave the vascular bed at the level of the high endothelial venules (HEV) located in the paracortical area.

Thus, lymph nodes can be considered as the anatomical fulcrum of the immune response. Soluble or particulate antigens reach the lymph nodes primarily through the lymphatic circulation. Once in the lymph nodes, antigen is concentrated on the antigen-retaining reticulum formed by the follicular dendritic cells. The antigen is retained for long periods by these cells in its unprocessed form, often associated with antibody (particularly during secondary immune responses), and the retained antigens are efficiently presented to B lymphocytes. The B lymphocytes recognize specific areas of the antigen known as epitopes or antigenic determinants but are also able to internalize and process the antigen, presenting antigen-derived peptides associated to MHC-II molecules to helper T lymphocytes, whose "help" is essential for the full activation and differentiation of the B cells presenting the antigen (see Chapters 3 and 4).

Spleen

The spleen is an organ with multiple functions. Its protective role against infectious diseases is related both to its filtering functions and to the presence of lymphoid structures able to support the initial stages of the immune response.

ANATOMICAL ORGANIZATION

Surrounded by a connective tissue capsule, the parenchyma of this organ is heterogeneous, constituted by the white and the red pulp. The white pulp is rich in lymphocytes, arranged in periarteriolar lymphatic sheaths that surround the narrow central arterioles, derived from the splenic artery after multiple branchings, and follicles, which lie more peripherally relative to the arterioles (Figure 2.5). T cells are concentrated in the periarteriolar lymphatic sheaths, whereas B lymphocytes are concentrated in the follicles. The follicles may or may not show germinal centers depending on the state of activation of the resident cells.

The red pulp surrounds the white pulp. Blood leaving the white pulp through the central arterioles flows into the penicillar arteries and from there flows directly into the venous sinuses. The red pulp is formed by these venous sinuses that are bordered by the splenic cords (cords of Billroth), where macrophages abound. From the sinuses, blood reenters the systemic circulation through the splenic vein.

Between the white and the red pulp lies an area known as the marginal zone, more sparsely cellular than the white pulp, but very rich in macrophages and B lymphocytes.

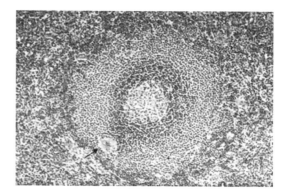

Figure 2.5 Morphology of the white pulp of the spleen. Lymphoid cells are concentrated around small arterioles (arrow), forming a diffuse periarteriolar lymphoid sheet, where T cells predominate, and large follicles with germinal centers (as seen in the picture) where B cells predominate. (Image courtesy of Professor Robert W. Ogilvie, Department of Cell Biology and Anatomy, Medical University of South Carolina, Charleston, South Carolina.)

PHYSIOLOGICAL ROLE

The spleen is the lymphoid organ associated with the clearing of particulate matter, infectious organisms, and aged or defective formed elements (e.g., spherocytes, ovalocytes) from the peripheral blood. The main filtering function is performed by the macrophages lining up the splenic cords. In the marginal zone, circulating antigens are trapped by the macrophages that will then be able to process the antigen, migrate deeper into the white pulp, and initiate the immune response by interacting with T and B lymphocytes.

Thymus

The thymus is the only clearly individualized primary lymphoid organ in mammals. It is believed to play a key role in determining the differentiation of T lymphocytes.

ANATOMICAL ORGANIZATION

The thymus, whose microscopic structure is illustrated in Figure 2.6, is located in the superior mediastinum, anterior to the great vessels. It has a connective tissue capsule from which emerge the trabeculae, which divide the organ into lobules. Each lobule has a cortex and medulla, and the trabeculae are coated with epithelial cells.

The cortex, an area of intense cell proliferation, is mainly populated by immunologically immature

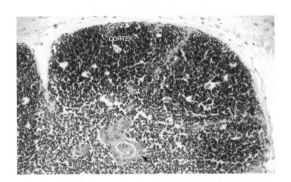

Figure 2.6 Morphology of a thymic lobe. The densely packed cortex is mostly populated by T lymphocytes and by some cortical dendritic epithelial cells and cortical epithelial cells. The more sparsely populated medulla contains epithelial and dendritic cells, macrophages, T lymphocytes, and Hassall's corpuscles. (Image courtesy of Professor Robert W. Ogilvie, Department of Cell Biology and Anatomy, Medical University of South Carolina, Charleston, South Carolina.)

T lymphocytes. A small number of macrophages and plasma cells are also present. In addition, the cortex contains two subpopulations of epithelial cells, the epithelial nurse cells and the cortical epithelial cells that form a network within the cortex.

Not as densely populated as the cortex, the medulla contains predominantly mature T lymphocytes and has a larger epithelial cell to lymphocyte ratio than the cortex. Unique to the medulla are concentric rings of squamous epithelial cells known as Hassall's corpuscles.

PHYSIOLOGICAL ROLE

The thymus is believed to be the organ where T lymphocytes differentiate during embryonic life and thereafter, although for how long the thymus remains functional after birth is unclear (recent data show that 30% of individuals aged 40 years or older retain substantial thymic tissue and function). The thymic cortex is an area of intense cell proliferation and death (only 1% of the cells generated in the thymus eventually mature and migrate to the peripheral tissues). The thymus epithelial cells are believed to produce hormonal factors (e.g., thymosin and thymopoietin) that may play an important role in the differentiation of T lymphocytes. Most T-lymphocyte precursors appear to reach full maturity in the medulla.

An important function of the thymus is to promote the differentiation of non-self reactive T cells while eliminating autoreactive cells. The elimination of autoreactive cells was classically attributed to a negative selection process involving the interaction of T-lymphocyte precursors with thymic epithelial cells. These interactions result in the elimination or inactivation of self reactive T-cell clones and in the differentiation of separate lymphocyte subpopulations with different membrane antigens and different functions. One such subpopulation is the central T-regulatory cells (T_{reg}) expressing the transcription factor forkhead box P3 (FOXP3) and expressing T-cell receptors that react with high avidity with MHC molecules carrying self-derived peptides, thus contributing to the functional elimination of autoreactive T lymphocytes.

Mucosal lymphoid tissues

The MALTs include the lymphoid tissues of the intestinal tract, genitourinary tract, tracheobronchial tree, and mammary glands. All of the mucosal-associated lymphoid tissues are noncapsulated and contain both T and B lymphocytes, the latter predominating.

GUT-ASSOCIATED LYMPHOID TISSUE

GALT designates all lymphatic tissues found along the digestive tract. Three major areas of GALT that can be identified are the tonsils, the Peyer's patches, located on the submucosa of the small intestine, and the appendix. In addition, scanty lymphoid tissue is present in the lamina propria of the gastrointestinal tract.

Tonsils, localized in the oropharynx, are predominantly populated by B lymphocytes and are the site of intense antigenic stimulation, as reflected by the presence of numerous secondary follicles with germinal centers in the tonsilar crypts (Figure 2.7).

Peyer's patches are lymphoid structures disseminated through the submucosal space of the small intestine (Figure 2.8). The follicles of the intestinal Peyer's patches are extremely rich in B cells, which differentiate into IgA-producing plasma cells. Specialized epithelial cells, known as M cells, abound in the dome epithelia of Peyer's patches, particularly at the ileum. These cells take up small particles, virus, bacteria, etc., and deliver them to submucosal macrophages, where the

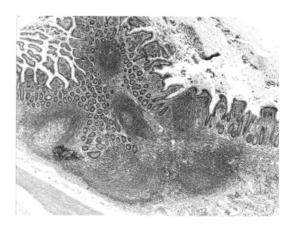

Figure 2.8 Morphology of a Peyer's patch. Well-developed follicles with obvious germinal centers are characteristic of the normal Peyer's patch. B lymphocytes are the predominant cell population. (Image courtesy of Professor Robert W. Ogilvie, Department of Cell Biology and Anatomy, Medical University of South Carolina, Charleston, South Carolina.)

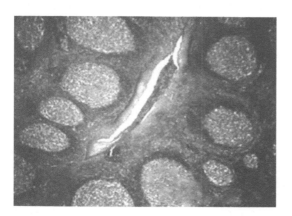

Figure 2.7 Morphology of the tonsils. The lymphoid tissue of these lymphoid organs is mostly constituted by primary and secondary follicles (characterized by the pale germinal centers), the later predominating as seen in this picture. The predominant cell population in the tonsillar follicles is B cells. (Image courtesy of Professor Robert W. Ogilvie, Department of Cell Biology and Anatomy, Medical University of South Carolina, Charleston, South Carolina.)

engulfed material will be processed and presented to T and B lymphocytes.

T lymphocytes are also diffusely present in the intestinal mucosa, the most abundant of them expressing membrane markers that are considered typical of memory helper T cells. This population appears to be critically involved in the induction of humoral immune responses. A special subset of T cells, with a different type of T-cell receptor (γ/δ T lymphocytes) is well represented on the small intestine mucosa. These lymphocytes appear to recognize generic bacterial products, particularly phosphorylated isoprenoids probably presented on the surface of APCs and recognized by the γ/δ T cells (see chapter 14), perhaps through an invariable T-cell receptor. That recognition would trigger local inflammatory responses against many different bacterial species capable of releasing those products. In the intestine and lungs, a set of innate T cells (mucosal-associated innate T cells [MAITs]) expressing CD8 and semi-invariant α/β T-cell receptors recognize and are activated by ligands derived from vitamin B12 metabolism, common to many different bacteria species, and expressed by B cells carrying an invariant MHC-related protein (MR-1).

GALT is also rich in T_{reg} cells (20%–30% of the CD4$^+$ T cells in the intestinal lamina propria are

T_{reg} cells), which are believed to maintain immune tolerance to dietary components and microbes colonizing the intestines.

LYMPHOCYTE TRAFFIC

The lymphatic and circulatory systems are intimately related (Figure 2.9a–c), and there is a constant traffic of lymphocytes throughout the body, moving from one system to another. Afferent lymphatics from interstitial spaces drain into lymph nodes that "filter" these fluids, removing foreign substances. "Cleared" lymph from below the diaphragm and the upper left half of the body drains via efferent lymphatics, emptying into the thoracic duct for subsequent drainage into the left innominate vein. "Cleared" lymph from the right side above the diaphragm drains into the right lymphatic duct with subsequent drainage into the origin of the right innominate vein. The same routes are traveled by lymphocytes stimulated in the lymph nodes or peripheral lymphoid tissues, which eventually will reach the systemic circulation.

Peripheral blood, in turn, is "filtered" by the spleen and liver, the spleen having organized lymphoid areas, while the liver is rich in Kupffer's cells, which are macrophage-derived phagocytes. Organisms and antigens that enter directly into the systemic circulation will be trapped in these two organs, predominantly by the spleen.

Lymphocyte recirculation and extravascular migration

One of the most important biological characteristics of B and T lymphocytes is their constant recirculation, entering the lymphoid tissues to circulate through the vascular system, just to enter again the lymphoid tissues, or to exit into the interstitial tissues if an inflammatory reaction is taking place.

Lymphocytes circulating in the systemic circulation eventually enter a lymph node, exit the systemic circulation at the level of the HEV, leave the lymph node with the efferent lymph, and eventually reenter the systemic circulation.

B lymphocytes of mucosal origin circulate between different segments of the MALTs, including the GALT, the mammary gland-associated lymphoid tissue, and the lymphoid tissues associated with the respiratory tree and urinary tract.

Cell adhesion molecules

The crucial step in the traffic of lymphocytes from the systemic circulation to a lymphoid tissue or to interstitial tissues is the crossing of the endothelial barrier by diapedesis at specific locations. Under physiological conditions, this seems to take place predominantly at the level of the HEV of lymphoid tissues. The crossing of the endothelial barrier involves cytoskeleton rearrangements on the lymphocytes that are induced by chemokines resulting in polarization of the cell followed by pseudopodia formation and ameboid migration. These specialized endothelial cells express surface molecules, selectins (e.g., endothelial-leukocyte adhesion molecule or E-selectin) that belong to an extensive family of cell-adhesion molecules (CAMs) that play important roles in the interaction of circulating lymphocytes and endothelial cells (Table 2.2). This initial interaction facilitates the interaction of chemokines expressed on the endothelial cell membrane with the corresponding receptors in lymphocytes, inducing the activation of lymphocyte integrins (e.g., LFA-1) that bind to cell adhesion molecules (e.g., intercellular adhesion molecule-1 [ICAM-1]). That interaction leads to transient tethering of lymphocytes and endothelial cells, followed by rolling along the endothelium. This facilitates interplay between additional endothelial and lymphocyte CAMs and homing of lymphocytes. Variations in the expression of CAMs and chemokines in different tissues are key to selective migration of lymphocytes and their subpopulations to the tissues where they play a key role.

Three main families of cell adhesion molecules have been defined (Table 2.2). The addressins or selectins are expressed on endothelial cells and leukocytes and mediate leukocyte adherence to the endothelium. The immunoglobulin superfamily of CAMs includes a variety of molecules expressed by leukocytes, endothelial cells, and other cells. The integrins are defined as molecules that interact with CAMs but also with cytoskeleton and tissue matrix compounds.

Regulation of lymphocyte traffic and homing

The regulation of lymphocyte traffic is complex and involves interactions between cell adhesion

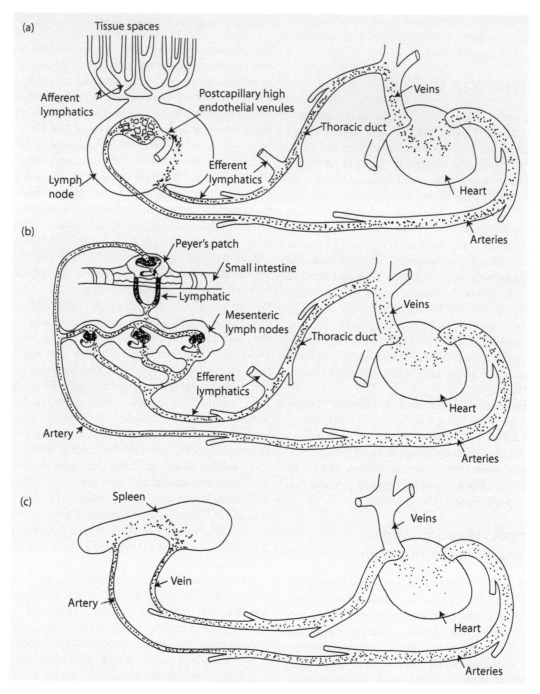

Figure 2.9 **Pathways of lymphocyte circulation:** (a) Blood lymphocytes enter lymph nodes, adhere to the walls of specialized postcapillary venules, and migrate to the lymph node cortex. Lymphocytes then percolate through lymphoid fields to medullary lymphatic sinuses and on to efferent lymphatics, which in turn collect in major lymphatic ducts in the thorax which empty into the superior vena cava. (b) The gut-associated lymphoid tissues (Peyer's patches and mesenteric lymph nodes) drain into the thoracic duct, which also empties into the superior vena cava. (c) The spleen receives lymphocytes and disburses them mainly via the blood vascular system (inferior vena cava). (Reproduced with permission from Hood LE, Weissman IL, Wood WB, Wilson JH. *Immunology*. 2nd ed. Benjamin-Cummings, Menlo Park, CA, 1984.)

Table 2.2 Main adhesion molecules, their families, ligands, and functions

Family	Members	Ligand	Function
Selectins	Endothelial-leukocyte adhesion molecule (ELAM-1, E-selectin)	Sialylated/fucosylated molecules	Mediates leukocyte adherence to endothelial cells in inflammatory reactions
	Leukocyte adhesion molecule-1 (L-Selectin, CD62L)	Immunoglobulin superfamily CAMs; mucins and sialomucins	Interaction with HEV expressing PNAd (lymphocyte homing); leukocyte adherence to endothelial cells in inflammatory reactions
	Intercellular adhesion molecule-1 (ICAM-1)	LFA-1 (CD11a/CD18), Mac-1 (CD11b)	Expressed by leukocytes, endothelial cells, dendritic cells, etc.; mediates leukocyte adherence to endothelial cells in inflammatory reactions
Immunoglobulin superfamily CAMs	ICAM-2	LFA-1	Expressed by leukocytes, endothelial cells, and dendritic cells; involved in control of lymphocyte recirculation and traffic
	Vascular CAM-1 (VCAM-1)	VLA-4	Expressed primarily by endothelial cells; mediates leukocyte adherence to activated endothelial cells in inflammatory reactions
	Peripheral lymph node addressin (PNAd)	L-selectin (CD62L)	Interacts with L-selectin in lymph nodes
	Mucosal addressin CAM-1 (MadCAM-1)	β_7, α_4, L-Selectin	Expressed by mucosal lymphoid HEV; mediates lymphocyte homing to mucosal lymphoid tissues
	Platelet/endothelial CAM-1 (PECAM-1)	PECAM-1	Expressed by platelets, leukocytes, and endothelial cells; involved in leukocyte transmigration across the endothelium in inflammation
Integrins VLA family	VLA-1 to 6	Fibronectin, laminin, collagen	Ligands mediating cell-cell and cell-substrate interaction
LEUCAM family	LFA-1	ICAM-1, ICAM-2, ICAM-3	Ligands mediating cell-cell and cell-substrate interaction
Other	Mac-1	ICAM-1, Fibrinogen, C3bi	HEV/Lymphocyte interactions in the lymph nodes
	CCR7	CCL19 and CCL21	Expressed on leukocytes;
	CD44	Hyaluronate, collagen, fibronectin	mediates cell-cell and cell-matrix interactions; involved in lymphocyte homing

molecules and chemokines expressed in HEV and the corresponding lymphocyte receptors. Homing to different tissues results both from differences in the expression of these CAMs and of differences in the nature of chemokines released in different tissues and the expression of the corresponding receptors in lymphocytes. The involvement of HEV as the primary site for lymphocyte egress from the systemic circulation is a consequence of the interaction between the peripheral lymph node addressin (PNAd), a specific CAM expressed in HEV, and L-selectin, expressed by naive T lymphocytes. Because PNAd is predominantly expressed by HEV, the opportunity for cell adhesion and extravascular migration is considerably higher in HEV than on segments of the venous circulation covered by flat endothelium. The migration of lymphocytes to peripheral lymph nodes requires the expression of L-selectin and of the chemokine receptor CCR7. L-selectin interacts with the PNAd, and the CCR7 interacts with the chemokines CC19 and CC21, expressed by endothelial cells on the lymph nodes. Different repertoires of CAMs and cytokines control migration of lymphocytes to different lymphoid organs.

As previously discussed, the lymphocyte constitution of lymphoid organs is variable (Table 2.1). T lymphocytes predominate in the lymph nodes, but B lymphocytes and IgA-producing plasma cells predominate in the Peyer's patches and the GALT in general. This differential homing is believed to be the result of the expression of specific addressins such as MadCAM-1 on the HEV of the perimucosal lymphoid tissues that are specifically recognized by the B cells and plasma cells resident in those tissues. Most B lymphocytes recognize specifically the GALT-associated HEV and do not interact with the lymph node–associated HEV, while most naive T lymphocytes recognize both the lymph node–associated HEV and the GALT-associated HEV. The differentiation of T-dependent and B-dependent areas in lymphoid tissues is a poorly understood aspect of lymphocyte "homing." It appears likely that the distribution of T and B lymphocytes is determined by their interaction with nonlymphoid cells. For example, the interaction between interdigitating cells and T lymphocytes may determine the predominant location of T lymphocytes in the lymph

node paracortical areas and periarteriolar sheets of the spleen, while the interaction of B lymphocytes with follicular dendritic cells may determine the organization of lymphoid follicles in the lymph node, spleen, and GALT.

The modulation of CAM expression at different states of cell activation explains changing patterns in lymphocyte recirculation seen during immune responses. Immediately after antigen stimulation, the recirculating lymphocyte appears to transiently lose its capacity to recirculate. This loss of recirculating ability is associated with a tendency to self-aggregate (perhaps explaining why antigen-stimulated lymphocytes are trapped at the site of maximal antigen density), due to the upregulation of CAMs involved in lymphocyte-lymphocyte and lymphocyte-accessory cell interactions.

After the antigenic stimulus ceases, a population of memory T lymphocytes carrying distinctive membrane proteins can be identified. This population seems to have a different recirculation pattern than that of the naive T lymphocyte, leaving the intravascular compartment at sites other than the HEV and reaching the lymph nodes via the lymphatic circulation. This difference in migration seems to result from the downregulation of the CAMs that mediate the interaction with HEV selectins and upregulation of other CAMs that interact with selectins located in other areas of the vascular tree.

B lymphocytes also change their recirculation patterns after antigenic stimulation. Most B cells will differentiate into plasma cells after stimulation, and this differentiation is associated with marked changes in the antigenic composition of the cell membrane. Consequently, the plasma cell precursors (plasmablasts) exit the germinal centers, move into the medullary cords, and, eventually, migrate to the bone marrow, where most of the antibody production in humans takes place. Another B-cell subpopulation—the memory B cells—retain B cell markers and reenter the circulation to migrate back to specific territories of the lymphoid tissues.

All memory lymphocytes, T or B, appear to home preferentially in the type of lymphoid tissue where the original antigen encounter took place, i.e., a lymphocyte that recognized an antigen in a peripheral lymph node will recirculate to another peripheral lymph node, while a lymphocyte that was stimulated at the GALT level will recirculate to the GALT. Memory B lymphocytes remain in the germinal centers, while memory T lymphocytes "home" in T-cell areas.

Inflammatory and immune reactions often lead to the release of mediators that upregulate the expression of adhesion molecules and chemokine receptors on lymphocytes and the expression of chemokines in the microvasculature near the area where the reaction is taking place. Under those conditions, the leukocytes slow down and start rolling along the endothelial surface. This stage is mediated primarily by selectins. Next, leukocytes adhere to endothelial cells expressing integrins such as VLA and CAMs of the immunoglobulin superfamily, such as ICAM and VCAM, and to chemokine receptors that vary in different populations of lymphocytes. Finally, the adherent leukocytes squeeze between two adjoining endothelial cells and move to the extravascular space.

The end result of this process is an increase in leukocyte migration to specific areas where those cells are needed to eliminate some type of noxious stimulus or to initiate an immune response. Some of the lymphocytes that migrate to a tissue where they can be stimulated by a specific antigen will differentiate in tissue resident memory T cells (T_{RM}), a different subpopulation than the central memory T cells (T_{CM}), which remain in circulation and are attracted to endothelial cells expressing inflammatory cytokines. Both subpopulations will contribute to inducing a potent and rapid immune response to the specific antigens that they have previously recognized.

BIBLIOGRAPHY

Agnello D, Lankford CS, Bream J, Morinobu A et al. Cytokines and transcription factors that regulate T helper cell differentiation: New players and new insights. *J Clin Immunol*. 2003;23:147–161.

Caramalho I, Nunes-Cabaço H, Foxhall R, Sousa AE. Regulatory T-cell development in the thymus. *Front Immunol*. 2015;6:395.

Fu H, Ward EJ, Marelli-Berg FM. Mechanisms of T cell organotropism. *Cell Mol Life Sci*. 2016;73:3009–3033.

Heesters BA, Myers, RC, Carroll MC. Follicular dendritic cells: Dynamic antigen libraries. *Nat Rev Immunol*. 2014;14:495–504.

Liuzzi AR, McLaren J, Price DA, Eberl M. Early innate responses to pathogens: Pattern recognition by unconventional human T cells. *Curr Opin Immunol*. 2015;36:31–37.

Mac Lennan IC. Germinal centers. *Annu Rev Immunol*. 1994;12:117–139.

Morice WG. The immunophenotypic attributes of NK cells and NK lineage lymphoproliferative disorders. *Amer J Clin Path*. 2007;127:881–886.

Muñoz MA, MBiro M, Weninger WT. Cell migration in intact lymph nodes in vivo. *Curr Opin Cell Biol*. 2014;30:17–24.

O'Garra A, Vieira P. Regulatory T cells and mechanisms of immune system control. *Nat Med*. 2004;10:801–805.

Sakaguchi S, Miyara M, Costantino CM, Hafler DA. FOXP3+ regulatory T cells in the human immune system. *Nat Rev Immunol*. 2010;10:490–500.

Tanoue T, Atarashi K, Honda K. Development and maintenance of intestinal regulatory T cells. *Nat Rev Immunol*. 2016;16:295–309.

3

Major histocompatibility complex

ELLEN KLOHE AND JANARDAN P. PANDEY

INTRODUCTION

The major histocompatibility complex (MHC) is a large group of closely linked genes that encode molecules involved in the induction and regulation of both innate and adaptive immune responses. In addition to these essential roles, molecules encoded by the MHC participate in functions as diverse as reproduction and central nervous system development.

The MHC is present in all jawed vertebrates studied so far but is best defined in mice and humans. The development of genetically identical inbred strains of mice laid the foundation for the discovery of the MHC. Studies conducted in the first half of the twentieth century demonstrated that tumors from one inbred strain were accepted by all mice of the same strain but failed to grow in different strains. Later, it was recognized that antigens present on the donor's tissues but absent from the recipient's tissues were responsible for tumor rejection. These and later experiments using autologous and allogeneic skin grafts in mice, humans, and rabbits demonstrated that the fate of transplanted tissues is under genetic control of codominantly expressed histocompatibility genes that differ between nonidentical members of the same species. Furthermore, it was recognized that tissue acceptance or rejection is subject to the general immunological rules of specificity and memory. Rejection occurred with grafts from non-identical donors, but not from identical or autologous donors. In addition, the speed and intensity of rejection were enhanced with a second graft from the first donor but not from a third-party nonidentical donor.

During the second half of the twentieth century, antibodies were discovered in the sera of parous females and blood transfusion recipients that agglutinated the leukocytes of other individuals. Patterns of antibody reactivity in different sera revealed a system of antigens that were recognized as products encoded by the human MHC. As a result, the human MHC was named the human leukocyte antigen (HLA) system. Intense research effort and collaboration through international workshops led to elucidation of the HLA system such that HLA typing and HLA antibody identification were possible. The ability to identify HLA-compatible donor-recipient pairs along with the development of immunosuppressive drugs led to the success of solid organ and hematopoietic stem cell transplants between nonidentical individuals.

During the 1970s, the MHC was found to play a central role in immune responses beyond transplantation. The discovery that virus-specific cytotoxic T cells from one mouse strain would kill infected cells only from mice that shared MHC determinants was one of a series of findings that revealed the role of the MHC in T-cell immunity.

It took until the end of the century when the crystal structures of the T-cell receptor and MHC molecules were resolved to fully unravel the molecular basis for this MHC restriction of T-cell responses. We now know that the main biological function of the MHC-encoded histocompatibility antigens is to present peptides (self or foreign) to αβ T cells for immune surveillance.

The MHC remains an area of intensive investigation in continuing efforts to fully understand immune responses to foreign antigens and immune tolerance to self antigens. From a clinical perspective, familiarity with MHC is important because of its association with transplant rejection, infectious diseases, and autoimmune diseases. In addition, there is a growing appreciation for its relevance in vaccine development, including cancer vaccines and T-cell immunotherapies as well as the prevention of adverse drug reactions.

MAJOR HISTOCOMPATIBILITY COMPLEX GENES

Chromosomal localization and gene arrangement

The MHC genes are located on chromosome 17 in mice and chromosome 6 in humans. The basic organizational structure of the MHC is largely conserved, but the number of genetic loci and alleles varies by species. The HLA region spans about four million base pairs and includes over 280 genetic loci, only about 15% of which encode the classical histocompatibility antigens. A simplified map of the HLA region is shown in Figure 3.1. A current comprehensive gene map can be found in the National Center for Biotechnology Information (NCBI) database (http://www.ncbi.nlm.nih.gov/gene/).

Gene classes, loci, and alleles

Like the MHC in other species, the HLA genes are categorized into three major classes. The class I and II regions include the **classical** genes that encode the histocompatibility antigens. The class I region also includes nonclassical genes whose encoded proteins facilitate interactions with T cells, natural killer (NK) cells, and NK T cells. The class II region includes other genes that encode proteins involved in antigen processing and transport. The classical class I and class II genes and their encoded gene products are the focus of the remainder of this chapter. The class III region includes a heterogeneous group of genes that are involved in stress responses, the complement cascade, inflammation, and immune regulation.

The class I histocompatibility antigens are composed of an HLA encoded α-chain and the β2-microglobulin chain encoded by a non-HLA gene located on chromosome 15. Genes at three distinct loci encode similar, yet distinct class I HLA-A, HLA-B, and HLA-C molecules. Genes that encode both the α- and β-chains of the class II histocompatibility antigens are found at six to nine different HLA loci, depending on the inherited haplotype. These genes give rise to analogous HLA-DP, HLA-DQ, and HLA-DR molecules.

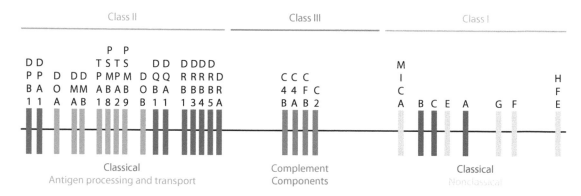

Figure 3.1 Simplified map of the HLA region on human chromosome 6. Classical class II genes are shown in dark blue. Class II genes involved in antigen processing and transport are shown in light blue. Class III complement genes are shown in orange. Classical class I genes are shown in dark purple. Nonclassical class I genes are shown in light purple. (Original drawing provided by Stephanie Skibby.)

An astonishing number of alleles have been identified at several HLA loci. Alleles are designated by a number that follows the relevant locus (e.g., HLA-A1, HLA-B8, or HLA-DR17). In fact, these are the most **polymorphic** structural gene loci in the entire human genome. Alleles may differ from each other by a single nucleotide or multiple nucleotides. Nucleotide substitutions may be either synchronous (no change to the amino acid in the encoded protein) or nonsynchronous (a different amino acid in the encoded protein). Many nonsynchronous substitutions are clustered in particular stretches of nucleotides in the gene sequence. This suggests that these differences did not arise by chance but rather were the result of natural selection. As of December 2017, 4,081 HLA-A, 4,950 HLA-B, and 3,685 HLA-C alleles have been identified. Many class II loci are also polymorphic, with 4,802 alleles currently identified. The IPD-IMGT/HLA Database is the repository for HLA DNA sequences and approved alleles and is located at https://www.ebi.ac.uk/ipd/imgt/hla/.

Inheritance

Genes across the entire HLA region are generally inherited *en bloc* so that extended maternal and paternal haplotypes are passed on through generations, with meiotic crossovers occurring at a lower frequency (1%) than in other parts of the genome. Population genetics theory predicts that over time in a panmictic population (random mating), the alleles at one locus will be randomly associated with alleles of other loci (linkage equilibrium). In this situation, the probability of co-occurrence of any two alleles will be the product of their individual frequencies. However, this is not the case for HLA, in that certain alleles are found together more often than would be expected. This phenomenon is termed *linkage disequilibrium*. For example, the HLA-A1 allele is found in the Caucasian population with a frequency of 0.158, and the HLA-B8 allele is found with a frequency of 0.092. Therefore, the A1, B8 haplotype should be found with a frequency of $0.158 \times 0.092 = 0.015$. In reality, it is found with a frequency of 0.072. The linkage disequilibrium is expressed as the difference (Δ) between the observed and expected frequencies of the alleles, i.e., $0.072 - 0.015 = 0.057$.

The extensive geographic variation in allele frequencies and linkage disequilibrium suggest that migration and demographic history have shaped HLA variation in humans. At the same time, natural selection is thought to be an important driver of HLA diversity in that throughout evolutionary history, new alleles and certain combinations of alleles may have been differentially selected because of their role in conferring immunity to particular infectious pathogens.

HLA alleles are inherited as autosomal codominant genes according to Mendelian laws. Therefore, alleles from both haplotypes that form the genotype will be expressed in the cells of that individual. This means that an individual who is homozygous at all loci may express as few as six different HLA molecules, whereas an individual who is heterozygous at all loci may express many as 18 different HLA molecules, depending on inherited haplotype and the ability of polymorphic class II α- and β-chains to pair in both *cis* or *trans* configurations.

Because of the high degree of polymorphism, it is unlikely that two unrelated individuals will share all their HLA alleles. As expected, related individuals share HLA haplotypes, and the proportion of shared genes depends on the degree of relatedness. Figure 3.2 shows possible haplotypes within a family. There is a 25% chance of two siblings being HLA identical, making them ideal donor-recipient candidates for organ and tissue transplantation. There is a 50% chance of two siblings sharing one haplotype and a 25% chance of two siblings sharing no haplotypes.

Human leukocyte antigen allele identification and nomenclature

Histocompatibility antigens were first identified serologically using panels of antisera with known antibody specificities directed against the HLA molecules expressed on lymphocytes. Now HLA alleles can be directly identified by DNA-based methods. The nucleotide sequences of the relevant exons can be sequenced or probed to identify different alleles. Another common method uses a panel of sequence-specific primers that amplify short stretches of nucleotide polymorphisms present in targeted alleles in polymerase chain reactions (PCRs). These DNA-based typing methods have identified even more HLA polymorphisms by detecting nucleotide differences between alleles that are not detected by serologic typing. For

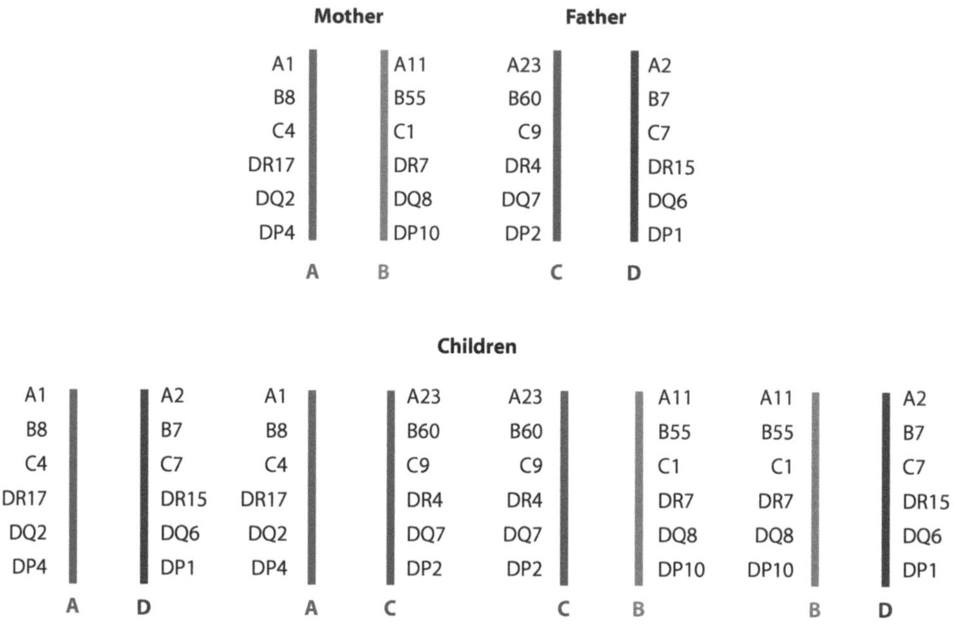

Mother

A1	A11
B8	B55
C4	C1
DR17	DR7
DQ2	DQ8
DP4	DP10

A   B

Father

A23	A2
B60	B7
C9	C7
DR4	DR15
DQ7	DQ6
DP2	DP1

C   D

Children

A1	A2	A1	A23	A23	A11	A11	A2
B8	B7	B8	B60	B60	B55	B55	B7
C4	C7	C4	C9	C9	C1	C1	C7
DR17	DR15	DR17	DR4	DR4	DR7	DR7	DR15
DQ2	DQ6	DQ2	DQ7	DQ7	DQ8	DQ8	DQ6
DP4	DP1	DP4	DP2	DP2	DP10	DP10	DP1

A   D   A   C   C   B   B   D

Figure 3.2 The genetic transmission of HLA haplotypes. Each parent has two haplotypes (one from each chromosome). Maternal haplotypes are designated A and B and paternal haplotypes C and D. Each offspring receives one maternal haplotype and one paternal haplotype. In a large family, 25% of the children share both haplotypes, 50% share one haplotype, and 25% have no haplotype in common. (Original drawing provided by Stephanie Skibby.)

instance, the serologically defined HLA-A2 antigen is associated with 573 different alleles based on DNA sequence analyses. All of these are collectively known as the HLA A*02 group alleles. By targeting the nucleotide polymorphisms that give rise to serologically defined epitopes, HLA low-resolution typing identifies allele groups that are basically equivalent to the serologic antigens. This is adequate for clinical applications such as platelet donor typing, and in most cases, solid organ transplantation. High-resolution typing at the allele level is required for hematopoietic stem cell transplantation, autoimmune disease, and drug hypersensitivity association studies. An individual's HLA type is simply a list of all the serologically defined antigens or alleles present at each HLA-A, HLA-B, HLA-C, HLA-DR, HLA-DQ, and HLA-DP. Table 3.1 compares the class I serologic,

low-resolution, and high-resolution typing results for one individual.

MHC PROTEIN STRUCTURE

Immunoglobulin superfamily receptor structure

MHC proteins are members of the immunoglobulin superfamily (IgSF). This superfamily includes many different receptors that mediate cell-to-cell interactions involved in immune responses, the most notable examples being the B-cell and T-cell antigen receptors. Most IgSF receptors share a basic heterodimer subunit structure. The extracellular domains form the receptors, while the transmembrane and cytoplasmic domains connect the receptor to the internal cellular environment

Table 3.1 Class I HLA type of an individual determined by different typing methods

Serology	A23	A31	B7	B44	C4	C7
Low-resolution DNA	A*23	A*31	B*07	B*44	C*04	C*07
High-resolution DNA	A*23:01	A*31:01	B*07:02	B*44:03	C*04:01	C*07:02

and facilitate signaling. Figure 3.3 illustrates the domain structure of the archetypal B-cell receptor compared to the T-cell receptor and the MHC class I and class II molecules. Each structure includes a membrane proximal region that consists of at least one typical immunoglobulin domain structure and a membrane distal variable region. Whereas the variable regions form the antigen receptors on B cells and T cells, the variable regions of MHC molecules form the peptide-binding site.

HLA class I and class II structures

The HLA class I heterodimers are formed by a 43,000–48,000 dalton α-chain encoded by the different alleles at the HLA-A, HLA-B, and HLA-C loci paired with β2-microglobulin, a 12,000 dalton protein encoded by a minimally polymorphic, non-HLA gene located on chromosome 15. The α-chain has a long extracellular region folded into three (α1, α2, and α3) domains, as well as transmembrane and intracellular segments. β2-microglobulin forms a single immunoglobulin-type domain that is noncovalently associated with the α-chain.

The amino acid sequences of different HLA α-chains reveal that stretches within the α1 and α2 domains are highly variable, whereas the α3 domain is much less polymorphic.

The resolution of the three-dimensional structures of HLA class I molecules by X-ray crystallography placed the most polymorphic residues on the floor and sides of a deep groove that also contained various peptides 8–11 amino acids in length. This peptide-binding groove was found atop a supporting frame formed by the α3 domain and β2-microglobulin (Figure 3.4). The α3 domain also has a binding site for the CD8 molecule expressed by cytotoxic T cells.

Although a remarkable degree of tertiary structure homology exists between class I and class II molecules, there are important differences in their primary structures. The class II molecules consist of two distinct polypeptide chains encoded by genes in the HLA region: a less polymorphic, heavier α-chain (33,000 daltons) and a highly polymorphic β-chain (28,000 daltons). Each chain has two extracellular domains (α1 and α2; β1 and β2). The extracellular domains include highly polymorphic α1 and β1 domains and less polymorphic α2 and β2 domains as well as both α-chain and β-chain transmembrane and intracellular segments. The class II three-dimensional

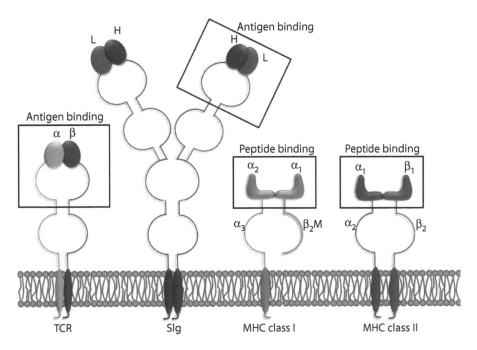

Figure 3.3 Immunoglobulin superfamily molecules, comparing surface immunoglobulin (sIg) and T-cell (TCR) antigen-binding receptors with MHC class I and class II peptide-binding molecules. (Modified from Leffell, MS et al. *Handbook of Human Immunology*, CRC Press, Boca Raton, FL, 1997.)

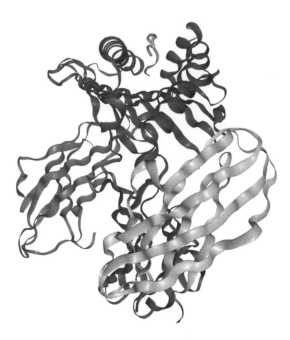

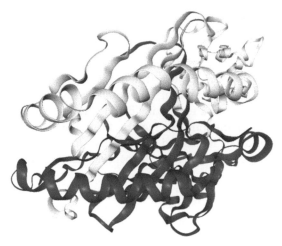

Figure 3.5 Ribbon diagram of the HLA-DQ8 molecule with bound peptide. This top view shows the polymorphic α1 and β1 domains that form the peptide binding groove with bound peptide. The native molecule has α2 and β2 domains, transmembrane and intracellular segments below that are not shown. (Obtained from the NGL viewer based on RCSB PDB [http://www.rcsb.org] PDB ID: 2 NNA. Henderson, K.N. et al., *Immunity*, 27, 23–34, 2007.)

Figure 3.4 Ribbon diagram of the HLA-A2 molecule with bound peptide. This side view shows the immunoglobulin-like domains (α3, β2m) at the bottom and the polymorphic domains (α1, α2) that form the peptide binding groove at the top. The native molecule has intramembrane and intracellular segments not shown. (Obtained from the NGL viewer based on RCSB PDB [http://www.rcsb.org] PDB ID: 1IM3. Gewurz, B.E. et al., *Proc. Natl. Acad. Sci. USA*, 98, 6794–6799, 2001.)

structure shows that the β1 domains resemble the α2 domains of their class I counterparts. The junction of α1 and β1 domains forms a groove similar to that of the class I molecule that permits binding of somewhat longer peptides from 15 to 25 amino acid residues in length (Figure 3.5). The β2 domain contains a receptor for the CD4 molecule of helper T lymphocytes.

Structural basis for MHC restriction

MHC class I and class II molecules act as restricting elements for foreign antigen recognition by the αβ CD8+ and CD4+ T-cell subsets, respectively. This means that T cells must recognize both the self MHC molecule and the foreign antigenic peptide that it binds. The polymorphic amino acids within and surrounding the peptide-binding groove form an allele-specific MHC-peptide complex that displays both the foreign antigenic

peptide and self MHC residues to T cells. The nature of T-cell recognition of the MHC-peptide complex was made crystal clear when trimolecular MHC-peptide/T-cell receptor complexes were resolved. A single T-cell receptor lies diagonally across the peptide-binding groove and makes contact with both the amino acids in the bound peptide and amino acids in the MHC molecule itself (Figure 3.6). The part of the HLA-peptide complex that interacts with the T-cell receptor is known as the **T-cell epitope**.

MHC PROTEIN FUNCTIONS

Protection against intracellular pathogens and abnormal cells

Antibodies and various immune cells protect against extracellular pathogens and toxins by recognizing their intact structures on cell surfaces or in body fluids. But cells infected by intracellular pathogens or neoplastic cells may be shielded from these defenses. The CD8+ and CD4+ αβ T-cell populations utilize peptide presentation by MHC class I and class II molecules, respectively, to

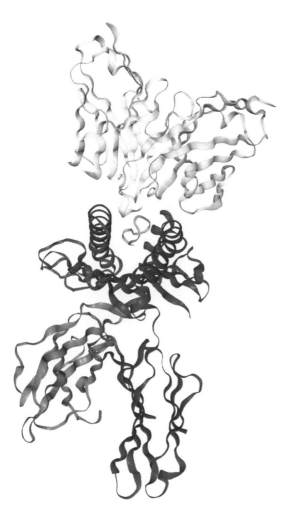

Figure 3.6 Ribbon diagram of the interaction between a T-cell receptor (top) and a HLA-A2 peptide complex (bottom). The peptide anchor residues bind to complementary allele-specific residues in the MHC peptide-binding groove. A combination of peptide and MHC residues forms a T-cell epitope consisting of contact residues for a T-cell receptor. (Obtained from the NGL viewer based on RCSB PDB [http://www.rcsb.org] PDB ID: 5ED9. Harris, D.T. et al., *Structure*, 24, 1142–1154, 2016.)

survey the internal contents of cells for microbial or abnormal self proteins. T cells whose antigen receptors recognize the combination of self MHC and foreign or altered self peptide are activated to carry out programmed effector functions that include direct killing of infected or aberrant cells and elaboration of cytokines that activate other immune cells and amplify their responses.

Cellular distribution and regulation of MHC expression

HLA class I molecules are expressed on all nucleated cells but are particularly abundant on the surfaces of lymphocytes (1,000–10,000 molecules/cell). The cell surface density varies with different cells and tissues and between the different HLA-A, HLA-B, and HLA-C loci. Because they are class I restricted, CD8$^+$ T cells are uniquely qualified to seek out and destroy infected or abnormal cells of any type in the body.

HLA class II molecules are constitutively expressed only on B cells and cells of the monocyte-macrophage family. The latter includes all **antigen-presenting cells** such as Langerhans cells in the skin, Kupffer cells in the liver, microglial cells in the central nervous system, and dendritic cells in the spleen and lymph nodes. Class II expression is induced on other cell types following activation, including T cells and endothelial cells.

The α- and β-interferons increase class I expression, whereas interferon γ upregulates the expression of both class I and class II molecules. Interferons are produced by cells of the innate immune system that encounter molecular signals from viruses or bacteria. Therefore, by increasing HLA expression on antigen-presenting cells and potentially infected cells, interferons amplify adaptive immune responses to invading organisms. The consequences of increased HLA class I and class II expression may be both beneficial and harmful. On the one hand, it facilitates the induction of T-cell responses against pathogens, but on the other hand, it may create optimal conditions for the activation of autoreactive T cells.

Antigen processing and presentation

Two major antigen-processing pathways are used to sample proteins derived from intracellular or extracellular sources. Intracellular proteins include normal self proteins in healthy cells, abnormal self proteins in neoplastic cells, and viral or intracellular parasitic proteins produced by conscripting the host cell's own protein-synthesizing machinery (Figure 3.7). Proteosome complexes degrade these proteins into short 8–10 amino acid peptide fragments in the cytosol. Interestingly, two subunits of the proteasome complex are encoded by the *PSMB8* and *PSMB9* genes located in the class II

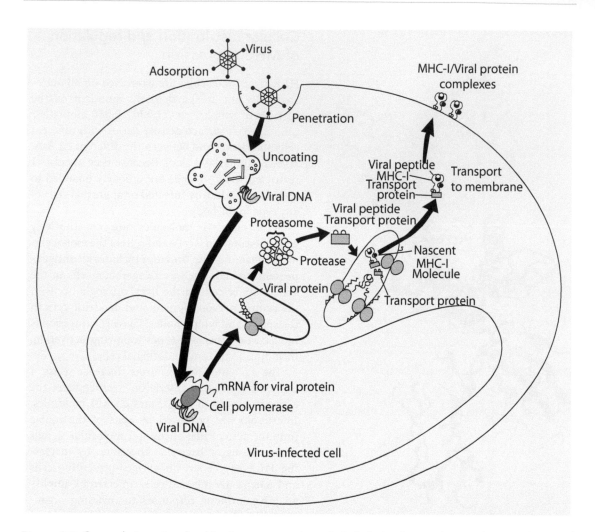

Figure 3.7 General steps involved in the presentation of viral-derived peptides on the membrane of virus-infected cells. The virus binds to membrane receptors and is endocytosed, its outer coats are digested, and the viral genome (in this case DNA) is released into the cytoplasm. Once released, the viral DNA diffuses back into the nucleus where it is initially transcribed into mRNA by the cell's polymerases. The viral mRNA is translated into proteins that diffuse into the cytoplasm, where some will be broken down into oligopeptides. Those small peptides are transported back into the endoplasmic reticulum where they associate with newly synthesized MHC-I molecules. The MHC-I/oligopeptide complex becomes associated to a second transport protein and is eventually inserted into the cell membrane. In the cell membrane, it can be presented to CD8+ T lymphocytes in traffic through the tissue where the viral-infected cell is located. A similar mechanism would allow a MHC-II synthesizing cell to present MHC-II/oligopeptide complexes to CD4+ lymphocytes.

region. The *TAP1* and *TAP2* transporter genes in the class II region encode proteins that escort these peptides to the endoplasmic reticulum where they encounter newly synthesized HLA class I molecules. Those peptides whose sequences are complementary to the amino acid sequences in the peptide-binding grooves of one or more of the different HLA-A, HLA-B, or HLA-C molecules bind within the groove. The stabilized HLA class I–peptide complex is then transported to the cell surface for scrutiny by CD8+ T cells.

Extracellular proteins, particles, or cells enter antigen-presenting cells through endocytosis of soluble proteins in body fluids or phagocytosis of particulate matter or whole cells (Figure 3.8). The internalized material is degraded within acidic

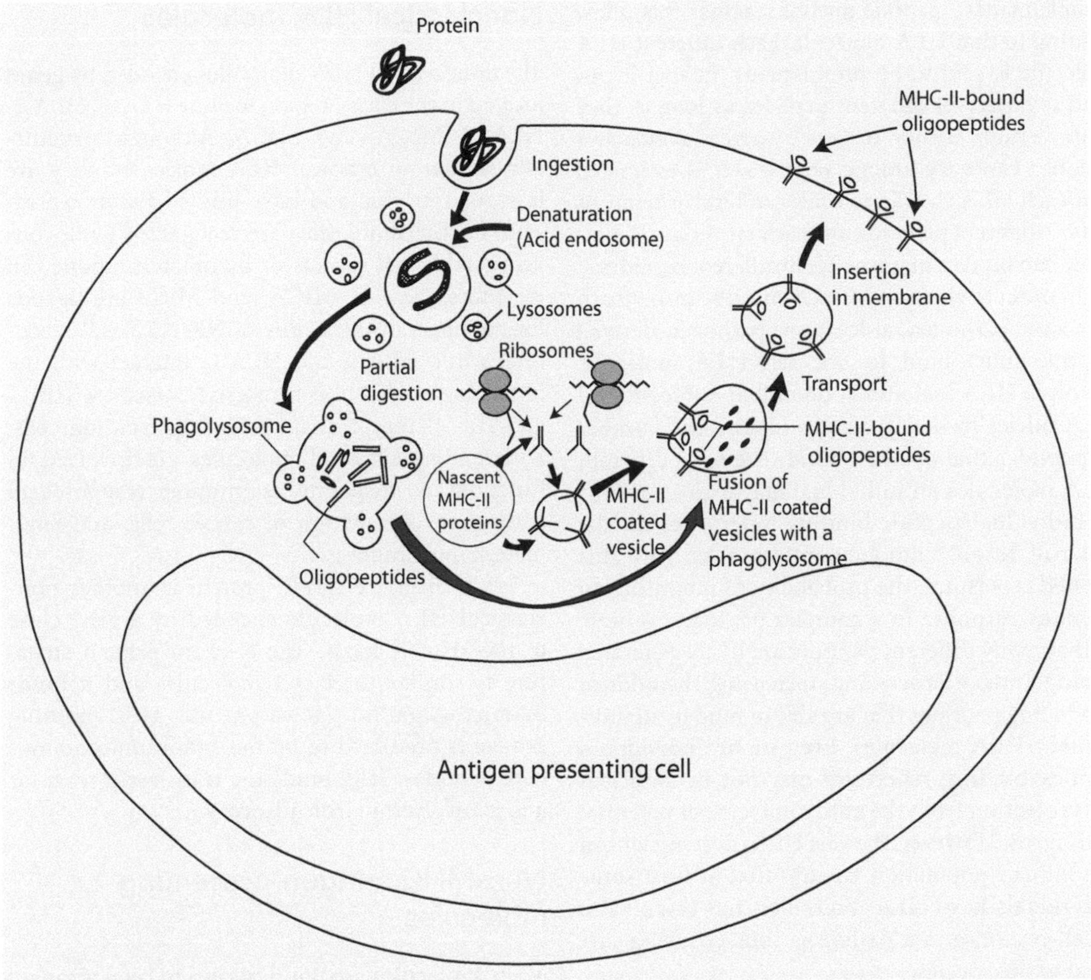

Figure 3.8 General steps in exogenous antigen processing. The antigen is ingested, partially degraded, and after vesicles coated with nascent MHC-II proteins fuse with the phagolysosomes, antigen-derived polypeptides bind to the MHC-II molecule. In this bound form, the oligopeptides seem protected against further denaturation and are transported together with the MHC-II molecule to the cell membrane, where they will be presented to CD4+ T lymphocytes in traffic through the tissue where the APCs are located.

endosomal-lysosomal compartments into slightly longer peptides of 15–25 amino acids. Meanwhile, newly synthesized class II molecules bind an invariant chain protein that blocks peptides from binding within the groove. After class II molecules are transported into the endosomal-lysosomal compartments, the invariant chain is degraded. The class II encoded DM and DO molecules are intracellular proteins that act as chaperones and regulators that facilitate the exchange of the invariant chain with extracellularly derived peptides that bind to one or more of the different HLA-DR, HLA-DQ, or HLA-DP molecules. Finally, the peptide-loaded

class II molecules are guided to the cell surface to be inspected by CD4+ T cells. Dendritic cells possess other antigen-processing pathways in which peptides derived from extracellular proteins can be cross-presented by class I molecules.

HLA binding specificity and αβ-T-cell immune response

Polymorphic amino acids encoded by a particular HLA allele form allele-specific pockets within its peptide-binding groove. The shape and charge of amino acids that line these pockets dictate the complementary peptide anchor residues that allow binding to that HLA molecule. Each different HLA molecule is said to be promiscuous, in that it can bind a variety of different peptides as long as they share certain anchor residues, whereas nonanchor residues can vary among peptides. It is estimated that each HLA class I molecule can bind as many as 10,000 different peptides, and each HLA class II molecule can bind as many as 2,000 different peptides.

In order to elicit a $\alpha\beta$-T-cell immune response to a specific pathogen, at least one pathogen-derived peptide must bind to one self HLA molecule. Multiple HLA loci and codominant expression of HLA alleles in heterozygotes expand the number of peptides that can be bound. The 6–18 different HLA molecules an individual may express results in individual peptide-binding repertoires on the order of 10^8–10^{10} unique peptides. Even with this limited repertoire, the probability of mounting an immune response to a complex pathogen is high, in that many different peptides are likely generated during antigen processing, increasing the odds of producing peptides that are able to bind to an individual's HLA molecules. Even so, an individual's peptide-binding repertoire may not be sufficient for protection from the entire universe of potential pathogens. However, the vast HLA diversity within the human population ensures that at least some individuals have HLA molecules that can elicit a T-cell response to a pathogen, thus ensuring survival of the species.

T-cell activation is governed by the interaction between the T-cell receptor and the MHC-peptide complex as well as by interactions between co-receptors and accessory molecules on the antigen-presenting cell and the T cell. But biophysical parameters such as binding affinity and kinetics between T-cell receptors and the MHC-peptide complex are thought to be major factors that determine the outcome of the interaction. Only a small fraction of the vast number of potential T-cell receptor–MHC-peptide complexes has been studied. Yet a clear hierarchy based on the peptide source is observed, with normal self peptides displaying the lowest affinities, followed by allo-peptides (normal polymorphic peptides derived from other individuals) and peptides from self cancer cells. The highest affinities are found for pathogen-specific peptides. This ranking is what is expected from an immune response that is designed to eliminate altered self and dangerous non-self.

Nonclassical HLA molecules

The nonclassical HLA molecules encoded by genes located in the class I region include HLA-E, HLA-F, HLA-G, MICA, and MICB. Although structurally similar to classical HLA molecules, they are less polymorphic and have limited tissue expression. Furthermore, they are recognized by unconventional T-cell subsets or by innate immune cell receptors. HLA-E, MICA, and MICB are ligands for members of the family of NK/NKT cell receptors, while HLA-F and HLA-G interact with the immunoglobulin-like transcript-2 and -4 (ILT-2 and ILT 4) receptors on antigen-presenting cells. Different nonclassical molecules are involved in functions as disparate as immune responses to pathogens, elimination of cancer cells, and fetal-maternal tolerance.

High (iron) Fe (HFE) protein is another nonclassical HLA molecule encoded by a gene close to the HLA-A locus. The α chain protein structure is similar to class I molecules and it binds β2-microglobulin. However, the HFE binding groove is predicted to be too small to accommodate peptides. HFE binds the transferrin receptor and is involved in iron adsorption.

Non-MHC antigen-presenting molecules

MHC molecules are not designed to bind strongly hydrophobic antigens such as lipids or carbohydrates. While the response to carbohydrates is elicited with minimal or no cooperation from helper T cells, (thus circumventing the need for MHC presentation), the response to lipids and glycolipids involves presentation by a family of MHC Class I-like proteins, named CD1. The human CD1a-e molecules are encoded by closely linked non-polymorphic genes on chromosome 1. These molecules are structurally similar to Class I molecules, with an α chain composed of α1, α2 and α3 domains that is non-covalently associated with β2-microglobulin. However, the α1 and α2 domains form a deep groove lined with hydrophobic residues that bind lipid structures, rather than peptides. The CD1 family binds a broad range of lipids, but each family member preferentially binds one or more lipid classes that may be derived from a host of different microbes, including *Mycobacterium tuberculosis*, the lipopolysaccharides from gram-negative bacteria or lipotechoic acid from gram-positive bacteria. The CD1a-c molecules present lipid antigens to diverse unconventional αβ or γδ T cells, while CD1d proteins present antigens to NKT cells.

HLA DISEASE ASSOCIATIONS

General considerations

There are two major approaches to determining the genetic etiology of a disease: linkage analysis and association analysis. These terms are often mistakenly used synonymously. **Linkage** implies that the gene under consideration and the putative gene responsible for the disease are on the same chromosome. It is determined by co-segregation of the disease with a particular genetic variant in families consisting of affected and unaffected individuals. This approach has been useful in the identification of genes for diseases that follow simple Mendelian inheritance. **Association** implies that a specific allele is found more or less often in a group of unrelated individuals with a disease than in subjects without that disease. This approach is more powerful than linkage in detecting the genes for complex diseases that are polygenetic or are strongly influenced by other factors as in many autoimmune diseases. In some cases, HLA allele-specified structural and functional differences have been identified and are postulated to play an important role in disease susceptibility or resistance as in the case of HIV control.

Hemochromatosis

Hemochromatosis is a disorder that increases the risk of iron overload. Family studies in Caucasians of western European descent demonstrated autosomal recessive inheritance in linkage with HLA-A3. Decades later, the HFE gene was discovered in close proximity to HLA-A. A common mutation within the HFE gene prohibits β2-microglobulin from binding to the HFE α-chain. This disrupts the binding of HFE to the transferrin receptor and alters iron absorption pathways.

Infectious disease

The association of HLA with HIV infection and progression to AIDS serves as an example of HLA infectious disease associations. HIV control as defined by low viremia and delayed onset of AIDS was originally associated with HLA-B57 alleles, whereas progression to AIDS was associated with HLA-B35 alleles. Fine mapping through genome-wide association studies identified polymorphisms at four amino acid sites in several different HLA-B molecules and provided a clear indication of the structural basis for the originally described HLA associations. Three of the four amino acids sites are within the groove and likely influence the HIV peptides that can bind and the conformations they adopt. The fourth amino acid is located in a region that is likely to impact binding to the CD8 co-receptor. Thus, all four sites are likely to influence the efficacy of CD8+ T-cell responses and, therefore, clinical outcomes.

Autoimmune disease

The prevailing theory of self tolerance states that T cells whose receptors do not bind self MHC die from neglect (negative selection), and T cells whose receptors bind strongly to self MHC + self peptides are killed (positive selection) during thymic development. Those T cells whose receptors have low to intermediate affinity for self escape the thymus and form the peripheral T-cell repertoire. These T cells can mount immune responses to foreign or abnormal peptides but have high enough activation requirements that they leave normal uninfected cells unscathed. However, this is not an error-proof process, as evidenced by the existence of more than 80 different autoimmune diseases. Some autoimmune diseases target specific cells or tissues, such as type I diabetes, whereas others are systemic, such as systemic lupus erythematosus. Autoimmune diseases are fairly common, with a prevalence approaching 10% worldwide. Most autoimmune diseases require predisposing genetic factors as well as environmental triggers. A lower threshold for self reactive T-cell activation may occur when the cellular environment signals danger in response to insults such as tissue damage, inflammation, or infections.

Many autoimmune diseases are known to be polygenetic, but HLA haplotypes and certain HLA alleles or binding motifs are strongly associated with autoimmune disease susceptibility or resistance. However, inheritance of a susceptibility gene does not necessarily portend disease development,

Table 3.2 Some HLA and disease associations

Disease	HLA allele(s)	Relative risk of developing the disease[a]	Description of the disease
Inflammatory diseases			
Ankylosing spondylitis	B27	100–200	Inflammation of the spine, leading to stiffening of vertebral joints
Reiter's syndrome	B27	40	Inflammation of the spine, prostate, and parts of eye (conjunctiva, uvea)
Juvenile rheumatoid arthritis	B27	10–12	A multisystem inflammatory disease of children characterized by rapid onset of joint lesions and fever
Adult rheumatoid arthritis	DR4	9	Autoimmune inflammatory disease of the joints often associated with vasculitis
Psoriasis	Cw6	7	An acute, recurrent, localized inflammatory disease of the skin (usually scalp, elbows, associated with arthritis)
Celiac disease	DQ2, DQ8	30	A chronic inflammatory disease of the small intestine; probably a food allergy to a protein in grains (gluten)
Multiple sclerosis	DQ6	12	A progressive chronic inflammatory disease of brain and spinal cord that destroys the myelin sheath
Endocrine diseases			
Addison's disease	DR3	5	A deficiency in production of adrenal gland cortical hormones
Diabetes mellitus	DQ8	14	A deficiency of insulin production; pancreatic islet cells usually absent or damaged
	DQ6	0.02	
Miscellaneous diseases			
Narcolepsy	DQ6	>40	A condition characterized by the tendency to fall asleep unexpectedly

Source: Modified from Hood, L.E. et al. *Immunology*, 2nd ed., Benjamin-Cummings, Menlo Park, CA, 1984.

[a] Numerical indicator of how many more times a disease is likely to occur in individuals possessing a given HLA allele relative to those who do not express the marker, determined by the following formula:

$$\text{Relative Risk} = \frac{\text{Number of patients with the marker} \times \text{Number of controls without the marker}}{\text{Number of patients without the marker} \times \text{Number of controls with the marker}}$$

(Epidemiologists term this value *odds ratio* (OR), which is usually accompanied by a 95% confidence interval (CI). The OR is considered significant if the CI does *not* include 1.)

nor does failure to inherit an identified susceptibility gene preclude disease development. Nevertheless, some HLA disease associations are strong enough to be of diagnostic assistance. For instance, virtually all patients with narcolepsy are positive for the HLA-DQB1*0602 allele. Hence, a diagnosis of narcolepsy can be excluded in a patient who does not have this allele. But one cannot predict the development of narcolepsy by typing for this allele, as it is frequently present in the general population in the absence of the disease. Table 3.2 lists strong HLA disease associations that have been confirmed by many studies and in different populations.

The mechanisms that underlie the associations between HLA and autoimmune diseases are not known. However, the onset of several diseases is temporally related to infection or vaccination. Molecular mimicry occurs when the structural similarity between a self peptide and a microbial peptide is recognized by cross-reactive, microbe-specific T cells. This mechanism has been postulated to explain diabetes development in genetically susceptible mice whose T cells exhibit cross-reactivity between an islet-specific protein and a transporter protein peptide of *Fusobacteria*.

Other potential mechanisms invoke self reactive T cells whose threshold for activation is lowered when they encounter higher concentrations of HLA-self peptide complexes than normal in specific tissues or under specific conditions, or self peptides derived from proteins that have undergone post-translation modifications and are therefore slightly structurally different than normal. These potential mechanisms all invoke allele-specific binding motifs that allow presentation of specific peptides (microbial, normal self, or modified self) to self T cells.

The HLA system is associated with the fate of transplanted tissues, pathogen-specific immunity, and autoimmunity. However, these seemingly disparate roles can be viewed as simply different manifestations of a common biologic function, which is to bind and present a diverse range of peptides for inspection by T cells. HLA provides an elegant example of the role of polymorphism, structure, and function on individual and population-wide immune responses.

BIBLIOGRAPHY

Berger M, Zhou R, Rizvi NA, et al. Patient HLA class I genotype influences cancer response to checkpoint blockade immunotherapy. *Science* 2018;359:582–587.

Berman HM, Westbrook J, Feng Z et al. The protein data bank. *Nucl Acids Res.* 2000;28:235–242.

Bettini L, Bettini M. Understanding autoimmune diabetes through the prism of the tri-molecular complex. *Front Endocrinol.* 2017;8:351.

Bjorkman J. MHC restriction in three dimensions: A view of T cell receptor/ligand interactions. *Cell* 1997;89:167–170.

Brent L. *A History of Transplantation Immunology.* San Diego, CA: Academic Press; 1997.

Bridgeman JS, Sewell AK, Miles JJ et al. Structural and biophysical determinants of αβ T-cell antigen recognition. *Immunology.* 2011;135:9–18.

Chowell D, Morris LGT, Grigg CM et al. HLA variation and disease. *Nat Rev Immunol.* 2018;18:325–339.

Gensterblum-Miller E, Wu W, Sawalha AH. Novel transcriptional activity and extensive allelic imbalance in the human MHC region. *J Immunol.* 2018;200:1496–1503.

Hammer C, Begemann M, McLaren PJ et al. Amino acid variation in HLA class II proteins is a major determinant of humoral response to common viruses. *Amer J Human Genet.* 2015; 97:738–743.

Martin MP, Naranbhai V, Shea PR et al. Killer cell immunoglobulin–like receptor 3DL1 variation modifies HLA-B*57 protection against HIV-1. *J Clin Invest.* 2018;128:1903–1912.

Matzaraki V, Kumar V, Wijmenga C et al. The MHC locus and genetic susceptibility to autoimmune and infectious diseases. *Genome Biol.* 2017;18:76.

Medawar PB. The immunology of transplantation. *Harvey Lect.* 1956–58 (series 52);144–176.

Pratheek BM, Nayak TK, Sahoo SS et al. Mammalian non-classical major histocompatibility complex I and its receptors: Important contexts of gene, evolution and immunity. *Indian J Human Genet.* 2014;20:129–141.

Rock K, Reits E, Neefjes J. Present yourself! by MHC class I and MHC class II molecules. *Trends Immunol.* 2016;37:724–737.

Rose AS, Bradley AR, Valasatava Y et al. Web-based molecular graphics for large complexes. *ACM Proceedings of the 21st International Conference on Web3D Technology (Web 3D'16)*; 2016:185–186.

Rose AS, Hildebrand PW. NGL Viewer: A web application for molecular visualization. *Nucl Acids Res.* 2015;43:W576–W579.

Rose PW, Prlić A, Altunkaya A et al. The RCSB protein data bank: Integrative view of protein, gene and 3D structural information. *Nucl Acids Res.* 2017;45:D271–D281.

Schneider-Hohendorfa T, Görlich D, Savolac P et al. Sex bias in MHC I-associated shaping of the adaptive immune system. *Proc Nat Acad Sci USA.* 2018;115:2168–2173.

Shiina T, Blancher A, Inoko H et al. Comparative genomics of the human, macaque and mouse major histocompatibility complex. *Immunology.* 2016;150:127–138.

Yin L, Scott-Browne J, Kappler JW et al. T cells and their eons-old obsession with MHC. *Immunol Rev.* 2012;250:49–60.

4

Adaptive immune response: Antigens, lymphocytes, and accessory cells

GABRIEL VIRELLA AND JOHN W. SLEASMAN

INTRODUCTION

The immune system has evolved to ensure constant surveillance of "non-self" structures. Both T and B lymphocytes have cell surface receptors able to recognize structures not normally presented or expressed by the organism. Once that recognition takes place, a complex series of events is triggered, leading to the proliferation and differentiation of immune-competent cells and to the development of immunological memory. These events will be directly or indirectly responsible for the elimination of the organism, cells, or molecules presenting non-self structures. Considerable effort has been applied to the study of *in vitro* and animal models allowing a detailed insight into the steps involved in the generation of an immune response.

ANTIGENICITY AND IMMUNOGENICITY

Antigenicity is defined as the property of a substance (antigen) that allows it to react with the products of a specific immune response (antibody or T-cell receptor). Immunogenicity is defined as the property of a substance (immunogen) that endows it with the capacity to provoke a specific immune response. From these definitions, it follows that all

immunogens are antigens; the reverse, however, is not true, as discussed later.

B-cell immunogens are usually complex, large molecules, able to interact with B-cell surface receptors (membrane immunoglobulins) and deliver by themselves the initial activating signal leading to clonal expansion and differentiation of antibody-producing cells. T-cell immunogens can be best defined as compounds that can be processed by antigen-presenting cells into short polypeptide chains that combine with major histocompatibility complex (MHC) molecules; the peptide-MHC complexes are able to interact with specific T-cell receptors and deliver activating signals to the T cells carrying such receptors.

Landsteiner, Pauling, and others discovered in the 1930s and 1940s that small aromatic groups, such as amino-benzene sulfonate, amino-benzene arsenate, and amino-benzene carboxylate, unable to induce antibody responses by themselves, could be chemically coupled to immunogenic proteins. The injection of these complexes into laboratory animals resulted in the production of antibodies specific for the different aromatic groups. The aromatic groups were designated as "haptens" and the immunogenic proteins as "carriers." The immune response induced by a hapten-carrier conjugate included antibodies able to recognize the hapten and the carrier as separate entities. The hapten-specific antibodies are also able to react with soluble hapten molecules, free of carrier protein. Thus, a hapten is an antigen but not an immunogen. In practical terms, it must be noted that the designations of *antigen* and *immunogen* are often used interchangeably.

Antigenic determinants

As noted previously, most immunogens are complex molecules (mostly proteins and polysaccharides). However, only a restricted portion of the antigen molecule—known as an antigenic determinant or epitope—is able to interact with the specific binding site of a B-lymphocyte membrane immunoglobulin, a soluble antibody, or a T-lymphocyte antigen receptor.

While B lymphocytes recognize epitopes expressed by unmodified native molecules, T lymphocytes recognize short peptides generated by antigen processing (i.e., intracellular cleaving of large proteins into short peptides) or derived from newly synthesized proteins cleaved in the cytoplasm. These oligopeptides are newly formed and have little or no three-dimensional homology with the epitopes expressed on native proteins.

Studies with X-ray crystallography and two-dimensional nuclear magnetic resonance have resulted in the detailed characterization of B-cell epitopes presented by some small proteins, such as lysozyme, in their native configuration. From such studies, the following rules have been derived for antigen recognition:

- Most epitopes are defined by a series of 15–22 amino acids located on discontinuous segments of the polypeptide chain, forming a roughly flat area with peaks and valleys that establish contact with the folded hypervariable regions of the antibody heavy and light chains.
- Specific regions of the epitope, the dominant epitopes, are constituted by a few amino acids that bind with greater affinity to specific areas of the antibody-binding site and, thus, are primarily responsible for the specificity of antigen-antibody interaction. The antibody-binding site has some degree of flexibility that optimizes the fit with the corresponding epitope (Figure 4.1).
- A polypeptide with 100 amino acids may have as many as 14–20 nonoverlapping epitopes.

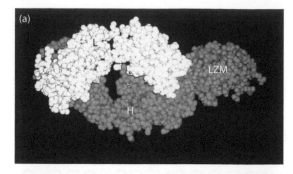

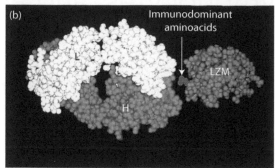

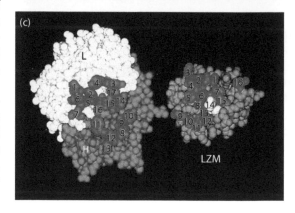

Figure 4.1 A space-filling model showing the fit between an epitope of lysozyme and the antigen-binding site on an anti-lysozyme antibody. The yellow and blue structures represent the heavy (H) and light (L) chain segments of an immunoglobulin molecule that define the antigen-binding site. The green structure represents the antigen, lysozyme. The amino acids depicted in red represent the dominant epitope of lysozyme. (a, b) The antigen-antibody complex is formed by lysozyme and its corresponding antibody. The fit of the immunodominant epitope to a pouch formed in the binding site of the antibody binding site is illustrated in panels (b) and (c). In panel (c) the immunodominant epitope is depicted in white. (Reproduced with permission from Amit A.G. et al., *Science*, 233, 747–753, 1986.)

However, a typical 100 amino acid globular protein is folded over itself, and most of its structure is hidden from the outside. Only surface epitopes will usually be accessible for recognition by B lymphocytes and for interactions with antibodies (Figure 4.1).

Determinants of immunogenicity

Many different substances can induce immune responses. The following characteristics influence the ability for a substance to behave as an immunogen:

- *Foreignness*: As a rule, only substances recognized as "non-self" will trigger the immune response. Microbial products and exogenous molecules are obviously "non-self" and are usually strongly immunogenic.
- *Molecular size*: The most potent immunogens are macromolecular proteins (molecular weight [M.W.] >100,000 daltons). Molecules smaller than 10,000 daltons are often only weakly immunogenic, unless coupled to an immunogenic carrier protein.
- *Chemical structure*: Proteins and polysaccharides are among the most potent immunogens, although relatively small polypeptide chains, nucleic acids, and even lipids can, given the appropriate circumstances, be immunogenic.

Proteins of high molecular weight express a wide diversity of antigenic determinants and are potent immunogens. It must be noted that the immunogenicity of a protein is strongly influenced by its chemical composition. Positively charged (basic) amino acids, such as lysine, arginine, and histidine, are repeatedly present in the antigenic sites of lysozyme and myoglobin, while aromatic amino acids (such as tyrosine) are found in two epitopes defined in albumin. Therefore, it appears that basic and aromatic amino acids may contribute more strongly to immunogenicity than other amino acids. Indeed, basic proteins with clusters of positively charged amino acids are strongly immunogenic.

Polysaccharides are among the most important antigens because of their abundant representation in nature. Pure polysaccharides, the sugar moieties of glycoproteins, lipopolysaccharides, glycolipid-protein complexes, etc., are all immunogenic. Many microorganisms have polysaccharide-rich capsules or cell walls, and a variety of mammalian antigens, such as the erythrocyte antigens (A, B, Le, H), are short-chain polysaccharides (oligosaccharides). As noted later in this chapter, polysaccharides and oligosaccharides stimulate B cells without T-cell help. In contrast, lipids and glycolipids can elicit immune responses with T-cell cooperation, as discussed in Chapter 3.

Nucleic acids (RNA and DNA) usually are not immunogenic but can induce antibody formation if coupled to a protein to form a nucleoprotein. The autoimmune responses characteristic of some of the autoimmune diseases (e.g., systemic lupus erythematosus) are often directed to DNA.

Polypeptides, such as insulin and other hormones, relatively small in size (M.W. 1500 for insulin), are usually able to induce antibody formation when isolated from one species and administered over long periods of time to an individual of a different species. Recombinant human insulin is considerably less immunogenic but still can be recognized as a foreign substance because it is not glycosylated.

- *Chemical complexity*: There is a direct relationship between antigenicity and chemical complexity; aggregated or chemically polymerized proteins are much stronger immunogens than their soluble monomeric counterparts.

Factors associated with induction of immune response

In addition to the chemical nature of the immunogen, other factors strongly influence the development and potency of an immune response, as discussed in the following sections.

Genetic background

Different animal species and different strains of one given species may show different degrees of responsiveness to a given antigen. In humans, different individuals can behave as "high responders" or "low responders" to any given antigen. The genetic control of the immune response is poorly understood but involves the repertoire of MHC molecules that bind antigen fragments and present them to the responding T-cell population. The affinity of the peptide for the MHC and of the peptide-MHC complex for the T-cell receptor will dictate, at least in part, the T-cell response. Data obtained in studies of gene expression in high- and low-responder humans to vaccinia virus and hepatitis B vaccine have revealed differences in gene expression, some genes being expressed in lower levels and others being expressed at higher levels in high responders. The genes in question, particularly those related to the expression of the killer cell immunoglobulin-like receptor (KIR), may be directly or indirectly involved in immunoregulatory processes that could be significantly different in high and low responders. These observations also underline the interactions between innate and adaptive immunity that may have significant implications in the magnitude of the adaptive immune response.

Method of antigen administration

The method of antigen administration has a profound effect on the immune response. A given dose of antigen may elicit no detectable response when injected intravenously, but a strong immune response is observed if injected intradermally. The presence of dendritic cells in the dermis (where they are known as Langerhans cells) may be a critical factor determining the enhanced immune responses when antigens are injected intradermally. This route of administration results in slow removal from the site of injection and in uptake and processing of the antigen by dendritic cells. The dendritic cells may present antigen to migrating T cells or may themselves migrate to the lymph node follicles, where the initial stages of the immune response take place. Thus, intradermal administration promotes prolonged antigenic stimulation and facilitates the involvement of one of the most specialized populations of antigen-presenting cells.

Use of adjuvants

Adjuvants are agents that when administered along with antigens enhance the specific response (Figure 4.2). In contrast to carrier proteins, adjuvants are often nonimmunogenic and are never chemically coupled to the antigens. Several factors seem to contribute to the enhancement of immune responses by adjuvants, including delayed release of antigen, nonspecific inflammatory effects, and the activation of monocytes and macrophages. Several microbial and inorganic compounds have been used effectively as adjuvants, both clinically and as investigational agents.

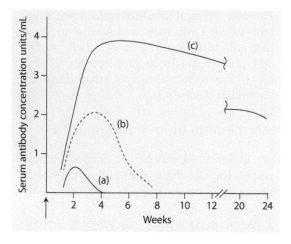

Figure 4.2 Quantities of antibodies formed by rabbits following a single injection of a soluble protein antigen (marked by arrow), (a) such as bovine γ-globulin in dilute physiologic saline solution, (b) adsorbed on precipitated alum, or (c) incorporated into Freund's complete adjuvant.

One of the most effective adjuvants is complete Freund's adjuvant (CFA), a water-in-oil emulsion with killed mycobacteria in the oil phase. This is the adjuvant of choice for production of antisera in laboratory animals. Bacillus Calmette-Guérin (BCG), an attenuated strain of *Mycobacterium bovis* used as a vaccine against tuberculosis, has also been used as an immunotherapeutic agent to boost the immune system in patients with some types of cancer (e.g., superficial bladder cancer, melanoma). Their use is limited, however, by side effects such as intense inflammatory reactions and discomfort. More recently, growth factors such as GM-CSF have been found to have adjuvant properties that may be clinically useful for the induction of cancer-specific immune responses.

Aluminum hydroxide, an inert compound that absorbs the immunogen, stimulates phagocytosis, and delays removal from the inoculation side, is an adjuvant frequently used with human vaccines. Aluminum hydroxide is not as effective as many of the adjuvants previously listed but is also considerably less toxic.

Exogenous and endogenous antigens

Most antigens to which we react are of exogenous origin and include microbial antigens, environmental antigens (such as pollens and pollutants), and medications. The objective of the immune response is the elimination of foreign antigens, but in some instances, the immune response may have a deleterious effect resulting in hypersensitivity or in autoimmune disease, discussed in later chapters of this book.

Endogenous antigens, by definition, are part of self, and the immune system is usually tolerant to them. The response to self antigens may have an important role in normal catabolic processes (i.e., antibodies to denatured IgG may help in eliminating antigen-antibody complexes from circulation). The loss of tolerance to self antigens, however, can also have pathogenic implications (autoimmune diseases).

A special type of endogenous antigens includes those that distinguish one individual from another within the same species and are termed *alloantigens*. Alloantigens elicit immune responses when cells or tissues of one individual are introduced into another. The alloantigens that elicit the strongest immune response are alleles of highly polymorphic systems, such as the erythrocyte A, B, O blood group antigens: some individuals carry the polysaccharide that defines the A specificity, others have B-positive red cells, AB-positive red cells, or red cells that express neither A nor B (O). Other alloantigenic systems that elicit strong immune responses are histocompatibility antigens of nucleated cells and tissues, the platelet (Pl) antigens, and the Rh erythrocyte blood group antigens. Examples of sensitization to exogenous alloantigens include the following:

- Women sensitized to fetal red cell antigens during pregnancy.
- Polytransfused patients who become sensitized against cellular alloantigens from the donor(s).
- Recipients of organ transplants who become sensitized against histocompatibility alloantigens expressed in the transplanted organ.

ACTIVATION OF HUMORAL IMMUNE SYSTEM

T- and B-cell cooperation in antibody responses

Experiments carried out with hapten-carrier complexes have contributed significantly to our understanding of the importance of T-B lymphocyte cooperation in the activation of humoral (antibody-mediated) immune responses. A specific example is illustrated in Figure 4.3. Mice primed with a hapten-carrier conjugate prepared by chemically coupling the 2-dinitrophenyl (2-DNP) radical to egg albumin (ovalbumin, OVA) produced antibodies both to DNP and OVA. Antibodies to the hapten (DNP) were not observed when mice were immunized with DNP alone or with a mixture of unlinked DNP and OVA. Secondary challenge of mice primed with DNP-OVA with the same hapten-carrier conjugate triggered an anamnestic or "recall" response of higher magnitude against both hapten and carrier. In contrast, if the DNP-OVA primed animals were challenged with the same hapten coupled to a different carrier, such as bovine γ-globulin (DNP-BGG), the ensuing response to DNP was of identical magnitude to that observed after the first immunization with DNP-OVA. The conclusion from these observations is that a "recall" response to the hapten can only be observed when the animal is repeatedly immunized with the same hapten-carrier conjugate (Figure 4.3).

Further experiments demonstrated that immunologic "memory" (defined as a response of higher magnitude, characteristic of a secondary response) to the hapten moiety of a hapten-carrier conjugate is exclusively dependent on a previous exposure to the carrier moiety by itself. In other words, the factors responsible for the secondary immune response were effective in enhancing the response to any hapten coupled to the carrier.

Additional hapten-carrier experiments were later repeated using sublethally irradiated inbred mice reconstituted with different cell subpopulations from immunocompetent animals of the same strain. They proved that both carrier and hapten-specific antibody-producing cells were "helped" by carrier-specific T lymphocytes (Figure 4.4). In other words, T-lymphocyte "help" is carrier specific, not antigen specific, since the T and B lymphocytes collaborating in the immune response may recognize antigenic determinants from totally unrelated compounds (hapten and carrier).

In the last two decades, the hapten-carrier concept has found significant applications in medicine. Hapten-carrier systems have been developed to raise antibodies to a variety of nonimmunogenic chemicals that are the basis for a variety of drug-level assays (e.g., plasma cyclosporine levels) and to enhance the response to polysaccharide vaccines. Last, the immune response to haptens coupled to

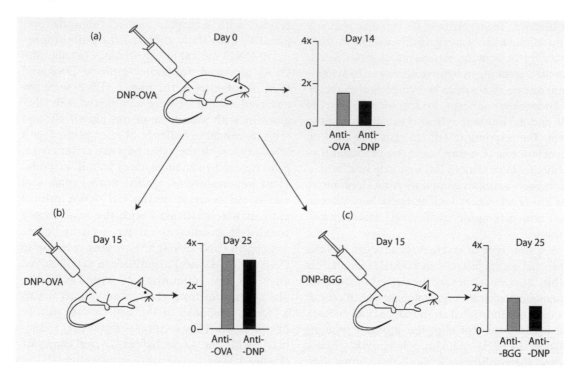

Figure 4.3 The hapten-carrier effect: In order to obtain a secondary immune response to the hapten (DNP), (a) the animal needs to be immunized and (b) challenged with the same DNP-carrier combination. (c) Boosting with a different DNP-carrier conjugate will result in an anti-DNP response of identical magnitude to that obtained after the initial immunization. The memory response, therefore, appears to be carrier dependent.

autologous carriers has been demonstrated to be the pathological basis for some abnormal immune reactions, including some drug allergies. For instance, the spontaneous coupling of the penicilloyl derivative of penicillin to a host protein is believed to be the first step toward developing hypersensitivity to penicillin. Hypersensitivity reactions to a number of drugs, chemicals, and metals are believed to result from spontaneous coupling of these nonimmunogenic compounds to endogenous proteins whose tertiary structure is modified as a consequence of the chemical reaction with the hapten. As a consequence, the conditions necessary for the elicitation of immune responses to nonimmunogenic compounds are created.

T-DEPENDENT AND T-INDEPENDENT ANTIGENS

Additional studies were performed with homozygous rodents sublethally irradiated after reconstitution of their immune systems with T lymphocytes,

B lymphocytes, or mixtures of T and B lymphocytes obtained from normal animals of the same strain. After reconstitution, the animals were challenged with a variety of antigens, and their antibody responses were measured.

For most antigens, including complex proteins, heterologous cells, and viruses, a measurable antibody response was only observed in animals reconstituted with mixtures of T and B lymphocytes. In other words, for most antigens, proper differentiation of antibody-producing cells required T-cell "help." The antigens that could not induce immune responses in T cell–deficient animals were designated as T-dependent antigens. Structurally, T-dependent antigens are usually complex proteins with large numbers of different, nonrepetitive, antigenic determinants.

Other antigens, particularly polysaccharides, can induce antibody synthesis in animals depleted of T lymphocytes, and are known as T-independent antigens. It should be noted that, in many species, there may be a continuous gradation of antigenic

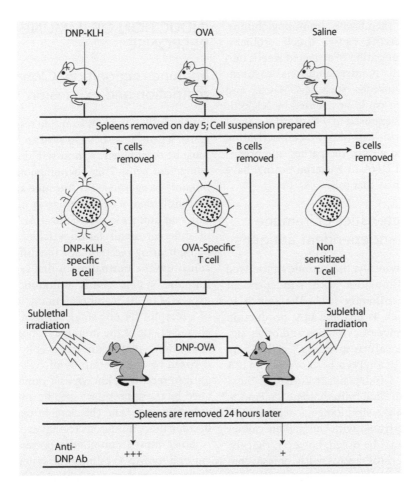

Figure 4.4 An experiment designed to determine the specificity of T-cell help in a classical hapten-carrier response. Sublethally irradiated mice were reconstituted with different combinations of T and B cells obtained from nonimmune mice or from mice immunized with DNP-OVA. T cells from mice pre-immunized with OVA "helped" B cells from mice pre-immunized with DNP-KLH to produce large amounts of anti-DNP antibodies, but the same B cells did not receive noticeable help from T cells separated from nonimmune mice. Thus, T cells with "carrier" memory efficiently stimulate B cells to produce higher concentrations of anti-DNP antibody without preexposure to DNP.

responses from T dependence to T independence, rather than two discrete groups of antigens. However, this differentiation is useful as a "working classification."

Biological basis of T independence

The basic fact that explains the inability of polysaccharides to behave as T-dependent antigens is that these compounds do not bind to MHC-II molecules and, therefore, cannot be presented to T cells. Immune responses elicited by T-independent antigens are mediated by different mechanisms that bypass the need for T-cell help.

Some T-independent antigens, such as bacterial lipopolysaccharides (LPSs), are mitogenic and can deliver dual signals to B cells, one by occupancy of the antigen-specific receptor (membrane immunoglobulin), while the mitogenic signal is delivered by the interaction of LPSs with the toll-like receptor 4 (TLR4). The engagement of these two receptors is sufficient to stimulate B cells and promote differentiation into antibody-producing cells. It is also a good example of synergism between innate and adaptive immunity.

Other T-independent antigens (such as polysaccharides) are not mitogenic but are composed of multiple sugar molecules, allowing extensive cross-linking of membrane immunoglobulins. Receptor cross-linking causes B-cell proliferation, but the differentiation of activated B cells into IgM-producing cells requires additional costimulatory signals. Cytokines, such as GM-CSF and interferon-γ, which could be released by NK cells or phagocytic cells exposed to the infectious agent with a polysaccharide capsule, or B cell–activating moieties contained within the pathogenic organism (e.g., bacterial DNA or bacterial porins) have been proposed to play that role.

Special characteristics of immune response to T-independent antigens

As mentioned previously, the antibody produced in response to stimulation with T-independent antigens is predominantly IgM. The switch to other isotypes, such as IgG and IgA, production requires the presence of cytokines and other signals delivered by locally responding T cells. There is, therefore, little (if any) synthesis of IgG and IgA after exposure to T-independent antigens. These antigens also fail to elicit immunological memory, which depends on the simultaneous activation of T cells, as demonstrated with the hapten-carrier experiments. It must be noted, however, that the exposure to infectious agents with polysaccharide capsules does elicit T-cell activation through the multiple T-dependent antigens contained in the organism. In those circumstances, given the fact that memory cells are not specific for a given antigen, the immune response to polysaccharides will proceed similarly to the response to a T cell–dependent immunogen, with switch to IgG synthesis and development of immunological memory.

Bacterial polysaccharides have been extensively used for immunization; however, the ontogenic development of the T-independent response is slow, and, as a rule, children younger than 1–2 years of age do not respond to polysaccharide immunization. A decade ago, it was discovered that poorly immunogenic polysaccharides induce the same type of immune responses associated with T-dependent immunogens when conjugated to immunogenic proteins. These conjugate vaccines act, essentially, as hapten-carrier complexes in which the polysaccharide plays the role of the hapten, and they are extremely effective in infants.

INDUCTION OF IMMUNE RESPONSE

Immune recognition: Clonal restriction and expansion

For the initiation of an immune response, an antigen or a peptide associated with an MHC molecule must be recognized as "non-self" by the immunocompetent cells. This phenomenon is designated *immune recognition*. The immune system of a normal individual may recognize as many as 10^6–10^8 different antigenic specificities. An equal number of different small families (clones) of lymphocytes, bearing receptors for the different antigens, constitute the normal germ-line repertoire of the immune system. Each immunocompetent cell expresses on its membrane many identical copies of a receptor for one single antigen. Thus, a major characteristic of the immune response is its clonal restriction—that is, one given epitope will be recognized by a single family of cells with identical antigen receptors, known as a clone. When stimulated by the appropriate specific antigen, each cell will proliferate, and the clone of reactive cells will become more numerous (clonal expansion).

Since most immunogens present many different epitopes to the immune system, the normal immune responses are polyclonal—that is, multiple clones of immunocompetent cells, each one of them specific for one unique epitope, are stimulated by any complex immunogen.

However, antibodies able to interact with epitopes of similar or unrelated nature have been well characterized and designated as "promiscuous" antibodies. Structural studies have shown that the flexibility and chemical characteristics of the binding sites of these antibodies result in their ability to recognize multiple epitopes. This can be beneficial by enabling a given antibody to react with closely related epitopes expressed as a result of mutations of the immunogenic organism, but this also may result in autoimmune reactivity if the promiscuous antibody can interact with epitopes expressed by self-tissues, cells, or secreted molecules.

Antigen receptor on B and T lymphocytes

In B lymphocytes, the antigen receptors (BCR) are membrane-inserted immunoglobulins, particularly IgD and monomeric IgM molecules. In T lymphocytes, T-cell receptors (TCR) are responsible for the recognition of non-self immunogens.

Two structurally different types of TCR have been identified. In differentiated T cells, the TCR most frequently found is constituted by two polypeptide chains, designated as α and β ($\alpha\beta$ TCR), with similar molecular weight (40–45,000). A second type of TCR, constituted by two different polypeptide chains known as γ and δ ($\gamma\delta$ TCR), is predominantly found in the submucosal lymphoid tissues.

The two chains of the $\alpha\beta$ TCR have extracellular segments with variable and constant domains, short cytoplasmic domains, and a transmembrane segment. A disulfide bridge joins them just outside the transmembrane segment.

The β chains are highly polymorphic and are encoded by a multigene family that includes genes for regions homologous to the V, C, D, and J regions of human immunoglobulins. The α-chains are encoded by a more limited multigene family with genes for regions homologous to the V, C, and J regions of human immunoglobulins. Similar polymorphisms have been defined for the $\gamma\delta$ chains. Together, the variable regions of $\alpha\beta$ and $\gamma\delta$ chains define the specific binding sites for peptide epitopes presented in association with MHC molecules. Peptides 7–15 amino acids in length are well recognized by CD4 and CD8 T cell receptors, although MHC-II molecules can accommodate larger peptides, up to 30 amino acids long. There is controversy about the degree of peptide specificity of the TCR. The TCR seems to have a high degree of flexibility, and the configuration of MHC-bound peptides appears to be subject to modifications after engagement with the TCR. As suggested by experimental studies, the combination of these two factors increases the number of peptides that can interact with a single TCR, but independent studies concerning the degree of cross-reactivity of the TCR have yielded contradictory data.

Antigen processing and presentation

Most immune responses to complex, T-dependent antigens involve the participation of several cell types, including T and B lymphocytes that are directly involved in the generation of effector mechanisms, and accessory cells that assist in the inductive stages of the immune response.

Antigen-presenting cells (APCs) are accessory cells that express MHC-II molecules on their membrane where antigen fragments can be bound and "presented" to lymphocytes. Additionally, they express ligands for costimulatory molecules and release cytokines that assist the proliferation and/or differentiation of T and B lymphocytes. As described in Chapter 2, several types of cells can function as APCs. The most effective are the dendritic cells found in the paracortical areas of the lymph nodes. The lymph node dendritic cells, largely derived from Langerhans cells and dendritic cells in the dermis and submucosae, are particularly well suited to initiate the immune response because they express MHC-II molecules constitutively at relatively high levels and because they can ingest microorganisms, dead cells, and proteins by endocytosis or phagocytosis mediated by interactions with several different constitutively expressed receptors. Once ingested, the infectious agents and soluble antigens are efficiently processed, and the resulting peptides can be presented in association with MHC-II molecules to resting T lymphocytes.

Tissue macrophages are also effective APCs because of their phagocytic and processing properties. However, the phagocytic properties of macrophages are only fully expressed after engagement of Fc and/or complement receptors by antigen molecules coated with IgG and/or complement, suggesting that their role may be more important in the late stages of the primary response and in secondary responses.

The sequence of events leading to antigen processing and presentation in a dendritic cell starts by endocytosis of antigens on membrane patches, transport to an acidic compartment (lysosome) within the cell that allows antigen degradation into small peptides. As antigens are broken down, vesicles coated with newly synthesized HLA-II molecules fuse with the lysosome. Some of the peptides generated during processing have high affinity for the binding site located within the MHC-II heterodimer that is initially occupied by an endogenous peptide (class II–associated invariant chain peptide [CLIP]), displaced by the antigen-derived peptide. The resulting MHC-peptide complexes are then transported to the APC cell membrane where they can interact with and activate CD4$^+$ T cells bearing receptors specific for the peptide.

Activation of helper T lymphocytes

The activation of resting T helper cells requires a complex and coordinated sequence of signals delivered from the T-cell receptor on the cell membrane to the nucleus of the cell. Of all the signals involved, the only antigen-specific interaction is the one that involves the T-cell receptor and the peptide–MHC-II complex. The binding of the peptide-MHC complex to the TCR is of low affinity, and other receptor-ligand interactions are required to maintain T-lymphocyte adhesion to APCs and for the delivery of required secondary signals.

The TCR on a helper T lymphocyte interacts with both the antigen-derived peptide and the MHC-II molecule (Figure 4.5). This selectivity of the TCR from helper T lymphocytes to interact with MHC-II molecules results from selection in the thymus. During thymic ontogeny, the differentiation of helper and cytotoxic T lymphocytes is based on the ability of their TCR to interact with MHC-II molecules (helper T lymphocytes) or with MHC-I molecules (cytotoxic T lymphocytes). The interactions between T lymphocytes and MHC-expressing cells are strengthened by cell surface

molecules, which also interact with constant (not peptide-loaded) regions of MHC molecules: the CD4 molecule on helper T cells interacts with MHC-II molecules, while the CD8 molecule on cytotoxic lymphocytes interacts with MHC-I molecules.

Several other cell-adhesion molecules (CAMs) can mediate lymphocyte-AC interactions, including lymphocyte function-associated antigen (LFA)-1 interacting with the intercellular adhesion molecules (ICAM)-1, -2, and -3, and CD2 interacting with CD58 (LFA-3). Unlike the interactions involving the TCR, these interactions are not antigen specific. Their role is to promote stable adhesion and signaling between T lymphocytes and APCs essential for proper stimulation through the TCR. Furthermore, T-cell activation requires sustained signaling achieved through the establishment of what is known as the immunological synapse, in which peptide–MHC-II complexes form clusters on the APC membrane, allowing aggregation and clustering of multiple TCR molecules on the opposing T-cell membrane. In the regions of contact, the two cells are separated by a narrow gap surrounded by other interacting

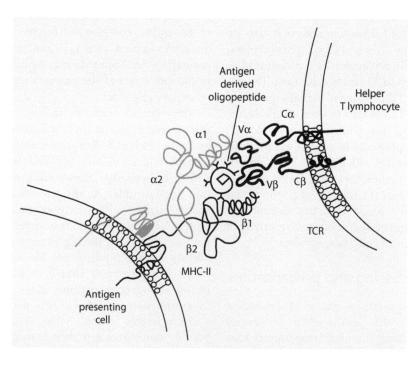

Figure 4.5 Interaction of an MHC-II–associated peptide with the TCR of a helper T cell. (Redrawn from Sinha, A.A., Lopez, M.T., McDevitt, H.O., *Science*, 248, 1380–1388, 1990.)

molecules such as CD2/CD58, LFA-1/ICAM-1, etc. The result is a stable and close apposition between APC and T cell, essential for sustained signaling (Figure 4.6).

It is important to stress that accessory cells participate in the activation of helper T lymphocytes through the delivery of signals involving cell-cell contact as well as by the release of soluble factors such as cytokines. The cell-cell interaction signals include signals mediated by CD4-MHC-II interactions and signals involving membrane molecules whose expression is increased after initial activation, including the following:

- CD2 (T cell): CD58 (APC)
- LFA-1 (T cell): ICAM-1, ICAM-2, ICAM-3 (APC)
- CD40 L (T cell): CD40 (APC)
- CD28 (T cell): CD80, CD86 (APC)

Signals mediated by interleukins include those mediated by interleukin-1 (IL-1) and interleukin-12 (IL-12). Interleukin-1 is a cytokine that promotes growth and differentiation of many cell types, including T and B lymphocytes. Both membrane-bound and soluble IL-1 are important in activating T lymphocytes *in vitro*. Membrane-bound IL-1 can only activate T lymphocytes in close contact with the APC. Interleukin-12 (IL-12) promotes Th1 cell differentiation as previously mentioned. However, all these costimulatory signals are not specific for any given antigen. The specificity of the immune response is derived from the essential and first activation signal delivered through the antigen-specific TCR.

Antigen presentation and activation of cytotoxic T lymphocytes

If an APC is infected by an intracellular organism (virus, bacteria, or parasite), the infecting agent will multiply in the cytosol. As described in Chapter 3, peptides derived from microbial proteins are loaded onto MHC-I molecules, transported to the cell surface, and presented to

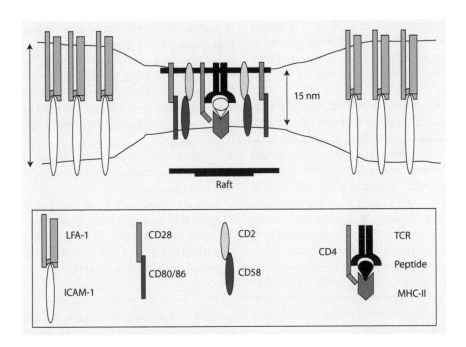

Figure 4.6 Topography of T-cell–APC cell interaction. In the areas where the T-cell receptors interact with peptide–MHC-II complexes, the cells are in very close apposition. The rafts designate cholesterol-rich membrane domains in the T-cell membrane where the TCR, CD4, and other costimulating molecules interact with their respective ligands in the APC. These interactions are primarily responsible for the close apposition of the T-cell and APC membranes and for assembling the early signaling complex. Other molecules, such as LFA-1 and ICAM-1, stabilize the interaction between T cells and APCs and are present outside the rafts. (Adapted from Dustin, M., Shaw, A.S., *Science*, 283, 649–650, 1999.)

Table 4.1 Functions of MHC-I and MHC-II molecules

MHC-I	MHC-II
Classical (HLA-A, B, C)	
• Present intracellular peptide antigens to cytotoxic CD8+ T cells (virus)	• Present processed peptides derived from extracellular antigens to CD4+ T cells
• Involved in intrathymic selection of CD8+ T cells	• Intrathymic selection of CD4+ T cells
Nonclassical (E, G, F)	
• Inhibit NK cell function	
• Protect fetus from maternal lymphocytes	

cytotoxic T lymphocytes (CTLs). CTLs are a special population of effector T cells capable of killing target cells bearing specific antigen and are largely CD8+.

The different roles of MHC-I and MHC-II molecules in the immune response and T-cell differentiation are summarized in Table 4.1. It should be noted that the MHC-I molecules designated as nonclassical play significant roles in maternal-fetal tolerance and in the control of natural killer cell activity.

The activation of cytotoxic T cells by MHC-I–peptide complexes requires peptide loading of MHC-I molecules, as described in Chapter 3. As a rule, MHC-I molecules are loaded by peptides derived from endogenously synthesized proteins, but it has also been demonstrated that MHC-I molecules can also be loaded with peptides generated from the processing of ingested exogenous proteins or cells, particularly in dendritic cells and macrophages. This phenomenon is known as cross-presentation and involves translocation of internalized antigens to the cytosol, where they are degraded by the proteasomes and the resulting fragments are transported to the endoplasmic reticulum by the TAP system.

The stimulation of cytotoxic T cells requires additional signals and interactions, some of which depend on cell-cell contact, such as those mediated by the interaction of CD8 with MHC I, CD2 with CD58, LFA-1 with ICAM family members, and CD28 with CD80 and CD86. The expansion of antigen-activated cytotoxic T lymphocytes

requires the secretion of IL-2. In experimental conditions, activated cytotoxic T lymphocytes can secrete sufficient quantities of IL-2 to support their proliferation and differentiation, and thus proceed without help from other T-cell subpopulations. Physiologically, it seems more likely that activated helper T lymphocytes provide the IL-2 necessary for cytotoxic T-lymphocyte differentiation. The simultaneous expression of immunogenic peptides in association with MHC-I and MHC-II molecules in dendritic cells and macrophages creates the necessary environment for activation of T-helper and T-cytotoxic lymphocytes in close proximity. In the case of viral infections, macrophages are often infected, and consequently, they will express viral peptides associated both with MHC-I (derived from newly synthesized proteins) and with MHC-II (derived from the degradation of endocytosed viral particles), thus becoming able to present viral-derived peptides both to T-helper and T-cytotoxic lymphocytes.

MIXED LYMPHOCYTE REACTION AND GRAFT REJECTION

Cytotoxic T lymphocytes also differentiate and proliferate when exposed to cells from an individual of the same species but from a different genetic background. *In vitro*, the degree of allostimulation between cells of two different individuals can be assessed by the mixed leukocyte reaction. Two recognition pathways have been proposed (Figure 4.7):

1. Direct allorecognition of non-self MHC molecules by lymphocytes expressing alloreactive T-cell receptors.
2. Indirect recognition of allogeneic peptides (probably resulting from ingestion and processing of dead donor cells or proteins) associated with MHC-II molecules by Th1 cells expressing receptors for non-self peptides.

This second pathway seems very important in the mixed leukocyte reaction because MHC-II-expressing cells must be present for the mixed leukocyte reaction to take place. This requirement suggests that activation of helper T cells by recognition of MHC-II–peptide complexes expressed by APCs is essential for the differentiation of cytotoxic CD8+ cells. The role of helper T cells in the mixed lymphocyte reaction is likely to be similar to the role of helper T cells that assist

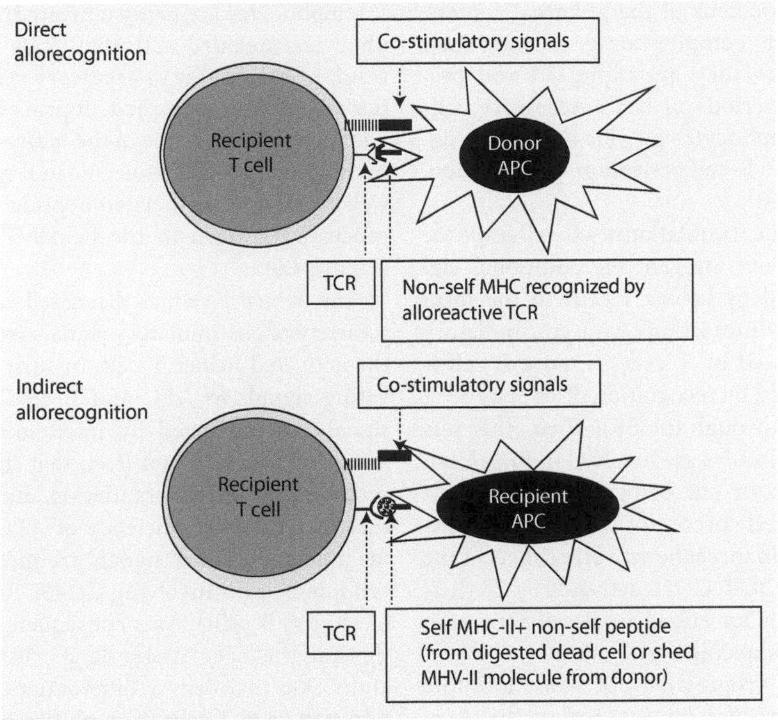

Figure 4.7 Two pathways involved in allostimulation between cells of two different individuals.

B-cell responses—that is, to provide cytokines and costimulatory signals essential for cytotoxic T-cell growth and differentiation.

In graft rejection, it is also believed that both pathways are involved. Graft rejection is more intense with increasing MHC disparity between donor and host. It seems intuitive that the strength of activation through the direct pathway should be directly related to the degree of structural differences between the nonshared MHC molecules. The transplanted tissues are likely to contain dying cells and activated cells shedding MHC-II molecules. Recipient APCs are likely to express allogeneic MHC-derived peptides as a consequence of either processing of phagocytized dead cells or endocytosis of soluble donor MHC molecules. Thus, MHC differences are likely to influence the rejection reaction, irrespective of which activation pathway is involved. As for what recipient T lymphocytes mediate the rejection, the indirect pathway can activate both CD4+ and CD8+ lymphocytes, because exogenous peptides can be loaded both to MHC-II and MHC-I molecules (through the cross-presentation pathway discussed earlier in this chapter). Thus, both activated Th1 and CD8 cytotoxic lymphocytes can be activated and become involved in graft rejection.

ALTERNATIVE PATHWAYS OF ANTIGEN PRESENTATION TO CYTOTOXIC T CELLS

The best characterized of these pathways involves CD1, a family of nonpolymorphic, MHC-I-related molecules that includes five different isomorphic forms (A to E). Antigen-presenting cells, including dendritic cells and B cells, express CD1A, B, and C molecules and have been shown to present mycobacterium-derived lipid and lipoglycan antigens to both γδ and αβ CD8+ cytotoxic T-lymphocytes. Both γδ and CD8+ αβ T cells stimulated by mycobacterial antigens presented in association with CD1 molecules cause the death of the presenting cells.

STIMULATION OF B LYMPHOCYTE RESPONSES TO T-DEPENDENT ANTIGENS

In contrast to T lymphocytes, B lymphocytes recognize external epitopes of unprocessed antigens, which do not have to be associated to MHC molecules. Some special types of APC, such as the follicular dendritic cells of the germinal centers, appear to adsorb complex antigens onto their membranes where they are expressed and presented for long periods of time. Accessory cells and helper T lymphocytes provide additional signals necessary for B-cell activation, proliferation, and differentiation.

In the case of the stimulation of a B-cell response with a T-dependent antigen, the additional signals are delivered by helper T cells in the form of cytokines and interactions with costimulatory molecules expressed by T cells. A naive B cell is initially stimulated by recognition of an epitope of the immunogen through the BCR. Two other sets of membrane molecules are involved in this initial activation, the main one being the CD19/CD21/CD81/Leu-13 B-cell coreceptor complex. The activation of CD19 enhances the activating effect of the occupancy of the BCR. CD21, activated by C3 fragments, is the basis for enhanced B-cell activation resulting from complement activation.

The proper progression of the immune response requires complex interactions between accessory cells, helper T lymphocytes, and B lymphocytes. In the same microenvironment where B lymphocytes are being activated, helper T lymphocytes are also activated. This could be the result of a dual role of accessory cells, presenting both membrane-absorbed, unprocessed molecules with epitopes reflective of the native configuration of the immunogenic molecule to B lymphocytes as well as MHC-II-associated peptides derived from processed antigen to the helper T lymphocytes (Figure 4.8).

The helper T cell, as discussed earlier, receives a variety of costimulatory signals from APCs, and the activated helper T cell, in turn, delivers activating signals to APC and B cells. Some of the signals are mediated by interleukins and cytokines, such as IL-2 and IL-4, that stimulate B-cell proliferation and differentiation, and interferon-γ, that increases the efficiency of APC, particularly macrophages. Other signals are mediated by cell-cell interactions involving CD40L (on T cells) and CD40 (on B cells). As a consequence of signaling through the CD40 molecule, B cells express CD80 and CD86 that deliver differentiation and activation signals to T cells through the CD28 family of molecules. That interaction is also a major determinant of the switch from IgM antibody synthesis

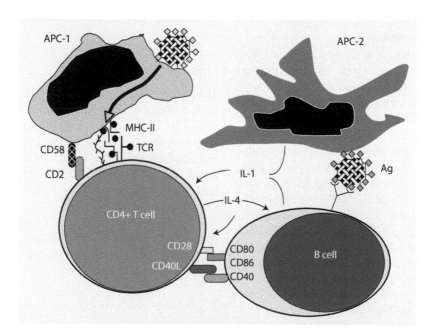

Figure 4.8 Interactions between APCs, T cells, and B cells in the early stages of an immune response. In this diagram, two separate APCs are involved in presentation of immunogenic peptides to Th2 cells (APC-1) and of adsorbed, unmodified antigen to B cells (APC-2). Costimulatory signals are exchanged between the interacting cells.

Table 4.2 Interleukins and cytokines released by Th1 and Th2 helper T lymphocytes

Th0/1 Interleukins/cytokines	Target cell/effect
Interleukin-2	Th0, Th1, and Th2 cells/expansion; B cells/expansion
Th1 Interleukins/cytokines	
Interferon-γ	Macrophages/activation; Th1 cells/differentiation; Th2 cells/downregulation
Lymphotoxin-α (LTα)	Th1 cells/expansion; B cells/homing
Th2 Interleukins/cytokines	
Interleukin-4	Th2 cells/expansion; B cells/differentiation; APC/activation
Interleukin-5	Eosinophils/growth and differentiation
Interleukin-6	B cells/differentiation; plasma cells/proliferation; Th1, Th2 cells/activation; CD8+ T cells/differentiation, proliferation
Interleukin-10	Th1, Th2 cells/downregulation; B cells/differentiation
Interleukin-13	Monocytes, macrophages/downregulation; B cells/activation, differentiation; mast cells, basophils/activation
Th1-Th2 Interleukins/cytokines	
Interleukin-3	B cells/differentiation; macrophages/activation
TNF	B cells/activation, differentiation
Granulocyte-monocyte CSF (GM-CSF)	B cells/differentiation

in the early stages of the immune response to IgG antibody synthesis characteristic of a sustained immune response.

T-helper lymphocyte subpopulations

The differentiation of helper T lymphocytes results in specialized functions to assist B-cell activation and differentiation (Th2 lymphocytes) and to assist in the proliferation and differentiation of cytotoxic T lymphocytes and KN cells (Th1 lymphocytes). These two subpopulations cannot be defined on the basis of expression of any specific membrane markers. Their definition is based on the repertoire of cytokines they release: Th1 cells predominantly release IFNγ and lymphotoxin α, and Th2 cells predominantly release IL-4, IL-5, IL-6, IL-10, and IL-13 (Table 4.2).

Several factors appear to control the differentiation of Th1 and Th2. The early stages of proliferation of Th0 cells (as the common precursors are often designated) are IL-2 dependent. IL-2 is the main cytokine released by activated Th0 as well as by activated Th1 and Th2 cells and has both autocrine and paracrine effects, thus promoting Th0 proliferation. As the cells continue to proliferate, IL-12 promotes Th1 differentiation, while IL-4 promotes Th2 differentiation. The cellular source of IL-12 is the APCs, and experimental work suggests that specific antigens or bacterial products with adjuvant properties may induce the release of IL-12 by those cells, especially in the DC1 subpopulation of dendritic cells, promoting the differentiation of Th1 cells. The initial source of IL-4 needed to determine the differentiation of Th2 cells is not clear. It is possible that APCs (possibly the DC2 subpopulation of dendritic cells) expressing NOTCH ligands may be critical for the activation of NOTCH, initiating a sequence that will result in the expression of a group of transcription factors, particularly GATA-3, which is associated with the differentiation of IL-4-producing T cells, thus creating an autocrine and paracrine microenvironment favorable to Th2 differentiation.

Several additional factors playing a role in determining Th1 or Th2 differentiation have been proposed, including the affinity of the interaction of the TCR with the MHC-II–associated peptide, the concentration of MHC-peptide complexes on the cell membrane, and signals dependent on cell-cell interactions (Table 4.3).

Cell-cell contact plays a significant role in promoting B-cell activation by delivering

Table 4.3 Signals involved in the control of differentiation of Th1 and Th2 subpopulations of helper T lymphocytes

Signals favoring Th1 differentiation	Signals favoring Th2 differentiation
Activation of T-bet transcription factor	Activation of GATA-3 transcription factor
Interleukin-12	Interleukin-4[a]
Interferon-γ[b]	Interleukin-1
Interferon-α[c]	Interleukin-10
CD28/CD80 interaction	CD28/CD86 interaction
High density of MHC-II–peptide complexes on the APC membrane	Low density of MHC-II–peptide complexes on the APC membrane
High-affinity interaction between TCR and the MHC-II – peptide complex	Low affinity interaction between TCR and the MHC-II–peptide complex

[a] IL-4 becomes involved in an autocrine/paracrine regulatory circuit that promotes the differentiation of Th2 cells and in paracrine regulation of B-cell differentiation.
[b] Interferon-γ does not act directly on Th2 cells but enhances the release of IL-12 by APCs, and as such has an indirect positive effect on Th2 differentiation.
[c] Interferon-α is released by dendritic cells and their circulating precursors.

costimulatory signals to the B cell and/or by allowing direct traffic of cytokines from helper T lymphocytes to B lymphocytes. Transient conjugation between T and B lymphocytes seems to occur constantly, due to the expression of complementary CAMs on their membranes. For example, T cells express CD2 and CD4, and B cells express the respective ligands, CD58 (LFA-3) and MHC-II; both T and B lymphocytes express ICAM-1 and LFA-1 that can reciprocally interact.

The continuing proliferation and differentiation of B cells into plasma cells is assisted by several soluble factors, including IL-4, released by Th2 cells, and IL-6 and IL-14, released by T lymphocytes and accessory cells, as well as by cell-cell interactions, particularly those mediated by CD40, expressed by B cells, and the respective ligand (CD40L), expressed by activated T cells. At the end of an immune response, the total number of antigen-specific T and B lymphocyte clones will remain the same, but the number of cells in those clones will be increased several-fold. The increased residual population of antigen-specific T cells is long-lived and is believed to be responsible for the phenomenon known as immunological memory. Immunological memory secures protection gains the eliciting antigen for an extended period of time. In most cases, the protection can last for 10 years or more, but the only vaccine that has been proven to induce life-long immunity is the smallpox vaccine using live vaccinia virus.

BIBLIOGRAPHY

Bottomly K. T cells and dendritic cells get intimate. Science. 1999;283:1124–1225.

Constant S, Pfeiffer C, Woodard A, Pasqualini T, Bottomly, K. Extent of T cell receptor ligation can determine functional differentiation of naive CD4+ T cells. J Exp Med. 1995;182:1591–1596.

Duronio V, Scheid M, Ettinger S. Downstream signaling events regulated by phosphatidylinositol 3-kinase activity. Cell Signal. 1998;10:233–239.

Dustin ML, Shaw AS. Costimulation: Building an immunological synapse. Science. 1999;283:649–650.

Farina MS, Lundgren KT, Bellmunt J. Immunotherapy in urothelial cancer: Recent results and future perspectives. Drugs. 2017;77:1077–1089.

Garcia K, Teyton L, Wilson I. Structural basis of T cell recognition. Annu Rev Immunol. 1999;17:369–397.

Garside P, Ingulli E, Merica RR, et al. Visualization of specific B and T lymphocyte interactions in the lymph node. Science. 1998;281:96–99.

Genestier L, Taillardet M, Mondiere P, et al. TLR agonists selectively promote terminal plasma cell differentiation of B cell subsets specialized in thymus-independent responses. J Immunol. 2007;178:7779–7786.

Good LM, Miller MD, High, WA. Intralesional agents in the management of cutaneous malignancy: A review. J Amer Acad Dermatol. 2011;64:413–422.

Heeger PS. T-cell allorecognition and transplant rejection: A summary and update. *Am J Transplant*. 2003;3:525–533.

Kaur H, Salunke DM. Antibody promiscuity: Understanding the paradigm shift in antigen recognition. *IUBMB Life*. 2015;67:498–505.

Kennedy RB, Oberg AL, Ovsyannikova IG, et al. Transcriptomic profiles of high and low antibody responders to smallpox vaccine. *Genes Immun*. 2013;14:277–285.

Krogsgaard M, Davis MM. How T cells "see" antigen. *Nature Immunol*. 2005;6:239–245.

Melhem NM, Mahfouz RA, Kreidieh K, et al. Potential role of killer immunoglobulin receptor genes among individuals vaccinated against hepatitis B virus in Lebanon. *World J Hepatol*. 2016;8:1212–1221.

Moll H. Antigen delivery by dendritic cells. *Int J Med Microbiol*. 2004;294:337–344.

Noelle RJ. The role of gp39 (CD40L) in immunity. *Clin Immunol Immunopath*. 1995;76:S203–207.

Shen L, Rock KL. Priming of T cells by exogenous antigen cross-presented on MHC class I molecules. *Curr Opin Immunol*. 2006;18:85–91.

Snapper CM, Mond JJ. A model for induction of T cell-independent humoral immunity in response to polysaccharide antigens. *J Immunol*. 1996;157:2229–2233.

Van Kooten C, Banchereau J. CD40-CD40 ligand. *J Leukoctye Biol*. 2000;67:2–17.

Wan YY. GATA-3: A master of many trades in immune regulation. *Trends Immunol*. 2014;35:233–242.

Wilson I, Garcia K. T-cell receptor structure and TCR complexes. *Curr Opin Struct Biol*. 1997;7:839–848.

Yan WL, Shen KY, Chen YA, Liu SJ. Recent progress in GM-CSF-based immunotherapy. *Immunotherapy*. 2017;9:347–360.

5

Immunoglobulins: Structure and diversity

GABRIEL VIRELLA

INTRODUCTION

Early studies of the characteristics of antibodies demonstrated that in serum electrophoresis, the γ-globulin fraction contained the majority of the proteins with antibody activity (Figure 5.1) and that two major types of antibodies could be defined by their sedimentation coefficient determined by analytical ultracentrifugation (7S and 19S antibodies), reflective of the molecular weight of monomeric and polymeric immunoglobulins. As protein fractionation techniques became available, complete immunoglobulins and their fragments were isolated in large amounts, particularly from the serum and urine of patients with multiple myeloma. These proteins were used both for studies of chemical structure and for immunological studies allowed to identify antigenic differences between proteins from different patients; this was the basis for the initial identification of the different classes and subclasses of immunoglobulins and the different types of light chains.

STRUCTURE OF IMMUNOGLOBULIN G

IgG is the most abundant immunoglobulin in human serum and in the serum of most mammalian species. It is also the immunoglobulin most frequently detected in large concentrations in multiple myeloma patients. For this reason, it was the first immunoglobulin to be purified in large quantities and to be extensively studied from the structural point of view.

The incubation of purified IgG with papain, a proteolytic enzyme extracted from the latex of *Carica papaya*, results in the splitting of the molecule into two fragments that differ in charge, antigenicity, biochemical characteristics, and biological functions. One of the fragments contains the binding site of the antibody and for that reason was designated as Fab, while the second fragment was found to be crystallizable and for that reason named Fc.

If the IgG molecule is incubated with a reducing agent containing free SH groups and fractionated

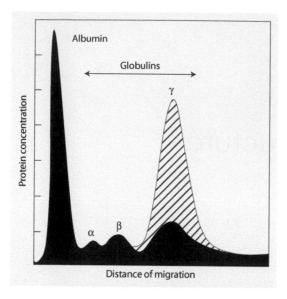

Figure 5.1 Demonstration of the γ-globulin mobility of circulating antibodies. The serum from a rabbit hyperimmunized with ovalbumin showed a very large γ-globulin fraction (shaded area) that disappeared when the same serum was electrophoretically separated after removal of antibody molecules by specific precipitation with ovalbumin. In contrast, serum albumin and the remaining globulin fractions were not affected by the precipitation step. (Redrawn after Tiselius A, Kabat EA. *J. Exp. Med.* 1939;69:119.)

by gel filtration or any other technique that separates proteins by size in conditions able to dissociate noncovalent interactions, two fractions are obtained. One of the fractions corresponds to polypeptide chains of M.W. 55,000 (heavy chains); the second corresponds to polypeptide chains of M.W. 23,000 (light chains) (Figure 5.2).

The sum of data obtained by proteolysis and reduction experiments resulted in the conception of a diagrammatic two-dimensional model for the IgG molecule (Figure 5.3).

The model shows that papain splits the heavy chains in the hinge region (so designated because this region of the molecule appears to be stereo flexible) and results in the separation of two Fab fragments and one Fc fragment per IgG molecule (Figure 5.4).

If the disulfide bond joining heavy and light chains in the Fab fragments is split, one can separate a complete light chain from a fragment, which comprises about half of one of the heavy chains,

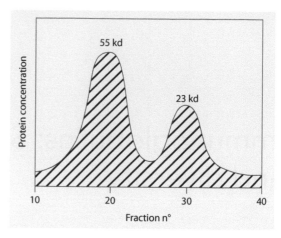

Figure 5.2 Gel filtration of reduced and alkylated IgG (M.W. 150,000) on a dissociating medium. Two protein peaks are eluted, the first corresponding to a M.W. 55,000 and the second corresponding to a M.W. 23,000. The 2:1 ratio of protein content between the high M.W. and low M.W. peaks is compatible with the presence of identical numbers of two polypeptide chains, one of which is about twice as large as the other.

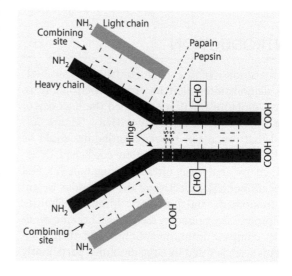

Figure 5.3 The IgG molecule. (Modified from Klein, J., *Immunology*, Blackwell Science, Boston, MA, 1990.)

the NH$_2$ terminal half. This portion of the heavy chain contained in each Fab fragment has been designated as an Fd fragment.

Pepsin, in contrast, splits the heavy chains beyond the disulfide bonds that join them at the

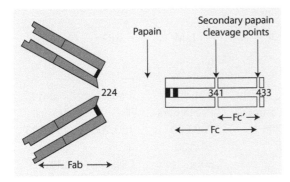

Figure 5.4 The fragments obtained by papain digestion of the IgG molecule. (Modified from Klein, J., *Immunology*, Blackwell Science, Boston, MA, 1990.)

hinge region, resulting in the production of F(ab′)$_2$ fragments but the Fc fragment is not recovered (Figure 5.5). The comparison of Fc, Fab, F(ab′)$_2$, and whole IgG molecules shows both important similarities and differences between the whole molecule and its fragments.

- Both Fab and F(ab′)$_2$ contain antibody binding sites, but while the intact IgG molecule and the F(ab′)$_2$ are bivalent, the Fab fragment is monovalent. Therefore, a Fab fragment can bind to an antigen but cannot cross-link two antigen molecules.
- An antiserum raised against the Fab fragment reacts mostly against light-chain determinants;

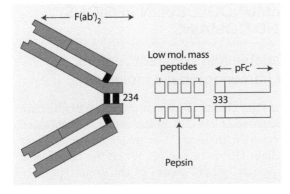

Figure 5.5 The fragments obtained by pepsin digestion of the IgG molecule. (Modified from Klein, J., *Immunology*, Blackwell Science, Boston, MA, 1990.)

the immunodominant antigenic markers for the heavy chain are located in the Fc fragment.
- The F(ab′)$_2$ fragment is identical to the intact molecule as far as antigen-binding properties but lacks most other biological properties of IgG, such as the ability to fix complement, bind to cell membranes, etc., which are determined by the Fc region of the molecule.

STRUCTURAL AND ANTIGENIC HETEROGENEITY OF HEAVY AND LIGHT CHAINS

As larger numbers of purified immunoglobulins were studied in detail, it became obvious that there was a substantial degree of structural heterogeneity, recognizable both by physicochemical methods as well as by antisera able to define different antigenic types of heavy and light chains.

Five classes of immunoglobulins were identified due to antigenic differences of the heavy chains and designated as IgG (the classical 7S immunoglobulin), IgA, IgM (the classical 19S immunoglobulin), IgD, and IgE. IgG, IgA, and IgM together constitute over 95% of the whole immunoglobulin pool in a normal human being and are designated as major immunoglobulin classes. Because they are common to all humans, the immunoglobulin classes can also be designated as isotypes. The major characteristics of the five immunoglobulin classes are summarized in Table 5.1.

The light chains also proved to be antigenically heterogeneous, and two isotypes were defined: kappa (κ) and lambda (λ). The majority of immunoglobulin molecules are homodimers constituted by a pair of identical heavy chains and a pair of identical light chains; hence, a given immunoglobulin molecule can have either κ or λ chains but not both. A normal individual will have a mixture of immunoglobulin molecules in his serum, some with kappa chains (e.g., IgGκ), and others with lambda chains (e.g., IgGλ). Normal serum IgG has a 2:1 ratio of κ over λ chain-bearing IgG molecules. In contrast, monoclonal immunoglobulins have a single heavy-chain isotype and a single light-chain isotype. This results from the fact that monoclonal proteins are the products of a large number of cells, all derived from a single mutant, constituting one large clone of identical cells producing identical molecules.

Antigenic differences between the heavy chains of IgG and IgA were later characterized, leading

Table 5.1 Major characteristics of human immunoglobulins

	IgG	IgA	IgM	IgD	IgE
Heavy-chain class	γ	α	μ	δ	ε
H-chain subclasses	γ 1,2,3,4	α 1,2	—	—	—
L-chain type	κ and λ	κ and λ	κ and λ	κ and λ	κ and λ
Polymeric forms	No	Dimers, trimers	Pentamers	No	No
Molecular weight	150,000	(160,000)n	900,000	180,000	190,000
Serum concentration (mg/dL)	600–1300	60–300	30–150	3	0.03
Intravascular distribution	45%	42%	80%	75%	51%

Table 5.2 IgG subclasses

	IgG1	IgG2	IgG3	IgG4
Percentage of total IgG in normal serum	60%	30%	7%	3%
Half-life (days)	21	21	7	21
Complement fixation[a]	++	+	+++	−
Segmental flexibility	+++	+	++++	++
Affinity for monocyte and PMN receptors	+++	+	++++	+

[a] By the classical pathway.

to the definition of IgG and IgA subclasses. In the case of IgG subclasses (Table 5.2), IgG1 and IgG3 are more efficient in terms of complement fixation and have greater affinity for monocyte receptors. Those properties can be correlated with a greater degree of biological activity, both in normal antimicrobial responses and in pathological conditions. Physiologically, these properties result in enhanced opsonization and bacterial killing. Pathologically, the assembly or deposition of extravascular immune complexes containing IgG1 and IgG3 antibodies activates pathways that induce tissue inflammation.

From the structural point of view, the IgG3 subclass has the greatest number of structural and biological differences relative to the remaining IgG subclasses. Most differences appear to result from the existence of an extended hinge region (which accounts for the greater M.W.), and with a large number of disulfide bonds linking the heavy chains together (estimates of their number vary between 5 and 15). This extended hinge region seems to be easily accessible to proteolytic enzymes, and this liability of the molecule is likely to account for its considerably shorter half-life.

Another interesting structural feature concerns the IgG4 molecules that are able to undergo a posttranslational modification known as Fab arm exchange, in which two IgG4 molecules exchange

among themselves one complete half of the molecule (both Fab and Fc), resulting in the generation of bi-specific antibodies. It is not clear whether this process results from the absence of interchain disulfide bonds replaced by intrachain bonds, or from relatively weak interchain bonds that can be easily broken in reducing conditions. It is also not clear whether the hybrid molecules can carry a different light-chain type (i.e., do the hybrid molecules remain κ or λ, or are they also κ and λ hybrids?).

IMMUNOGLOBULIN REGIONS AND DOMAINS

Variable and constant regions of immunoglobulin molecule

The light chains of human immunoglobulins are composed of 211–217 amino acids. As mentioned previously, there are two major antigenic types of light chains (κ and λ). When the amino acid sequences of light chains of the same type were compared, it became evident that two regions could be distinguished in the light-chain molecules: a variable region, comprising the portion between the amino terminal end of the chain and residues of 107–115, and a constant region, extending from

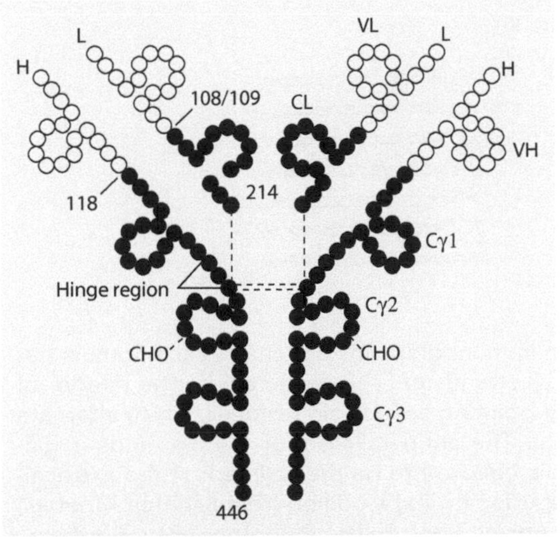

Figure 5.6 Primary and secondary structures of a human IgG. The light chains are constituted by about 214 amino acids and two regions, variable (first 108 amino acids, white beads in the diagram) and constant (remaining amino acids, black beads in the diagram). Each of these regions contains a loop formed by intrachain disulfide bonds and containing about 60 amino acids, which are designated as variable domain and constant domain (VL and CL in the diagram). The heavy chains have slightly longer variable regions (first 118 amino acids, white beads in the diagram), with one domain (VH) and a constant region that contains three loops or domains (Cγ1, Cγ2, and Cγ3), numbered from the NH2 terminus to the COOH terminus.

the end of the variable region to the carboxyl terminus (Figure 5.6).

The light-chain constant regions were found to be almost identical in light chains of the same type but differ markedly in κ and λ chains. It is assumed that the difference in antigenicity between the two types of light chains is directly correlated with the structural differences in constant regions.

In contrast, the amino acid sequence of the light-chain variable regions is different even in proteins of the same antigenic type, and early workers thought that this sequence would be totally individual to any single protein. With increasing data, it became evident that some proteins shared similarities in their variable regions, and it has been possible to classify variable regions into three groups: Vκ, Vλ, and VH. Each group has been further subdivided into several subgroups. The light-chain **V region subgroups** (Vκ, Vλ) are

"type" specific, i.e., Vκ subgroups are only found in κ-proteins, and Vλ subgroups are always associated with λ-chains. In contrast, the heavy-chain V region subgroups (VH) are not "class" specific. Thus, any given VH subgroup can be found in association with the heavy chains of any of the known immunoglobulin classes and subclasses.

The heavy chain of IgG is about twice as large as a light chain; it is constituted by approximately 450 amino acids, and a variable and a constant region can also be identified. The variable region of the IgG heavy chain is constituted by the first 113–121 amino acids (counted from the amino terminal end), and subgroups of these regions can also be identified. The constant region of the IgG heavy chain is almost three times larger than the variable region; for most of the heavy chains, it starts at residue 116 and ends at the carboxyl terminus (Figure 5.6). The maximal degree of homology is found between constant regions of IgG proteins of the same subclass.

Immunoglobulin domains

The immunoglobulin molecule contains several disulfide bonds formed between contiguous residues. Some of them join two different polypeptide chains (interchain disulfide bonds), keeping the molecule together. Others (intrachain bonds) join different areas of the same polypeptide chain, leading to the formation of "loops." These "loops" and adjacent amino acids constitute the immunoglobulin domains, which are folded in a characteristic β-pleated sheet structure (Figure 5.7).

The variable regions of both heavy and light chains have a single domain, which is involved in antigen binding. Light chains have a single constant region domain (CL), while heavy chains have several constant region domains (three in the case of IgG, IgA, and IgD; four in the case of IgM and IgE). The constant region domains are generically designated as CH1, CH2, CH3, and, if existing, CH4. To be more specific, the constant region domains can be identified as to the class of immunoglobulins to which they belong, by adding the symbol for each heavy-chain class (γ, α, μ, δ, ε). For example, the constant region domains of the IgG molecule can be designated as Cγ1, Cγ2, and Cγ3. Different functions have been assigned to the different domains and regions of the heavy chains. For instance, Cγ2 is the domain involved in complement fixation, while both Cγ2 and Cγ3

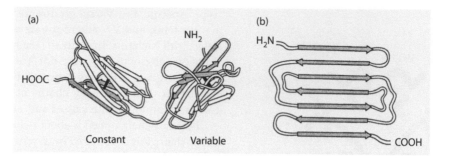

Figure 5.7 Model for the V and C domains of a human immunoglobulin light chain. Each domain has two β-pleated sheets consisting of several antiparallel β strands of 5–10 amino acids. The interior of each domain is formed between the two β sheets by in-pointing amino acid residues, which alternate with out-pointing hydrophilic residues, as shown in (a). The antiparallelism of the β-strands is diagrammatically illustrated in (b). This β-sheet structure is believed to be the hallmark of the extracellular domains of all proteins in the immunoglobulin superfamily. ([a] Modified from Schiffer, M. et al., *Biochemistry*, 12, 4620–4231, 1973. [b] Modified from Amzel, L.M., Poljak, R.J., *Annu. Rev. Biochem.*, 48, 961–997, 1979.)

are believed to be involved in the binding to phagocytic cell membranes.

The "hinge region" is located between the CH1 and CH2 domains, and its name is derived from the fact that studies by a variety of techniques, including fluorescence polarization, spin-labeling, electron microscopy, and X-ray crystallography, have shown that the Fab fragments can rotate and waggle, coming together or moving apart. As a consequence, IgG molecules can change their shape from an "Y" to a "T" and vice versa, using the region intercalated between Cγ1 and Cγ2 as a "hinge." The length and primary sequence of the hinge regions play an important role in determining the segmental flexibility of IgG molecules. For example, IgG3 has a 12-amino acid hinge amino terminal segment and has the highest segmental flexibility. The hinge region is also the most frequent point of attack by proteolytic enzymes. In general, the resistance to proteolysis of the different IgG subclasses is inversely related to the length of the hinge amino terminal segments—IgG3 proteins are the most easily digestible, while IgG2 proteins, with the shortest hinge region, are the most resistant to proteolytic enzymes.

Immunoglobulin superfamily of proteins

The existence of globular "domains" is considered as the structural hallmark of immunoglobulin structure. A variety of other proteins exhibit amino acid sequence homology with immunoglobulins, and their molecules also contain Ig-like domains (Figure 5.8). Such proteins are considered as members of the immunoglobulin superfamily, based on the assumption that the genes that encode them must have evolved from a common ancestor gene coding for a single domain, much likely the gene coding for the Thy-1 molecule found on murine lymphocytes and brain cells.

The majority of the membrane proteins of the immunoglobulin superfamily seem to be functionally involved in recognition of specific ligands, which may determine cell-cell contact phenomena and/or cell activation. The T-cell antigen receptor molecule, the major histocompatibility antigens, the polyimmunoglobulin receptor on mucosal cells (see later discussion), and the CD2 molecule on T lymphocytes are a few examples of proteins included in the immunoglobulin superfamily.

ANTIBODY-COMBINING SITE

As mentioned earlier, the binding of antigens by antibody molecules takes place in the Fab region and is basically a noncovalent interaction that requires a good fit between the antigenic determinant and the antigen-binding site on the immunoglobulin molecule. The antigen-binding site appears to be formed by the variable regions of both heavy and light chains, folded in close proximity and forming a pouch (paratope) where an antigenic determinant or epitope will fit (Figure 5.9).

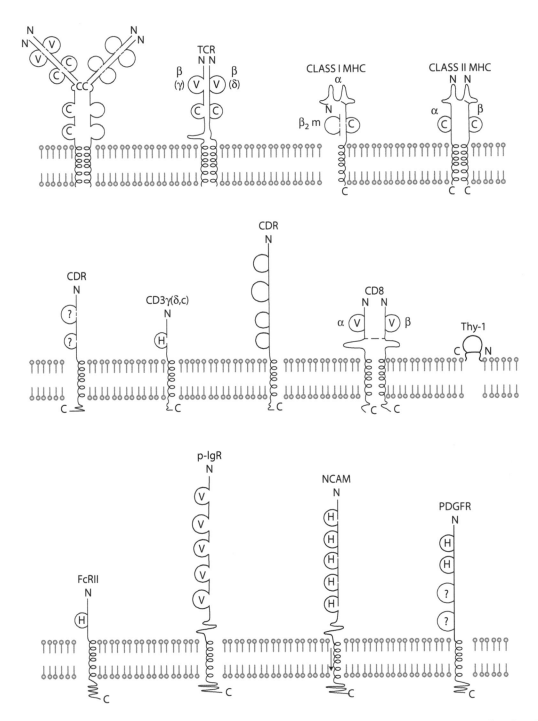

Figure 5.8 Model representations for some proteins included in the immunoglobulin superfamily. This includes several molecules that participate in the immune response and show similarities in structure, causing them to be named the immunoglobulin supergene family. Included are CD2, CD3, CD4, CD7, CD8, CD28, T-cell receptor (TCR), major histocompatibility complex (MHC) class I and class II molecules, leukocyte function associated antigen 3 (LFA-3), the IgG receptor, the Poly Ig receptor, and several other proteins. These molecules have in common an immunoglobulin-like domain with a length of approximately 100 amino acid residues and a central disulfide bond that anchors and stabilizes antiparallel β-strands into a folded structure resembling immunoglobulin.

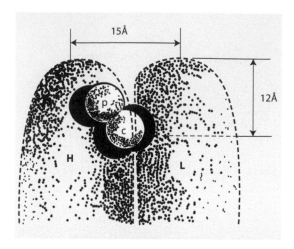

Figure 5.9 Hypothetical structure of an antigen-binding site. The variable regions of the light and heavy chains of a mouse myeloma protein, which binds specifically the phosphorylcholine hapten, form a pouch in which the hapten fits. In this particular example, the specificity of the binding reaction depends mostly on the structure of the heavy-chain V region. (Modified from Padlan, E. et al., In: Sercarz, E., Williamson, A., Fox, C., eds., *The Immune System: Genes, Receptors, Signals*, Academic Press, New York, 1975.)

Actually, certain sequence stretches of the variable regions vary widely from protein to protein, even among proteins sharing the same type of variable regions. For this reason, these highly variable stretches have been designated as hypervariable regions (Figure 5.10). The structure of hypervariable regions is believed to play a critical role in determining antibody specificity, since these regions are believed to be folded in such a way that they determine the three-dimensional structure of the "pouch" where a given epitope of an antigen will fit. In other words, the hypervariable regions will interact to create a paratope whose configuration is *complementary* to that of a given epitope. Thus, these regions can be also designated as complementarity-determining regions (CDRs). A paratope is determined by three CDR regions (1, 2, 3). CD1 and CD2 are mainly formed by hypervariable regions, while CDR3, the most variable of them, is formed by hypervariable regions but also by other regions of light- and heavy-chain molecules known as diversity and joining regions, described in detail in Chapter 7.

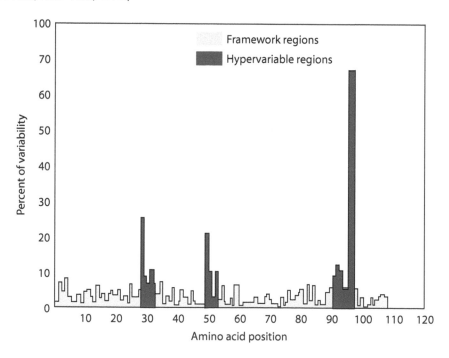

Figure 5.10 Graphical demonstration of the extent of variability at individual amino acid residue positions in immunoglobulin variable regions. In this Wu-Kabat plot, the percentage variability is plotted at each residue position, demonstrating that the most variable residues of immunoglobulin light chains are clustered in three hypervariable regions. The same clustering is observed in the heavy chains.

IMMUNOGLOBULIN M: A POLYMERIC MOLECULE

Serum IgM is basically constituted by five subunits (monomeric subunits, IgMs), each one of them constituted by two light chains (κ or λ) and two heavy chains (μ). The heavy chains are larger than those of IgG by about 20,000 daltons, corresponding to an extra domain on the constant region (Cμ4). A third polypeptide chain, the J chain, can be revealed by adequate methodology in IgM molecules. This is a small polypeptide chain of 15,000 daltons, also found in polymeric IgA molecules. A single J chain is found in any polymeric IgM or IgA molecule, irrespective of how many monomeric subunits are involved in the polymerization. It has been postulated that this chain plays a key role in the polymerization process.

IMMUNOGLOBULIN A: A MOLECULARLY HETEROGENEOUS IMMUNOGLOBULIN

Serum IgA is molecularly heterogeneous, constituted by a mixture of monomeric, dimeric, and larger polymeric molecules. In a normal individual, over 70%–90% of serum IgA is monomeric. Monomeric IgA is similar to IgG, constituted by two heavy chains (α) and two light chains (κ or λ). Two subclasses of IgA have been defined: IgA1 and IgA2.

IgA1 predominates in serum, and IgA2 predominates in secretions. The dimeric and polymeric forms of IgA found in the mucosal secretions and in circulation are covalently bonded synthetic products containing J chains.

IgA of the IgA2 subclass is the predominant immunoglobulin in secretions. Secretory IgA2 molecules are most frequently dimeric, contain J chains as do all polymeric immunoglobulin molecules, and in addition, contain a unique polypeptide chain, designated as a secretory component (SC) (Figure 5.11). A single polypeptide chain of approximately 70,000 daltons, with five homologous immunoglobulin-like domains constitutes this unique protein. It is synthesized by epithelial cells in the mucosa and by hepatocytes, initially as a larger membrane molecule known as polyimmunoglobulin receptor, from which the secretory component is derived by proteolytic cleavage that separates it from the intramembrane and cytoplasmic segments of its membrane form.

MINOR IMMUNOGLOBULIN CLASSES: IgD AND IgE

IgD and IgE were the last immunoglobulins to be identified, due to their low concentrations in serum and low frequency of patients with multiple myeloma producing them. Both are monomeric immunoglobulins, similar to IgG, but their heavy chains are larger than γ-chains. IgE has five domains in the heavy chain (one variable and four constant); IgD has four heavy-chain domains (as most other monomeric immunoglobulins).

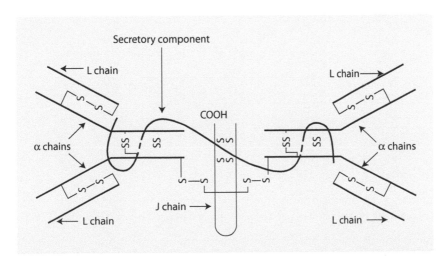

Figure 5.11 Structural model of the secretory IgA molecule. (From Turner, M.W.: *Immunochemistry: An Advanced Textbook.* 1977. Copyright Wiley-VCH Verlag GmbH & Co. KGaA. Reproduced with permission.)

IgD and IgM are the predominant immuno-globulin classes in the B-lymphocyte membrane, where they are the antigen-binding molecules in the antigen-receptor complex. Membrane IgD and IgM are monomeric. The heavy chains of membrane IgD and IgM (δm, μm) differ from those of the secreted forms at their carboxyl termini, where the membrane forms have a hydrophobic transmembrane section and a short cytoplasmic tail, which are lacking in the secreted forms. In contrast, a hydrophilic section is found at the carboxyl termini of heavy chains of secreted immunoglobulins. The membrane immunoglobulins form a membrane complex with several other membrane proteins including Igα and Igβ, which have sequence motifs in their cytoplasmic portions that are required for signal transduction. No other biological role is known for IgD besides existing as a membrane immunoglobulin.

IgE has the unique property of binding to Fc$_\varepsilon$ receptors on the membranes of mast cells and basophils. The binding of IgE to those receptors has an extremely high affinity (7.7×10^9 L/M^{-1}), about 100-fold greater than the affinity of IgG binding to monocyte receptors. The high-affinity binding of IgE to basophil membrane receptors depends on the configuration of Cε3 and Cε4 domains. In allergic individuals, if those IgE molecules have a given antibody specificity and react with the antigen while attached to the basophil or mast cell membranes, they will triggering the release of histamine and other substances that cause the symptoms of allergic reactions.

BIBLIOGRAPHY

Day ED. *Advanced Immunochemistry*. 2nd ed. New York, NY: Wiley-Liss; 1990.

Johansen FE, Braathen R, Brandtzaeg P. Role of J chain in secretory immunoglobulin formation. *Scand J Immunol*. 2000;52:240–248.

Murre C, ed. Molecular Mechanisms That Orchestrate the Assembly of Antigen Receptor Loci. New York, NY: Academic Press; 2015. *Advances in Immunology*; vol 128.

Nezlin R. Internal movements in immunoglobulin molecules. *Adv Immunol*. 1990;48:1–40.

Polonelli L, Pontón J, Elguezabal N, et al. Antibody complementarity-determining regions (CDRs) can display differential antimicrobial, antiviral and antitumor activities. *PLOS ONE*. 2008;3(6): e2371.

Schroeder HW Jr, Cavacini L. Structure and function of immunoglobulins. *J Allergy Clin Immunol*. 2010;125(2 Suppl 2):S41–S52.

van der Neut Kolfschoten M, Schuurman J, Losen M, et al. Anti-inflammatory activity of human IgG4 antibodies by dynamic Fab arm exchange. *Science*. 2007;317:1554–1557.

Van Oss CJ, van Regenmortel MHV. *Immunochemistry*. New York, NY: Marcel Dekker; 1994.

Williams AF, Barclay AN. The immunoglobulin superfamily—Domains for cell surface recognition. *Annu Rev Immunol*. 1988;6:381–405.

6

Immunoglobulins: Metabolism and biological properties

GABRIEL VIRELLA

IMMUNOGLOBULIN BIOSYNTHESIS

Immunoglobulin synthesis is the defining property of B lymphocytes and plasma cells. Resting B lymphocytes synthesize only small amounts of immunoglobulins that mainly become inserted into the cell membrane. Plasma cells, considered as end-stage cells arrested at the late G1 phase with very limited mitotic activity, are specialized to produce and secrete large amounts of immunoglobulins. The synthetic capacity of the plasma cell is reflected by its abundant cytoplasm, which is extremely rich in endoplasmic reticulum (Figure 6.1).

Normally, heavy and light chains are synthesized in separate polyribosomes of the plasma cell. The amounts of H and L chains synthesized on the polyribosomes are roughly balanced so that both types of chains will be combined into complete IgG molecules, without surpluses of any given chain. The assembly of a complete IgG molecule can be achieved by (1) associating one H and one L chain to form an HL hemimolecule, joining in the next step two HL hemimolecules to form the complete molecule (H_2L_2) or by (2) forming H_2 and L_2 dimers that later associate to form the complete molecule.

The synthesis of light chains is usually slightly unbalanced, so that plasma cells secrete a small amount of excess free light chains, which are eliminated in the urine, in very small concentrations. When plasma cells undergo malignant transformation, this unbalanced synthesis of light chains may be grossly aberrant, and this is reflected by the elimination of the excessively produced light chains of a single isotype in the urine, traditionally known as Bence Jones protein. In contrast, free heavy chains are generally not secreted. The heavy chains are synthesized and glycosylated in the endoplasmic reticulum, but secretion requires association to light chains to form a complete immunoglobulin molecule. If light chains are not synthesized or heavy chains are synthesized in excess, the free heavy chains associate via their C_H1 domain with a heavy-chain binding protein, which is believed to be responsible for their intracytoplasmic retention. In rare cases, the free heavy chains are structurally abnormal and are secreted. Free heavy chains are usually retained in circulation because their molecular weight, about twice as large as that of light chains, exceeds the glomerular filtration limit.

Synthesis of polymeric immunoglobulins (IgM, IgA)

All polymeric immunoglobulins have one additional polypeptide chain, the J chain. This chain is synthesized by all plasma cells, including those

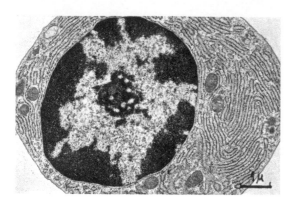

Figure 6.1 Ultrastructure of a mature plasma cell. Note the eccentric nucleus with clumped chromatin, the large cytoplasm containing abundant, distended endoplasmic reticulum. (Electron microphotograph courtesy of Professor P. Groscurth, MD, Institute of Anatomy, University of Zurich, Switzerland.)

that produce IgG. However, it is only incorporated to polymeric forms of IgM and IgA. It is thought that the J chain has some role in initiating polymerization. IgM proteins are assembled in two steps. First, the monomeric units are assembled. Then, five monomers and one J chain will be combined via covalent bonds to result in the final pentameric molecule. This assembly seems to coincide with secretion in some cells, in which only monomeric subunits are found intracellularly. However, in other cells, the pentameric forms can be found intracellularly and secretion seems linked to glycosylation.

Synthesis of secretory IgA

Secretory IgA is also assembled in two stages, but each one takes place in a different cell. Dimeric IgA, containing two monomeric subunits and a J chain joined together by disulfide bridges, is predominantly synthesized by submucosal plasma cells, although a minor portion may also be synthesized in the bone marrow. Secretory component (SC), on the other hand, is synthesized in the epithelial cells, where the final assembly of secretory IgA takes place. Two different biological functions have been postulated for the secretory component:

1. SC is responsible for secretion of IgA by mucosal membranes. The process involves uptake of dimeric IgA, assembly of IgA-SC complexes, and secretion by the mucosal cells.

The uptake of dimeric IgA by mucosal cells is mediated by a glycoprotein related to SC, called polyimmunoglobulin receptor (Poly-IgR). The Poly-IgR is constituted by a single polypeptide chain of approximately 95,000 daltons, composed of an extracellular portion with five immunoglobulin-like domains, a transmembrane domain, and an intracytoplasmic domain. It is expressed on the internal surface of mucosal cells and binds J chain–containing polymeric immunoglobulins.

The binding of dimeric IgA to Poly-IgR seems to be the first step in the final assembly and transport process of secretory IgA. Surface-bound IgA is internalized, and Poly-IgR is covalently bound to the molecule, probably by means of a disulfide-interchanging enzyme that will break intrachain disulfide bonds in both IgA and Poly-IgR and promote their rearrangement to form interchain disulfide bonds joining Poly-IgR to an α-chain.

After this takes place, the transmembrane and intracytoplasmic domains of the receptor are removed by proteolytic cleavage, and the remaining five domains remain bound to IgA, as SC, and the complete secretory IgA molecule is secreted (Figure 6.2).

The same transport mechanisms are believed to operate in the liver at the hepatocyte level. The hepatocytes produce Poly-IgR, bind and internalize dimeric IgA reaching the liver through the portal circulation, assemble complete secretory IgA, and secrete it to the bile. Secretory IgA must also flow back to the bloodstream, because small amounts are found in the blood of normal individuals. Higher levels of secretory IgA in blood are found in some forms of liver disease, when the uptake of dimeric IgA backflowing from the gut through the mesenteric lymph vessels takes place, but its secretion into the biliary system is compromised. Under those circumstances, secretory IgA assembled in the hepatocyte backflows into the systemic circulation.

Among all J chain-containing immunoglobulins, the poly-IgR has higher binding affinity for dimeric IgA. In IgA-deficient individuals, IgM coupled with SC can be present in external secretions. It is believed that the same basic transport mechanisms are involved, starting by the binding of pentameric IgM to the Poly-IgR

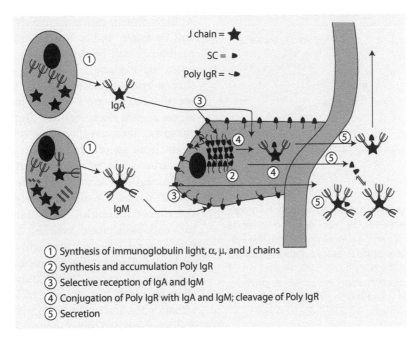

① Synthesis of immunoglobulin light, α, μ, and J chains
② Synthesis and accumulation Poly IgR
③ Selective reception of IgA and IgM
④ Conjugation of Poly IgR with IgA and IgM; cleavage of Poly IgR
⑤ Secretion

Figure 6.2 Mechanisms involved in the synthesis and external transfer of dimeric IgA. According to this model, a polyimmunoglobulin receptor is located at the membrane of mucosal cells and binds polymeric immunoglobulins in general and dimeric IgA with the greatest specificity. The Poly-IgR-IgA complexes are internalized, and in the presence of a disulfide interchanging enzyme, covalent bonds are established between the receptor protein and the immunoglobulin. The transmembrane and intra-cytoplasmic bonds of the Poly-IgR are cleaved by proteolytic enzymes, and the extracellular portion remains bound to IgA, constituting the secretory component. The IgA-SC complex is then secreted to the gland lumen. If the individual is IgA deficient, IgM may become involved in a similar process. (Reprinted from Brandzaeg, P., Baklien, K., *Immunology of the Gut, Ciba Fdtn. Symp. 46 (new series)*, Copyright 1977, with permission from Elsevier.)

on a mucosal cell, and proceeding along the same lines outlined for the assembly and secretion of dimeric IgA. The fact that secretory IgM, with covalently bound SC, is detected exclusively in secretions of IgA-deficient individuals is believed to reflect the lower affinity of the interaction between poly-IgR and IgM-associated J chains (perhaps this is a consequence of steric hindrance of the binding sites of the J chain). Therefore, the interaction between IgM and poly-IgR would only take place in the absence of competition from dimeric IgA molecules.

2. A function proposed for SC is that of a stabilizer of the IgA molecule. This concept is based on experimental observations showing that secretory IgA or dimeric IgA to which SC has been non-covalently associated *in vitro* are more resistant to the effects of proteolytic enzymes than monomeric or dimeric IgA

molecules devoid of SC. One way to explain these observations would be to suggest that the association of SC with dimeric IgA molecules render the hinge region of the IgA monomeric subunits less accessible to proteolytic enzymes. From a biological point of view, it would be advantageous for antibodies secreted into fluids rich in proteolytic enzymes (both of bacterial and host origin) to be resistant to proteolysis.

IMMUNOGLOBULIN SYNTHETIC AND CATABOLIC RATES

All proteins produced by an organism will eventually be degraded or lost through the excreta. However, the speed of the metabolic elimination, and the fractional turnover rate (which is the fraction of the plasma pool catabolized and cleared into urine in a day) and the synthetic rate vary

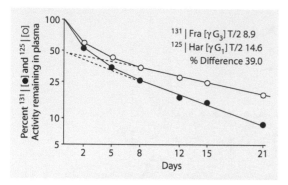

Figure 6.3 Plasma elimination curves of two IgG proteins, one typed as IgG1 (Har) and the other as IgG3 (Fra). The T 1/2 can be determined from the stable part of the curve and its extrapolation (dashed line) as the time necessary for a 50% reduction of the circulating concentration of labeled protein. (Reproduced with permission from Spiegelberg, H.L. et al., *J. Clin. Invest.*, 47, 2323–2330, 1968.)

considerably from protein to protein. Within the immunoglobulin group, different immunoglobulin isotypes have different synthetic rates and different catabolic rates.

One of the most commonly used parameters to assess the catabolic rate of immunoglobulins is the half-life (T 1/2) that corresponds to the time elapsed for a reduction to half of the IgG concentration after equilibrium has been reached. This was originally determined by injecting an immunoglobulin labeled with a radio-isotope (^{131}I is preferred for the labeling of proteins to be used for metabolic studies due to its fast decay rate) and following the plasma activity curve. Figure 6.3 reproduces an example of a metabolic turnover study. After an initial phase of equilibration, the decay of circulating radioactivity follows a straight line in a semilogarithmic scale. From this graph, it is easy to derive the time elapsed between concentration n and $n/2$, i.e., the half-life.

Following is a summary of the metabolic properties of immunoglobulins:

- IgG is the immunoglobulin class with the longest half-life (21 days) and lowest fractional turnover rate (4%–10%/12 hours) with the exception of IgG3 which has a considerably shorter half-life (7 days), close to that of IgA (5–6 days) and IgM (5 days).
- IgG catabolism is uniquely influenced by its circulating concentration of this immunoglobulin.

At high protein concentrations, the catabolism will be faster, and at low IgG concentrations, catabolism will be slowed down. These differences are explained, according to Brambell's theory, by the protection of IgG bound to IgG-specific Fc receptors in the internal aspect of endopinocytotic vesicles from proteolytic enzymes. These receptors are structurally different from all other known Fc receptors and are structurally related to MHC-I molecules (FcRn). IgG is constantly pinocytosed by cells able to degrade it, but at low IgG concentrations most molecules are bound to FcRn on the endopinocytotic vesicles, and the fraction of total IgG degraded will be small. The undegraded molecules are eventually released back into the extracellular fluids. At high IgG concentrations, the majority of IgG molecules remain unbound in the endopinocytotic vesicle and are degraded, resulting in a high catabolic rate (Figure 6.4).

- While most immunoglobulin classes and subclasses are evenly distributed among the intra- and extravascular compartments, IgM, IgD, and to a lesser extent, IgG3, are predominantly concentrated in the intravascular space, and IgA2 is predominantly concentrated in secretions.
- The synthetic rate of IgA1 (24 mg/kg/day) is not very different from that of IgG1 (25 mg/kg/day), but the serum concentration of IgA1 is about one-third of the IgG1 concentration. This is explained by a fractional turnover rate three times greater for IgA1 (24%/day).
- The highest fractional turnover rate and shorter half-life are those of IgE (74%/day and 2.4 days, respectively).
- The lowest synthetic rate is that of IgE (0.002 mg/kg/day compared to 20–60 mg/kg/day for IgG).

BIOLOGICAL PROPERTIES OF IMMUNOGLOBULINS

The antibody molecules have two major functions: binding to the antigen, a function that basically depends on the variable regions located on the Fab region of the molecule, and several other extremely important functions, listed in Table 6.1, which depend on the Fc region. Of particular physiological interest are placental transfer, complement fixation, and binding to Fc receptors.

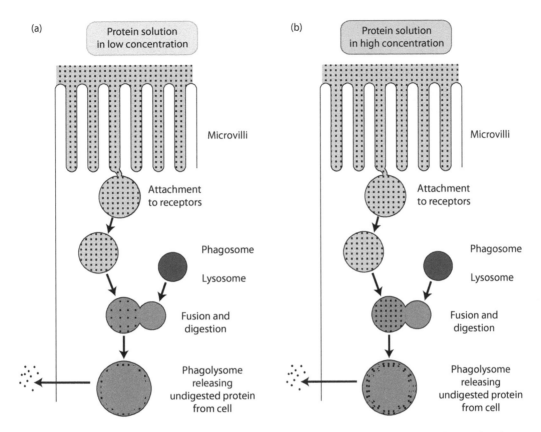

Figure 6.4 Brambell's theory concerning the placental transfer of IgG and the relationship between concentration and catabolism of IgG. (a) shows that pinocytotic IgG will be partially bound to phagosome wall receptors and protected from proteolysis, being later released undigested. This mechanism would account for transplacental transfer. (b) shows that if the concentration of IgG is very high, the number of IgG molecules bound to phagosome receptors will remain the same as when the concentration is low, while the number of unbound molecules will be much greater, and those will be eventually digested, resulting in a higher catabolic rate.

Placental transfer

In humans, the only major immunoglobulin transferred from mother to fetus across the placenta is IgG. The placental transfer of IgG is an active process; the concentration of IgG in the fetal circulation is often higher than the concentration in matched maternal blood. It is also known that a normal fetus synthesizes only trace amounts of IgG, depending on placental transfer for acquisition of passive immunity against common pathogens.

The selectivity of IgG transport has been explained by Brambell's receptor theory for IgG catabolism. The trophoblastic cells on the maternal side of the placenta would endocytose plasma containing all types of proteins but would have receptors in the endopinocytotic vesicles for the Fc region of IgG, and not for any other immunoglobulin. IgG bound to Fcγ receptors would be protected from catabolism, and through active reverse pinocytosis would be released into the fetal circulation. The receptors involved are FcRn, identical to those described earlier, which protect IgG from degradation in endocytic vesicles.

Complement activation

The complement system can be activated by three distinct pathways (see Chapter 9). All immunoglobulins have been found able to fix complement by either the classical or the alternative pathway. IgG1, IgG3, and IgM molecules are the most efficient in fixing complement, all of them through the more powerful classical pathway. Complement activation is an extremely important amplification

Table 6.1 Biologic properties of immunoglobulins

	IgG1	IgG2	IgG3	IgG4	IgA1	IgA2	IgM	IgD	IgE
Serum concentration (mg/dL)[a]	460–1140	80–390	28–194	2.5–16	50–200	0–20	50–200	0–40	0–0.2
Presence in normal secretions	−	−	−	−	+	+++	+	−	+
Placental transfer	+	+	+	+	−	−	−	−	−
Complement fixation									
Classic pathway	+++	+	+++	−	−	−	+++	−	−
Alternative pathway[b]	+	+	+	+	+	+	?	+	+
Reaction with Fc receptors on									
Macrophages	+	−	++	−	+	+	−	−	−
Neutrophils	+	−	++	−	−	−	−	−	−
Basophils/mast cells	−	−	−	−	−	−	−	−	+++[c]
Platelets	+	+	+	+	−	−	−	−	−
Lymphocytes	++	?	++	?	−	−	+	−	−

[a] IgG subclass values. Adapted from Shakib F, et al. *J Immunol Methods*. 1975;8:17–28.
[b] After aggregation.
[c] High-affinity receptors.

mechanism, which enhances antibody-dependent neutralization and elimination of infectious agents, and also plays an important role in inducing inflammatory reactions that may be responsible for a variety of pathological diseases, as discussed in later chapters.

Binding to Fc receptors

Virtually every type of cell involved in the immune response has been found to be able to bind one or more immunoglobulin isotypes through Fc receptors (Table 6.2). These receptors have been classified according to the isotype of immunoglobulin that they preferentially bind as FcγR (receptors for IgG), FcαR (receptors for IgA), FcεR (receptors for IgE), and FcμR (receptors for IgM). The Fcγ receptors are the most diverse, since they exist in three major types:

- FcγRI (CD64), a high-affinity receptor, able to bind monomeric IgG, expressed exclusively by monocytes and macrophages.
- FcγRII (CD32), a low-affinity receptor for IgG expressed by phagocytic cells, platelets, and B lymphocytes. Two functionally distinct forms of FcγRII have been identified: FcγRIIa and FcγRIIb.
- FcγRIII (CD16), a second low-affinity IgG receptor expressed by phagocytic and NK cells.

Fc receptors are constituted by one or several polypeptide chains. The extracellular domains responsible for interaction with the Fc region are located on the α-chain, represented in all Fc receptors. While FcγRII is constituted exclusively by an α-chain, Fcα, FcγRI and FcγRIII receptors have an additional polypeptide chain (γ), and FcεRI has a third chain, β.

Table 6.2 Different types of Fc receptors described in the cells of the immune system

Fc receptor	Characteristics	Cellular distribution	Function
FcγRI (CD64)	Transmembrane and intracytoplasmic domains; high affinity; binds both monomeric and aggregated IgG	Monocytes, macrophages	ADCC (monocytes)
FcγRIIa (CD32) FcγRIIb	Transmembrane and intracytoplasmic domains; low affinity	Monocytes/macrophages; Langerhans cells; granulocytes; platelets; B cells (FcγRIIb)	IC binding; phagocytosis; degranulation; ADCC (monocytes); downregulation (FcγRIIb)
FcγRIII (CD16)	Glycosyl-phosphatidyl inositol anchor in neutrophils; transmembrane segment in NK cells; low affinity	Macrophages; granulocytes; NK and K cells	IC binding and clearance; "priming signal" for phagocytosis and degranulation; ADCC (NK cells)
FcαR	Transmembrane and intracytoplasmic segments; low affinity	Granulocytes, monocytes/ macrophages, platelets, T and B lymphocytes	Phagocytosis, degranulation
FcεRI	High affinity	Basophils, mast cells	Basophil/mast cell degranulation
FcεRII (CD23)	Low affinity	T and B lymphocytes; monocytes/macrophages; eosinophils; platelets	Mediate parasite killing by eosinophils

The binding of free or complexed immunoglobulins to their corresponding Fc receptors has significant biological implications. The catabolic rate and the selective placental transfer of IgG depend on the interaction with FcγR on pinocytic vesicles. IgG also mediates phagocytosis by all cells expressing FcγR on their membranes (granulocytes, monocytes, macrophages, and other cells of the same lineage). Thus, IgG is also considered as an opsonin. IgA (particularly its dimeric form) has been shown to mediate phagocytosis, but by itself, it seems to be a weak opsonin, and complement activation by the alternative pathway seems to significantly enhance this activity. In reality, IgG and C3b have synergistic opsonizing effects, and their joint binding and deposition on the membrane of an infectious agent are the most effective ways to promote its elimination.

A significant property of Fcγ receptors is their ability to deliver activating signals to the cells where they are inserted. Activation is mediated by immunoreceptor tyrosine-based activation motifs (ITAMs) located either in the α-polypeptide chain (FcγRIIa) or in one or both of the associated chains (γ and β). The activation of ITAMs requires cross-linking of Fc receptors by Ag-Ab complexes containing at least two antibody molecules.

One notable exception to the ability to induce cell activation is the opposite effect mediated by FcγRIIb receptors. These receptors have mmunoreceptor tyrosine-based inhibitory motifs (ITIM) in their intracellular portion. These receptors are expressed on B lymphocytes and may play a critical role in the downregulation of humoral immune responses as a consequence of the formation of circulating immune complexes.

An important consequence of complement activation and Fc-mediated cell activation is the induction of inflammatory reactions that are a significant component in infectious and autoimmune diseases. As stated previously, IgG antibodies (mostly of the IgG1 and IgG3 subclasses) are most effective in both counts. Conversely, IgG4 antibodies are weak complement activators and because of their tendency to form heterodimers, they often have two different valences and are unable to cross-link antigens and to form pro-inflammatory antigen-antibody complexes. It has been proposed with an experimental basis that IgG4 antibodies can downmodulate autoimmune and allergic reactions and could be valuable immunotherapeutic tools. However, a recent study in patients with rheumatoid arthritis (RA) and systemic lupus erythematosus (SLE) showed that IgG4 antibodies can have a beneficial impact in SLE, but the opposite was the case in RA, where IgG1 autoantibodies reacting with the CH2 region of IgG4 would generate large-sized, highly pro-inflammatory immune complexes. Other undesirable effects of Ig4 antibodies are related to the inhibition of protective immune responses, for example, in melanoma, and the loss of efficiency of vaccination, demonstrated in patients receiving experimental HIV vaccines.

Antibody-dependent cellular cytotoxicity

Granulocytes, monocytes/macrophages, and NK cells can destroy target cells coated with IgG antibody (antibody-dependent cellular cytotoxicity [ADCC]). In this case, the destruction of the target cell does not depend on opsonization, but rather on the release of toxic mediators.

The specific elimination of target cells by opsonization and ADCC depends on the binding of IgG antibodies to those targets. The antibody molecule tags the target for destruction; phagocytic or NK cells mediate the destruction. Not all antibody molecules are able to react equally with the $Fc\gamma$ receptors of these cells. The highest binding affinities for any of the three types of $Fc\gamma$ receptor known to date are observed with IgG1 and IgG3 molecules.

Fcε receptors

Two types of Fcε receptors specific for IgE have been defined. One is a low-affinity receptor (FcεRII), present in most types of granulocytes. It mediates ADCC reactions directed against helminths, which typically elicit IgE antibody synthesis (see Chapter 14). The other is a high-affinity Fcε receptor (FcεRI) expressed by basophils and mast cells. The basophil/mast cell–bound IgE functions as a true cell receptor. When an IgE molecule bound to a high-affinity FcεRI membrane receptor interacts with the specific antigen against which it is directed, the cell is activated, and as a consequence, histamine and other mediators are released from the cell. The release of histamine and a variety of other biologically active compounds is the basis of the immediate hypersensitivity reaction.

BIBLIOGRAPHY

Brandtzaeg P. Molecular and cellular aspects of the secretory immunoglobulin system. *APMIS.* 1995;103:1–19.

Burton DR, Wilson IA. Square-dancing antibodies. *Science.* 2007;317:1507–1508.

Davies AM, Sutton BJ. Human IgG4: A structural perspective. *Immunol Rev.* 2015;268:139–159.

Djistelnloem HM, van de Winkel J, Kellenberg CGM. Inflammation in autoimmunity: Receptors for IgG revisited. *Trends Immunol.* 2001;22:510–516.

Firan M, Bawdon R, Radu C, et al. The MHC class I-related receptor, FcRn, plays an essential role in the maternofetal transfer of γ-globulin in humans. *Int Immunol.* 2001;13:993–1002.

Ghetie V, Ward ES. Multiple roles for the major histocompatibility complex class I-related receptor FcRn. *Annu Rev Immunol.* 2000;18: 739–766.

Janoff EN, Fasching C, Orenstein JM, et al. Killing of *Streptococcus pneumoniae* by capsular polysaccharide-specific polymeric IgA, complement, and phagocytes. *J Clin Invest.* 1999; 104:1139–1147.

Karagiannis P, Gilbert AE, Josephs DH, et al. IgG4 subclass antibodies impair anti-tumor immunity in melanoma. *J Clin Invest.* 2013;123:1457–1474.

Karnasuta C, Akapirat S, Madnote S, et al. Comparison of antibody responses induced by RV144, VAX003, and VAX004 vaccination regimens. *AIDS Res Hum Retroviruses.* 2017;33: 410–423.

Nezlin R. Immunoglobulin structure and function. In: van Oss CJ, van Regenmortel MHV, eds. *Immunochemistry.* New York, NY: Marcel Dekker; 1994.

Pan Q, Lan Q, Peng Y, et al. Nature, functions and clinical implications of IgG4 autoantibodies in systemic lupus erythematosus and rheumatoid arthritis. *Discov Med.* 2017;23:169–174.

Parkhouse RME. Biosynthesis of immunoglobulins. In: Glynn LE, Steward MW, eds., *Immunochemistry: An Advanced Textbook.* New York, NY: John Wiley and Sons; 1977.

Ravetch JV, Bolland S. IgG Fc receptors. *Annu Rev Immunol.* 2001;19:275–290.

Schroeder HW, Cavacini L. Structure and function of immunoglobulins. *J Allergy Clin Immunol.* 2010;125(Suppl. 2):S41–S52.

Waldmann TA, Strober W. Metabolism of immunoglobulins. *Prog Allergy.* 1969;13:1–110.

7

Genetics of immunoglobulins: Ontogenic, biological, and clinical implications

JANARDAN P. PANDEY

INTRODUCTION

Human immunoglobulin (Ig) molecules are coded by three unlinked gene families: two for light (L) chains located on chromosomes 2 (κ-chains) and 22 (λ-chains), and one for heavy (H) chains located on chromosome 14. As mentioned in the preceding chapters, everyone can produce billions of antibody molecules with different antigenic specificities, and this diversity corresponds to the extreme heterogeneity of the variable (V) regions in those antibody molecules, implying that everyone must possess a large number of structural genes for Ig chains. The allotypic determinants on the constant (C) region (see following discussion), in contrast, segregate as a single Mendelian trait, suggesting that there may be only one gene for each of the several Ig chain C regions. To reconcile these seemingly contradictory observations, Dreyer and Bennet, in 1965, proposed that two separate genes that are brought together by a translocation event during lymphocyte development encode the V and C regions. Employing recombinant DNA technology, Hozumi and Tonegawa, in 1976, obtained conclusive proof of this hypothesis (for his seminal studies, Tonegawa was awarded the 1987 Nobel Prize in Medicine and Physiology).

IMMUNOGLOBULIN GENE REARRANGEMENT

It is well established that an immunoglobulin polypeptide chain is coded by multiple genes scattered along a chromosome of the germ-line genome. These widely separated gene segments are brought together (recombined) during B-lymphocyte differentiation to form a complete immunoglobulin gene.

The V regions of the immunoglobulin light chains are coded by two gene segments, designated as V and J (J for joining, because it joins V and C region genes). Three gene segments are required for the synthesis of the V region of the heavy chains: V, J, and D (D for diversity, corresponds to the most diverse region of the H chain). To form a functional light- or heavy-chain gene, one or two gene rearrangements are needed. On chromosomes 2 or 22, a V gene moves next to a J gene. On chromosome 14, first the D and J regions are joined, and next one of the V genes is joined to the DJ complex. The VJ segments and one of the L chain C regions (Cκ or Cλ) or VDJ segments and one of the CH-gene complexes (Cμ, Cδ, Cγ3, Cγ1, Cα1, Cγ2, Cγ4, Cε, or Cα2) are then transcribed into nuclear RNA that contains these sequences as well as the interconnecting noncoding sequences. The intervening noncoding sequences are then excised making a contiguous VJC mRNA for an L chain and a contiguous VDJC mRNA for an H chain (Figures 7.1 and 7.2). Gene rearrangements occur in a sequential order: usually heavy chain genes rearrange first, followed by κ-chain genes, and last by λ-genes.

The VDJ joining is regulated by two proteins encoded by two closely linked **recombination-activating genes**, RAG-1 and RAG-2, localized on the short arm of human chromosome 11.

These genes have at least two unusual characteristics not shared by most eukaryotic genes: they are devoid of introns and, although adjacent in location and synergistic in function, they have no sequence homology. The latter implies that, unlike the immunoglobulin and major histocompatibility complex genes, RAG-1 and RAG-2 did not arise by gene duplication. Recent studies suggest that these genes may be evolutionarily related to transposons, genetic elements that can be transposed in the genome from one location to the other. Conserved recombination signal sequences (RSSs) serve as substrate for the enzymes coded by the RAG genes. These enzymes introduce a break between the RSS and the coding sequence. Mechanisms involved in subsequent rejoining to form a mature coding segment are not completely understood.

The transcription of Ig genes, like other eukaryotic genes, is regulated by *promoters* and

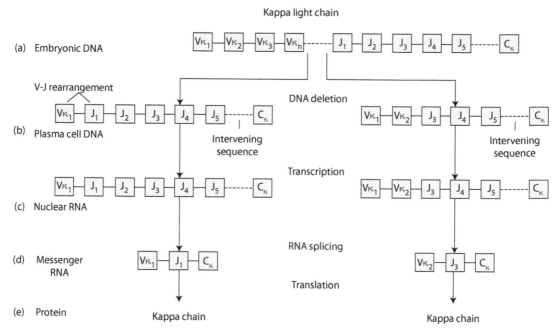

Figure 7.1 The embryonic DNA of chromosome 2 contains over 300 V genes, 5 J (joining) genes, and a C (constant) gene (a). The V and J gene code for the κ chain's variable region, C for its constant region. In the left pathway, differentiation of the embryonic cell to a plasma cell results in deletion of the intervening V genes so that $V\kappa_1$ is joined with the J_1 gene (b). The linked $V\kappa_1 J_1$ segment codes for one of over 1,500 possible κ light-chain variable regions. The plasma cell DNA is transcribed into nuclear RNA (c). Splicing of the nuclear RNA produces messenger RNAs with the $V\kappa 1$, J_1, and C genes linked together (d), ready for translation of a κ light-chain protein (e). The alternate pathway at right (b–d) shows another of the many possible pathways leading to a different κ light chain with a different variable region specificity. (Modified from David, J.R., In: *Scientific American Medicine*, Scientific American Inc., New York, 1980.)

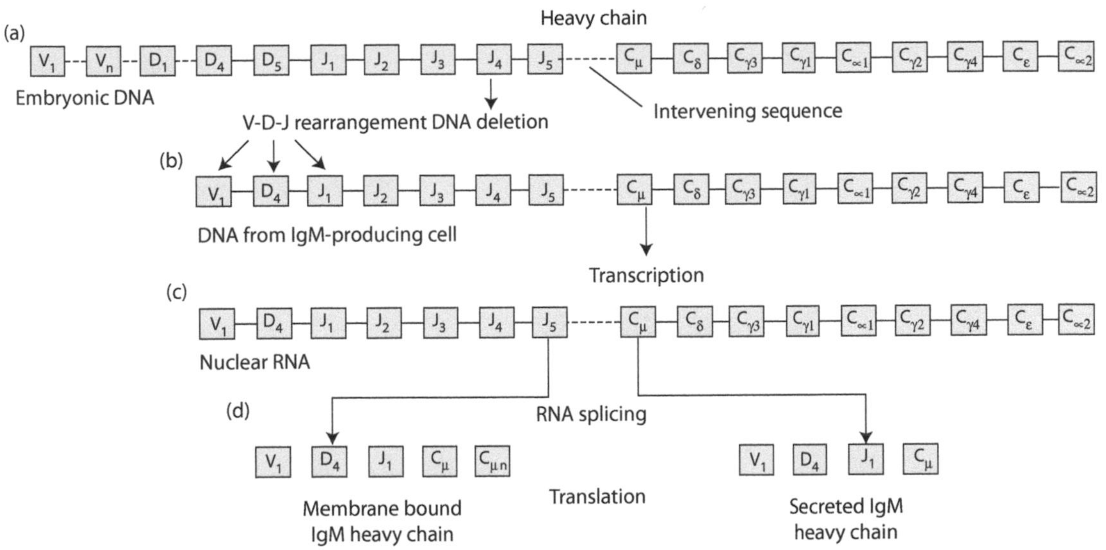

Figure 7.2 A stretch of embryonic DNA in chromosome 14 contains a section coding for the heavy-chain variable region; this DNA is made up of at least 100 V genes, 50 D genes, and 4–6 J genes. The section coding for the constant region is formed by nine C genes (a). In the pathway shown, when the embryonic cell differentiates into a plasma cell, some V and D genes are deleted so that V_1, D_4, and J_1 are joined to form one of many possible heavy-chain genes (b). The plasma cell DNA is then transcribed into nuclear RNA (c). RNA splicing selects the C gene and joins it to the V_1, D_4, and J_1 genes (d). The resulting messenger RNAs will code for IgM heavy chains. If RNA splicing removes the Cμm piece from the Cμ gene, the IgM will be secreted. If the piece remains, the IgM will be membrane bound. (Modified from David, J.R., In: *Scientific American Medicine*, Scientific American Inc., New York, 1980.)

enhancers. Promoters, located 5′ of the V segments, are necessary for transcription initiation. Enhancers, located in the introns between J and C segments, increase the rate of transcription. For this reason, immunoglobulin synthesis (H or L chains) is only detected after the VDJ or VJ rearrangements, which bring the promoter in close proximity to the enhancer.

During ontogeny and functional differentiation, the H chain genes may undergo further gene rearrangements that result in **immunoglobulin class switching**. As the B lymphocytes differentiate into plasma cells, one heavy-chain C gene segment can be substituted for another without alteration of the VDJ combination (Figure 7.3). In other words, a given variable region gene can be expressed in association with more than one heavy-chain class or subclass, so that at the cellular level, the same antibody specificity can be associated with the synthesis of an IgM immunoglobulin (characteristic of the early stages of ontogeny and of the primary response) or with

an IgG immunoglobulin (characteristic of the mature individual and of the secondary response). Immunoglobulin class switching is the result of an intrachromosomic recombination between the switch region of Cμ and one of the downstream switch regions. This recombination event leads to looping-out deletion of the intervening DNA segment and joins the rearranged V region to a different C region (Cγ, Cε, Cα).

GENETIC BASIS OF ANTIBODY DIVERSITY

It has been estimated that an individual can produce up to 10^9 different antibody molecules. How this vast diversity is generated from a limited number of germline elements has long been one of the most intriguing problems in immunology. There are two possible mechanisms for this variability: either the information is transmitted from generation to generation in the germ line, or it is generated somatically during B-lymphocyte

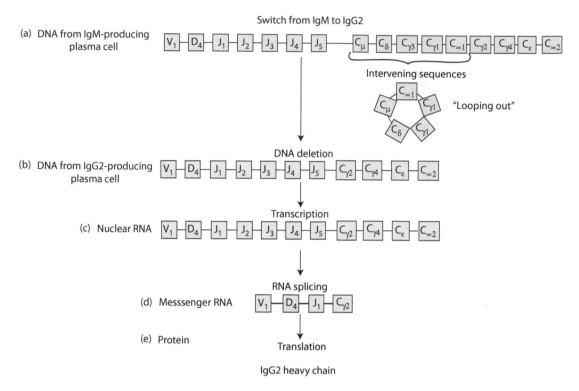

Figure 7.3 In the secondary response, a plasma cell switches from IgM production (a) to IgG2 production by deleting a DNA loop containing the constant-region genes Cμ, C∂, Cγ3, Cγ1, and Cμ1 from the IgM heavy-chain gene (b). This DNA is now transcribed into nuclear RNA (c). RNA splicing links the Cγ2 gene with the J_1 gene (d), and then the mRNA is translated into an IgG2 heavy chain (e). (Modified from David, J.R., In: *Scientific American Medicine*, Scientific American Inc., New York, 1980.)

differentiation. The following genetic mechanisms have been shown to contribute to the generation of antibody diversity:

- *V gene number*: There are a large number of V genes and a smaller set of D and J segments in the germline DNA, which have probably been generated during evolution because of environmental pressure. The human V_H locus comprises approximately 105 V, 27 D, and 9 J segments.
- *Combinatorial association*: As previously mentioned, there are at least 105 V region genes for the heavy chain, and this is probably a conservative estimate. The total number of possible V genes is probably higher because any V segment can combine, in principle, with any J and D segments. Imprecise joining of various V gene segments, creating sequence variation at the points of recombination, augments diversity significantly. In the case of the light chain,

the number of V region genes is estimated as 300, and they can also recombine with different J region genes. Last, random association of L and H chains plays an important role in increasing diversity. For example, random association of 1,000 H chains and 1,000 L chains would produce 10^6 unique antibodies.

- *Somatic mutations*: In the 1950s, these were proposed to be a source of antibody diversity. Experimental support for this hypothesis, however, was only obtained three decades later. Comparison of nucleotide sequences from murine embryonic DNA and DNA obtained from plasmacytomas revealed several base changes, suggesting the occurrence of mutations during lymphocyte differentiation. There appear to be some special mutational mechanisms involved in immunoglobulin genes since the mutation sites are clustered around the V genes and not around the C genes. In addition to these point mutations, certain enzymes can randomly insert and/or delete DNA bases. Such changes can shift the reading frame for translation (frameshift mutations) so that all codons distal to the mutation are read out of phase and may result in different amino acids, thus adding to the antibody diversity. A large-scale sequencing of H and L chain genes found a much higher proportion of somatically introduced insertions and deletions than previously recognized. These insertions and deletions were clustered around the antigen-binding site, thus constituting a major mechanism of antibody diversity.

Somatic mutations (sometimes termed *hypermutations*) play a very important role in affinity maturation—production of antibodies with better antigen-binding ability. During the initial exposure to an antigen, rearranged antibodies with appropriate specificity bind to the antigen. Late in the response, random somatic mutations in the rearranged V genes result in the production of antibodies of varying affinities. By a process analogous to natural selection, B cells expressing higher-affinity antibodies are selected to proliferate, and those with the lower-affinity antibodies are eliminated.

Additionally, gene conversion, a nonreciprocal exchange of genetic information between genes, has also been shown to contribute to antibody diversity.

The discovery of the enzyme activation-induced cytidine deaminase (AID) has revolutionized research aimed at delineating the molecular mechanisms underlying various processes that amplify genomic information. AID appears to be an essential catalyst for somatic hypermutation, class switch recombination, and gene conversion, and thus a unifier at the molecular level of three apparently disparate mechanisms of antibody diversity. Its mode of action is under active investigation.

ANTIGENIC DETERMINANTS OF IMMUNOGLOBULIN MOLECULES

Three main categories of antigenic determinants are found on immunoglobulin molecules:

Isotypes: These determinants are present on all molecules of each class and subclass of immunoglobulin heavy chains and on each type of light chain; they are defined serologically by antisera directed against the constant regions of H and L chains. The antisera are produced in animals, which, upon injection of purified human immunoglobulins, recognize the structural differences between constant regions of H and L chains. Isotypic determinants are common to all members of a given species; hence, they cannot be used as genetic markers. Their practical importance results from the fact that they allow the identification of classes and subclasses of immunoglobulins through the heavy-chain isotypes and types of light chains (κ, λ). All classes and subclasses of normal immunoglobulins share the two light-chain isotypes.

Idiotypes: The antigen-combining site in the V region of the immunoglobulin molecule, in addition to determining specificity for antigen binding, can also act as an antigen and induce production of antibodies against it. Such antigenic determinants, usually associated with hypervariable regions, are known as idiotypes.

Allotypes: These are hereditary antigenic determinants of Ig polypeptide chains that may differ between individuals of the same species. The loci controlling allotypic determinants are codominant (i.e., both are expressed phenotypically in a heterozygote) autosomal genes that follow Mendelian laws of heredity. All allotypic markers that have so far been identified on human immunoglobulin molecules, with one exception (see later), are present in the C regions of H chains of IgG, IgA, IgE, and on κ-type L chains. Since different individuals of the same species may have different allotypes, these determinants can be used as genetic markers.

Isoallotypes: As the term implies, these determinants possess properties of both allotypes and isotypes. They behave as alleles in one IgG subclass (allotype) but are also expressed in all molecules of at least one other IgG subclass (isotype). For instance, the codon 409 of the $\gamma4$ chain codes for either arginine or lysine amino acids. In a heterozygous individual, half of the $\gamma4$ molecules will have arginine, and the other half will have lysine at position 409. In other words, these determinants behave as alleles of each other in $\gamma4$. However, the arginine residue is present in all $\gamma1$ and $\gamma3$ molecules, and the lysine is present in all $\gamma2$ proteins. Therefore, these determinants behave as isotypes in these subclasses.

This simple arginine/lysine substitution in IgG4 appears to have important biological/clinical implications. The arginine409 allele enables the Fab-arm exchange (Chapter 5), while the lysine409 allele abrogates it. Therefore, while manufacturing therapeutic IgG4 antibodies, one must make sure that the arginine409 allele has been mutated/stabilized, for an arms exchange between the infused therapeutic antibody and the native IgG4 would result in the loss of specificity.

IgG heavy-chain allotypes (GM allotypes)

Allotypes have been found on γ1, γ2, and γ3 heavy chains, but not yet on γ4 chains. They are denoted as G1M, G2M, and G3M, respectively (G for IgG; the numerals 1, 2, and 3 identify the subclass; the letter M for marker). At present, 18 GM specificities can be serologically defined (Table 7.1): 4 associated with IgG1 (G1M), 1 associated with IgG2 (G2M), and 13 associated with IgG3 (G3M). G1M 3 and G1M 17 are localized in the Fd portion of the IgG molecule, while the rest are in the Fc portion. The amino acid/nucleotide substitutions responsible for some allotypes are

Table 7.1 Currently testable GM allotypes

Heavy-chain subclass	Numeric	Alphameric
γ1	G1M 1	a
	2	x
	3	f
	17	z
γ2	G2M 23	n
γ3	G3M 5	b1
	6	c3
	10	b5
	11	b0
	13	b3
	14	b4
	15	s
	16	t
	21	gl
	24	c5
	26	u
	27	v
	28	g5

known. For instance, G1M 3 heavy chains have arginine at position 214, and G1M 17 heavy chains have lysine at this position. A single heavy chain may possess more than one GM determinant; G1M 17 and G1M 1 are frequently present on the Fd and Fc portions of the same H chain in Caucasians.

The four C-region genes on human chromosome 14 that encode the four IgG subclasses are very tightly linked. Because of this tight linkage, GM allotypes of various subclasses are transmitted as a group called **haplotype**. Also, because of almost absolute linkage disequilibrium between the alleles of various IgG C-region genes, certain allotypes of one subclass are always associated with certain others of another subclass. For example, the IgG1 gene controls G1M 3, whereas the IgG3 gene controls G3M 5 and G3M 21. We should expect to find G1M 3 associated with G3M 5 as often as with G3M 21; in fact, in Caucasians, a haplotype carrying G1M 3 is almost always associated with G3M 5 and not with G3M 21. Every major ethnic group has a distinct array of several GM haplotypes. GM* 3 23 5,10,11,13,14,26 and GM* 1,17 5,10,11,13,14,26 are examples of common Caucasian and Negroid haplotypes, respectively. In accordance with the international system for human gene nomenclature, haplotypes and phenotypes are written by grouping together the markers that belong to each subclass, by the numerical order of the marker and of the subclass; markers belonging to different subclasses are separated by a space, while allotypes within a subclass are separated by commas. An asterisk is used to distinguish alleles and haplotypes from phenotypes.

IgA heavy-chain allotypes (AM allotypes)

Two allotypes have been defined on human IgA2 molecules: A2M 1 and A2M 2. They behave as alleles of one another. No allotypes have been found on IgA1 molecules yet. Individuals lacking IgA (or a particular IgA allotype) have in some instances been found to possess anti-IgA antibodies directed either against one of the allotypic markers or against the isotypic determinant. In some patients, these antibodies can cause severe anaphylactic reactions, following blood transfusion containing incompatible IgA.

IgE heavy-chain allotypes (EM allotypes)

Only one allotype, designated as EM 1, has been described for the IgE molecule.

κ-type light-chain allotypes (KM allotypes)

Three KM allotypes have been described so far: KM 1, KM 2, and KM 3. (About 98% of the subjects positive for KM 1 are also positive for KM 2.) They are inherited via three alleles, KM* 1, KM* 1,2, and KM* 3 on human chromosome 2. No allotypes have yet been found on the λ-type light chains.

Heavy-chain V-region allotype (HV 1)

So far, HV 1 is the only allotypic determinant described in the V region of human immunoglobulins. It is located in the V region of H chains of IgG, IgM, IgA, and possibly also on IgD and IgE.

Traditionally, Ig allotypes have been characterized serologically by a hemagglutination-inhibition method, using serum or plasma. Briefly, the method employs human blood group ORh+ erythrocytes coated with anti-Rh antibodies of known allotypes and a panel of monospecific anti-allotype sera. Test sera containing immunoglobulin of a particular allotype inhibit hemagglutination by the monospecific anti-allotype antibody, whereas negative sera do not. Most of the older literature on allotypes is based on the serologically determined markers. The availability of anti-allotype sera for serological typing is now extremely scarce; for some markers, they are no longer available. In the past few years, several DNA-based methods for allotyping have been developed, such as direct DNA sequencing, PCR-restriction fragment length polymorphisms, and the TaqMan genotyping assay from Applied Biosystems Inc., using allotype-specific DNA primers and probes.

ALLELIC EXCLUSION

One of the most fascinating observations in immunology is that immunoglobulin heavy-chain genes from only one of the two homologous chromosomes 14 (one paternal and one maternal) are expressed in each B lymphocyte. Recombination of VDJC genes described earlier usually takes place on one of the homologues. Only if this rearrangement is unproductive (i.e., it does not result in the secretion of an antibody molecule), does the other homologue undergo rearrangement. Consequently, of the two H chain alleles in a B cell, one is productively rearranged, and the other is either in the germline pattern or is aberrantly rearranged (in other words, *excluded*). Involvement of the chromosomes is random; in one B cell, the paternal allele may be active, and in another, it may be a maternal allele. (Allelic exclusion is reminiscent of the X-chromosome inactivation in mammals, although it is genetically more complex.)

Two models have been proposed to explain allelic exclusion: *stochastic* and *regulated*. The main impetus for proposing the *stochastic model* was the finding that a high proportion of VDJ or VJ rearrangements are nonproductive, i.e., they do not result in transcription of mRNA. Therefore, according to this model, allelic exclusion is achieved because of a very low likelihood of a productive rearrangement on both chromosomes. According to the *regulated model*, a productive H or L chain gene arrangement signals the cessation of further gene rearrangements (feedback inhibition).

Results from experiments with transgenic mice (mice in which foreign genes have been introduced in the germline) favor the regulated model. It appears that a correctly rearranged H-chain gene not only inhibits further H-chain gene rearrangements but also gives a positive signal for the κ-chain gene rearrangement. The rearrangement of the λ gene takes place only if both alleles of the κ gene are aberrantly rearranged. (Although in some cases, it appears that the λ gene rearrangement is autonomous, that is, it does not depend on the prior deletion and/or nonproductive rearrangement of both κ alleles.) This mutually exclusive nature of a productive L gene rearrangement results in **isotypic exclusion**, i.e., a given plasma cell contains either κ or λ chains, but not both.

Allelic exclusion is evident at the level of the GM system. A given plasma cell from an individual heterozygous for G1M* 17/G1M* 3 will secrete IgG carrying either G1M 17 or G1M 3, but not both. Since the exclusion is random, serum samples from such an individual will have both G1M 17 and G1M 3 secreted by different immunoglobulin-producing cells.

The process of allelic exclusion results in the synthesis of Ig molecules with identical V and C regions in each single plasma cell because all expressed mRNA will have been derived from a single rearranged chromosome 14 and from a single rearranged chromosome 2 or 22. Therefore, the antibodies produced by each B lymphocyte will be of a single specificity.

GM ALLOTYPES AND IgG SUBCLASS CONCENTRATIONS

Studies from several laboratories have found a correlation between certain GM allotypes or phenotypes and the concentration of the four subclasses of IgG. The results vary; however, virtually all studies report a significant association between the GM 3 5,13 phenotype and a high IgG3 concentration and the G2M 23 allotype and an increased concentration of IgG2. These associations imply that a determination of whether a person's IgG subclass level is in the "normal" range should be made in the context of the individual's GM phenotype.

IMMUNOGLOBULIN ALLOTYPES, IMMUNE RESPONSE, AND DISEASES

Numerous studies have shown that immune responsiveness to a variety of self and non-self antigens, as well as susceptibility/resistance to many autoimmune, infectious, and malignant diseases, are influenced by GM and KM allotypes. How can C-region allotypes influence immune responsiveness thought to be exclusively associated with the V-region genes? Contrary to the prevalent paradigm in immunology, these constant-region determinants could directly influence antibody affinity and specificity by causing conformational changes in the antigen-binding site in the immunoglobulin variable region. There is convincing evidence that the immunoglobulin constant region can influence antibody affinity and specificity. Thus, constant regions expressing different GM allotypes, even when combined with identical variable region sequences, can generate new antibody molecules with new functions.

Recent mechanistic studies have shown that GM allotypes interact with γ-receptors (FcγRs) expressed on effector cells (e.g., natural killer cells and neutrophils) and influence the magnitude of antibody-dependent cell-mediated cytotoxicity (ADCC). ADCC, which links the specific humoral responses to the vigorous innate cytotoxic effector responses, is a major host defense mechanism against tumors and virally infected cells as well as a leading mechanism underlying the clinical efficacy of therapeutic antibodies against malignant diseases.

The biological role and reasons for the extensive polymorphism of Ig allotypes remain unknown. The marked differences in the frequencies of Ig allotypes among races, strong linkage disequilibrium within a race, and racially restricted occurrence of GM haplotypes, all suggest that differential selection over many generations may have played an important role in the maintenance of polymorphism at these loci. One mechanism could be the possible association of these markers with immunity to certain lethal infectious pathogens implicated in major epidemics, and different races may have been subjected to different epidemics throughout our evolutionary history. As first suggested by JBS Haldane, high-mortality infectious diseases have probably been the principal selective forces of natural selection in humans. After a major epidemic, only individuals with genetic combinations conferring immunity to the pathogen would survive. In this context, it is interesting to note that GM genes have been shown to influence the chance for survival in certain typhoid and yellow fever epidemics. Like infectious diseases, malignant diseases might also have exerted adaptive pressure on GM, KM, and FcγR polymorphisms. It is important to keep in mind that approximately two-thirds of the human population remain free of cancer, making it reasonable to speculate that particular ligand-receptor combinations of Fc (GM) and FcγR genes could have been evolutionarily selected because of their contribution—through ADCC and other Fc-mediated protective immunosurveillance mechanisms—to survival from malignant diseases.

BIBLIOGRAPHY

Casadevall A, Pirofski LA. A new synthesis for antibody-mediated immunity. Nat Immunol. 2011;13:21–28.

Moraru M, Black LE, Muntasell A, et al. NK cell and Ig interplay in defense against herpes simplex virus type 1: Epistatic interaction of CD16A and IgG1 allotypes of variable affinities modulates antibody-dependent cellular cytotoxicity and susceptibility to clinical reactivation. *J Immunol.* 2015;195:1676–1684.

Oxelius VA, Pandey JP. Human immunoglobulin constant heavy G chain (IGHG) (Fcγ) (GM) genes, defining innate variants of IgG molecules and B cells, have impact on disease and therapy. *Clin Immunol. 2013*;149:475–486.

Pandey JP. Immunoglobulin GM genes, cytomegalovirus immunoevasion, and the risk of glioma, neuroblastoma, and breast cancer. *Front Oncol.* 2014;4:236. doi: 10.3389/fonc.2014.00236.

Pandey JP, Namboodiri AM, Elston RC. Immunoglobulin G genotypes and the risk of schizophrenia. *Hum Genet.* 2016;135:1175–1179.

Pandey JP, Namboodiri AM, Wolf B, et al. Endogenous antibody responses to mucin 1 in a large multiethnic cohort of patients with breast cancer and healthy controls: Role of immunoglobulin and Fcγ receptor genes. *Immunobiology.* 2018;223:178–182.

Ternant D, Arnoult C, Pugnière M, et al. IgG1 allotypes influence the pharmacokinetics of therapeutic monoclonal antibodies through FcRn binding. *J Immunol.* 2016;196:607–613.

8

Antigen-antibody reactions

GABRIEL VIRELLA

GENERAL CHARACTERISTICS OF THE ANTIGEN-ANTIBODY REACTION

The reaction between antigens and antibodies involves complementary binding sites on the antibody and on the antigen molecules. The antigen molecules usually have numerous epitopes sites that combine with the binding site (paratope) of an antibody. In the same way that the binding site is determined by different segments on the variable regions of heavy and light chains that come in close proximity due to the folding of those regions, the epitopes are also formed by discontinuous segments of an antigen molecule. Some subsets of amino acids within the epitope contribute most of the binding energy with the antibody, while the surrounding residues provide structural complementary, which may play a stabilizing role when antigens and antibodies interact.

Chemical bonds responsible for the antigen-antibody reaction

The interaction between the antibody binding site and the epitope involves exclusively noncovalent bonds, in a similar manner to that in which proteins bind to their cellular receptors or enzymes bind to their substrates. The binding is reversible and can be prevented or dissociated by high ionic strength or extreme pH. The following intermolecular forces are involved in antigen-antibody binding:

- *Electrostatic bonds*: Electrostatic bonds result from the attraction between oppositely charged ionic groups of two protein side chains, for example, an ionized amino group (NH^{4+}) on a lysine in the antibody, and an ionized carboxyl group (COO^-) on an aspartate residue in the antigen.
- *Hydrogen bonding*: When the antigen and antibody are in very close proximity, relatively weak hydrogen bonds can be formed between hydrophilic groups (e.g., OH and C=O, NH and C=O, and NH and OH groups).
- *Hydrophobic interactions*: Hydrophobic groups, such as the side chains of valine, leucine, and phenylalanine, tend to associate due to van der Waals bonding and coalesce in an aqueous environment, excluding water molecules from their surroundings. Therefore, the distance between them decreases, enhancing the energies of attraction involved. This type of interaction is estimated to contribute up to 50% of the total strength of the antigen-antibody bond.
- *Van der Waals bonds*: These forces depend on interactions between the "electron clouds" that surround the antigen and antibody molecules. The interaction has been compared to that

which might exist between alternating dipoles in two molecules, alternating in such a way that at any given moment oppositely oriented dipoles will be present in closely apposed areas of the antigen and antibody molecules.

All of these types of interactions depend on the close proximity of the antigen and antibody molecules. For that reason, the "fit" between an antigenic determinant and an antibody combining site determines the stability of the antigen-antibody reaction.

Antibody specificity

Most of the data concerning this topic was generated in studies of the immune response to closely related haptens. Using a conjugate of protein-p-benzoate (haptenic group) with an immunogenic carrier protein, it was noticed that an animal inoculated with this conjugate would produce an antibody that reacted strongly with the protein-p-benzoate conjugate, but also with p-benzoate and with benzoate in which chlorine occupied the p position, but not with p-benzoate with chlorine substitutions at positions *ortho* or *meta* (Figure 8.1). These and other experiments of the same type led to the conclusions that specificity is mainly determined by the overall degree of complementarity between antigenic determinant and antibody binding site, and that differences in the degree of complementarity determine the "affinity" of the antigen-antibody reaction.

Antibody affinity and avidity

Antibody affinity can be defined as the attractive force between the complementary configurations of the antigenic determinant and the antibody-combining site. Experimentally, the reaction is best studied with antibodies directed against monovalent haptens. The reaction, as previously mentioned, is reversible and can be defined by the following equation:

$$Ab + Hp \underset{k_2}{\overset{k_1}{\rightleftarrows}} Ab \cdot Hp$$

where k_1 is the association constant and k_2 the dissociation constant.

This equation can be rewritten as

$$K = \frac{k_1}{k_2} = \frac{[Ab \cdot Hp]}{[Ab][Hp]}$$

where K is the affinity constant that measures how much antibody-antigen complex exists at the point of equilibrium. High values for K will reflect a predominance of *the* association constant over the dissociation constant, or, in other words, a tendency for the antigen-antibody complex to be stable and not to dissociate. The affinity constant can be measured in the laboratory by a variety of methods, usually based on determining the ratio of free versus bound antigen in a system designed to allow such determination. The determinations are more exact when haptens are used because there is a single epitope in play. Purified antibodies against polyvalent antigens will contain a mixture of antibodies of different affinities recognizing several epitopes; therefore, only an average affinity can be determined.

Based on data generated in a system in which the antibody concentration remains constant but the concentration of hapten is variable, a Scatchard plot can be generated, in which the quotient between moles of hapten bound per moles of antibody (r/c) and the concentration of free hapten (c) are plotted against the concentration of hapten bound per mole of antibody (r). The slope of the plot of r/c versus r values corresponds to $-K$. As illustrated in Figure 8.2, with high-affinity antibodies, r will reach saturation (r = n) at relatively low concentrations of hapten, and the plot will have a steep slope, as shown in Figure 8.2a. With low-affinity antibodies, the stable occupancy of the antibody binding sites will require higher concentrations of free hapten, so the slope is considerably less steep and r/c value significantly lower, as shown in Figure 8.2b. Since the reactants (antibodies and haptens) are expressed as moles-liter^{-1}, the affinity constant is expressed as liters mole^{-1} (L mol^{-1}).

From the Scatchard plot, it is obvious that at extremely high concentrations of unbound hapten (c), r/c becomes close to 0, and the plot of r/c versus r will intercept r on the horizontal axis (the interception corresponds to n, the antibody *valency*). For an IgG antibody and all other monomeric antibodies, the value of n is 2; for IgM antibodies, the theoretical valency is 10, but the functional valency is usually 5, suggesting that steric hindrance effects

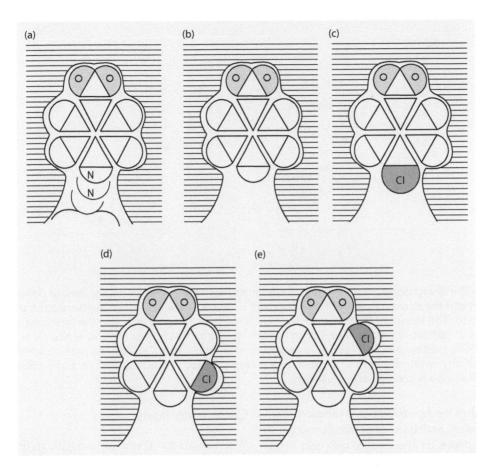

Figure 8.1 The "closeness of fit" between antigenic determinants and antibody binding sites. Antibodies were raised against the **p**-azobenzoate group of a protein-p-benzoate conjugate. The resulting anti-**p**-benzoate groups react well with the original protein-p-benzoate conjugate (a) and with **p**-benzoate itself (b). If a chlorine atom (Cl) is substituted for a hydrogen atom at the **p** position, the substituted hapten will react strongly with the original antibody (c). However, if chlorine atoms are substituted for hydrogen atoms at the **o** or **m** positions (d,e), the reaction with the antibody is disturbed, since the chlorine atoms at those positions cause a significant change in the configuration of the benzoate group. (Redrawn from Van Oss, C. In: Rose N, Milgrom F, Van Oss C, eds. *Principles of Immunology*. 2nd ed. Macmillan, New York, 1979.)

prevent simultaneous occupation of the binding sites of each subunit.

High-affinity antibodies have K_0 values as high as 10^{10} liters mole^{-1}. The same principles can be applied to measurements using human antigens and the corresponding antibodies, with the previously mentioned caveat that the obtained values are reflective of the average affinity or, in other words, avidity (see later in chapter) of specific antibodies reacting with several epitopes of a complex antigen. But, if a monoclonal antibody is tested for its reactivity with a complex antigen, the values will be closely reflective of true affinity, because the antibody interacts with a single epitope.

In humans it has been noted that autoantibodies are usually of low affinity, while induced antibodies are of high affinity. For example, the affinity of induced anti-keyhole limpet hemocyanin (a very strongly immunogenic protein isolated from mollusks known as keyhole limpets) IgG antibodies was measured as 7.6 mol/L $\times$ E^{-10}, while the average affinity of 30 isolated human autoantibodies formed spontaneously against oxidized LDL was 1.02 ± 1.1 mol/L $\times$ E^{-8}.

Antibody avidity can be defined as the strength of the binding of the several different antibodies that are produced in response to an immunogen, which presents several different epitopes to the immune system.

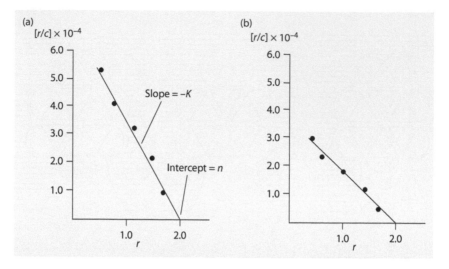

Figure 8.2 The Scatchard plots correlating the quotient between moles of hapten bound per moles of antibody (r) and the concentration of free hapten (c) with the concentration of hapten bound per mole of antibody (r). The slopes of the plots correspond to the affinity constants, and the intercept with the horizontal axis correspond to the number of hapten molecules bound per mole of antibody at a theoretically infinite hapten concentration (n or valency of the antibody molecule). The plot (a) corresponds to a high-affinity antibody, and the slope is very steep; the plot (b) corresponds to a low-affinity antibody, and its slope is considerably less steep.

The strength of the Ag·Ab reaction is enhanced when several different antibodies bind simultaneously to different epitopes on the antigen molecule, cross-linking antigen molecules very tightly. Thus, a more stable bonding between antigen and antibody will be established, due to the "bonus-effect" of multiple antigen-antibody bonds (Figure 8.3); the increased stability of the overall antigen-antibody reaction corresponds to an increased avidity.

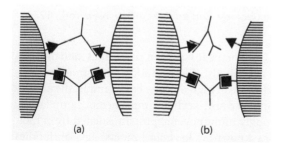

Figure 8.3 The avidity concept. The binding of antigen molecules by several antibodies of different specificities (a) stabilizes the immune complex, since it is highly unlikely that all Ag·Ab reactions dissociate simultaneously at any given point of time (b). (Redrawn from Roitt I. *Essential Immunology*. 4th ed. Blackwell Publishing, Hoboken, NJ; 1980.)

Cross-reactions

When an animal is immunized with an immunogen, its serum will contain several different antibodies directed to the various epitopes presented by the immunizing molecule, reflecting the polyclonal nature of the response. Such serum from an immune animal is known as an antiserum directed against the immunogen.

Antisera containing polyclonal antibodies can often be found to *cross-react* with immunogens partially related to that used for immunization, due to the existence of common epitopes or of epitopes with similar configurations. Less frequently, a cross-reaction may be totally unexpected, involving totally unrelated antigens that happen to present epitopes whose whole spatial configuration may be similar enough to allow the cross-reaction. The avidity of a cross-reaction depends on the degree of structural similarity between the shared epitopes; when the avidity reaches a very low point, the cross-reaction will no longer be detectable (Figure 8.4). The differential avidity of given antiserum for the original immunogen and for other immunogens sharing epitopes of similar structure is responsible for the "specificity" of the antiserum, i.e., its ability to recognize only a

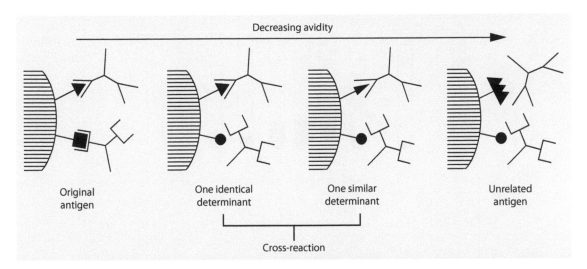

Decreasing avidity

| Original antigen | One identical determinant | One similar determinant | Unrelated antigen |

Cross-reaction

Figure 8.4 The concept of cross-reaction between complex antigens. An antiserum containing several antibody populations to the determinants of a given antigen will react with other antigens sharing common or closely related determinants. The avidity of the reaction will decrease with decreasing structural closeness, until it will no longer be detectable. The reactivity of the same antiserum with several related antigens is designated as a cross-reaction. (Redrawn from Roitt I. *Essential Immunology*. 4th ed. Blackwell Publishing, Hoboken, NJ; 1980.)

single immunogen, or a few, very closely related immunogens.

An exception to those general rules is the existence of "promiscuous antibodies" that show reactivity with a variety of unrelated antigens with structurally unrelated epitopes. Those are usually germline antibodies that show a greater degree of flexibility and high frequency of aromatic acids and β-pleated sheets in the complementarity determining variable regions of the heavy chains. These molecular features are believed to be the basis for their ability to interact with multiple unrelated epitopes presented by totally unrelated antigens.

SPECIFIC TYPES OF ANTIGEN-ANTIBODY REACTIONS

Antigen-antibody reactions may be revealed by a variety of physical expressions, depending on the nature of the antigen and on the conditions surrounding the reaction.

Precipitation

When antigen and antibody are mixed in a test tube in their soluble forms, one of two things may happen: both components will remain soluble, or variable amounts of Ag·Ab precipitate will be formed.

If progressively increasing amounts of antigen are mixed with a fixed amount of antibody, a **precipitin curve** can be constructed (Figure 8.5). There are three areas to consider in a precipitin curve:

- *Antibody excess*: Free antibody remains in solution after centrifugation of Ag·Ab complexes.
- *Equivalence*: No free antigen or antibody remains in solution. The amount of precipitated Ag·Ab complexes reaches its peak at this point.
- *Antigen excess*: Free antigen is detected in the supernatant after centrifugation of Ag·Ab complexes.

The **lattice theory** was created to explain why different amounts of precipitation are observed at different antigen-antibody ratios. At great antibody excess, each antigen will tend to have its binding sites saturated, with antibody molecules bound to all its exposed determinants. Extensive cross-linking of antigen and antibody is not possible. But if one can determine the number of antibody molecules bound to one single antigen molecule, a rough indication of the valency (i.e., number of epitopes) of the antigen will be obtained. At great antigen excess, single antigen molecules will saturate the binding sites of the antibody molecule, and not much cross-linking will take place. If the antigen is very small

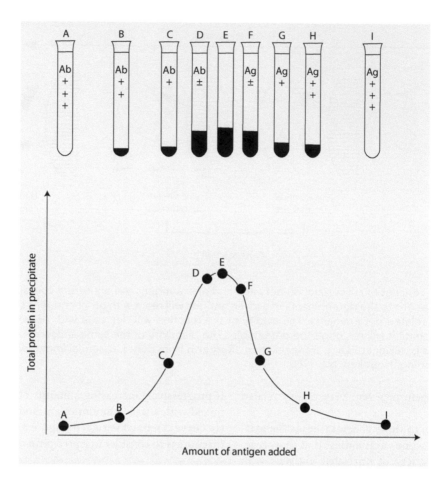

Figure 8.5 The precipitin curve. When increasing amounts of antigen are added to a fixed concentration of antibody, increasing amounts of precipitate appear as a consequence of the antigen-antibody interaction. After a maximum precipitation is reached, the amounts of precipitate begin to decrease. Analysis of the supernatants reveals that at low antigen concentrations, there is free antibody left in solution (antibody excess); at the point of maximal precipitation, neither antigen nor antibody are detected in the supernatant (equivalence zone); with greater antigen concentrations, antigen becomes detectable in the supernatant (antigen excess).

and has no repeating epitopes, calculation of the number of antigen molecules bound by each antibody molecule will indicate the antibody valency, as discussed earlier in this chapter. When the concentrations of antigen and antibody reach the **equivalence point**, maximum cross-linking between Ag and Ab will take place, resulting in formation of a large precipitate that contains all antigen and antibody present in the mixture (Figure 8.6).

When antigens and antibodies are present in circulation, the same general rules apply, except that circulating antigen-antibody complexes do not precipitate. If the concentration of antigen is in excess of the binding capacity of circulating antibodies, the free antigen can be easily detected by conventional tests. The inverse is also true; if the concentration of antibody exceeds the binding capacity of the antigen, free antibody will be easily detected. But when the concentrations of antigen and antibody are roughly equivalent, neither antigen nor antibody may be detectable by conventional assays. One classical example is the "window" period in hepatitis serology when the virus surface antigen and the corresponding antibodies circulate as immune complexes and are undetectable. Similar problems have been reported in both infectious and autoimmune diseases.

Agglutination

When bacteria, cells, or large particles in suspension are mixed with antibodies directed to their

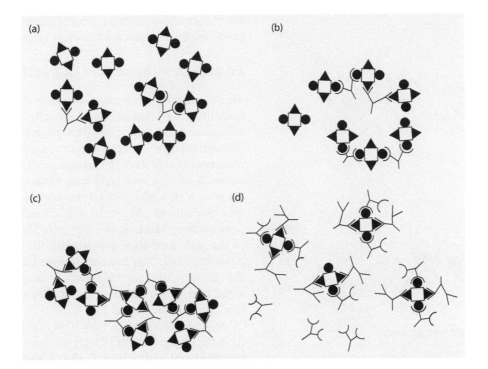

Figure 8.6 The lattice theory explaining precipitation reactions in fluid media. At great antigen excess (a), each antibody molecule has all its binding sites occupied. There is free antigen in solution, and the antigen-antibody complexes are very small ($Ag_2 \cdot Ab_1$, $Ag_1 \cdot Ab_1$). The number of epitopes bound per antibody molecule at great antigen excess corresponds to the antibody valency. With increasing amounts of antibody (b), larger Ag·Ab complexes are formed ($Ag_3 \cdot Ab_2$, etc.), but there is still incomplete precipitation and free antigen in solution. At equivalence, large Ag·Ab complexes are formed, in which virtually all Ab and Ag molecules in the system are cross-linked (c). Precipitation is maximal, and no free antigen or antibody is left in the supernatant. With increasing amounts of antibody (d), all antigen-binding sites are saturated, but there is free antibody left without binding sites available for it to react. The Ag·Ab complexes are larger than at antigen excess [$Ag_1 \cdot Ab_{4,5,6 \, (n)}$] but usually soluble. The number of antibody molecules bound per antigen molecule at great antibody excess allows an estimate of the antigen valency.

surface determinants, one will observe the formation of large clumps; this is known as an agglutination reaction.

Agglutination reactions result from the cross-linking of cells and insoluble particles by specific antibodies. Due to the relatively short distance between the two Fab fragments, 7S antibodies (such as IgG) are usually unable to bridge the gap between two cells, each of them surrounded by an electronic "cloud" of identical charge that will tend to keep them apart. IgM antibodies, in contrast, are considerably more efficient in inducing cellular agglutination (Figure 8.7).

The visualization of agglutination reactions differs according to the technique used for their study. In slide tests, the nonagglutinated cell or particulate antigen appears as a homogeneous suspension, while the agglutinated antigen will appear irregularly clumped (Figure 8.8). In red cell agglutination assays carried out on microtiter plates, agglutinated red cells sediment fast and cover the whole bottom, while nonagglutinated red cells roll and sediment in compact buttons at the very bottom of the well (Figure 8.9).

BIOLOGICAL CONSEQUENCES OF THE ANTIGEN-ANTIBODY REACTION

Opsonization

After binding to particulate antigens or after forming large molecular aggregates, antibodies unfold and may interact with Fc receptors on phagocytic cells. Such interaction is followed by ingestion by

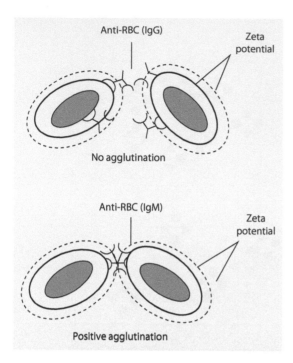

Figure 8.7 IgM antibodies are more efficient in inducing red cell agglutination. Red cells remain at the same distance from each other due to their identical electrical charge (zeta potential). IgG antibodies are not large enough to bridge the space between two red cells, but IgM antibodies, due to their polymeric nature and size, can induce red blood cell agglutination with considerable ease.

the phagocytic cell (phagocytosis). Substances that promote phagocytosis are known as opsonins.

Fc-receptor–mediated cell activation

The interaction of antigen-antibody complexes containing IgG antibodies (especially those of subclasses IgG1 and IgG3) with phagocytic cells through their Fcγ receptors results in the delivery of activating signals to the ingesting cell. The activation is usually associated with enhancement of the phagocyte's microbicidal activity. A less favorable outcome of phagocytic cell activation is an inflammatory reaction, often triggered by spillage of the toxic mediators generated in the activated phagocytic cell. This outcome is more likely when the antigen-antibody complex is immobilized along a basement membrane or a cellular surface (see Chapters 18, 20, and 23).

Another adverse reaction is one that results from the engagement of Fc receptor–bound IgE on basophils and mast cells with their corresponding antigen. The result of this reaction is the release of the potent mediators that trigger an allergic reaction (see Chapter 21).

Complement activation

One of the most important consequences of antigen-antibody interactions is the activation (or

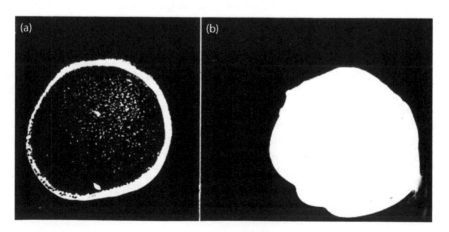

Figure 8.8 Latex agglutination assay for rheumatoid factor. Latex particles coated with human IgG were suspended in a dilution of the serum of a patient with rheumatoid arthritis positive for rheumatoid factor (a) and on a dilution with saline (b). Rheumatoid factor is an autoantibody that reacts with human IgG. The reaction of rheumatoid factor with the IgG-coated latex particles results in visible clumping (agglutination), while no clumping is seen on the particles suspended in saline.

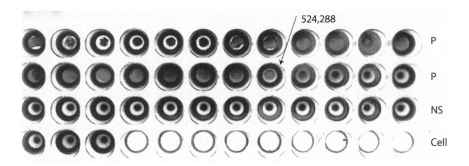

524,288

P
P
NS
Cell

Figure 8.9 Reproduction of a hemagglutination reaction performed in a microtiter plate. In the top two rows, red blood cells were added to a series of doubling dilutions of a serum sample containing anti–red cell antibodies, starting at 1:2. In the third row, red cells were added to an identical series of doubling dilutions of serum obtained from a normal healthy volunteer, also starting at 1:2. The three wells to the left on the fourth row were filled with red cells added to saline to show how red cells sediment as a round compact button in the absence of antibody. An identical pattern is observed in the red cells mixed with normal serum, indicating that the serum does not contain antibody. On the top row the sedimentation pattern is different, the bottoms of the wells to the left are diffusely covered by sedimented red cells, and normal sedimentation is only seen on the wells to the extreme right, where the sample has been diluted the most and the antibody is no longer present in sufficient concentrations to cause visible agglutination. The sedimentation pattern in the first six dilutions of the patient's serum is irregular compared to the perfectly round cell buttons in row 4. This phenomenon is due to antibody excess and defines what is known as the prozone.

"fixation") of the complement system. The activation sequence induced by antigen-antibody reactions is known as the "classical" pathway and is described in detail in Chapter 9. This pathway is initiated by the binding of C1q to the CH_2 domain of the Fc region of IgG and equivalent regions of IgM. It must be noted that the complement-binding sequences in IgG and IgM are usually not exposed in free antibody molecules, thus avoiding unnecessary and potentially deleterious activation of the complement system. The antigen-antibody interaction causes configurational changes in the antibody molecule, and the complement-binding regions become exposed. The activation of C1q requires simultaneous interaction with two complement-binding immunoglobulin domains. This means that when IgG antibodies are involved, relatively large concentrations are required, so that antibody molecules coat the antigen in very close apposition allowing C1q to be fixed by IgG duplets. In contrast, IgM molecules, by containing five closely spaced monomeric subunits, can fix complement at much lower concentrations. One IgM molecule bound by two subunits to a given antigen will constitute a complement-binding duplet.

After the binding of C1q, a cascade reaction takes place, resulting in the successive activation of eight additional complement components. Some of the components generated during complement activation are recognized by receptors on phagocytic cells and promote phagocytosis. C3b is the complement fragment with greater opsonizing capacity. Phagocytic cells take up an antigen coated with opsonizing antibodies and C3b with maximal efficiency. Others, particularly the terminal complement components, induce cell lysis.

The activation of the complement system may also have adverse effects, if it results in the destruction of host cells or if it promotes inflammation, which is beneficial with regard to the elimination of infectious organisms but always has the potential of causing tissue damage and becoming noxious to the host.

Neutralization

Another very important defense mechanism mediated by antibodies is neutralization of infectious agents. As discussed in greater detail in Chapters 12 and 14, the binding of antibodies to bacteria, toxins, and viruses has protective effects because it prevents the interaction of the microbial agents or their products with the receptors that mediate their infectiveness or toxic effects. As a consequence, the infectious agent or the toxin becomes harmless, or, in other words, is neutralized.

BIBLIOGRAPHY

Day ED. *Advanced Immunochemistry*. 2nd ed. New York, NY: Wiley-Liss; 1990.

Eisen HN. Antibody-antigen reactions. In: Davis BD, Dulbecco R, Eisen HN, Ginsberg HS, eds. *Microbiology*. Philadelphia, PA: Lippincott; 1990.

Foxman B. A primer of molecular biology. In: *Molecular Tools and Infectious Disease Epidemiology*. New York, NY: Academic Press/ Elsevier Science; 2011.

Laffy JMJ, Dodev T, Macpherson JA et al. Promiscuous antibodies characterised by their physico-chemical properties: From sequence to structure and back. *Progr Biophys Mol Biol*. 2017;128:47–56.

Landsteiner K. *The Specificity of Serological Reactions*. New York, NY: Dover Publications; 1962.

Laver WG, Air GM, Webster RG, Smith-Gill SJ. Epitopes on protein antigens: Misconceptions and realities. *Cell*. 1990;61:553–556.

Mironova M, Lopes-Virella MF, Virella G. Isolation and characterization of human anti-oxidized LDL auto-antibodies. *Arterioscler Thromb Vasc Biol*. 1996;16:222–229.

Neri D, Montigiani S, Kirkham PM. Biophysical methods for the determination of anti-body-antigen affinities. *Trends Biotechnol*. 1996;14:465–470.

Reverberi R, Reverberi L. Factors affecting the antigen-antibody reaction. *Blood Transfus*. 2007;5:227–240.

Van Oss CJ, van Regenmortel MHV. *Immuno-chemistry*. New York, NY: Marcel Dekker; 1994.

Virella G, Lopes-Virella MF. Lipoprotein autoan-tibodies: Measurement and significance. *Clin Diagn Lab Immunol*. 2003;10:499–505.

9

The complement system in health and disease

CARL ATKINSON

INTRODUCTION

The complement system is an evolutionary conserved member of the innate immune system that plays central roles in protective immune processes, including pathogen clearance, recognition of foreign antigens, modulation of cellular immune responses, noninflammatory removal of self-antigens derived from apoptotic processes, and immune complex removal. In addition to these inflammatory driving and immune regulatory functions, less well-appreciated functions of the complement system are that complement promotes autoinflammatory responses to injured self-tissues, indirectly regulates the growth of tumors, contributes to angiogenesis, can shape natural antibody repertoires, and unexpectedly enhances tissue regeneration following ischemia reperfusion injury following liver resection or transplantation. Finally, although largely considered an effector system of the innate immune response, recent studies have demonstrated that

complement is essential for immune cell health, priming both cellular and humoral immunity, and bridging innate and adaptive immune responses.

The complement system consists of approximately 30 serum and membrane-bound proteins that are found in the circulation and in tissues, most of which exist in a nonactive state. Upon activation, these complement components are rapidly converted to their active form, unleashing a potent sequential cascade leading to the formation of multiprotein membrane-spanning complexes and membrane receptor engagement of bioactive complement fragments, both of which exert substantial biological effects. Activation of the complement cascade occurs via three main activation pathways: classical, alternative, and lectin (Figure 9.1). Although the pathways of activation differ in how they are initiated, all of them generate complexes that result in the cleavage of the most abundant complement protein, C3, and as such, all pathways converge at this point.

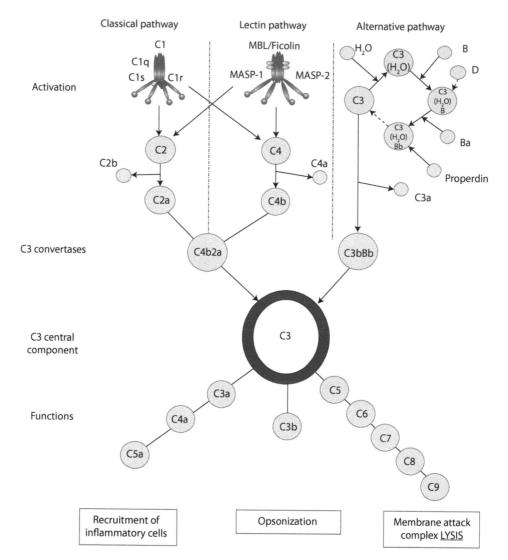

Figure 9.1 Overview of the complement activation system. The complement system can be initiated by three distinct, but interrelated pathways, the classical, lectin, and alternative pathways. Each pathway has its own distinct activating signals resulting in the formation of C3 convertase molecules that cleave and activate the central component of the complement system, C3, into C3b and C3a. The consequences of this activity are the liberalization of biologically active complement fragments that can promote inflammation, opsonization, and the assembly of the C5 convertase complex entry into the late steps of the complement pathway which leads to C5a generation and assembly of the cell lytic membrane attack complex. (MASP-1, Mannan-binding lectin (MBL) and associated protease-1, MASP-2, MBL and associated protease-1.)

COMPLEMENT ACTIVATION MECHANISMS AND PATHWAYS

The classical complement pathway is predominantly initiated by antibody-dependent mechanisms, although a number of other antibody-independent mechanisms have been described

(Tables 9.1 and 9.2). Immunoglobulins and native complement components are normally found in the serum and in the lymph, but these molecules do not interact with each other until the antibodies interact with their corresponding antigens and undergo the necessary secondary and tertiary conformational changes (Figure 9.2). These immunoglobulin

Table 9.1 Complement pathway specific activators

Pathways		
Classical	**Alternative**	**Lectin**
Immune complexes (IgM, IgG)	"Tick-over"	Repeating simple sugars
C-reactive protein	Amplification pathway	G0 carbohydrate glycoforms
Apoptotic bodies	Endotoxin	Cytokeratin-1
β-amyloid fibrils	IgA immune complexes	
Serum amyloid P	Polysaccharides	
Mitochondrial products	C3 nephritic factor	
C4 nephritic factor		
PMX3		

Table 9.2 Complement activation pathway proteins

Component	Approximate serum concentrations (μg/mL)	Approximate molecular weight
Classical pathway		
C1q	70	410,000
C1r	34	170,000
C1s	31	85,000
C4	600	206,000
C2	25	117,000
Alternative pathway		
Factor D	1	24,000
C3	1300	195,000
Factor B	200	95,000
Lectin pathway		
MBL	150 (very wide range)	600,000
MASP-1	6.0	83,000
MASP-2	0.5	76,000
MASP-3	–	95,000
Membrane attack complex (MAC)		
C5	80	180,000
C6	60	128,000
C7	55	120,000
C8	65	150,000
C9	60	79,000

conformational changes are required and the basis for specific activation of the very powerful classical complement pathway. While antibodies are central to this activation, not all immunoglobulin activate complement equally. The general order of complement-activating activity is IgM > IgG3 > IgG1 > IgG2 >> IgG4. IgA can activate the alternative pathway, and IgE generally has no complement fixing activity except under unusual inflammatory situations. For immunoglobulins to promote complement fixation, IgM and IgG are required to bind to antigen, and this binding induces conformational changes in the antibody that facilitate binding of the first complement component, C1.

Upon binding to multimeric antigen, IgM undergoes conformational changes described as "stapling down," which is essential for the binding of complement recognition components (Figure 9.2).

While a single IgM molecule can bind C1, a single native IgG molecule cannot bind C1 and activate the complement pathway. However, if IgG antibodies form aggregates as a consequence of antigen binding, their Fab arms move about the hinge region in order to bind to antigenic determinants and therein expose the C_H2 region on their Fc, which will result in C1 binding (fixation) and activation. This hinge region exposure in part explains differences in the ability of IgG subclasses to activate complement. A longer hinge region allows movement of the Fab arms farther away from the Fc so as to more fully expose the C_H2 region. Thus, IgG3, upon binding antigen, is by far the most efficient subclass of IgG in activating complement, followed by IgG1 and weakly by IgG2.

The first component of the complement pathway that interacts with bound antibody is C1. C1 is a large, multimeric, protein complex composed of C1q, C1r, and C1s subunits, that each has distinct roles in the activation cascade. Under normal physiological conditions, the subcomponents of

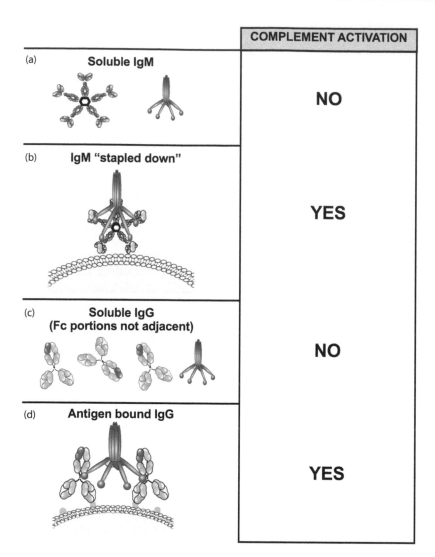

Figure 9.2 **C1q binds to the Fc portions of IgM and IgG only when bound antibodies are bound to antigen.** For the C1 complex (consisting of C1q, C1r², and C1s²) to bind to antibody, the antibodies must be bound to antigen. This requirement prevents fluid-phase activation of the classical pathway and serves as a mechanism to control complement activation. Once antigen binding IgM staples down, this conformation change exposes C1q binding domains, leading to C1 activation and initiation of complement activation. Similarly, for C1 to bind to IgG, at least two or more Fc portions of the antibody must be exposed by binding to antigen for C1 to bind and activate. IgG molecules in fluid phase will not activate C1 because each IgG molecule has only one Fc region.

C1 (C1q, C1r$_2$, and C1s$_2$) associate, which prevents spontaneous C1 activation. C1q contains several distinct portions: a collagen-like stem region that branches into a six-branched umbrella shape. Within the umbrella portion of the stem, an association with the two C1r and two C1s pro-enzymes occurs. Each of the six collagen-like branches of C1q terminates in a single globular head region. It is these globular head regions that have the potential to associate with the exposed Fc regions of the antibodies present on immune complexes (Figure 9.2). After the C1q globular head regions interact with the exposed C$_H$2 of adjacently deposited IgG3 or IgG1 antibodies, C1q undergoes significant conformational changes that result in self-activation of the two C1r pro-enzymes by one another to form two activated C1r enzymes within the macromolecular C1 complex. Each of the activated $C1r_2$ enzymes has a protease activity that cleaves a peptide bond within the two adjacent C1s molecules, which in turn become activated enzymes. Activated $C1s_2$ enzymes (within the C1 macromolecular complex) are then able to cleave and activate the next component in the series, C4.

As native C4 molecules come into contact with the C1-immune complex, they bind and are cleaved by activated C1s into a small fragment, which remains soluble (C4a), and a larger fragment, C4b. As a helpful rule, fragments released into the fluid phase are often designated by the letter **a,** while those fragments that remain bound to membranes are designated by the letter **b.** However, the nomenclature of C2 fragments is reversed, i.e., the bound fragment is designated as C2a, and the soluble fragment as C2b. Each activated C1 is able to cleave and convert many C4 molecules to C4a and C4b. The second fragment derived from C4, C4b, has a very short-lived and highly reactive binding site, an acylating group. This active binding site allows C4b to bind covalently to the nearest hydroxy or amino group, which is usually located on the antigenic surface. Antibody-coated viral envelopes or antibody-coated bacterial membranes serve as excellent sites for C4b deposition. Any activated C4b molecules that do not reach the nearby antigenic surface within a few nanoseconds (unable to bind covalently to the antigen) will lose their short-lived active binding site and undergo conformational changes that facilitate binding to a serum factor termed *C4-binding protein.* Binding of C4b to C4 binding protein causes rapid loss of C4b function and is a very important control mechanism to protect the host's tissues from "bystander attack" by the C4b molecules being formed in areas of infection.

The activated C1s within the bound C1 macromolecular complex are also responsible for the activation of C2, the next complement component to be activated in the classical pathway. In the presence of magnesium ions (Mg^{2+}), C2 interacts with antigen-bound C4b and is, in turn, split by C1s into two fragments, termed *C2b* and *C2a*. C2b fragments are released into the fluid phase, and C2a binds to C4b. Thus, appropriate concentrations of Ca^{2+} ions are needed for optimal C1q-$C1r_2$-$C1s_2$ interactions, and Mg^{2+} ions are required for C4b-C2a formation. In the absence of Ca^{2+} and/or Mg^{2+} (due to the addition of metal chelators such as EDTA), the classical activation pathway is interrupted. An excessive level of Ca^{2+} can also disrupt the association of C1q-$C1r_2$-$C1s_2$.

The major consequence of this sequential activation is the assembly of the multiprotein complex, C4b2a, which serves as a classical pathway C3 convertase activating enzyme (Figure 9.3). Once active, C4b2a complexes are deposited on the antigenic membrane surface surrounding each of the immune complexes. Each bound C4b2a complex is capable of rapidly activating many C3 molecules into C3a and C3b, until the C4b2a complex is disrupted or the enzymatic activity of C2a decays. The newly formed C3b must bind to an amino group or hydroxyl group on the antigen (via its very short-lived active binding site) to remain active. If this fails to happen, the fluid-phase C3b associates with Factor H in the serum and is quickly digested by a serum protease, Factor I. Some of the C3b molecules generated by the classical pathway C3 convertase complex (C4b2a) bind to the convertase and form C4b2a3b complex. Binding of C3b to form this complex renders it capable of binding to C5, switching it from a C3 convertase to a C5 convertase complex. The C2a within the C4b2a3b complex then has the potential to cleave C5 into C5b and C5a.

Thus, given these details, a general rule of the complement system is that as each additional component is added to the complex, the growing complexes acquire the information needed for binding and activating the next component in the series. The activities expressed at each stage of the sequence are regulated by several mechanisms, including the spontaneous decay of C2a activity with time, the short-lived active binding sites on activated complement fragments, the effects of membrane-bound complement inhibitors, and the effects of the normally occurring serum complement inhibitors/regulators (which are discussed in detail later in this chapter).

ALTERNATIVE COMPLEMENT PATHWAY

The alternative pathway does not require specific activation. Instead, in a process termed *tick-over*," C3 undergoes conformational changes and spontaneous activation resulting in deposition of C3b to microbial surfaces without the need for antibody assistance. The C3 protein contains a reactive thioester bond that is buried deep in a large domain

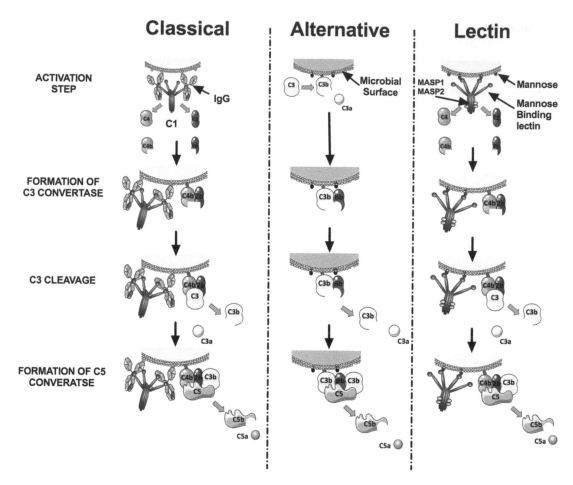

Figure 9.3 Early steps of the complement activation pathway. The classical pathway is initiated by the binding of C1 to IgM or IgG (as shown) antigen-bound antibody complexes. The alternative pathway is activated by C3b binding to activating surfaces, such as microbial polysaccharides. The lectin pathway is activated by plasma lectins binding to microbes. Activation of each pathway results in C3b deposition and the formation of a membrane-bound C3 convertase complex, which in turns cleaves C3 and leads to the formation of the C5 convertase. The late steps of the activation of the complement system are the same irrespective of the activating pathway and are outlined in Figure 9.4. (MASP-1, MBL and associated protease-1, MASP-2, MBL and associated protease-1.)

known as the thioester domain. When C3 is cleaved, the C3b protein undergoes a distinct conformational change resulting in the exposure of the primarily hidden reactive thioester bond. Under normal physiological conditions, C3b fragments are formed slowly during normal plasma C3 "tickover." Once formed, C3b may become covalently attached to the surface of cells, or microbes, via the thioester bond reacting to amino or hydroxyl groups of surface proteins or polysaccharides to form amide or ester bonds (Figure 9.3). Some of the most significant activators of the alternative pathway are the bacterial membrane lipopolysaccharides characteristic of Gram-negative bacteria and the peptidoglycans and teichoic acids from the cell walls of certain Gram-positive bacteria. These substances fix to their surfaces a group of several plasma glycoproteins, including C3b, which constitute the initial portion of the alternative pathway sequence. The generation of a "protected" (i.e., nondegraded and stable) bound form of C3b must first occur in order for the alternative complement pathway/amplification loop to be initiated. By definition, if the surface is an activator of the alternative pathway, then C3b upon binding to the substance will not be rapidly inactivated by natural inhibitory systems and will survive on the activating surface long enough to recruit the next component of the alternative pathway.

When C3b undergoes its conformational change, it exposes a binding site for a plasma protein called Factor B. Bound Factor B is then in turn cleaved by a plasma serine protease called Factor D, releasing Ba and generating Bb that remains attached to the C3b, forming a C3bBb complex, which is also known as the alternative pathway C3 convertase (Figure 9.3). Not unlike the classical C3 convertase (C4b2b), the alternative pathway C3 convertase (C3bBb) functions to promote more C3b deposition on the activating surface, thus setting up an amplification loop. Even when C3b is generated by classical or lectin pathway, Factor B can associate and generate alternative pathway convertases amplifying complement activity and deposition. The amplification loop of the alternative pathway was long thought to be a relatively minor contributor to inflammation; however, recent studies have shown the alternative pathway to be a major contributor to tissue injury and disease and as such has become a focus for therapeutic modulation.

The alternative pathway begins with at least one stable C3b covalently bound to a surface and proceeds with the cleavage of many additional C3 molecules to form more bound C3b and fluid-phase C3a. The nature of the surface to which the C3b binds regulates to a great extent C3b survival time. The absence of a C3b degradation system on the surface to which C3b is bound "allows" bound C3b to remain intact and, consequently, the alternative pathway/amplification loop to be activated. If stable C3bBb is formed on the mammalian cells, it is rapidly inactivated by Factor I, acting in concert with several cofactors present, such as membrane cofactor protein (CD46) and decay accelerating factor (CD55). These cofactors are most effective in binding and regulating C3b that inadvertently binds to bystander host cells (discussed later in the chapter). A lack of regulatory proteins on the microbial surface permits C3b binding and activation of the alternative pathway. Further, another plasma glycoprotein of the alternative pathway, properdin, can bind and associate with C3bBb complex stabilizing the C3 convertase,

and forming C3bBbP. Properdin attachment to C3bBb is favored on microbial surfaces as compared to mammalian cells and is thus the only known positive regulator of complement activation. In keeping with the classical pathway, C3 convertase C3b molecules generated by the alternative pathway can bind to the C3bBb complex itself, forming the C3bBbC3b, which functions as the alternative pathway C5 convertase.

The biological significance of the alternative pathway can be understood if we consider, as an example, an infection with a hypothetical bacterium. Since all normal individuals have low levels of antibody to most bacteria, some limited classical pathway activation occurs. Theoretically, in the presence of large numbers of bacteria, the relatively low levels of specific antibody may be effectively absorbed by antigens present on the proliferating bacteria, allowing uncoated bacteria to escape destruction by the more effective classical pathway. While optimal classical pathway function is awaiting production of large amounts of specific antibody, C3b molecules (produced via normal C3 turnover) are slowly (inadvertently) deposited on the bacteria, initiating the alternative complement sequence. Most bacteria, fungi, and viruses will activate the alternative pathway, but with varying efficiencies. That is, there is a large variability in the avidity and degree of the interaction with this pathway, depending on the species and strain of microorganism. Perhaps aiding the activation of the alternative pathway are the proteolytic enzymes being produced by microorganisms, which directly activate components like C3. If a higher rate of C3 conversion to C3b and C3a occurs near the membrane of the organism, C3b molecules will more rapidly deposit on the foreign surface via their highly reactive C3b binding site, and the alternative complement pathway will be more effectively initiated. On another note, large levels of powerful broad-spectrum proteases located on bacterial surfaces could protect the bacteria from the effects of complement by simply degrading the complement components as they deposit.

In summary, the alternative pathway of complement activation is important, especially during the early phase of the infection, when the concentrations of specific antibody are very low. After the antibody response is fully developed, the classical and alternative pathways work synergistically, with the alternative pathway functioning as an amplification loop of the classical pathway.

LECTIN PATHWAY OF COMPLEMENT ACTIVATION

The lectin pathway is initiated by target recognition through the binding of circulating lectins, such as plasma mannan-binding lectin (MBL) and Ficolins 1–3. These protein components belong to the collectin family, structurally resemble C1q, and are involved with the recognition of foreign organisms such as bacteria and virus. Mannan, a constituent of the polysaccharide capsules of many pathogenic fungi and yeasts (e.g., *Cryptococcus neoformans* and *Candida albicans*), is one of several polysaccharide substances to which MBL binds via Ca^{2+}-dependent interactions, while bacterial lipoteichoic acid and peptidoglycan associate with serum Ficolins. In addition to carbohydrate motifs of microorganisms, MBL can bind to glycoproteins on the envelope of several types of viruses. The activation of the lectin pathway does not involve antigen-antibody interactions. Like the alternative complement pathway, the lectin pathway is an innate system designed to activate the complement system independently of specific antibodies, and as such requires no adaptive immune system help. Both mannan-binding lectin and ficolins are acute-phase reactants, meaning that their concentration increases during infection and inflammation. Both types of lectins stay associated with serum serine proteases, and upon binding initiation proceeds through the activations of processes mediated by MBL-associated serine proteases (MASPs) such as MASP-1, MASP-2, and MASP-3. These proteases form a tetrameric complex similar to the one formed by C1r and C1s of the classical pathway, and MASP-2 subsequently cleaves C4 and C2, and then subsequently C3 in the same manner as that of the classical pathway (Figure 9.3).

The activation of C4 and C2 generates deposition of C4b2a and subsequent C3b deposition and terminal component activation. Thus, the initiation of the lectin pathway has several features that somewhat parallel the classical complement pathway. It is important to realize that under normal conditions, the classical pathway activation by immune complexes is much more efficient and powerful than activation by the lectin pathway.

LATE STEPS OF COMPLEMENT ACTIVATION

The full effect of the activation of the later complement components is evident when the activated complement components are deposited on a cell membrane. C5 molecules can be activated by antigen-bound (membrane-associated) C4b2a3b complexes or by alternative pathway/amplification loop enzymes as described previously. Activation of C5 is mediated by C5 convertases generated by the classical, alternative, and lectin pathways and culminates in formation of a cytocidal complex. C5 convertases cleave C5 into a small fragment (C5a), which is released into the fluid phase, and a large fragment (C5b). Unlike other complement fragments previously discussed, C5b does not bind immediately to the nearest cell membrane. A complex of C5b, C6, and C7 is first formed, and then the C5b67 complex attaches to the cell membrane through hydrophobic amino acid groups of C7, which become exposed as a consequence of the binding of C7 to the C5b-C6 complex (Figure 9.4, Table 9.3). The membrane-bound C5b-6-7 complex acts as a receptor for C8 and then C9. C8, on binding to the complex, will stabilize the attachment of the complex to the foreign cell membrane through the transmembrane insertion of its α and β chains and attracts C9. The entire C5b-9 complex is known as the membrane attack complex (MAC). This designation is due to the fact that on binding to C5b-8, C9 molecules undergo polymerization, forming a transmembrane channel of 100 Å diameter, whose external wall is believed to be hydrophobic, while the interior wall is believed to be hydrophilic. This transmembrane channel will allow the free exchange of ions between the cell and the surrounding medium. Due to the rapid influx of ions into the cell and their association with cytoplasmic proteins, the osmotic pressure rapidly increases inside the cell. This results in an influx of water, swelling of the cell, and for certain cell types, rupture of the cell membrane and lysis.

Less than 20 seconds is required for lysis of 1 million sheep erythrocytes coated with excess IgG antibody when they are mixed with 1 mL of fresh undiluted human serum as a source of complement. In contrast, many Gram-positive bacteria are not susceptible to damage by the MAC, as long as their membrane is covered by an intact cell

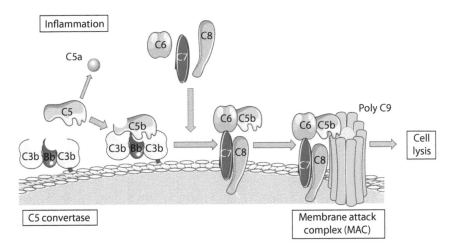

Figure 9.4 Terminal pathway of complement activation and the formation of the membrane attack complex (MAC). Membrane-associated C5 convertases generate C5b, which then becomes associated with C6. This association leads to the binding and formation of a complex that includes C5b6-7 that directly inserts into the membrane, and which is stabilized by C8 binding. Up to 15 C9 molecules can be polymerized around the complex leading to the generation of the pore-forming membrane attack complex, which can induce cell lysis. During this part of the activation pathway, the cleavage of C5 results not only in the generation of C5b, but also C5a, which is a potent inducer of inflammation.

Table 9.3 Proteins of the late steps of complement activation

Protein	Structure	Serum concentration (μg/mL)	Function
C5	190-kD dimer or 115- and 75-kD chains	80	C5b initiates assembly of the membrane attack complex (MAC) C5a stimulates inflammation (anaphylatoxin)
C6	110-kD monomer	45	Component of the MAC: binds to C5b and accepts C7
C7	100-kD monomer	90	Component of the MAC: binds to C5b,6 and inserts into lipid membranes
C8	155-kD trimer of 64-, 64-, 22-kD chains	60	Component of the MAC: binds to C5b,6,7 and initiates the binding and polymerization of C9
C9	79-kD monomer	60	Component of the MAC: binds to C5b,6,7,8 and polymerizes to form membrane pores

wall. For these organisms, complement-mediated, enhanced phagocytosis is of prime importance.

COMPLEMENT RECEPTORS

Activation of the complement system by whichever pathway leads to the generation of proteolytic cleavage fragments that have distinct biological functions. In a way, each step of the complement activation pathway is designed to elicit the help and support of other immune mediators to deal with the infectious agent. While the complement system is thought to be a key effector system of innate immunity, the generation of many of the complement fragments enables it to bridge, prime, and activate mechanisms of the adaptive immune response (Table 9.4). The cleavage fragments interact with high-affinity complement receptors

Table 9.4 Complement receptors

Receptors	Structure	Ligands	Distribution	Major activities
Complement receptor 1 (CR1, CD35)	190–250 kD; Multiple CCPRs	C3b > C4b > iC3b	Mononuclear phagocytes, neutrophils, B and T cells, erythrocytes, eosinophils, FDCs	Immune complex transport (E); phagocytosis (PMN, Mac); immune adherence (E); cofactor and decay-acceleration; secondary Epstein–Barr virus receptor
Complement receptor 2 (CR2, CD21)	145 kD Multiple CCPRs	C3d, C3dg > iC3b	B lymphocytes, FDCs, nasopharyngeal epithelium	B-cell coactivator, primary Epstein–Barr virus receptor, CD23 receptor
Complement receptor 3 (CD11b, CD18)	Integrin, with 165 kD α chain and 95 kD β2 chain	iC3b, ICAM-1; also binds microbes	Mononuclear phagocytes, neutrophils, NK cells	Leukocyte adherence, phagocytosis of iC3b-bound particles
Complement receptor 4 (CD11c, CD18)	Integrin, with 150 kD α chain and 95 kD β2 chain	iC3b	Mononuclear phagocytes, neutrophils, NK cells	Leukocyte adherence
C5a receptor (CD88)	50 kD	C5a	Mononuclear phagocytes, neutrophils, B and T cells, erythrocytes, eosinophils, FDCs	Cell activation, immune polarization, chemotaxis
C5L2	50 kD	C5a	Mononuclear phagocytes, neutrophils, B and T cells, eosinophils, DCs, SMC, EC	Modulates C5a functions which include cytokine production, vasodilation, smooth muscle cell constriction
C3a receptor	75 kD	C3a	Mononuclear phagocytes, neutrophils, B and T cells, eosinophils, DCs, SMC, EC	Modulates C3a functions, which include cytokine production, vasodilation, smooth muscle cell constriction

Abbreviations: CCPRs, complement control protein repeats; CRIg, complement receptor of the immunoglobulin superfamily; DCs, dendritic cells; E, erythrocyte; ECs, endothelial cells; FDCs, follicular dendritic cells; ICAM, intercellular adhesion molecule; Mac, macrophage; PMN, polymorphonuclear; SMC, smooth muscle cells.

present on the surface of innate and adaptive immune cells and are further present on parenchymal cells to promote processes such as vascular permeability and vasoconstriction. There are five distinct receptors that have been described to interact with different fragments of C3. Complement receptor type 1 (CR1, CD35) is a widely distributed molecule found on erythrocytes, neutrophils, mononuclear phagocytes, B cells, and some T cells. CR1 binds to both C4b and C3b ligands, which are the initial degradation products of C4 and C3 that are covalently bound to the membrane surface. Engagement of CR1 leads to a variety of functional outcomes dependent largely on the cell type on which it is expressed. For example, CR1 present on erythrocytes is important for processing immune complexes, whereas expression on neutrophils and macrophages acts to promote phagocytosis. On B lymphocytes, CR1 serves as a processing molecule to convert C3b to iC3b, and as a competitive receptor to complement receptor 2 (CR2) to downregulate responses to C3b-coated antigen.

Degradation of C3b by factor I and cofactors, such as CR1, results in the formation of two fragments, iC3b and C3dg. C3dg can be further degraded into C3d via nonspecific proteases, and all of these fragments are ligands for CR2. CR2 has primary binding specificity for a molecular site on the α-chain of C3 that is exposed during proteolytic cleavage of C3 to iC3b, C3dg, and C3d. B lymphocytes have both CR2 and CR1 molecules on their surface. Follicular dendritic cells (important in antigen presentation) have CR2, CR3, and CR1 on their surface. Antibody production is greatly enhanced by complement-coated antigens, which stimulate B cells via their CR2 and CR1. In animal models, when C3d was chemically linked to an antigen, and added to specific B cells *in vivo*, a thousand-fold enhancement of antibody production occurred. CR2 not only stimulates the B cells directly but also associates with CD19, another B-cell membrane protein that is known to greatly stimulate antibody production. Interestingly, CR2 is also the primary receptor for the immunoregulatory molecule CD23, an interaction that promotes the production of IgE, as well as the receptors for Epstein–Barr virus, involved in the induction of B-cell malignancies.

CR3 and CR4 are cell surface glycoprotein receptors that via Ca^{2+}-dependent interactions bind to site(s) exposed predominantly on the C3-degradation product iC3b. CR3 and CR4 are expressed on tissue macrophages, mononuclear phagocytes, polymorphonuclear cells (PMNs), and follicular dendritic cells. The final receptor for C3 is the complement receptor of the immunoglobulin superfamily (CRIg), which is expressed on liver Kupffer cells and plays a key role in the removal of opsonized infectious organisms, complement-coated particles, and large complexes in the circulation.

The small complement fragments, C5a and C3a, are released into the fluid phase and recognized by neutrophils, promoting the migration of these phagocytes in the direction from which these small fragments originated. The term for this chemical attraction is *chemotaxis*, and its main biological function is to attract phagocytes into a tissue where complement-activating reactions are taking place. Once the PMNs reach the area, by moving toward the highest concentration of freshly generated chemoattractants, the PMNs bind to the C4b and C3b coated antigenic substances via their CR1 receptors (and to iC3b via their CR3 receptors) and proceed to phagocytize the foreign material.

Besides their role as chemokines, C5a and C3a activate the phagocytic cells that carry C5a and C3a receptors. In the case of neutrophils, such activation leads to the expression of cell adhesion molecules and facilitates extravascular migration. In the case of circulating basophils and of mast cells associated with the epithelial and mucosal tissues, C5a and C3a stimulate the release of biologically active mediators such as heparin and vasoactive amines (e.g., histamine). Histamine, when released into the tissues, results in increased capillary permeability and smooth muscle contraction. Fluid is released into the tissue, causing edema and swelling. The end result is very similar to the classical anaphylactic reaction that takes place when IgE antibodies bound to the membranes of mast cells and basophils react with the corresponding antigens. For this reason, C3a and C5a are known as anaphylatoxins.

In addition to priming innate immune responses, C3a and C5a receptors have been shown to be present on endothelial cells, parenchymal cells, and immune T and B cells. Interaction of C3a and C5a on endothelial cells can promote cytokine and chemokine release and induce endothelial call activation that facilitate immune cell adhesion and migration and also cause increased vascular permeability. The expression of C3a and C5a receptors on immune lymphocytes is somewhat controversial, in part due to differences seen between rodents and humans. However, available data suggest that C3a and C5a play important roles in tuning T-cell effector and regulatory functions and promoting T-cell homeostasis.

REGULATION OF COMPLEMENT ACTIVATION

Given its potential to cause significant self-injury and inflammation, the complement system is tightly regulated so that it prevents damage to self-tissues (Table 9.5). Regulation is achieved at each stage of the sequence by several mechanisms:

1. Spontaneous decay, e.g., decreasing C2a activity with time
2. Short-lived active binding sites on activated complement fragments, e.g., hydrolysis of the C3 thioester bond
3. Effects of specific membrane-bound and plasma complement inhibitors

The effects of specific membrane-bound and plasma complement inhibitors are achieved by inhibiting protease activity, competitive inhibitors/disassociation factors, cofactor proteases, and subtraction of specific proteases. Figure 9.5 illustrates the points at which complement activation by host membrane and serum inhibitors act upon the complement system to exert control. Given the scope of these inhibitory mechanisms, it is clear to see that the complement system lives in a balance between activation and inhibition, and that loss of that balance can have broad-reaching implications in health and disease, discussed later in the chapter.

Regulatory mechanisms of the early stages

Soon after antigen and antibody react, high levels of C4b and especially C3b accumulate on the antigenic surface, at such high levels that they begin to deposit onto the specific antigenic determinants recognized by the antibody molecules. C4b and especially C3b molecules also bind to the Fab region (CH1) of the bound antibodies. Both

of these phenomena interfere with the ability of antibodies to remain associated with specific epitopes in the antigen. This partial dissolution of the immune complex results in the loosening of the C1 macromolecule from the immune complex, as the antibody molecule recovers its native configuration and the sites on the CH2 region (that interact with C1q) become less accessible. As C1 begins to separate from the immune complex, the $C1q$-$C1r_2$-$C1s_2$ macromolecular complex tends to return to its loosely associated form. At that point, the activated $C1r_2$ and $C1s_2$ enzymes are extremely susceptible to irreversible inhibition by C1 inhibitor (C1 INH), a normal serum glycoprotein. C1 INH forms covalent C1-INH-C1r and C1-INH-C1s complexes, most of which are separated from the bound C1q unless the initial attachment of C1 to the immune complexes was weak, in which case C1-INH removes the entire $C1q$-$C1r_2$-$C1s_2$ macromolecular complex. Activated C1, once having performed its function while bound to the immune complex, is now irreversibly inhibited from unnecessarily consuming more native C4 and C2. Importantly, a rate-limiting factor in classical complement pathway activation under normal physiological conditions is not the level of any early complement component, but rather the controlling function of C1-INH.

Inhibition of C3 and C5 convertases

Inhibition of the assembly of C3 and C5 convertases is achieved by the binding of regulatory proteins to C4b and C3b deposited on host membrane surfaces. This inhibition is mediated by several membrane or membrane-associated proteins, including type 1 complement receptor (CR1), decay accelerating factor (DAF, or CD55), membrane cofactor protein (MCP, or CD46), and a plasma protein called factor H.

CR1 is a receptor glycoprotein, which in binding to activated C3b, blocks C3b function in the complement sequence by causing C3b to be rapidly cleaved to inactivated C3b (iC3b), by a serum enzyme known as Factor I. Obviously, once the phagocyte is actively engulfing the complement-coated particle, there is no reason to continue consuming additional complement or risk inadvertently damaging the phagocyte by depositing C3b and/or MAC complexes on its surface. Therefore, cell surface CR1 molecules after binding

Table 9.5 Complement regulatory proteins

Soluble regulatory proteins	Concentrations/ distribution	Approximate molecular weight (kD)	Major functions
Positive regulation			
Properdin	Plasma protein; 25 µg/mL	220	Stabilizes alternative pathway C3/C5 convertases
Negative regulation			
C1-INH	Plasma protein; 200 µg/mL	105	Inhibits C1r/C1s, MAPSs
C4-bp	Plasma protein; 250 µg/mL	550	Inhibition of classical pathway C4b2a C3 convertase by decay acceleration and cofactor activity for C4c cleavage by Factor I
Factor H	Plasma protein; 500 µg/mL	150	Decay-acceleration; inhibition of alternate pathway C3 convertase by decay-acceleration and cofactor activity for C3b cleavage by Factor I
Factor I	Plasma protein; 34 µg/mL	90	Cleavage of C3b/C4b
Anaphylatoxin inactivator-carboxypeptidase	Plasma protein; 35 µg/mL	280	Generates C3a/C5a desArg
S protein (vitronectin)	Plasma protein; 500 µg/mL	80	Blocks MAC formation
SP-40,40 (clusterin)	Plasma protein; 60 µg/mL	80	Blocks MAC formation
Membrane regulatory proteins			
Decay-accelerating factor (CD55)	Blood cells, endothelial cells, epithelial cells	70	Inhibition by decay acceleration of the classical and alternative pathway C3 convertases
Membrane cofactor protein (MCP, also known as CD46)	Leukocytes, epithelial cells, endothelial cells	45–70	Inhibition by cofactor activity for classical and alternative pathway proteins C4b and C3b, respectively
CD59	Blood cells, endothelial cells, epithelial cells	20	Blocks C8-C9 and C9

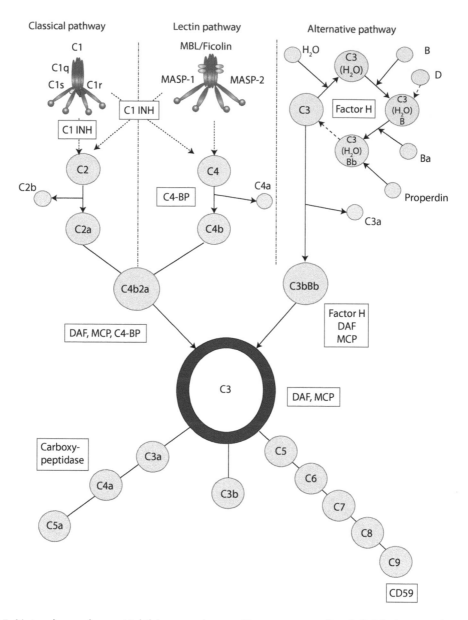

Figure 9.5 Natural complement inhibitory pathways. The presence of both fluid-phase and membrane-associated complement inhibitory proteins aim to prevent host cell bystander damage. (C1-INH, C1 inhibitor; C4-BP; C4b-binding protein; DAF, decay accelerating factor [also known as CD55]; MCP, membrane cofactor protein [also known as CD46]; MASP-1, MBL and associated protease-1, MASP-2, MBL and associated protease-1.)

to C3b have two independent functions: (1) to enhance phagocytosis of C4b/C3b coated particles by phagocytes and (2) to inactivate C4b/C3b, including those complexes that may become inadvertently deposited on host cells.

Decay-accelerating factor (DAF, CD55) is a complement-inhibitory protein widely expressed on host cell membranes. The name of this factor derives from the fact that it can accelerate the dissociation of active C4b2a complexes, turning off their ability to continue activating C3. In addition, DAF attaches to membrane-bound C4b and C3b and prevents the subsequent interaction of C4b with C2 and of C3b with factor B, respectively. As a consequence, the two types of C3 convertases, C4b2a and C3bBb, will not be formed or will become dissociated, and the rate of additional C3 activation is significantly limited. Thus, the host cell will be spared from complement-mediated membrane damage.

Membrane cofactor protein (MCP, CD46) is also widely distributed on host cells and acts a cofactor on the membrane for C3 or C4 cleaving them into their inactive forms, iC3b and iC4b, respectively. Thus, by binding C4b and C3b, these membrane proteins inhibit the binding of other components to these C3 convertases, such as C2a and Bb of the classical and alternative pathways, respectively, thus inhibiting further progression of the complement pathway. In addition to these membrane-bound inhibitors, plasma protein inhibitors of the complement system similarly inhibit C3 and C4 activity. C4-binding protein (C4BP) inactivates C4b by serving as a cofactor for factor I mediated cleavage, and serves to accelerate the spontaneous decay of C2a from C4b. Factor H serves the binding of Bb to C3b, by membrane association, and thus is a specific regulator of the alternative pathway.

Inhibition of anaphylatoxins

Once the complement cascade is activated, the complement components are under very tight regulation and control. An important aspect of this regulation is the constant presence of plasma inhibitors for the activated complement components. For each type of activated fragment, there is at least one inhibitor or inhibitory mechanism. The tight regulation and rapid neutralization of the active fragments limit their range of action.

In the case of C3a and C5a, there are several serum inhibitors, one of which is believed to be a serum protease that removes the carboxy-terminal arginine residue of the peptides and limits their ability to stimulate PMNs, leukocytes, basophils, and mast cells.

Inhibition of the membrane attack complex

CD59 is another membrane-bound complement inhibitor that is widely expressed on mammalian cells. It binds to C8 in the C5b-8 complex and blocks the binding and incorporation of C9 into the complex. Further, CD59 also binds directly to C9 stopping the addition of additional C9 to the complex, inhibiting its polymerization, and therefore stops the complex from forming a transmembrane pore. In addition to this membrane regulator of membrane attack complex formation, additional soluble proteins can inhibit assembly or membrane insertion. Clusterin and vitronectin are widely distributed intracellular matrix proteins that can incorporate into the C5b-7 complex rendering them nonmembrane-binding inactivated complexes. Finally, normal human cells have the ability to eliminate the membrane attack complex from their surface either by endocytosis or by direct emission/release of membrane vesicles (ectocytosis).

FUNCTIONS OF THE COMPLEMENT SYSTEM

Under normal physiological conditions, the complement system has three primary functions: (1) opsonization and phagocytosis, (2) stimulation of inflammatory responses, and (3) complement-mediated cytolysis. Additionally, recent studies have shown that the complement system bridges innate and adaptive immunity by facilitating B-cell antibody production, skewing T-cell effector responses, and augmenting antigen presentation.

Opsonization and phagocytosis

Prior to its decay or its inactivation, each one of the activated membrane-bound C4b2a enzyme complexes activates C3 molecules, until one or two of the C3b molecules associate with the C4b2a complex. The normal concentration of serum C3 is about 130 mg/dL, which is relatively high and indicates the importance of C3 in the complement activation pathways. C3 is converted through a process that involves its proteolytic cleavage and release of a small biologically active peptide, termed C3a. The larger C3b fragment upon activation behaves very much like the C4b fragment, in that it also has a short-lived, highly reactive binding site, which binds irreversibly to the nearest membrane surface, which is usually the complement activating antigen.

C3b associates with the bound C4b2a complexes. However, other C3b molecules bind independently to the antigenic membrane. The independently deposited C3b molecules also participate in a tremendous amplification of additional C3b deposition via the alternative pathway amplification loop. It is important to understand that the irreversible (covalent) binding of C4b and of C3b molecules to the antigen actually *changes the nature of the antigen*. In the case of endotoxin, C4b and C3b deposition abrogates the toxicity of the molecule. Similarly, C4b and C3b contribute to antibody-mediated neutralization of viruses, rendered incapable of properly binding and infecting host cells.

Of great biological significance is the fact that after C4b and C3b successfully bind to the antigenic surface, they undergo conformational changes that result in the exposure of regions of these two molecules that extend away from the antigenic membrane. These exposed parts of C4b and C3b are biologically important because they contain molecular segments that are able to bind to C3b/C4b receptors (currently designated as CR1, complement receptor 1) located on host phagocytic cells. Additional types of receptors for other regions on bound C3b play a significant role in enhancing phagocytosis. Some of those receptors recognize interior (cryptic) regions of C3b exposed as this component is further catabolized (with time) to form inactivated C3b (iC3b), then C3dg and finally C3d.

Polymorphonuclear leukocytes, like other phagocytic host cells, have thousands of complement receptors on their membranes allowing them to bind, with high avidity, to particles coated with C3b and C4b and/or with breakdown products of bound C3b (i.e., iC3b and C3d). This increased avidity of phagocytic cells for complement-coated particles is known as enhanced immune adherence, and its main consequence is a significant potentiation of the phagocytosis process. In this process, the phagocyte is stimulated to engulf the complement-coated particle because of the interactions with complement receptors on the phagocytic cell membrane. Once engulfed, antigens are digested in phagolysosomes, vesicles that result from the fusion of phagosomes, containing phagocytosed particles, and lysosomes, which contain a large variety of degradative enzymes. The phagocytic process is one of the most important fundamental defense mechanisms, because it provides a direct way for the host to eliminate foreign substances.

Stimulation of inflammatory responses

Cleavage of C4, C3, and C5 generates complement fragments, C4a, C3a, and C5a. These peptides are discussed earlier in the chapter and are important for the activation of neutrophils, mast cells, macrophages, and T cells. C3a and C5a are chemotactic peptides that can stimulate endothelial cell activation, respiratory burst, and the promotion of reactive oxygen species. The combined effects of these diverse functions are the ability to promote immune cell migration, directly and indirectly, through the promotion of endothelial adhesion, increased vascular permeability, and cytokine production, thus promoting inflammation at sites of complement activation and enhancing the ability to defend the host against invading pathogens.

Complement-mediated cytolysis

Complement-mediated lysis of microbes is mediated through the formation of MAC on the cell surface. While MAC can be deposited on many pathogenic surfaces, the evolution of pathogens with thick cell walls or capsules impedes the efficacy of MAC and resistance from lysis. MAC-mediated lysis is, however, essential for defense against *Neisseria*-mediated infections, and thus people with genetic deficiency in MAC proteins are susceptible to infections from this genus of bacteria.

COMPLEMENT AND DISEASE

The complement system is a potent tissue-destructive and immune-activating system that for obvious reasons is tightly regulated. Therefore, it stands to reason that loss of this regulation or activation that overwhelms these regulatory mechanisms is likely to lead to injury, inflammation, and disease. Rodent models and the application of complement therapeutics have yielded important insights into the role of complement in human disease. While genetic deficiency in complement is largely associated with infectious disease, there are a growing number of diseases in which excessive complement activity has been shown to play a significant role in their pathobiology. While genetic deficiencies are covered in Chapter 29, here we focus on diseases caused by mutations in complement regulatory proteins.

Hereditary angioedema

This is a rare genetic disorder due to a genetically inherited C1-INH deficiency, of which two main variants are known. In the most common, the genetic inheritance of a silent gene results in a significantly lower level of C1-INH. The second variant is characterized by normal levels of C1-INH protein, but 75% of the molecules are dysfunctional, i.e., will not inhibit activated C1r or C1s because of an aberrant amino acid substitution. While the lack of C1-INH can be easily detected by a quantitative assay, the synthesis of dysfunctional C1-INH can only be revealed by a combination of quantitative and functional tests. An acquired form of C1-INH deficiency can be detected in certain malignant diseases. Individuals with congenital C1-INH deficiency may present clinically with a disease known as hereditary angioedema, characterized by spontaneous swelling of the face, neck, genitalia, and extremities, often associated with abdominal cramps and vomiting. The disease can be life threatening if the airway is compromised by laryngeal edema, and tracheotomy is a lifesaving measure in those cases. This anaphylactoid reaction is due not to IgE-mediated reactions, but rather to spontaneous uncontrolled activation of the complement system by C1 and other systems controlled by C1-INH. The complement reaction is usually self-limiting and will cease after all C4 and C2 have been consumed. However, in vivo there is not a substantial consumption of the remaining complement sequence (C3-9) due to the action of several other regulatory mechanisms that are especially effective against the unbound (free) forms of C4b and C3b (i.e., C4b and C3b that are not bound to any antigen).

Attacks in patients with C1-INH deficiency occur after surgical trauma, particularly after dental surgery, or after severe stress. It is notable that activated Hageman factor, kallikrein, and plasmin are also controlled (in part) by binding to C1-INH. After surgical trauma, binding to each of the previous enzymes further depletes the available C1-INH in deficient patients. In the absence of sufficient C1-INH, spontaneous activation of a limited number of C1 molecules and the other substances controlled by C1-INH will gradually accentuate the depletion of C1-INH to the point that activated unbound activated C1 and other activated enzymes controlled by C1-INH are present in the circulation. These blood enzymes controlled by C1-INH become much less restricted. For example, the continued presence of activated, uninhibited fluid-phase C1s will cause spontaneous and continuous activation of the next two components in the sequence, C4 and C2, until their complete consumption.

Low C4 levels are considered diagnostic of C1-INH deficiency, and they remain low even when the patients are not experiencing an attack, probably due to a continuously exaggerated C4 catabolism by activated C1. Loss of control over unbound (fluid-phase) activated C1 results in total depletion of C4 and C2 and a further rapid depletion of any residual C1-inhibitor. At the same time, there is a reduction in control by C1-inhibitor over activated kallikrein. Plasma prekallikrein circulates complexed with high molecular weight kininogen, and uncontrolled activated kallikrein cleaves kininogen to release bradykinin. There is mounting evidence to suggest that the major angioedema-producing substance is bradykinin, although earlier reports suggest a role for a fragment of C2 (C2a) liberated by the action of C1 on C2 followed by the cleavage of C2 by unrestricted plasmin. While it is generally accepted that serum C3 levels are not significantly altered during attacks of angioedema, in vitro evidence has shown that if appropriate levels of antibody to human C1-INH are added to whole human serum, 100% C3 conversion occurs. This complete C3 conversion can only be achieved when the function of C1-INH is blocked. Thus, minor participation of low levels of C3a in angioedema cannot be ruled out when localized C1-INH levels approach zero. Recently, recombinant C1-INH has been developed and is U.S. Food and Drug Administration approved for prophylactic therapy in this at-risk population.

Paroxysmal nocturnal hemoglobinuria

Paroxysmal nocturnal hemoglobinuria (PNH) is an acquired disorder on the surface of selected hemopoietic stem cell lines and their erythrocyte progeny. The patients develop hemolytic anemia manifested by the intermittent passage of dark urine (due to hemoglobinuria), which usually is more accentuated at night. The spontaneous hemolysis is due to an increased susceptibility of the abnormal population of erythrocytes to complement-mediated lysis. The erythrocytes are not responsible for the activation of the complement system; rather, they are lysed as innocent bystanders when complement is activated.

Detailed studies of the circulating erythrocytes in PNH patients have demonstrated the existence of three erythrocyte subpopulations with varying degrees of sensitivity to complement. The reason for the existence of these subpopulations was elucidated when the molecular basis of PNH was established. Several membrane proteins are attached to cell membranes through phosphatidylinositol "anchors." The red cell membrane contains two such proteins: the DAF, which prevents or disrupts the formation of C4b2a and C3bBb, and CD59 that prevents the proper assembly of the membrane attack complex by binding to C8 or C9 or both. These two proteins (together with CR1 and MCP) have an important protective role for "bystander" erythrocytes by controlling the rate of complement activation on the erythrocyte membrane. The deficiency of the phosphatidylinositol anchoring system is reflected by deficiencies of DAF and CD59. Type I PNH red cells have normal or slightly lowered levels of these two proteins and usually show normal resistance to complement-mediated hemolysis; type III PNH red cells lack both proteins and are very sensitive to hemolysis; type II PNH red cells lack DAF and have intermediate sensitivity to hemolysis. Although deficiency of the phosphatidylinositol leads to a loss of all phosphatidylinositol-linked proteins from the membranes, PNH is a complement-mediated disorder as inhibition of complement ameliorates disease. Treatment of PNH with eculizumab, an anti-C5 monoclonal antibody, significantly inhibits hemolysis and its associated disease pathology (Figure 9.6). The successful clinical application of eculizumab in PNH has led to an increased confidence in the application of complement inhibitors, and many new complement therapeutics are under development.

Atypical hemolytic uremic syndrome

Atypical hemolytic uremic syndrome (aHUS) is a rare disease that causes blood clots that, over time, reduce significantly the blood flow in the kidneys, impairing its ability to remove waste products, which ultimately leads to kidney failure. aHUS is associated with mutations in proteins of the alternative pathway, primarily factor H, that lead to uncontrolled complement activation. Recent clinical trials have shown that eculizumab therapy improves outcomes, which has led to the approval of its use in aHUS.

Other diseases associated with the complement system

With improved access to complement therapeutics and genetic rodent models, the role of the complement system in disease is being rigorously investigated. Genome-wide association studies have shown that complement plays a role in rheumatoid arthritis, neurodegenerative diseases, sepsis, and even cancer metastasis. Further, complement plays a key role in ischemia reperfusion-induced injuries and as such is being extensively studied in myocardial infarction, stroke, and organ transplantation. Given the huge disease scope presented, it is clear that the investigation and application of complement pharmacotherapeutics will likely increase in clinical medicine in the coming years.

COMPLEMENT LEVELS IN DISEASE

Complement proteins have some of the highest turnover rates of any of the plasma components. At any one time, the level of a complement component is a direct function of its catabolic and synthetic rates. Over 90% of complement components are generated by the liver. However, there is a growing appreciation that complement produced within the local microenvironment by parenchymal and immune cells can influence complement activity. Further, while complement is thought of as an extracellular system, recent studies have shown that some cells, most notably T and B cells, and epithelial cells, cannot only produce complement but can store intracellular activated complement components within the cell cytoplasm as a means to influence local complement signaling and intracellular responses. There are many factors that cause the increased production of complement components by the liver, and from cells present at local sites of inflammation. In vitro studies have shown that the addition of cytokines, such as interleukin-1β, interferon-γ, and tumor necrosis factor (TNF), can upregulate C3 synthesis. Interleukin-1β, interleukin-6, and interferon-γ also regulate factor B synthesis. Interestingly, TNF and interferon-γ concomitantly increase DAF expression on host cells (e.g., vascular endothelial cells) in order to protect the host from bystander complement attack, especially in areas where the membrane attack complex is inadvertently being deposited (e.g., on the vascular endothelium) during localized inflammation.

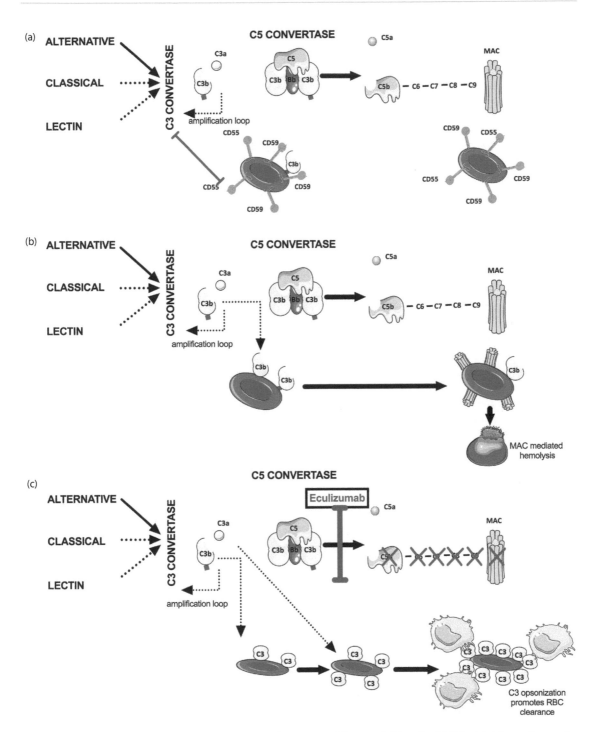

Figure 9.6 Role of complement in paroxysmal nocturnal hemoglobinuria (PNH). (a) Normal steady-state alternative pathway tick-over shows that the presence of membrane-bound phosphatidylinositol complement inhibitors, CD55 and CD59, which prevent the accumulation of C3 and formation of MAC on normal red blood cells (RBCs). (b) In patients with PNH, the lack of CD55 and CD59 on the surface of RBCs leads to exacerbated C3 tick-over, formation of the MAC, and MAC-mediated intravascular hemolysis. (c) Intravascular hemolysis is prevented by the anti-C5 monoclonal antibody, Eculizumab, through inhibition of MAC formation and promotion of C3-mediated RBC clearance by macrophages in the spleen and liver.

The catabolic rates of the serum complement system are primarily a function of the extent of complement activation by all the pathways involved. Therefore, the levels of complement proteins are influenced by the levels of complement activators (i.e., immune complexes), the class and subclass of immunoglobulin within the immune complexes, the release of direct complement-activating bacterial products, and, in certain chronic inflammatory diseases, the presence of autoantibody to complement components. The synthetic rates of complement glycoproteins vary widely in disease states and during the course of a given disease. In the end, the level of a complement component is a function of its metabolic rate (synthesis versus catabolism) and the type and course of the inflammatory reaction. Elevated levels of a given complement component in a disease state probably means that there is both a rapid synthetic and catabolic rate. Lower overall complement levels indicate that consumption is greater than synthesis at that particular time, usually in association with acute inflammation or an exacerbation of a chronic inflammatory process. Severe complement depletion, in contrast, is usually associated with impaired hepatic synthesis (e.g., as in liver failure).

Hypocomplementemia and clearance of immune complexes

The development of immune complex diseases is believed to be favored by the inability to properly eliminate immune complexes from the kidney and/or from the basement membrane of dermal tissues. This phenomenon is due to the deposition of large complement fragments such as C4b and C3b on the antigen and on the Fab region of the antibody, which interferes with the antigen-antibody binding reaction. If a deficiency in the early complement components exists, there will likely be a corresponding defect in the production and binding of C4b and C3b to the immune complex. As a result, the rate of formation of new immune complexes surpasses the inefficient rate of immune complex dissolution and/or phagocytic clearance, and the generation of pro-inflammatory complement fragments will be possible for a longer period of time. The reasons for the lower levels of early complement components (i.e., C1q, C4, and/or C2) are multiple and include not only genetic factors

but also a variety of metabolic control mechanisms as previously mentioned.

In patients with systemic lupus erythematosus (SLE), a reduction in the levels of CR1 on erythrocyte has been reported. As previously discussed, the binding of complement-coated immune complexes to erythrocytes is an important physiological mechanism of immune complex removal from the circulation. Small to medium-sized immune complexes are not taken up as efficiently by CR1 and tend to persist longer in circulation. However, when the number of CR1 receptors on erythrocyte membranes is decreased, even large-sized (complement coated) immune complexes may persist for longer periods in circulation and may have a greater opportunity to be deposited in organs and tissues, thereby causing inflammation. The depleted number CR1 per erythrocyte may be due in part to the overwhelming utilization of the erythrocyte CR1 in SLE and subsequent CR1 catabolism as the complement coated immune complexes are presented to phagocytic cells in the liver and spleen.

Complement deficiencies

Primary complement deficiencies, discussed in detail in Chapter 29, are associated with two types of clinical situations: chronic bacterial infections, caused by capsulated organisms such as *Neisseria* species, and autoimmune disease, mimicking SLE.

MICROBIAL ANTICOMPLEMENTARY MECHANISMS

In general, complement-mediated phagocytosis is the most effective mechanism for elimination of infectious microorganisms. However, pathogenic organisms have evolved several mechanisms to circumvent either effective complement activation or effective complement deposition on their outer surface. These evasion strategies are most efficient during the early stages of an infection, when the levels of specific antibody are low. In some cases, the microorganisms (e.g., *Candida* spp.) have on their surface a structural protein that mimics the protective effect of DAF or other complement regulators.

Streptococcus pyogenes, *Neisseria gonorrhoeae*, and *Candida albicans* have surface structures that attract host serum Factor H and promote host serum Factor I-mediated cleavage of any deposited

C3b to form iC3b. Inactivated C3b (iC3b) does not participate in the amplification loop. As a result, less C3b is deposited on these organisms. Interestingly, HIV acquires membrane DAF (CD55) upon leaving the infected host cell, and during the infectious process appears to adsorb Factor H from serum. In these situations, if insufficient levels of high-affinity antibody fail to deposit on the pathogen, a reduced deposition of complement components leads to a less effective neutralization/elimination.

Other less-sophisticated complement-restrictive mechanisms that different microorganisms have acquired include the shedding of MAC-coated pili, destruction of C3b by proteases on the bacterial surface, and protection of the cytoplasmic membrane from the dissolving effect of the MAC by slime layers, peptidoglycan layers, and polysaccharide capsules. With the deposition of sufficient levels of high-affinity antibodies, these protective mechanisms are usually overridden, and the microorganisms are properly phagocytosed, although some bacteria have acquired antiphagocytic capsules that further complicate the job of the immune system, as discussed in Chapter 14.

BIBLIOGRAPHY

Alawieh A, Langley EF, Tomlinson S. Targeted complement inhibition salvages stressed neurons and inhibits neuroinflammation after stroke in mice. *Sci Transl Med*. 2018; 10(441):eaao6459.

Bayly-Jones C, Bubeck D, Dunstone MA. The mystery behind membrane insertion: A review of the complement membrane attack complex. *Philos Trans R Soc Lond B Biol Sci*. 2017;372(1726). doi: 10.1098/rstb.2016.0221

Cao M, Leite BN, Ferreiro T et al. Eculizumab modifies outcomes in adults with atypical hemolytic uremic syndrome with acute kidney injury. *Am J Nephrol*. 2018;48:225–233.

Chen JY, Cortes C, Ferreira VP. Properdin: A multifaceted molecule involved in inflammation and diseases. *Mol Immunol*. 2018;102:58–72.

Clarke EV, Tenner AJ. Complement modulation of T cell immune responses during homeostasis and disease. *J Leukoc Biol*. 2014;96:745–756.

DiScipio RG, Schraufstatter IU. The role of the complement anaphylatoxins in the recruitment of eosinophils. *Int Immunopharmacol*. 2007;7:1909–1923.

Dobo J, Kocsis A, Gal P. Be on target: Strategies of targeting alternative and lectin pathway components in complement-mediated diseases. *Front Immunol*. 2018;9:1851.

Ehlers MR. CR3: A general purpose adhesion-recognition receptor essential for innate immunity. *Microbes Infect*. 2000;2:289–294.

Erdei A, Sandor N, Macsik-Valent B et al. The versatile functions of complement C3-derived ligands. *Immunol Rev*. 2016;274:127–140.

Freeley S, Kemper C, Le Friec G. The "ins and outs" of complement-driven immune responses. *Immunol Rev*. 2016;274:16–32.

He S, Atkinson C, Qiao F et al. A complement-dependent balance between hepatic ischemia/reperfusion injury and liver regeneration in mice. *J Clin Invest*. 2009;119:2304–2316.

He S, Atkinson C, Evans Z et al. A role for complement in the enhanced susceptibility of steatotic livers to ischemia and reperfusion injury. *J Immunol*. 2009;183:4764–4772.

Heesterbeek DAC, Angelier ML, Harrison RA, Rooijakkers SHM. Complement and bacterial infections: From molecular mechanisms to therapeutic applications. *J Innate Immun*. 2018;10:455–464.

Hill A, Hillmen P, Richards SJ et al. Sustained response and long-term safety of eculizumab in paroxysmal nocturnal hemoglobinuria. *Blood*. 2005;106:2559–2565.

Hovingh ES, van den Broek B, Jongerius I. Hijacking complement regulatory proteins for bacterial immune evasion. *Front Microbiol*. 2016;7:2004.

Jager NM, Poppelaars F, Daha MR, Seelen MA. Complement in renal transplantation: The road to translation. *Mol Immunol*. 2017;89:22–35.

Kemp JG, Craig TJ. Variability of prodromal signs and symptoms associated with hereditary angioedema attacks: A literature review. *Allergy Asthma Proc*. 2009;30:493–499.

Kim DD, Song WC. Membrane complement regulatory proteins. *Clin Immunol*. 2006;118:127–136.

Kolev M, Le Friec G, Kemper C. The role of complement in CD4(+) T cell homeostasis and effector functions. *Semin Immunol*. 2013;25:12–19.

Kraiczy P, Wurzner R. Complement escape of human pathogenic bacteria by acquisition of complement regulators. *Mol Immunol*. 2006;43:31–44.

Macor P, Capolla S, Tedesco F. Complement as a biological tool to control tumor growth. *Front Immunol*. 2018;9:2203.

Manthey HD, Woodruff TM, Taylor SM, Monk PN. Complement component 5a (C5a). *Int J Biochem Cell Biol*. 2009;41:2114–2117.

Panagiotou A, Trendelenburg M, Osthoff M. The lectin pathway of complement in myocardial ischemia/reperfusion injury-review of its significance and the potential impact of therapeutic interference by C1 esterase inhibitor. *Front Immunol*. 2018;9:1151.

Reddy YN, Siedlecki AM, Francis JM. Breaking down the complement system: A review and update on novel therapies. *Curr Opin Nephrol Hypertens*. 2017;26:123–128.

Thurman JM, Holers VM. The central role of the alternative complement pathway in human disease. *J Immunol*. 2006;176:1305–1310.

Tomlinson S. Complement defense mechanisms. *Curr Opin Immunol*. 1993;5:83–89.

10

Monocyte and lymphocyte membrane markers: Ontogeny and clinical significance

SCOTT SUGDEN, DAMIEN MONTAMAT-SICOTTE, KAREN K. YAM, JOSEPH MURPHY, BADER YASSINE DIAB, AND VIRGINIA LITWIN

INTRODUCTION

This chapter describes the differentiation process of human monocytes and lymphocytes as well as the membrane markers expressed on the mature cells. Membrane markers include a wide variety of functional proteins, including antigen-specific receptors, co-stimulatory molecules, adhesion molecules, inhibitory receptors, growth factor receptors, cytokine receptors, chemokine receptors, and receptors that mediate cell death. Membrane markers can be shared by various cell types and can be pan lineage specific or lineage subset specific.

HEMATOPOIETIC STEM CELLS

In humans, hematopoietic activity begins when the fetal liver receives stem cells from the yolk sac at the sixth week of gestation. In the 12th week, a minor contribution is made to the production of blood cells by the spleen. At 20 weeks of gestation, thymus, lymph node, and bone marrow begin hematopoietic activity. The bone marrow becomes the sole hematopoietic center after 38 weeks.

All blood cell types are derived from pluripotent precursors known as hematopoietic stem cells (HSCs). HSCs are found primarily in the fetal liver and bone marrow but persist throughout adult life. By definition, a stem cell must be capable of both self-renewal and differentiation. Self-renewal is the ability to give rise to at least two daughter cells at the same stage of development as the parent and is dependent on growth factors such as GM-CSF, G-CSF, IL-3, and IL-5. Differentiation of HSC along the various hematopoietic lineages is progressive in that cells develop first into multipotent progenitors and then into precursors with decreasing pluripotency and increasing commitment to a single differentiation pathway. This progression was once thought to be an orderly sequence of events; however, this view may be oversimplified. As research in this field continues, new questions emerge. For example, it is not clear whether lymphoid progenitors are discrete, homogeneous populations or overlapping populations. Nor is it clear whether lineage commitment occurs via a continuum of differentiation with a progressive loss of lineage options or abrupt events resulting in the acquisition of certain properties. Whatever the precise mechanism, HSCs give rise to progeny with progressively more restricted myeloid, erythroid, or lymphoid developmental potential, which is accompanied by the silencing of some genes and the activation of others. Changes in the expression levels of cytokine receptors, signal transduction molecules, and transcription factors are key components in lymphoid differentiation.

Hematopoietic stem cell markers

The markers of HSCs include both membrane and functional markers. HSCs are characteristically described as lacking CD135 (Flt3) and the markers specific to discrete lymphoid lineages (Lin), but expressing high levels of CD117 (c-kit). HSCs also express CD44, low levels of CD90 (Thy1), but no CD127 (IL-7Rα) or CD27. Thus, the phenotype of HSCs can be expressed as Lin⁻, CD117/c-kit^{high}, CD44⁺, CD90/Thy1^{low}, CD27⁻, or CD127/IL-7Rα⁻. Progression of HSC differentiation and lineage commitment is indicated by changes in this phenotype, as described in the following and as summarized in Figure 10.1.

- **Flt3 (CD135)** is a cytokine tyrosine kinase receptor that is important in early lymphoid development and plays a major role in maintaining B lymphoid and dendritic cell progenitors.
- **CD27** plays a role in lymphoid proliferation, differentiation, and apoptosis. The acquisition of CD27 and CD135/Flt3 by the HSC coincides with the loss of long-term repopulating potential. At this stage, the cells retain both lymphoid and myeloid potential and are referred to as multipotent progenitors.
- **Stem cell growth factor receptor or c-kit (CD117)**, a cytokine tyrosine kinase receptor, is expressed at high levels **in stem cells** but progressively declines with lineage commitment and thus can be used to distinguish general categories of lymphoid progenitors. In the bone marrow, HSC and early lymphoid progenitors are CD117/c-kit^{high}, as are the early thymocyte progenitors, the most primitive cells in the thymus. A population of CD117/c-kit^{low} cells in the bone marrow called pro-lymphocytes has limited self-renewal capacity and has lymphoid but not myeloid potential.

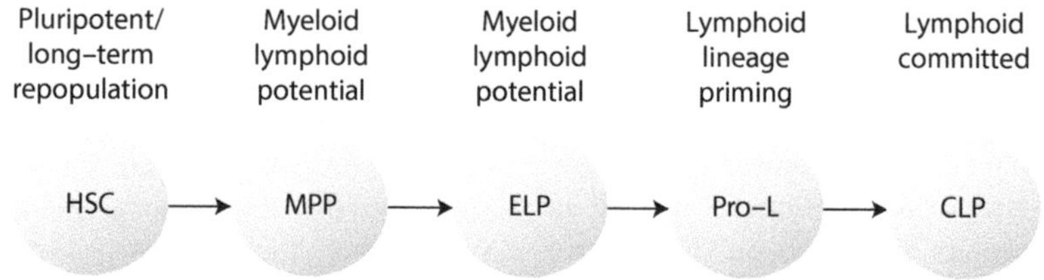

	Pluripotent/ long–term repopulation	Myeloid lymphoid potential	Myeloid lymphoid potential	Lymphoid lineage priming	Lymphoid committed
	HSC →	MPP →	ELP →	Pro–L →	CLP
c–kit	H	H	H	L	L
Thy1	L	L	L	L	L
CD44	+	+	+	+	+
FLt3	–	+	+	+	+
CD27	–	+	+	+	+
TdT	–	–	L	+	+
RAG	–	–	L	+	+
IL–7Rα	–	–	–	+/–	+
γC	–	–	–	–	+

Figure 10.1 Model of lymphopoiesis. The differentiation of the pluripotent, self-renewing, hematopoietic stem cells (HSC) in the bone marrow is progressive. First cells develop into multipotent progenitors (MPPs) and then into early lymphoid progenitors (ELPs), into pro-lymphocytes (Pro-L), and finally into the common lymphoid progenitor (CLP), which is fully committed to the lymphoid lineage. Changes in the expression of the hallmark surface markers and intracellular proteins that typify each stage of differentiation are shown.

- **Terminal deoxynucleotidyl transferase (TdT)** is a template independent DNA polymerase believed to play an important role in the generation of antigen receptor diversity both in B cells and T cells. The expression of this enzyme is restricted to lymphoid precursors and transformed cells in patients with acute lymphoblastic leukemia.
- **Recombinase-activation genes 1 and 2 (RAG-1, RAG-2)** are transposases. The absence of the RAG affects both T- and B-cell differentiation and results in severe combined immunodeficiency (see Chapter 29).
- **The common γ chain (γc, CD132)** is a subunit shared by the membrane-bound receptors for IL-2, IL-4, IL-7, IL-9, IL-13, IL-15, and IL-21. A common lymphoid progenitor cell exists within the pro-lymphocyte population and is defined on the basis of upregulation of CD127/IL-7Rα and CD132/γc. These progenitor cells have the ability to give rise to all lymphoid lineages—T cells, B cells, natural killer (NK) cells, and dendritic cells (DC), but not myeloid cells. Patients with CD132/γc chain gene deficiency (see Chapters 11 and 29) display defects in T, B, and NK cell development and suffer from X-linked severe combined immunodeficiency (SCID).

MONOCYTES

Previously, monocytes were considered simply as development intermediates between bone marrow precursors and tissue macrophages, destined to differentiate into either macrophages or DCs; but it is now known that they play a pivotal role in protective immunity and carry out specific effector functions.

Monopoiesis

HSCs give rise to the common myeloid progenitors (CMPs), which in turn give rise to the monocyte/dendritic cell progenitors (MDPs) or the granulocyte/monocyte progenitors (GMPs). Maturation then occurs in three stages: monoblast, promonocyte, and monocyte. Monoblasts expressing CD64, CD33, HLA-DR, CD34, and CD4 are derived from both MDP and GMP. As differentiation progresses transition toward promonocytes, there is a loss of CD34 expression and increased expression of CD4 (Figure 10.2). Changes in the expression levels of CD34, HLA-DR, CD117/c-kit, CD64, CD45, CD36, CD14, and CD300 are used to delineate monocyte maturation stages (Table 10.1). Monocytic-myeloid-derived suppressor cells (M-MDSCs) are also differentiated from MDPs.

One of the key players of monopoiesis is the transcription factor PU.1. High expression of PU.1 will lead to the activation of different myeloid specific factors such as interferon regulatory factor-8 (IRF8), kruppel-like factor 4 (KLF-4), and Erg1. PU.1 expression is also indispensable to the expression of macrophage colony stimulating factor receptor (M-CSFR, CD115). Macrophage colony stimulating factor (M-CSF) and IL-34 are two ligands for CD155 crucial to monocyte development.

Monocyte membrane markers

Three populations of mature monocytes are distinguished by the expressions HLA-DR, CD14, and CD16: classical (HLA-DR$^+$, CD14^{bright}, CD16$^-$); intermediate (HLA-DR$^+$, CD14^{bright}, CD16^{dim}); pro-inflammatory (HLA-DR$^+$, CD14^{dim}, CD16^{bright}). Intermediate and classical monocytes

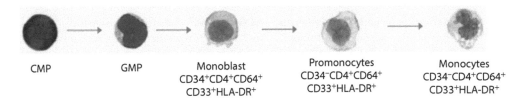

CMP GMP Monoblast
CD34$^+$CD4$^+$CD64$^+$
CD33$^+$HLA-DR$^+$

Promonocytes
CD34$^-$CD4$^+$CD64$^+$
CD33$^+$HLA-DR$^+$

Monocytes
CD34$^-$CD4$^+$CD64$^+$
CD33$^+$HLA-DR$^+$

Figure 10.2 Model of monopoiesis. Common progenitor cells (CMP) differentiate into granulocyte monocyte progenitors and then into monoblasts, which start expressing CD34, CD4, CD64, CD33, and HLA-DR. As monoblasts mature into promonocytes, CD34 expression is lost. Promonocytes can then differentiate into monocytes; however, discerning between the two requires a more complex phenotyping.

Table 10.1 Monocyte maturation

Maturation stage	Phenotype
Stage 1—Immature Monocytic Precursors	CD34+ HLA-DR^{high} CD117+ CD64^{low} CD45^{low} CD36- CD14- CD300E-
Stage 2—Monoblasts	CD34- HLA-DR^{high} CD117- CD64^{high} CD45+ CD36± CD14- CD300E-
Stage 3—Monocytic Precursors	CD34- HLA-DR^{high} CD117- CD64^{high} CD45+ CD36^{low} CD14^{int} CD300E-
Stage 4—Monoblasts	CD34- HLA-DR^{high} CD117- CD64^{high} CD45+ CD36^{high} CD14^{high} CD300E-
Stage 5—Mature Monocytes	CD34- HLA-DR^{high} CD117- CD64^{high} CD45+ CD36^{high} CD14^{high} CD300E+

are potent producers of pro-inflammatory signals such as tumor necrosis factor (TNF), nitric oxide, and reactive oxygen species. They are rapidly recruited to sites of infection where they differentiate into monocyte-derived dendritic cells (MDDCs).

CD47 is expressed at higher levels on leukemia cells than on healthy cells. The surface protein targets signal regulatory protein α (SIRPα) on the surface of myeloid cells. CD47-SIRPα interaction inhibits macrophage phagocytosis, allowing cancer cells to escape immune surveillance. Current focus in immunotherapy has been targeted toward inhibiting CD47-SIRPα interaction via anti-CD47 antibodies. This activates innate immunity, promoting cancer cell destruction by macrophages. It also activates adaptive immunity by promoting antigen presentation, mostly by DCs, leading to antitumor cytotoxic reactions.

DENDRITIC CELLS

DCs represent a group of specialized antigen presenting cells (APCs), which are members of the mononuclear phagocyte system, a group of myeloid cells including monocytes and macrophages, which modulate innate and adaptive immune functions. In addition to antigen presentation, DCs are producers of type 1 interferons (α and β) and play an important role in the maintenance of immunological tolerance.

There are three major subsets of DCs, myeloid DCs 1 (mDC1), myeloid DCs 2 (mDC2), and plasmacytoid DCs (pDCs) (Figure 10.3). Subsets are based on location (resident or circulating), surface phenotype, morphology, specialized functions, transcription factors, and gene expression profiles.

DC ontogeny

DCs (with the exception of Langerhans cells) are differentiated in the bone marrow from HSCs. The differentiation of HSCs after two intermediate progenitors leads to the appearance of DC progenitor cells, the common DC progenitors, which under the control of CD135/Flt3-mediated signaling can be polarized into mDC1, mDC2, or pDC. DCs are localized in the lymphoid organs (thymus, liver, lymph nodes, or mucous membranes associated with lymphoid ganglia) or nonlymphoid organs (pancreas, heart, liver, kidneys, skin). DCs have a half-life of a few days (between 3 and 5 days) and are continually being replaced by precursors from the bone marrow. This regeneration depends on the Flt3L cytokine.

DC membrane markers

Immature mDC express C-type lectin (CLEC) and DC-SIGN. **Mature mDC** are defined by the co-expression of CD11c and HLA-DR, and the lack of CD14 or CD16 (Table 10.2).

mDC1 represent the majority of mDC and express CD1c (BDCA1), CD11b, CD13, CD33, CD172, and CD45RO. mDC1 present in tissues express more activation markers (CD80, CD83, CD86, CD40) than those found in the circulating mDC1. They regulate the expression of chemokine receptors, i.e., decreasing the expression of two homing receptors: cutaneous lymphocyte-associated antigen (CLA) and CD62L, and by increasing the expression of the CD197 (CCR7) promote their migration to the lymph nodes. mDC secrete TNF, IL-8, IL-10, IL-23, and IL-12p70, allowing them to act on the cell differentiation during the T cell immune response.

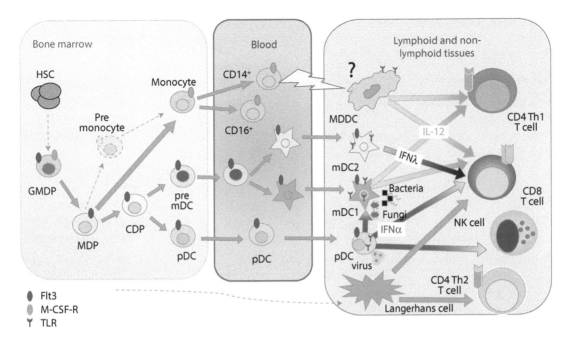

Figure 10.3 Model of dendritic cell ontogeny. Proposed ontogeny and differentiation of DC subsets and their interactions with the immune system.

mDC2, defined by the expression of CD141, are abundant in the bone marrow and in secondary lymphoid organs but rare in peripheral blood. mDC2 express the c-type lectin domain containing 9A (CLEC9A) molecule that recognizes dead cells and produce cytokines that inhibit viral replication (IFNα, IFNλ IL-29, IL-28A, and IL-28B).

pDC (CD11c⁻, CD123bᵇʳⁱᵍʰᵗ, CD45RA⁺, CD303⁺/BDCA-2, CD304⁺/BDCA-4) constitute half of all peripheral blood DC and express several receptors related to endocytosis of pathogens such as CD205 (DEC-205), Sialic acid-binding immunoglobulin-type lectins H (Siglec-H), FcγRIIa, and DC ImmunoReceptor (DCIR). While they are primarily localized in the secondary lymphoid organs, pDC are rapidly recruited to sites of inflammation. They are potent producers of type 1 interferons in response to a viral infection and selectively express TLR-7 and TLR-9, which detect nucleic acids from viruses, bacteria, or dead cells.

Langerhans cells (LCs) are DCs of the skin but can also be found in other tissues, such as lymph nodes, particularly in association with the condition known as Langerhans cell histiocytosis. LCs overregulate the expression of MHC-II molecules, as well as the expression of co-stimulatory molecules and CD197/CCR7.

LYMPHOCYTES

There are three major types of lymphocytes: T cells, B cells, and NK cells. T cells and B cells comprise the cellular arm of the adaptive immune system.

The immune system is controlled by balance of stimulatory and inhibitory signals mediated by lymphocyte membrane markers. Engagement of activation receptors on lymphocytes can induce cellular migration, proliferation, differentiation, anergy, or apoptosis. Several factors that influence the outcome include antigen concentration, binding avidity, duration of antigen recognition, association with co-stimulatory molecules, cytokines, and the developmental stage of the lymphocyte. Engagement of cellular inhibitory receptors will inhibit functional responses. In most cases, conserved sequences within the cytoplasmic domains of the receptors and/or association with intracellular adapter proteins mediate the activation or inhibitory cascade.

Most inhibitory receptors contain one or more copies of the conserved tyrosine-based inhibitory motif (ITIM) within the cytoplasmic domain. Upon receptor ligation, inhibitory signaling is mediated by tyrosine phosphorylation within this region and the subsequent recruitment of the tyrosine-specific phosphatases, SHP-1 and SHP-2

Table 10.2 Dendritic cells

DC subsets	Frequency	Localization	Cytokine production upon stimulation	Phenotype
Plasmacytoid DCs	~1% PBMC	Blood	IFN-I+, IFN-III (IFN-λ)+	CD123high, CD303+, CD304+, CD85g+, CD11clow CD11b− CD14−
		Lymph node T cell zone	IL-6+, IL-8+	
		Tonsil	IP-10 (CXCL10)+	
			TNF+	
CD1c+ Myeloid DCs	~1% PBMC	Blood	IL-1β+, IL-6+, IL-8+	CD1c+, CD172a+, CLEC6A+, CD11b+/low, CD11c+ CX3CR1+ CD14low−
		Nonlymphoid tissues: skin, liver, lung, and gut	IL-10+, IL-12+ IL-23+	
		Lymphoid tissues: spleen, lymph nodes	TNF+ IL-15+ (skin)	
CD141+ Myeloid DCs	0.03% PBMC	Lymph node, tonsil, spleen, bone marrow	IFN-I+, IFN-III (IFN-λ)+	CD141high, CD370+, NECL2+, CD11c+/low, CD14−
		Nonlymphoid tissues: skin, lung, liver, intestine	CXCL-10 (IP-10)+ TNF+	
Langerhans cells		Stratified squamous epithelia	IL-15+	CD207+, CD324+, CD326+, CD11blow, CD11c+, CD14−
		Draining lymph nodes		
Inflammatory DCs		Inflammatory sites	IL-1β+, IL-6+	CD16+, CD64+
			IL-10+, IL-12+, IL-23+	
			TNF+	

or the phospholipid-specific phosphatases, SHIP. In general, these phosphatases work by degrading phosphatidylinositol triphosphate or decreasing the phosphorylation of intracellular signaling proteins such as ZAP70, Syk, and phospholipase Cγ.

In a similar fashion, activation receptors share common signaling pathways mediated by the transmembrane association with adapter proteins containing the conserved tyrosine-based activation motif (ITAM). Upon tyrosine phosphorylation of ITAM, the tyrosine kinases Syk and ZAP70 are recruited via their SH2 domains and stimulate the activation of intracellular signaling proteins. ITAM-containing adapter proteins include FcεRIγ and CD3ζ.

Several important membrane markers are common to more than one type of lymphocyte:

- **CD45**, expressed by all leukocytes, is a major cell surface component occupying up to 10% of the surface. The most remarkable feature of CD45

is its cytoplasmic domain that comprises 705 amino acids and is the largest intracytoplasmic domain of all known membrane proteins. This intracytoplasmic domain has intrinsic tyrosine phosphatase activity and plays an essential role in lymphocyte activation.

- **CD69** is a lectin receptor encoded in a region of chromosome 12 known as the "NK gene complex." CD69 is expressed on a variety of hematopoietic cells. CD69 is absent on resting lymphocytes but rapidly upregulated during activation of T, B, and NK cells. Because monoclonal antibodies directed against CD69 can activate lymphocytes, a role for CD69 in signal transduction has been suggested.

- **Membrane markers of the tumor necrosis factor receptor (TNFR) family.** Several members of the TNFR family (CD27, CD30, CD137, CD154) have co-stimulatory effects on T cells. With regulated and transient expression, these molecules are key mediators of survival signal induction and the generation of effector/memory populations. Members of the TNF family are involved in cancer, infectious diseases, autoimmunity, and transplantation and thus are attractive therapeutic targets.

- **CD154 (CD40 ligand, CD40L)** is one of the first activation-induced cell surface molecules expressed on T cells. It is expressed on all activated CD4$^+$ cells and a small population of CD8$^+$ cells and $\gamma\delta$ T cells. CD154 interacts with CD40, expressed on B cells. This interaction is required for the development and maturation of T-dependent B-lymphocyte responses. As discussed in Chapter 29, the lack of expression of CD154 is the molecular basis of most cases of a unique immunodeficiency disease known as hyper IgM syndrome.

- **CD27** is a co-stimulatory molecule expressed on most T and NK cells and is induced on primed B cells. Its activity is regulated by the transiently expressed TNF-like ligand CD70 expressed on T cells, B cells, and DCs. The **CD27-CD70** system acts by increasing cell survival and is important in effector and memory cell formation.

- **CD137 (4-1BB)** is transiently expressed on activated T cells. 4-1BB ligand is expressed on DC, B cells, and macrophages. Signaling through 4-1BB can activate T cells, but the major effect is to prolong survival in activated cells. Interest in 4-1BB as a cancer therapeutic comes from the fact that antibodies to 4-1BB have been found to enhance CD8 expansion and IFN-γ production.

- **CD30** is expressed on activated T cells, NK cells, and B cells. The CD30 ligand (CD153) is expressed on activated T cells, resting B cells, and macrophages. Like other members of the TNFR family, CD30 activation results in enhanced proliferation and cytokine secretion. CD30 is also expressed in a variety of hematological malignancies.

- **CD2** is expressed on all thymocytes, T cells, and NK cells. The heterotypic interaction between CD2 and its major ligand, leukocyte function-associated antigen 3 (LFA-3), enhances T cell antigen recognition. **CD58/LFA-3** is expressed on about half of the circulating T and B cells, APCs, and erythrocytes.

- **LFA-1 and ICAM-1** are expressed by T, B, and NK cells and are responsible for homotypic adhesion. An LFA-1 expressing cell will bind with the counter-receptor on another cell type and vice versa. LFA-1 is a heterodimer composed of CD11a and CD18, which is expressed on APC and other leukocytes. CD54 (ICAM-1), CD102 (ICAM-2), and CD50 (ICAM-3) are all co-receptors for the integrin LFA-1. CD54/ICAM-1 is expressed by both hematopoietic and non-hematopoietic cell types. The expression on leukocytes is upregulated during activation. Similarly, the expression on the endothelium is upregulated during inflammation. CD54/ICAM-1 also binds to other related integrins that share CD18 but express unique CD11 chains such as Macrophage-1 antigen (MAC-1) which consists of CD11b and CD18; and p150,95 which consists of CD11c and CD18.

- **CD38** is a type II transmembrane glycoprotein, which is expressed on immature B and T cells, but not on most mature, resting peripheral lymphocytes.

Lymphopoiesis

Lymphocytes start to differentiate early in fetal life. NK cells are the first functionally active lymphocytes in the developing fetus; they can be isolated from the fetal liver, prior to formation of the thymic rudiment. There is also evidence of extrathymic T cell development in the fetal liver early in fetal development. At about 38 weeks, differentiated T and B lymphocytes appear in the circulation.

Natural killer cells

NK cells, part of the innate immune system, are considered one of the first lines of defense against infection. NK cells, active in the naive, or non-immunized host, do not require prior antigen exposure, or priming, nor do they express the exquisitely specific antigen receptors found on T and B cells. They possess potent cytolytic activity and produce an array of immunoregulatory cytokines and chemokines (IFN-γ, TNF, GM-CSF, MIP-1α, MIP-1β, RANTES). Given that NK cell produced cytokines are important regulators of the adaptive immune system, NK cells provide a bridge between adaptive and innate immunity.

NK CELL ONTOGENY

Although considered part of the innate immune system, NK cells are more closely related to T cells than to other cells of the innate immune system. NK cells not only share many surface markers and functional activities in common with T lymphocytes, they also arise from a common bipotential progenitor (the T/NK precursor).

Although committed NK progenitors can be found in the thymus, the thymus is not required for NK development. It is believed that NK cells can develop in a variety of organs; however, the major site of NK cell development has yet to be identified. NK cells require IL-15 for differentiation and c-kit ligand and Flt3 ligand for the expansion of functionally active NK cells (Figure 10.4). In addition, γc and IL-21 are critical for NK cell development and maturation.

In humans, the majority (85%–90%) of the NK cells are CD56+, CD16+, surface CD3− and have a high cytolytic capacity. A smaller subset (10%–15%) that expresses high levels of CD56, little or no CD16, CD25 (IL-2Rα), CD117/c-kit, and lymph node homing receptors is responsible for cytokine production and exhibits enhanced survival capacity. In the lymph nodes, they differentiate into functionally mature CD56+, CD16+, CD3− NK cells that express killer cell immunoglobulin-like receptors (KIRs), natural cytotoxicity receptors (NCRs), and critical adhesion molecules.

NK CELL MEMBRANE MARKERS

NK cells distinguish normal and abnormal cells through a sophisticated repertoire of stimulatory and inhibitory receptors, which are invariant and constitutively expressed (Table 10.3). NK cell

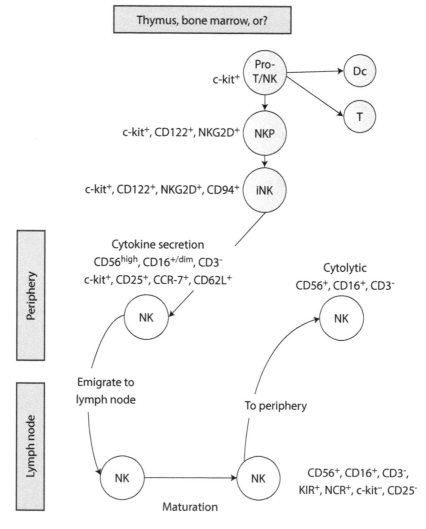

Figure 10.4 Model of NK ontogeny. Proposed ontogeny and differentiation of NK cell.

activation, proliferation, and effector functions are controlled by the competition between signals resulting from stimulatory and inhibitory receptors, the affinity of the receptor for the ligand, as well as the level of ligand expression on the target cell. Positive stimuli are required to activate NK cell effector function, while cytokines and inhibitory receptors control specificity and regulation. In essence, cells lacking the ligands for the inhibitory receptors or overexpressing the ligands for the activation receptors activate NK cells.

- **CD16** is a low-affinity IgG Fc receptor (FcγRIII) expressed on most NK cells, activated monocytes, and a subset of T cells. CD16 engagement on NK results in antibody-dependent cellular cytotoxicity (ADCC) and cytokine secretion. The transmembrane anchored CD16 isoform is complexed with the CD3ζ chain or the FcϵRγ chain. Receptor ligation results in the phosphorylation of tyrosine residues within the ITAM in the cytoplasmic domains of the CD3ζ chain or the FcϵRγ chain.
- **CD2** is expressed on all thymocytes, T cells, and NK cells. CD2 activation by CD58/LFA-3 induces NK cell mediated cytotoxicity and induces a similar cascade of intracellular signaling events as CD16. CD2 is both a primary activation receptor on NK cells as well as a co-stimulatory receptor that augments NK cell activation.
- **Natural cytotoxicity receptors (NKp46, NKp3, NKp44)** are selectively expressed on NK cells at varying surface densities. They associate with different ITAMs such as CD3ζ, FcϵRIγ, or DAP12 and play a major role in activating lysis of tumor and virally infected targets.
- **NKG2D** is a lectin-like, homodimer activation receptor constitutively expressed on NK and CD8$^+$ T cells. It forms a transmembrane association with the ITAM-bearing adapter protein DAP-10. NKG2D is involved in tumor and viral immunity and recognizes two families of stress-induced, MHC class I–like molecules.
- **CD226 (DNAM-1)** activation results in enhanced NK cell activity (lysis and cytokine production). Receptors for DNAM-1 include two members of the nectin family, the CD155 (poliovirus receptor, PVR) and CD112 (nectin-2), highly expressed on many tumors and normal cells and tissues.

- **CD161 (NKR-P1)**, a member of the C-type lectin superfamily, is expressed on subsets of NK cells, $\gamma\delta$TCR$^+$ T cells, and on about 25% of CD4$^+$ and CD8$^+$ T cells, primarily of the effector/memory phenotype. These receptors interact with glycoproteins resulting in the delivery of activating signals to the NK cells.
- **CD244 (NK receptor 2B4)** is present on all NK cells, most $\gamma\delta$TCR$^+$ T cells and CD8$^+$ T cells. The interaction with its ligand, CD48, results in the activation of the cytolytic properties of the NK cell.

NK-CELL INHIBITORY MARKERS

Historically, NK cells were defined as mediators of MHC non-restricted cytolysis because of their ability to lyse allogeneic as well as autologous virally infected or transformed targets. However, the observation that NK cells preferentially lyse target cells that expressed low levels or no MHC class I antigens precipitated the study of MHC class I receptors on NK cells. Two distinct MHC class I receptor families have been described in humans: the **KIRs** and **CD94/NKG2A**, each of which rely on ITIM sequences in the cytoplasmic domains to mediate inhibitory signaling. NK cell proliferation, cytotoxicity, and cytokine production are downregulated as a consequence of MHC class I–NK receptor interaction.

- **KIR** family members recognize classical MHC class I and are expressed on overlapping subsets of human NK cells, $\gamma\delta$TCR$^+$ T cells, and memory/effector $\alpha\beta$TCR$^+$ T cells. There are 15 genes in the KIR family coding for type I transmembrane glycoproteins containing two or three Ig-like domains. Variability also exists within the cytoplasmic domains. The KIRs family members with the longer cytoplasmic tails contains one to two ITIM sequences. The KIRs with the shorter cytoplasmic region do not contain ITIM and form a transmembrane association with ITAMs bearing the DAP12 adapter protein, delivering activation rather than inhibitory signals.
- **CD94 and NKG2** are type II membrane proteins of the C-type lectin-like family, which form disulfide-linked heterodimers. They recognize the nonclassical MHC molecule HLA-E. CD94 associates with human NKG2 proteins (NKG2A or NKG2C) and is expressed on most NK cells,

Table 10.3 NK cell receptors

Receptor	Function	Ligand
CD85J (ILT2LIR-1)	Inhibitory	Different HLA-1 alleles
CD159a NKG2a	Inhibitory	HAL-E
CD158a, b, d, f (KIR2DL)	Inhibitory	HLA-C
	Inhibitory	HLA-Bw4
CD279 PD-1	Inhibitory	CD274 (PD-L1)
		CD273 (PD-L2)
CD328 Siglec7	Inhibitory	Ganglioside DSGb5
CD300a IRP60	Inhibitory	α-Herpesviruses
		Pseudorabies virus
		Phosphatidylserine
		Phosphatidylethanolamine
TIGIT	Inhibitory	CD155 (PVR0)
CD159C NKG2c	Activation	HLA- E Inhibitory
CD158 g, h, i, j (KIR2DS)	Activation	HLA-C
CD158E2 (KIR3DS)	Activation	HLA-Bw4
		HLA-F?
CD59	Activation	CD2
NKp46	Activation	?
NKp30	Activation	B7-H6- BAG6/BAT3
NKp44	Activation	21spe-MLLS
NKG2D	Activation	MICA- MIVB - ULPBs
DNAM1	Activation	CD112 NECTIN - 2/CD155 PVR
NKp80KLRF1	Activation	AICL
CD244 2B4	Activation	CD48
CD352 NTB-A	Activation	CD352 NTB-A
CD2	Activation	CD58
CD319 CRACC/CS1	Activation	CD319 CRACC/CS1
CD96 Tactile	Activation	CD155 PVR
CD16 (FcγRIII)	Activation	IgG Fc

γδTCR⁺ T cells, and a subset memory/effector CD8⁺αβTCR⁺ T cells. CD94-NKG2A contains an ITIM in its cytoplasmic domain and functions as an inhibitory receptor, whereas CD94-NKG2C functions as an activation receptor when associated with DAP-12. IL-15, Il-2, and TGF-β induce CD94-NKG2 expression.

Antigen-specific T cell and B cell receptors

A critical step in T and B lymphopoiesis is the complex process of forming functional, but not autoreactive, antigen-specific T cell (TCR) and B cell (BCR) receptors (Figures 10.5 and 10.6). A diverse array of receptors is generated from the recombination of a limited number of germline gene segments (variable [V], diversity [D], and joining [J]) (Figures 7.1 and 7.2). The initiation V(D) J recombination requires the expression of RAG genes, which are restricted to lymphocyte progenitors and developing lymphocytes. In addition, lineage-specific, cis elements control the accessibility of DNA regions to RAG-1 and RAG-2. This and other control processes ensures that TCR genes are only rearranged to completion in T lymphocytes and BCR genes are only rearranged to completion in B lymphocytes.

Due to the random nature of gene rearrangement, a productive V(D)J rearrangement occurs only about a third of the time. If rearrangement of one allele is nonproductive, the process will proceed on the second allele. However, by allelic exclusion, the generation of a functional protein will result in RAG inactivation and thus gene rearrangement on the second allele will not occur. Consequently, only one functional antigen-specific receptor will be expressed per developing T or B lymphocyte.

A major difference between TCR and BCR is that once the rearrangements are completed in the thymus, the TCR will not change, whereas the BCR will undergo additional gene modifications such as class switching and affinity maturation in the secondary lymphoid organs. The estimated diversity of $\alpha\beta$TCR (10^{15}–10^{18}) exceeds the potential diversity of immunoglobulins (10^9–10^{11}) by several orders of magnitude.

TCR and BCR are similar in structure, composed of highly diverse, antigen-specific variable regions and conserved constant regions (Figures 10.5 and 10.6). Their short intracytoplasmic regions are not capable signal transduction but are associated with co-receptor molecules that lend signal transduction capacity to the mature receptor complex.

T cells

T CELL LYMPHOPOIESIS

T cells are often referred to as "directors" of the adaptive-immune response and are discussed in detail in Chapters 2 and 4. Upon antigen-specific activation, they can provide help to B cells, influence the type of immune response via their cytokine secretion profile or engage in cytolytic activity.

The key transcriptional components that drive precursor cells toward the T lineage are the levels of NOTCH1, E proteins, and GATA-3. When activated, the intracellular domain of NOTCH1 is cleaved off and translocates to the nucleus where

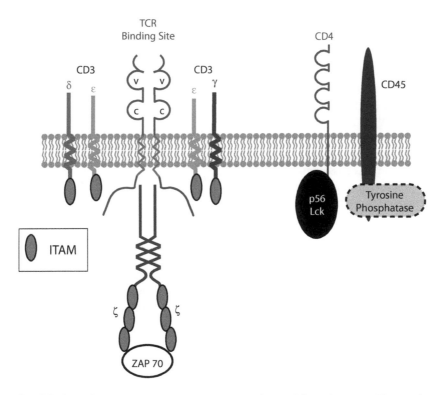

Figure 10.5 The TCR2 and its coreceptors on a mature CD4+ T lymphocyte. The $\alpha\beta$ heterodimer is associated with the CD3γδεζ complex, which contains tyrosine-based activation motifs (ITAMs). It is believed that activating signals are transmitted by the ζ chain. Coreceptors also contribute to initial T cell activation. CD45 has intrinsic phosphatase activity, and CD4 is associated to a p56lck tyrosine kinase. At least two more tyrosine kinases—p59fyn and ζ-associated p70 (ZAP70) appear to play a role in the initial signaling cascade.

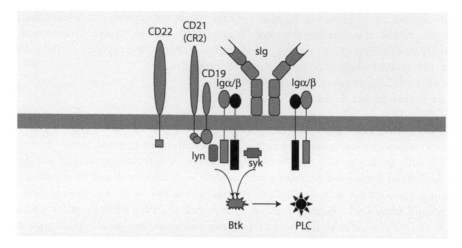

Figure 10.6 B-cell receptor complex. The BCR constituted by a membrane immunoglobulin molecule closely associated with Igα and Igβ molecules. Three additional molecules, CD19, CD21, and CD22, are associated with the BCR complex and play a role in B-cell signaling.

it activates T cell–specific gene expression. The transcription factor GATA-3 is expressed in a T cell–specific manner and is required for T cell development. During T cell development, GATA-3 is important in the β selection and positive selections stages by regulating the expression of RAG-2, TCR gene enhancers, and CD4. E proteins, such as E2A, are important in the regulation of CD4, RAG-1/RAG-2, and GATA-3.

T-cell development occurs almost exclusively in the thymus and requires signals generated from the thymic stromal cells (Figure 10.7). A complex set of regulatory and growth factors acting in various combinations drives T cell developmental choice-points. Several stages at which specific regulators are required in order for T cell development to proceed have been defined. Later in T cell development and maturation, these same regulatory factors influence T cell specialization. T cells are unique among the lymphocyte populations in their ability to further specialize as mature cells.

Stage one: Thymic migration

Multipotent precursors enter the T cell pathway as they immigrate to the thymus. The most primitive cells in the thymus are the early thymocyte progenitors that retain all lymphoid and myeloid potential but exist only transiently, rapidly differentiating into T and NK lineages, via the intermediate stage—the common lymphoid precursor.

Stage two: Proliferative expansion and T cell lineage commitment

Final commitment to the T cell lineage occurs within the thymic microenvironment. The CD117/c-kit+, IL-7R+ precursor cells proliferate rapidly once they reach the thymus, where IL-7 and CD117/c-kit ligand are plentiful. As development proceeds, thymocytes express several enzymes of the purine salvage pathway, such as ADA and PNP, as well as Tdt.

NOTCH1 is a member of a highly conserved Notch family of signaling receptors that feature an extracellular domain containing epidermal growth factor–like repeats and an intracellular signaling domain. When early thymoctyes upregulate NOTCH1 and engage thymic stromal cells expressing NOTCH1 ligands, they become restricted to the T cell lineage. Higher levels of NOTCH1 signaling are thought to favor T lymphocytes expressing αβTCR lineage over T lymphocytes expressing γδTCR.

Early thymocytes do not express CD4 or CD8 and are known as double-negative (DN) thymocytes (Figure 10.7). Within the thymic cortex, the most primitive DN1 T cells (CD117/c-kit+, CD44+, CD25−) retain multipotential ability and can differentiate into cells of the myeloid or lymphoid lineages. More differentiated DN T cells (DN2; CD117/c-kit−, CD44+, CD25+) have more limited potentiality but are not yet fully restricted to the T cell lineage (could develop into DC, T cells, or NK

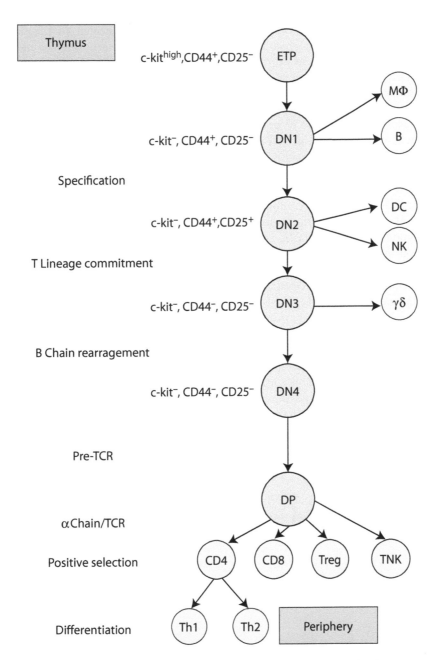

Figure 10.7 Model of T cell lymphopoiesis. Intrathymic T lymphopoiesis. Early thymocyte progenitors (ETPs) give rise to double-negative thymocytes (DN), which become increasingly committed to the T cell lineage in thymic cortex. DN1 retain myeloid and B cell potential. DN2 retain dendritic cell (DC) and natural killer cell potential. DN3 are T cell lineage committed. DN4 give rise to double positive (DP) thymocytes expressing the $\alpha\beta$ T cell receptor (TCR) cells and both CD4 and CD8. In the thymic medulla, mature single positive CD4 and CD8 T cells emerge as well as natural killer T (NKT) cells and regulatory T (Treg) cells emerge from the DP population. Further differentiation into T helper (Th1) 1 and T helper 2 (Th2) occurs in the periphery.

cells). DN3 cells (CD117/c-kit⁻, CD44⁻, CD25⁺) are fully committed to the T cell lineage, which translates to induction of T cell–specific gene expression and initiation of TCR gene rearrangement.

Productive rearrangement of the TCRα, β, γ, and δ genes can result in the generation of either of two types of receptors, TCR1 (γδTCR) or TCR2 (αβTCR). TCR gene rearrangement occurs in an ordered and sequential fashion. Due to the chromosomal organization of the TCR genes, the TCRγ and TCRδ genes are rearranged before the TCRα and TCRβ genes. TCR gene V(D)J recombination is mediated by RAG and involves the transposition of noncontiguous segments of DNA and the deletion of intervening and noncoding sequences (Figure 10.8).

The β- and γ-chain genes are located in distant regions of chromosome 7, whereas the α- and δ-chain genes are located on chromosome 14. The generation of the extensive diversity needed for a complete TCR repertoire relies primarily in the D regions where random nucleotide addition occurs, particularly at the DJ junction. Only the β and δ genes contain D regions, and thus, they display hypervariability as compared to the α and γ chains.

The δ gene is located in the middle of the α-chain gene, between the Vα and Jα regions. When RAG transposes the elements of the δ genes to form a VδJδ complex, it eliminates the V and J regions of the α gene. The rearranged δ chain will pair with the γ chain. T cells expressing TCR1 (γδ TCR) will leave the thymus to migrate to the skin and mucosae.

Stage three: β-Selection

Rearrangement of TCRβ genes occurs in two steps. First, Dβ-to-Jβ rearrangement, followed by the Vβ-to-DβJβ rearrangement. Finally, the Cβ region gene is added to the VβDβJβ.

The productively rearranged β chain will be present in the cytoplasm for several days prior to TCRα gene rearrangement. During that period, the β chain will associate with a protective polypeptide, known as the pre-Tα. When the β chain/pre-Tα associates with CD3 molecules and is transported to the cell membrane, the pre-TCR is formed. CD3 is a complex of five unique subunits designated γ, δ, ε, ζ, and η (note that the γ and δ chains of the CD3 unit are distinct from the γδ chains of the TCR1). The CD3γδε trimolecular complex is synthesized first and remains intracytoplasmic, where

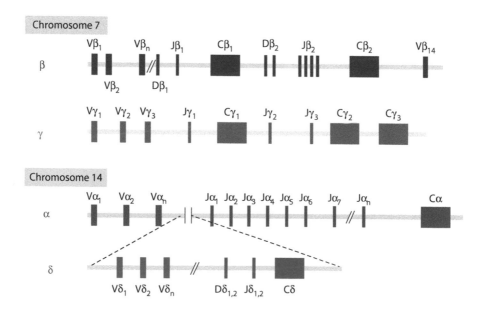

Figure 10.8 Genomic organization of the T cell receptor genes. The genes for the β- and γ-chains rearrange independently at their own end of chromosome 7. The δ genes are in the middle of the α-gene locus on chromosome 14. Rearrangement of the α genes leads to removal of the δ genes that are found as extrachromosomal DNA in cells that have productive rearrangements of the α and β genes yielding a TCR2⁺ T cell. In TCR1⁺ (γδ) T lymphocytes, the α and β genes are deleted.

it becomes associated with pre-Tα molecules. Soon thereafter, the CD3ζ chains are synthesized and become associated to the CD3 complex. Once the ζ chain has been added to the CD3 molecule, the whole CD3-pre-Tα complex is transported from the Golgi apparatus to the cell membrane. A critical characteristic of the ζ chain is its long intracytoplasmic tail, which has affinity for the ζ-associated protein kinase (ZAP70). The association of ZAP70 to the ζ chain is critical for further differentiation of the T cell. The congenital absence of ZAP70 is associated with a block at the DN stage of T cell development.

Signaling through the pre-TCR generates activation signals, which lead to a cascade of proliferation and differentiation, such as the co-expression of CD4 and CD8, characteristic of the double-positive thymocyte population. These cells re-express their *RAG* genes and undergo TCRα gene rearrangement. Rearrangement of the TCRα gene results in the deletion of the δ gene, which will appear as extrachromosomal circular DNA in germline configuration. Upon successful rearrangement of the VαJαCα chain, the pre-Tα chain of the pre-TCR is replaced by the newly synthesized α chain, and the TCR2 (αβ) with a full complement of CD3 molecules, is inserted in the T cell membrane (Figure 10.5).

Stage four: TCR selection

TCR selection occurs in the thymic medulla where the double-positive thymocytes encounter epithelial cells expressing MHC class I and class II molecules. Only 2%–3% of the differentiating thymocytes, those that express TCR capable of interaction with MHC molecules, but tolerant to self-peptides, survive the selection process. Many newly formed thymocytes are subject to negative selection, probably as a consequence of several different sets of circumstances. Some are eliminated because the TCR is abnormal (the recombination process resulted in out-of-frame rearrangements), or because the resulting TCR is unable to interact with MHC molecules. A small percentage of double-positive thymocytes are thought to die from apoptosis because their interaction with the MHC peptide complexes is too strong (they would be activated by self-peptides). The recognition of self-peptides in the thymus is likely to involve both thymic-derived peptides and peptides of extrathymic origin. During the time T cells are differentiating,

extensive development of most other tissues is taking place; hence, large numbers of cells are undergoing apoptotic death. This results in the extensive release of self-antigens, which are eventually captured by the thymic epithelial cells and presented to the pre-T cells in the context of self-MHC. The thymocytes whose TCR interact strongly with MHC-peptide complexes receive apoptotic signals and are eliminated. This negative selection process is critical to the development of self-tolerance during embryonic differentiation.

Positive selection results in the selection of thymocytes that express a TCR capable of interaction with MHC molecules but fails to recognize the self-peptides associated to the MHC molecules. If the TCR is MHC class I restricted, CD8 must also associate with MHC class I. The CD8-TCR-MHC class I interaction results in the activation of repressor genes that turn off CD4 expression. Conversely, double-positive T cells that have MHC class II–restricted TCR engage CD4, and the expression of CD8 is turned off. The single positive CD4 or CD8 T cells emerging from the medulla leave the thymus and colonize the peripheral lymphoid organs.

The positive signal delivered to the double-positive thymocytes through these TCR-MHC interactions involves CD45 and the lymphocyte-specific tyrosine kinase, p56lck. Both CD4 and CD8 T cells utilize these molecules. As the TCR interacts with MHC, the phosphatase activity of CD45 is upregulated, and ZAP70 is activated. Both activities contribute to the dephosphorylation of p56lck, which becomes activated. The activation of p56lck is critical for further T cell differentiation and proper expression of MHC molecules.

Stage five: Continuing differentiation in the periphery

Several factors may contribute to the supply of T cells in adult life: generation in the thymus, extrathymic differentiation, and the fact that memory T cells are long lived and survive for decades.

UNCONVENTIONAL T CELLS

The thymus also gives rise to T cell populations, collectively referred to as unconventional T cells, which do not fit into the established categories of "adaptive" and "innate" immune cells. In contrast to the TCR gene rearrangements previously described, the TCRs expressed by unconventional T cells have undergone limited gene rearrangement. These TCRs recognize ubiquitous antigens such as pathogen-associated molecular patterns (PAMPs) or self antigens presented in the nonclassical MHC molecules (MHC-Ib molecules, MR1, CD1d). The innate-like properties of these T cell subsets, such as limited repertoire and rapid activation, suggest that they represent a vestige of the primordial adaptive immune systems.

γδ T cells

γδ *T cells* express TCR complexes at their cell surface composed of the TCRδ and TCRγ proteins. They represent only 1%–5% of peripheral blood T cells but constitute the majority of T cells in the mucosa and skin. They are primarily associated with immune homeostasis, wound repair, and clearing of microbial infection. γδ T cells can expand to up to 50% of circulating T cells during microbial infection. They recognize a broad spectrum of antigens; however, the nature of presentation to γδ T cells remains ill defined.

Several differences between αβ and γδ T cell development have been described. γδ T cells do not pass through the critical CD4/CD8 double-positive stage of the αβ T cells, they are positively rather than negatively selected on cognate self antigen, and they emigrate the thymus in "waves" of clonal populations, which home to discrete tissues.

There are two major subsets of γδ T cells (Vd1γ/δ and Vd2γ/δ). The Vd1γ/δ T cells express TRDV1 coupled with TCRγ chains containing variable TRGV2 regions and localize to the skin and gut. They recognize lipid and metabolite antigens presented by MHC-like molecules such as CD1c, CD1d, MICA, and ULBP. ULBP and MICA are also stress-induced antigens, and thus, Vd1γδ T cells may respond to antigen-independent host stress signals.

The Vd2γδ T cells express TRDV2, which predominantly pairs with TCRγ chains containing TRGV9. The majority of γδ T cells in peripheral blood circulation are Vd2γδ T cells that primarily recognize bacterial phosphoantigens.

NKT cells

NKT cells express a semi-invariant form of the αβ TCR receptors (TCR2) along with NK cell markers such as CD56 and various KIR molecules. They recognize glycolipid antigens presented in association with CD1. NKT cells are thought to play an important role in tumor immunity and immunoregulation. NKT cells can be separated into two groups based on ligand usage.

GROUP 1 NKT CELLS

Group 1 NKT cells recognize antigens presented in the context of the molecules CD1a, CD1b, and CD1c. CD1a is expressed at high levels in the skin epidermis and on Langerhans cells, CD1b on mDCs, and CD1c on B cells. CD1d is expressed by a broad variety of APC. The group 1 NKT cells therefore seem to act in cell-type/tissue-specific antigen recognition, perhaps as a means of providing tissue-specific immune responses. Many Group 1 CD1-restricted T cells are autoreactive, with IL-22-producing CD1a autoreactive T cells.

GROUP 2 NKT CELLS

Group 2 NKT cells recognize lipid antigens presented in the context of CD1d molecules and are further divided into two types. Type I CD1d-restricted T cells, also referred to as invariant NKT (iNKT cells), express invariant α-chains and semi-invariant β-chains. iNKT cells are rapidly activated by the bacterial lipid antigen, αGalCer. Activated iNKT cells stimulate several parts of the immune system, particularly dendritic cells (DCs), which in turn promote the accelerated activation of classical CD4+ and CD8+ T cells.

Type II CD1d-restricted NKT cells recognize a wider range of antigens including glycolipids, phospholipids, and hydrophobic peptides. Type II CD1d-restricted NKT cells function as a counterbalance to type I CD1d-restricted NKT cells and express a dominantly immunosuppressive phenotype.

Mucosal-associated invariant T (MAIT) cells

Mucosal-associated invariant T (MAIT) cells develop in the periphery but localize preferentially to the mucosa in the genital tract, lung, and liver. They display invariant TCRα along with a TCRβ chain with limited variability and primarily recognize products of microbial metabolism presented by the MHC-I-like molecule MR1. MAIT cells are believed to function primarily in a negotiator role between microbial flora and the host at the interface separating host and environment. Most of the circulating MAIT cells are CD4 and CD8 double negative, a small percentage of which express low levels of CD8 or CD4. They also express CD161, CD218a (IL-18Rα), and CD26, but lack CD45RA.

T-regulatory cells

CD4+, CD25+ regulatory T cells (Tregs) are also referred to as naturally occurring regulatory T cells. Tregs comprised about 5% of the circulating CD4+ T cells. These cells are thought to be important to autoimmunity by regulating autoreactive T cells in the periphery. The transcription factor **Foxp3** appears to correlate with the Tregs activity.

Unconventional T cells in health and disease

Recently, particular interest has been drawn to invariant T cell populations as possible effectors of vaccine-induced antitumor immunity. Over the course of tumor development, many tumors downregulate both highly immunogenic tumor-associated peptides as well as the peptide-presenting MHC molecules from the surface of tumor cells, and thereby circumvent traditional cell-mediated adaptive immune responses. By recognizing antigens, including nonpeptide antigens, presented in the context of nontraditional MHC-like molecules, unconventional T cells may be less affected by traditional immunoevasive strategies. In addition, expression of invariant/semi-invariant TCR molecules on the many unconventional TCR populations renders them ideal vectors for allogeneic implants. For example, invariant T cell populations such as MAITs and NKTs that recognize tumor-associated antigens in the context of MHC-like molecules (CD1 and MR1) circumvent the challenge of the polymorphic nature of MHC-I and MHC-II molecules.

T LYMPHOCYTE MARKERS

Approximately three-quarters of peripheral blood mononuclear cells are T lymphocytes, and among T lymphocytes, CD4+ cells, often referred to as T helper cells, predominate over CD8+ cells, or cytotoxic T lymphocytes (CTL), by a 2:1 ratio.

- **CD4** is expressed on most thymocytes, two-thirds of T cells, and monocytes. CD4 defines the T-helper cell population and binds to MHC class II antigens during antigen-specific TCR binding. CD4 is also the binding receptor for HIV-1.

- **CD8** is expressed on most thymocytes, a third of T cells, and some NK cells. CD8, which binds to MHC class I antigens during antigen-specific TCR binding, can be expressed as a CD8αβ heterodimer or as a CD8αα homodimer. CD8αβ is only found on αβTCR T cells (cytotoxic T lymphocytes). CD8αα can be found on NK cells, γδT cells, or αβT cells.

Markers associated with T cell downregulation

- **CD3** is first expressed during thymic differentiation and continues to be expressed by all mature T cells in the periphery. CD3 is a complex of five unique, invariant chains (γδεζη) . The cytoplasmic domains of the CD3ζ chain contain ITAM motifs and are responsible for signaling. The ζ chain also associates with CD16 and functions as the signaling domain of that receptor expressed on NK cells. Phosphorylated ITAM motifs of the CD3ζ chain bind to SH2 domains of the intracellular signaling molecules, e.g., ZAP70.

- **CD28** is the dominant co-stimulatory pathway in T cell activation resulting from the interaction of CD28 with the APC antigens CD80 and CD86 (see Chapter 11).

- **CD25** the α chain of the IL-2 receptor is expressed at low levels by about 30% of resting lymphocytes, and is upregulated upon activation. Thus, CD25 expression is an indicator of T cell activation.

- **CD2** engagement by CD58/LFA-3 expressed on an APC and other cells stimulates T cell proliferation and differentiation.

- **CD45** exists in three isoforms (CD45RA, CD45RB, CD45RO), generated by alternate splicing of nuclear RNA. These isoforms share the intracellular domains but vary in their extracellular domains. The ontogenic development of the CD45 isoforms is not clear, but in mature lymphocytes, their expression becomes restricted. CD45RA is expressed both by naive and memory CD4+ T cells. In the case of naive populations, CD45RA is co-expressed with CD62L and CD197/CCR7, while memory T cells either express CD45RA only, or switch from CD45RA to CD45RO. CD45RO+ T cells are considered either as primed T lymphocytes or as memory

T lymphocytes (the expression of this marker seems to be maintained long after the primary response has waned). Other markers associated with mature T cells are shown in Table 10.4.

- **CD71**, the transferrin receptor, is a type II membrane glycoprotein that is upregulated during leukocyte activation. The CD71 homodimer associates with CD3ζ, suggesting a role in signal transduction. The CD71 controlled supply of iron to the cell is important during proliferative responses.

Markers associated with T cell exhaustion

At the time of finalizing this chapter, the 2018 Nobel Prize in Physiology or Medicine was awarded to James P. Allison (CD152/CTLA-4) and Tasuku Honjo (CD279/PD-1) for discoveries that led to the development of cancer therapies that work by harnessing the body's own immune system.

- **Cytotoxic T cell Late Antigen 4 (CTLA-4, CD152)** binds CD80 and CD86, the same ligands as CD28, but with a much higher affinity. Unlike CD28, which is constitutively expressed, CD152/CTLA-4 is upregulated on activated T cells. CD152/CTLA-4 engagement results in downregulation of T cell responses induced by CD28 signaling and thus plays a role in establishing peripheral T cell tolerance.

  Immunotherapies that block CD152/CTLA-4 essentially remove the inhibition of antitumor immune responses by allowing the activation and proliferation of tumor-specific T cells to proceed. Ipilimumab (Yervoy), an anti-CTLA-4 monoclonal antibody, has received U.S. Food and Drug Administration (FDA) approval, and others are in development and may provide the unique benefits of immunotherapy to a broader population of cancer patients.

- The **programmed cell death (PD-1, CD279)** on T and B lymphocytes plays a negative regulatory role in response to antigen and is upregulated on DCs by various inflammatory stimuli. A vast amount of work has demonstrated the antitumor efficacy of CD279/PD-1 blockade. There are currently two FDA-approved anti-PD-1 therapies (nivolumab and pembrolizumab) and others in development.

- **Programed cell death ligand 1 (PD-L1, CD274)** facilitates apoptosis of activated T cells. It also stimulates IL-10 production in human peripheral blood T cells, thus mediating immune suppression. CD274/PD-L1 can also induce T cell dysfunction through a variety of mechanisms such as promoting T cell anergy. CD274/PD-L1 serves as a receptor on cancer cells and can induce intrinsic resistance to T cell killing upon interaction with CD279/PD-1. These CD274/PD-L1 functions result in a "molecular shield" on cancer cells that prevents effector immune cells from killing cancer cells. CD274/PD-L1 immunotherapeutics are in development.

- **Lymphocyte activation gene 3 (LAG3;CD223)** is in many ways a T cell activation marker, expressed

Table 10.4 **Mature T cell subsets**

Population	Phenotype
Total T cells	CD3+
CD4 T cells	CD3+ CD4+ CD8-
CD4 Naïve	CD3+ CD4+ CD8- CD45RA+ CCR7+
CD4 Central memory	CD3+ CD4+ CD8- CD45RA- CCR7+
CD4 Effector memory	CD3+ CD4+ CD8- CD45RA- CCR7-
CD4 Terminally differentiated effector memory (TEMRA)	CD3+ CD4+ CD8- CD45RA+ CCR7-
CD8 T cells	CD3+ CD4- CD8+
CD4 Naïve	CD3+ CD4- CD8+CD45RA+ CCR7+
CD4 Central memory	CD3+ CD4- CD8+CD45RA- CCR7+
CD4 Effector memory	CD3+ CD4- CD8+ CD45RA- CCR7-
CD4 Terminally Differentiated effector memory (TEMRA)	CD3+ CD4- CD8+ CD45RA+ CCR7-

on both CD4 and CD8 T cells 3–4 days post-activation. It is also expressed on NK cells and is required to control overt activation and prevent the onset of autoimmunity. Persistent antigen exposure in the tumor microenvironment results in sustained CD223/LAG3 expression, contributing to a state of exhaustion resulting in impaired proliferation and cytokine production. The synergy between CD223/LAG3 and CD279/PD-1 observed in multiple settings, coupled with the contrasting intracellular cytoplasmic domain of CD223/LAG3 as compared with other immune regulators, highlights the potential uniqueness of CD223/LAG3. Several CD223/LAG3-targeted therapies are in development.

- **Inducible T cell Costimulator (ICOS; CD278)** is weakly expressed on naive T cells and is quickly upregulated on activated T cells. Constitutive expression of CD278/ICOS by Treg$_s$ has also been reported. CD275 (ICOS ligand; ICOS-L) is expressed by professional APC. The ICOS-ICOS-L pathway provides a key co-stimulatory signal for T cell proliferation and T cell survival. CD278/ICOS regulates development and response of T follicular helper (Tfh), Th1, Th2, and Th17 cells and plays roles in the maintenance of memory effector T cells and Tregs homeostasis. Given its role in sustaining T cell activation and effector functions, targeting ICOS-ICOS-L potentially represents a feasible approach to enhance antitumor immunity.
- **Tumor necrosis factor receptor superfamily, member 4 (TNFRSF4; CD134; OX40)** is a member of the TNFR superfamily of receptors. CD134/OX40 is a secondary co-stimulatory immune checkpoint molecule, expressed following 24–72 hours of activation. Expression of CD134/OX40 is dependent on full activation of the T cell; without CD28, expression of CD134/OX40 is delayed and of fourfold lower levels.
- **T-cell immunoglobulin and mucin-domain containing-3 (TIM-3, CD366)** is a negative regulator of antitumor immunity. It is preferentially expressed on intra-tumoral T cells and can both enhance and inhibit proximal signaling in T cells, depending on the cellular context. Therefore, the distinctive expression and intracellular signaling suggest a great potential for targeting CD366/TIM-3 alone or in combination with current CD279/PD-1 and CD152/CTLA-4-based immunotherapy of cancer.

B CELLS

B cells are the cellular mediators of humoral immune responses and are identified by the presence of surface immunoglobulin (sIg). After antigenic stimulation, B cells differentiate into plasma cells that secrete large quantities of immunoglobulins. Within a single cell or a clone of identical cells, the antibody binding sites of membrane and secreted immunoglobulins are identical.

B lymphopoiesis

B lymphopoiesis occurs exclusively in the bone marrow (Figure 10.9). B lymphocytes are made continuously throughout life in the human bone marrow. The microenvironment in the bone marrow is composed of stromal cells, extracellular matrix, cytokines, and growth factors, which are critical for proliferation, differentiation, and survival of early lymphocyte and B-lineage precursors.

B lymphopoiesis requires three transcription factors, E proteins (E2A and EBF), and Pax5. E2A and EBF act in concert to drive the differentiation of common lymphocyte precursors toward the B-lineage pathway by activating B cell–restricted gene expression and μIgH chain gene rearrangements. Commitment to the B cell lineage is orchestrated by Pax5, which simultaneously represses the transcription of B cell lineage-inappropriate and activates the expression of B cell lineage-specific genes. Terminal differentiation of B cells to memory cells and plasma cells depends on the transcriptional repressor Blimp-1.

The relative proportion of precursor B cells in the bone marrow remains constant throughout life in a healthy individual. Pre-B-I cells comprise about 5%–10% of the total. Pre-B-II cells represent 60%–70%, while the remaining 20%–25% are immature B cells. Immature B cells then migrate to the spleen where they go through transitional stages before final maturation.

B lymphopoiesis can be divided into distinct stages based on the sequential expression, or loss, of cell surface or intracellular proteins, and immunoglobulin (Ig) gene rearrangement. Deregulation of B lymphopoiesis can lead to autoimmunity, leukemia, or lymphoma. The most critical aspects in B lymphopoiesis are the Ig gene rearrangement and expression of the pre-B cell receptor (pre-BCR) and the BCR. Pre-BCR and BCR receptor signaling plays a crucial role at developmental checkpoints

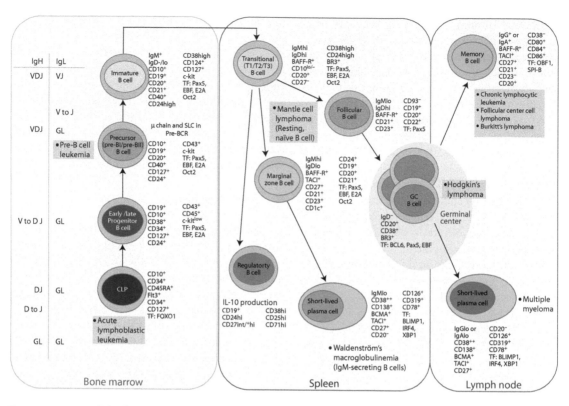

Figure 10.9 Model of B-cell lymphopoiesis. B-lymphopoiesis and maturation in the bone marrow, spleen, and lymph nodes. For each B-cell subset, surface expression of immunoglobulin (Ig) or key feature of the subset is indicated along with the typical phenotype and associated transcription factors (TF). Overall, steps of the rearrangement of V, D, and J-gene segments, or expression from the germline (GL), of the immunoglobulin heavy-chain genes (IgH) and light-chain genes (IgL) are shown. From the common lymphoid progenitor (CLP), rearrangement of the IgH D to J gene segments from the GL initiates the progenitor B cell stage. The completion of the IgH D to J rearrangement marks the transition from progenitor B cells to precursors (Pre-B) B cells. Pre-B-I B cells express a pro-B cell receptor (BCR), while pre-B-II express cytoplasmic IgHμ chain and the pre-BCR with a surrogate light chain (SLC). After IgL chain rearrangement, the complete BCR is expressed as IgM on the immature B cells, which migrate to the spleen. Selection and maturation of immature B cells occurs through a series of transitional B cells, (T1/T2/T3). Transitional B cells differentiate into circulating follicular B cells and give rise to germinal center B cells, which undergo isotype switching and affinity maturation, to generate high-affinity, class-switched plasma and memory B cells. A small percentage of transitional B cells differentiate into marginal zone B cells, which are uniquely located in the marginal zone of the spleen. Once activated, marginal zone B cells become short-term plasma cells. Finally, regulatory B cells are hypothesized to be generated in response to environmental stimuli or may develop from a dedicated lineage of B cells. Pathologies associated with B-cell subsets are described in gray boxes. (Adapted from Pieper, K. et al., *J. Allergy Clin. Immunol.*, 131, 959–971, 2013.)

such as negative selection, anergy, receptor editing, and positive selection.

PROGENITOR B CELLS (PRO-B CELLS)

In the bone marrow, the earliest cells in B lymphopoiesis are referred to as the progenitor B cells (pro-B cells), which express CD117/c-kit, CD135/Flt3, TdT, RAG, CD34, and CD45RA, but no lineage-specific markers. Coincident with the onset of RAG expression, μIg heavy (μIgH) gene rearrangements begin. The D to J gene segment rearrangement on both alleles is initiated, but not completed, at the pro-B cell stage. At this stage, the pro-B cell is not fully committed to the B-cell lineage.

Like TCR gene rearrangement, Ig genes rearrangement occurs in an ordered fashion. μIgH genes are the first to be rearranged, followed by Igκ, and, finally, by Igλ. μIgH variable region exons are assembled from component V, D, and J gene segments; Igκ and Igλ light-chain variable regions are assembled from component V and J gene segments. Most B cells express the functional product of only one IgH allele and one IgL allele as a consequence of allelic exclusion, as discussed in Chapter 7. Cells in which the first V(D)J rearrangement at the μIgH, Igκ, or Igλ locus is nonproductive will proceed with V to (D)J rearrangement of the second allele.

B-CELL PRECURSORS

B-cell precursors (pre-B cells) exist in two distinct stages, pre-B-I and pre-B-II. The pre-B I cells still express CD117/c-kit and have a unique capacity for self-renewal (extended proliferation at the same stage of differentiation). During the pre-B-I stage, the μIgH D to J gene segment rearrangement on both alleles is completed. Rearrangement of the V region gene segments has been initiated, but the immunoglobulin heavy chain (μIgH chain) is not yet expressed in the cytoplasm. Pre-B-I cells have downregulated TdT and CD34. They express genes specific to the B-lineage (CD19, CD20, CD79a/Igα, CD79b/Igβ) and are committed to the B-lineage. A surrogate light chain associates with other proteins to form the pro-B cell receptor that is expressed on the surface or the pre-B-I cells.

Pre-B-II cells downregulate CD117/c-kit and upregulate CD2, CD25, and CD72. In addition, μIgH rearrangement is completed during the pre-B-II stage. The resultant VDJ variable region exon is then linked to the μ constant region exon via RNA splicing to form a cytoplasmic μIgH chain. The product of a functionally rearranged μIgH chain from the first allele prevents initiation of V to DJ gene rearrangement on the second allele, and RAG expression is terminated. The expression of the μIgH chain on the cell membrane is required for allelic exclusion to occur.

Successful VDJ rearrangements of the μIgH chain gene result in the high levels of cytoplasmic μIgH chain expression. The μIgH chain associates with surrogate light chains and the signaling components CD79a (Igα) and CD79b (Igβ) to form the pre-BCR, which is expressed on the membrane of the pre-B-II cells. The physiological role of surrogate light chains seems to be that of a stabilizer, protecting nascent μIgH chains from degradation, until light-chain synthesis is turned on. The expression of surrogate light chains is critical to normal B-cell development. Patients defective in the genes coding for surrogate light chains have a severe form of B-cell deficiency.

Although the pre-BCR is only transiently expressed on the pre-B cell, signaling through the pre-BCR is essential for the selection, proliferation, and differentiation of pre-B cells. Pre-BCR expression serves as a checkpoint that monitors for functional μIgH chain rearrangement, and triggers clonal expansion and developmental progression of surface IgM$^+$ pre-B cells. The pre-BCR is not activated in an antigen-specific manner, but via interaction with stromal cells. Pre-BCR signaling regulates the pre-B cell proliferative phase by a negative feedback mechanism. The interaction of the surrogate light chains with complementary proteins induces internalization of the pre-BCR and subsequent suppression of surrogate light-chain synthesis, followed by re-expression of the *RAG* genes. During the second wave of *RAG* expression, further arrangements of the μH loci are prevented, as the chromatin is no longer accessible to RAG. Because these pre-B-II cells are cycling, they are also referred to as large pre-B cells. After cellular proliferation has subsided, the pre-B-II cells are also referred to as small pre-B cells. These cells no longer express the pre-BCR and μIgH chain accumulates in the cytoplasm. The small pre-B-II cells express CD2, CD22, CD45RA, and MHC class II. The second wave of RAG expression occurs in the small pre-B-II cells and promotes the rearrangement of the immunoglobulin light (IgL) chain ($V_L J_L$), resulting in synthesis of IgL chains. Only cells that fail to generate a productive Igκ chain will go on to rearrange the Igλ locus. Once a productive IgL is formed, it will pair with the previously rearranged μIgH chain to create a mature BCR. After a complete BCR is expressed, the cell is considered an immature B cell.

In the bone marrow, the majority of the cells are CD19$^+$, membrane IgM$^+$, characteristics shared by pre-B-II cells and immature B cells. The pre-BCR and BCR control cell fate decisions at specific antigen-independent checkpoints. There are many similarities as well as significant differences in the signaling by the pre-BCR and the BCR. Notably, the pre-BCR is able to stimulate proliferative expansion in a cell-autonomous fashion. Activation signals from the pre-BCR and BCR involve the phosphorylation of ITAMs present in

Ig-α and Ig-β. This complex contains three classes of activated protein tyrosine kinases (PTKs)—Src family kinase, Lyn, the Syk/Zap70 kinase, and the Tec-family kinase (Btk); as well as other proteins including the adapter molecule, phosphoinositide 3-kinase (PI3K), and phospholipase C-γ2.

B-cell maturation

Immature B cells are characterized as resting cells (not cycling) that express CD19, sIgM, CD79a/Igα, and CD79b/Igβ, but are sIgD$^-$. Like the small pre-B-II cells, RAG-2 expression is high in the immature B cells, indicating that additional IgL gene rearrangement can still occur. Final differentiation occurs when RAG expression is terminated.

Immature B cells leave the bone marrow and emigrate to the spleen where they advance through several developmental stages, including negative and positive selection, before final maturation. Signaling through the BCR plays a key role in inducing the elimination of self-reactive B cells during the final stages of differentiation (negative selection). Immature and transitional B cells expressing BCR reactive with self-antigens are either eliminated by selective death or become anergic and thus fail to progress through subsequent developmental stages. Cell fate, death (by apoptosis), or anergy are determined by the strength of the BCR signal, ligand density, as well as other factors. This negative selection in the immature B cells may occur in the bone marrow or in the periphery (spleen). Positive selection requires that a subthreshold survival signal be generated through the BCR and leads to the survival and subsequent development of transitional B cells. Failure to receive such antiapoptotic signals will result in cell death; positive selection occurs in the periphery.

The immature B cells are CD19+, sIgM^{high}, sIgD^{low}, CD21$^-$, CD23$^-$. They most likely undergo clonal deletion or anergy as evident by their lack of expression of survival factor, Bcl-2, and high expression of the pro-apoptotic molecule, CD95 (FAS). The surviving cells display a phenotype close to that of a mature B cell, CD19+, sIgM^{high}, sIgD^{low}, CD21^{high}, and CD23^{high}. BCR signaling of these cells results in extensive proliferation.

Mature B cells express phenotype CD19, sIgM, and sIgD. These transitional B cells (T1, T2/T3) further develop into circulating follicular B cells in the lymph nodes. About 80% of adult B cells are found in the lymph node follicle (follicular B cells), and this population gives rise to germinal center B cells, memory B cells, and plasma cells (terminally differentiated). A small percentage of transitional B cells will differentiate into the marginal zone (MZ) B cells, which is uniquely located in the MZ of the spleen. These cells exist in a pre-activated state, enabling them to respond rapidly.

B-cell activation

Activation of B cells can occur through two different routes based on the type of stimulating antigen. T cell or thymus-independent (T-independent) antigens are non-protein antigens such as lipids, nucleic acids, and polysaccharides. In comparison, T cell or thymus-dependent (T-dependent) antigens are protein antigens that induce long-lasting responses that involve both B and T cells.

MZ B cells are key players in T-independent responses and are responsible for early antibody production in primary T-dependent responses. MZ B cells can become activated through toll-like receptors or through the direct cross-linking of BCR by polysaccharide antigens. Since activation occurs without T cell help, these responses do no induce efficient isotype switching or affinity maturation. These short-lived plasma cells usually produce IgM antibodies, and the majority will die off within 2–3 weeks. Typically, MZ B cells display a phenotype of sIgM^{high}, sIgD^{low}, CD19+, CD21+, and CD23$^-$. Because of their role in rapid antibody production and the fact that they express toll-like receptors, MZ B cells are thought to be cells that bridge the innate and the adaptive immune systems.

Activation of follicular B cells by T-dependent antigens is initiated by the binding of antigen to the surface BCR or Ig receptor leading to expression of co-stimulatory molecules on the B cells and antigen-BCR internalization. Protein antigens are processed within the B cell and will be presented on MHC class II molecules on the cell surface, which will lead to activation of cognate T cells. This B- and T cell interaction leads to the transcription of Ig genes and the production of cytokines that will induce B- and T cell proliferation. Clustering of proliferating B cells at borders of B-cell follicles and T cell zones in the lymph nodes and spleen form germinal centers (GCs). The formation of each GC contains cells from a single or a few antigen-specific B-cell clones. Within these temporary structures, germinal center B cells undergo isotype switching and affinity maturation to generate high-affinity, class-switched plasma cells, and memory B cells. This generation of memory B cells and plasma cells results in long-lived humoral immunity. Typically, GC B cells display a phenotype of CD20$^+$, CD38$^+$, BR3$^+$, and IgD$^-$.

Isotype switching and affinity maturation. Around birth, mature, resting B cells co-express sIgM and sIgD on their membranes. The sIgM and sIgD expressed on individual B-cell clones have the same antigenic specificity. These mature, naive B lymphocytes home to secondary lymphoid organs where, upon antigenic challenge, they downmodulate sIgD and, less constantly, sIgM. Activated B cells undergo subsequent heavy-chain constant region gene rearrangements or isotype switching by a process called class switch recombination (Figure 7.3). Hence, the same variable region can be associated with a different heavy-chain isotype (IgG, IgE, or IgA). The resultant sIg of different isotypes are expressed on nonoverlapping B-cell subsets, sometimes in association with sIgM. In addition to isotype switching, activated B cells undergo antibody affinity maturation by a process called somatic hypermutation, which results in the emergence and selection of B-cell clones producing antibodies of similar specificity but higher affinity, as discussed in Chapters 7 and 12.

Memory B cells. It is currently unknown how some GC B cells are selected to differentiate into either memory B cells or long-lived plasma cells. Memory B cells return into circulation and are distributed throughout lymphoid tissues, bone marrow, mucosal epithelium, and spleen, and may return to sites of infection to become tissue-resident memory B cells.

Some studies have shown that antigen-specific memory B cells can persist for decades without the presence of cognate antigen. Human memory B cells are characterized by CD27 expression and typically display a phenotype of CD20$^+$, CD38$^-$, CD27$^+$, CD80$^+$, CD84$^+$, and CD86$^+$. Since these cells have high affinity for antigen and elevated expression of co-stimulatory molecules, once reactivated by antigen encounter and T cell help, they exhibit a greater capacity to rapidly proliferate and differentiate into antibody-secreting cells compared to naïve B cells. The hyper-response of memory B cells following reexposure to antigen results in the generation of high titers of high-affinity antibodies and promotes clearance of the antigen.

Plasma cells. Long-lived plasma cells are terminally differentiated cells that function to secrete large amounts of immunoglobulins and can persist for years. Most plasma cells home to the bone marrow, and, to a lesser extent, in the spleen, and peripheral tissues. Specialized niches of the BM allow the long-term survival of plasma cells, and the cellular population of plasma cells is hypothesized to be maintained through the continuous, antigen-driven differentiation of memory B cells. Plasma cells typically display a phenotype of CD20$^-$, CD38^{high}, CD27^{high}, CD138$^+$, TACI$^+$ and/or BCMA$^+$, CD126$^+$, CD319$^+$, and CD78$^+$.

Regulatory B cells. Recently, suppressive B cells were identified that negatively regulate immune responses, known as regulatory B cells (Bregs). The main function of Breg is the suppression of pro-inflammatory lymphocytes such as Th1 cells, cytotoxic CD8 T cells, and pro-inflammatory monocytes and dendritic cells through the production of cytokines IL-10, TGF-ß, and IL-35. Bregs are hypothesized to be generated in response to environmental stimuli, rather than develop from a dedicated lineage of B cells. Immature B cells, mature B cells, and short-term plasma cells were all shown to be able to differentiate into IL-10-producing Breg cells. Various phenotypes of Bregs were published and display a phenotype of CD19$^+$, CD24^{high}, CD27$^{int/+/high}$, CD38^{high}, CD25^{high}, and CD71^{high}.

Markers associated with B cell activation and proliferation

The **B cell receptor (BCR)** complex is constituted by sIg associated with CD79a/Igα) and CD79b/Igβ (Figure 10.3). Antigen recognition occurs though the sIg, whereas Igα and Igβ mediate signal transduction. After antigen binding, the recruitment of tyrosine kinase to the cytoplasmic domains of Igα and Igβ initiates the activation cascade. The major kinase that is recruited to the BCR complex is Bruton's tyrosine kinase (Btk). Congenital Btk deficiency is associated with a block in B-cell differentiation, demonstrating that signals delivered through the fully assembled BCR and associated kinases are necessary for B cell development during ontogeny.

Three cellular receptors of the TNFR family are involved in proliferation and maturation of B cells: the B cell maturation antigen (BCMA), the transmembrane activator and calcium modulator and cyclophilin ligand interactor (TACI), and the BLyS receptor 3 (BR3). BAFF (for B-cell activating factor) and a proliferation inducing ligand (APRIL) are soluble ligands belonging to a TNF subfamily that interacts with those receptors.

BAFF has a co-stimulatory effect in B-cell activation but alone is not sufficient to induce B-cell activation. Co-stimulation through BAFF allows a greater proportion of cells to be activated and induces anti-apoptotic members of the Bcl-2 gene family, which allows for longer post-activation survival.

- **CD19** is expressed on all B-lineage cells with the exception of plasma cells. It is also found on most malignancies of B-lymphocyte origin. CD19 contains potential phosphorylation sites in the cytoplasmic domain and associates with CD21 and other molecules. The formation of this molecular complex lowers the activation threshold for the BCR and results in early activation events such as modulating Ca^{2+} influx.
- **CD21** is expressed at high levels on mature, resting B cells but is lost upon activation. The cytoplasmic domain of CD21 contains potential phosphorylation sites. CD21 is also known as CR2, because this molecule functions as a receptor for the iC3b and C3d fragments of complement. The interaction between antigen bound C3d and CD21 can deliver a co-stimulating signal to the B cell that results in amplification of humoral immune responses. CD21 is also the receptor used by the Epstein–Barr virus to infect B lymphocytes.
- **CD20** is an antigenic cluster associated with the first membrane marker to be found on a developing B lymphocyte. It is detectable on pre-B lymphocytes expressing cytoplasmic μ chains and remains expressed during maturation on the mature B lymphocyte, but it is not expressed on plasma cells. It is a highly unusual molecule in that it crosses the membrane several times and both the N-terminal and the C-terminal residues are intracellular. The extracellular domain contains only 42 amino acids. The carboxyl terminal end has 15 serine and threonine residues, the hallmark of a protein susceptible to phosphorylation by protein kinases, which occurs after mitogenic stimulation. This suggests that CD20 may play an important role in the activation and proliferation of mature B lymphocytes.

- **CD38** disappears from the membrane of memory B cells differentiated in the mantle zone of the lymph nodes, which subsequently leave the nodes as $CD20^+$, $CD38^-$ memory B cells, and migrate to different lymphoid organs. Antibodies to CD38 induce T- and B-cell proliferation.
- **CD80 (B7.1) and CD86 (B7.2)**, expressed at low levels on resting B cells and other APCs, are upregulated upon activation. They bind CD28 and CTLA-4, expressed on T lymphocytes.
- **CD40** interacts with the CD154 (CD40 ligand, CD40L). CD40 is expressed on all mature B cells but is absent on plasma cells. It is also present on some epithelial, endothelial, DC, and activated monocytes. The interaction of CD40 and its co-receptor expressed on helper T cells is required for B lymphocyte maturation and isotype switching. The interaction of CD40:CD154 results in signaling, which leads to the upregulation of antiapoptotic members of the Bcl-2 family increasing cell survival.

Markers associated with B-cell downregulation

- **CD22**, an integral part of the B-cell receptor complex, is first detected in the cytoplasm of pre-B-II cells containing cytoplasmic μ chains. Later, it is found on the surface of 75% of $sIgM^+$ immature B cells, and on 90% of $sIgM^+$, $sIgD^+$ mature, resting cells. In the adult, CD22 is expressed at relatively high levels in tissue B cells (e.g., in the tonsils and lymph nodes) but not in circulating B cells. CD22 is upregulated during activation but is lost in the terminally differentiated plasma cells. CD22 binds to sialylated carbohydrate ligands (e.g., CD45RO) and plays an important regulatory role in B-cell activation by raising the B-cell activation threshold. CD22-deficient mice produce excessive antibody responses to antigen stimulation, as well as increased levels of autoantibodies. In contrast, cross-linking of CD22 suppresses the response of B cells to antigenic stimulation because the intracytoplasmic segment has numerous ITIM motifs that function as docking sites for SHP-1. The binding of SHP-1 to CD22 prevents phosphorylation of the kinases needed for further B-cell activation. In this way, CD19 and CD22 cross-regulate each other because activation through CD22 inhibits the CD19 pathway.

- **CD32 (FcγRII)** is expressed on a range of leukocytes, including monocytes, macrophages, Langerhans cells, granulocytes, B cells, and platelets. CD32 is one of two low affinity IgG Fc receptors, which only binds aggregated IgG. The cytoplasmic domains are associated with SHP-1 and other down-regulatory kinases. Co-ligation of CD32 with membrane Ig (a situation that emerges during the immune response, due to the formation of antigen-antibody complexes in antigen excess, as described in Chapter 12), leads to the binding and activation of SHIP. This is followed by inhibition of inositol 1,4,5 triphosphate (IP3), thus blocking the pathways activated after BCR occupation.
- **CD72** is a type II transmembrane protein of the C-type lectin family. CD72 is expressed on B cells, dendritic cells, and a subpopulation of T cells and macrophages. CD72 contains intracellular ITIMs and is known to have an inhibitory role in B-cell signaling.
- **CD100** has recently been identified as a ligand for CD72. CD100 is expressed at high levels on T cells and at low levels on B cells and dendritic cells, but it is upregulated upon activation.

Other B-cell membrane markers

- **CD10** is expressed on precursor and immature B cells, pre-T cells, neutrophils, and bone marrow stromal cells. CD10 is a commonly used marker for pre-B acute lymphocytic leukemias and some lymphomas. This molecule is a member of the type II membrane metalloproteinases and has neutral endopeptidase activity. CD10 on bone marrow stromal cells appears to regulate B-cell development, since inhibition of CD10 *in vivo* enhances B-cell maturation.
- **CD5** is expressed on most T lymphocytes and on a small subpopulation of B lymphocytes. CD5 is found on most chronic lymphocytic leukemias. However, there is no apparent correlation between disease activity and the numbers of circulating CD5$^+$ cells; thus, the precise role of these cells remains speculative.
- **Major histocompatibility complex (MHC) antigens**, both MHC-I and MHC-II, are expressed at high levels by B lymphocytes. The presence MHC-II enables B lymphocytes to serve as antigen-presenting cells. B lymphocytes are unique in that they express antigen-specific receptors and are capable of antigen presentation.

BIBLIOGRAPHY

Andrews LP, Marciscano AE, Drake CG, Vignali DA. Lag3 (Cd223) as a cancer immunotherapy target. *Immunol Rev*. 2017;276:80–96.

Dong H, Zhu G, Tamada K, Chen L. B7-H1, A third member of the B7 family, co-stimulates T cell proliferation and interleukin-10 secretion. *Nat Med*. 1999;5:1365–1369.

Du W, Yang M, Turner A Xu C, Ferris RL, Huang J, Kane LP, Lu B. TIM-3 as a target for cancer immunotherapy and mechanisms of action. *Int J Mol Sci*. 2017;18(3). doi: 10.3390/ijms18030645

Du W, Yang M, Turner A, et al. Tim-3 as a target for cancer immunotherapy and mechanisms of action. *Int J Mol Sci*. 2017 Mar 16;18(3). doi: 10.3390/ijms18030645

Folkes As, Feng M, Zain Jm, Abdulla F, Rosen St, Querfeld C. Targeting CD47 as a cancer therapeutic strategy: The cutaneous T cell lymphoma experience. *Curr Opin Oncol*. 2018;30: 332–337.

Guilliams M. Dendritic cells, monocytes and macrophages: A unified nomenclature based on ontogeny. *Nat Rev Immunol*. 2014;14:571–578.

Godfrey DI, Le Nours J, Andrews DM et al. Unconventional T cell targets for cancer immunotherapy. *Immunity* 2018;48(3):453–473.

Godfrey DI, Uldrich AP, McCluskey J et al. The burgeoning family of unconventional T cells. *Nat Immunol*. 2015;16:1114–1123.

Melchers F. Checkpoints that control B cell development. *J Clin Invest*. 2015;125:2203–2210.

Pieper K, Grimbacher B, Eibel H. B-cell biology and development. *J Allergy Clin Immunol*. 2013;131:959–971.

Schattgen SA, Thomas PG. Bohemian T cell receptors: Sketching the repertoires of unconventional lymphocytes. *Immunol Rev*. 2018;284: 79–90.

Vermijlen D, Gatti D, Kouzeli A et al. γδ T cell responses: How many ligands will it take till we know? *Semin Cell Dev Biol*. 2018;84:75–86. doi: 10.1016/j.semcdb.2017.10.009

11

Cell-mediated immunity

JOSÉ C. CRISPÍN AND GABRIEL VIRELLA

INTRODUCTION

Adaptive immune responses have been traditionally divided into humoral (antibody-mediated) and cellular (cell-mediated) immune responses. Humoral (B cell–mediated) immune responses function predominantly in the elimination of soluble antigens and the destruction of extracellular microorganisms, while cell-mediated (T cell) immunity is more important for the elimination of intracellular organisms (such as viruses). Both humoral and cellular immunity are coordinated by T lymphocytes, and there is significant interplay between these two arms of the immune response. The humoral response to proteins depends on "help" provided by T lymphocytes in the form of cytokines and other ancillary signals, and cell-mediated immunity involves T cell–directed recruitment and activation of multiple types of immune cells for antigen clearance. In this chapter, we discuss how T lymphocytes become activated after encountering antigen, how they differentiate into effector cells, and the multiple consequences of this effector response in coordinating antigen clearance. We also discuss how T-cell activation can culminate in a memory immune response that can persist for the lifetime of an individual, and how T-cell subsets also play central roles in immunoregulation.

T-CELL ACTIVATION

Initial recognition of antigen-derived peptides by T-cell receptors

A major distinction between antigen recognition by T versus B lymphocytes is the inability of T cells to recognize free, soluble antigen through the T-cell receptor (TCR), as B cells do via surface immunoglobulin. T cells recognize antigen-derived peptides associated to self major histocompatibility complex (MHC) molecules (see Chapters 3 and 4), but the tertiary structure of these peptides often has no resemblance to their structure within the native molecule, because they have been generated by processing in antigen-presenting cells (APCs). As a result, T and B lymphocytes bind antigenic determinants that are structurally distinct.

The antigen-derived peptides that fit into the binding sites of class I or class II MHC molecules interact with TCRs of different T-cell subpopulations. MHC-II/peptide complexes expressed on the surface of APCs are recognized by the T-cell receptor of $CD4^+$ lymphocytes, while MHC-I/peptide complexes, expressed by a large variety of cells, are recognized by the T-cell receptor of $CD8^+$ lymphocytes. This dichotomy of recognition between CD4 and CD8 T cells is due to the specific interaction of the CD4 and CD8 coreceptors with MHC class II and class I, respectively. This trimolecular complex of the TCR/MHC-peptide and CD4 or CD8 coreceptor form a focal point of contact between the T cell and the APC. The CD4 molecule on the lymphocyte membrane interacts with nonpolymorphic areas of the class II MHC molecules on the APC, and CD8 interacts with analogous regions of MHC class I. This interaction stabilizes the contact between the MHC and the TCR but is also involved in signal transduction in the early stages of T lymphocyte activation, as discussed later in this chapter.

In addition to the TCR-coreceptor/MHC interaction, other interactions between T cells and APCs are necessary for the proper T-cell engagement that is required for full T-cell activation and differentiation. These additional interactions include both adhesive molecular contacts that strengthen the bond between T cells and APCs, and costimulatory molecules that convey positive and negative signals and thus modulate T-cell activation in a qualitative manner. Both of these interactions are described in detail in the next sections.

Adhesive interactions between T cells and APC

Activation of a T lymphocyte requires a close and prolonged interaction with an APC. For this to occur, the natural electrostatic repulsions between two cell membranes must be overcome. The interaction between the TCR and the MHC-peptide is not sufficient to keep the cells together, so other molecular interactions between the cells are required to stabilize their contact. Adhesion molecules fulfill this requirement. Two sets of adhesion molecules (CD2/CD58 and LFA-1/ICAM-1) play a primary role in T lymphocyte–APC adhesion. CD2 molecules, expressed by essentially all T lymphocytes, bind to CD58 (LFA-3) molecules expressed by most cells. The initial interaction between the MHC-peptide complex and the TCR causes a conformational change on the CD2 molecule that increases its affinity for CD58 on the APC. In addition to its role in stabilizing cell-cell contact, the interaction between CD2 and CD58 delivers an activating signal to the T lymphocyte.

The leukocyte function antigen-1 (LFA-1), an integrin that interacts with the intercellular adhesion molecule 1 (ICAM-1), also undergoes conformational changes in the early stages of T-cell activation. Both APCs and T cells express LFA-1 and ICAM-1, and the heterotypic interaction between pairs of these molecules results in the formation of strong intercellular bonds. The strengthening of the adhesive interaction between ICAM-1 and LFA-1 occurs due to contact of the TCR with MHC-peptide complexes and is referred to as integrin "inside-out signaling" (Figure 11.1).

The establishment of APC-T lymphocyte interactions brings the membranes of the two cells into close proximity (immunological synapse, see Chapter 4). Such close contact is critical for the delivery of additional activating signals to the T cell and allows for high local concentrations and maximal effects of the interleukins and cytokines released by APCs and T lymphocytes.

Costimulatory interactions between T cells and APCs

The recognition of antigen, presented as an MHC-peptide complex, is central to T-cell activation, because it provides specificity to the immune response. The aforementioned adhesive molecules stabilize the T cell–APC interaction and contribute to intracellular signaling. However, an additional element, called costimulatory signal, is necessary for T-cell activation to occur. Costimulatory signals not only allow T-cell activation but also modulate the activation process. A large number of costimulatory (and coinhibitory) molecules exist on APCs that have corresponding receptors on T cells (Table 11.1). Through their differential expression, APCs are able to convey functional messages to the T cell that determine the qualitative characteristics of the effector T cell that will arise from the process of antigen presentation.

The first characterized costimulatory interaction is the one between CD28 on T cells and its two ligands, CD80 and CD86, on APCs. CD28 is expressed by all T cells, and its engagement is required for activation of naive CD4 T cells and for IL-2 production. Antigen encountered in the absence of costimulation via CD28 results in the inactivation of the naïve T cell through a process called *anergy*. This is because only activated APCs express CD80 and CD86, and antigen presentation in the absence of these ligands is interpreted by the T cell as a negative signal. The continuous presentation of self antigens in the absence of costimulation inactivates self-reactive T cells. This constitutes a

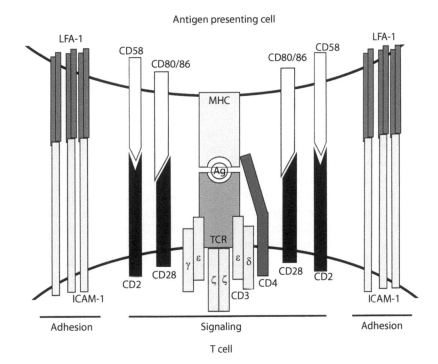

Figure 11.1 The immunological synapse. T cells recognizing an MHC-peptide complex presented by an antigen-presenting cell interact through a variety of membrane proteins, some primarily involved in promoting attachment of the two cells, and others delivering activating signals to the T cell.

mechanism of peripheral tolerance. The presence of infection or other cellular stressors activates APCs and induces their expression of high levels of CD80 and CD86. Activated APCs will then convey a positive pro-inflammatory signal to T cells recognizing infection-associated antigens.

While the CD28-CD80/CD86 interaction is the most important costimulatory pathway for activation of naive T cells, these molecules are but a few in the growing family of costimulatory proteins that function to both positively and negatively regulate T-cell activation (Table 11.1). CD28 is the main costimulatory molecule on resting T cells, but activation induces upregulation of additional members of the costimulatory family, such as inducible costimulator (ICOS) for positive regulation of effector functions, and CD154 (also called CD40 ligand) for promoting the interaction

Table 11.1 Costimulatory receptor-ligand interactions between T cells and APC

T-cell receptor	APC ligand	T-cell effects
CD28	CD80 (B7–1) CD86 (B7–2)	Naïve T-cell activation, proliferation, survival, and memory; IL-2 production
CTLA-4	CD80 (B7–1) CD86 (B7–2)	Inhibition of T-cell proliferation and effector function
CD40L (CD154)	CD40	Costimulation; T-cell:B-cell interactions
ICOS	ICOSL (B7-H2)	CD4 cell proliferation, differentiation, and effector functions; T-cell survival, and memory
PD-1	PD-L1 PD-L2	Inhibition of T-cell proliferation and effector function
CD2	CD48 CD58	Naïve T-cell activation, proliferation

between the T cell and APCs and for promoting T-B cell cooperation. Importantly, there are additional regulatory molecules that are upregulated following activation that serve critical roles in curbing T-cell activation and cytokine production. CTLA-4, upregulated on T cells upon activation, also binds CD80 and CD86, but with higher affinity than CD28. CTLA-4 plays an essential role as a negative regulator of T-cell activation, and its deficiency in mice is associated with severe lymphoproliferation and autoimmune manifestations. CTLA-4 is constitutively expressed by FoxP3$^+$ regulatory T cells, and the phenotype observed in *Ctla4*$^{-/-}$ mice is probably due to the lack of negative regulation in T cells and also to functional defects in regulatory T cells.

Programmed death-1 (PD-1) is another coinhibitory molecule that is upregulated on T cells following activation. It has two known ligands, PD-L1 and PD-L2. Whereas expression of PD-L2 is largely confined to APCs, PD-L1 is also present on the surface of nonimmune cells. Signaling through PD-1 maintains immune tolerance, as its deficiency or blockade unleashes autoimmune phenomena. In some instances, for example in cancer and chronic viral infections, PD-1 signaling inhibits potentially beneficial T-cell effector responses, and its blockade has been used therapeutically to reinvigorate the cellular immune response.

A large number of molecules can act as costimulators or coinhibitors, depending on the cellular context where they are expressed. Because they modulate the immune response in a quantitative and qualitative manner, currently they are the focus of intense research.

Intracellular events associated with CD4 T cell activation

The signals described in the preceding section exert their effects by altering the cell cycle and the gene expression profile of CD4 and CD8 T cells. For this to occur, the events that take place at the cell membrane have to trigger cascades of intracellular signals that deliver the messages at the nuclear level.

The intracellular portion of the TCR heterodimer is very short and lacks signal transduction capacity. However, the TCR is associated with a complex of molecules that transmit its signal when it recognizes an antigen on an APC. This molecular complex consists of four proteins (CD3γ, δ,

ε, and ζ) equipped with immunoreceptor tyrosine-based activation motifs (ITAMs) that contain tyrosine residues (two per ITAM) that become phosphorylated by tyrosine kinases. This represents the initial intracellular event triggered by T-cell antigen recognition.

TCR-initiated signaling can be divided into three distinct phases: proximal, linker/adapter, and distal (Figure 11.2). TCR engagement triggers the proximal phase, which consists on the phosphorylation of the ITAMs of the CD3 complex by the src-related tyrosine kinase Lck, which is noncovalently associated with the cytoplasmic domains of CD4 and of CD8. The cell surface molecule CD45, expressed by all leukocytes, contains an intracytoplasmic phosphatase that in T cells regulates the activity of src family kinases, including Lck. Phosphorylation of the ITAMs located in the CD3ζ subunit allows the coupling of a third tyrosine kinase, called ZAP-70 (for ζ-associated protein of 70 KDa). When ZAP-70 associates with the CD3 complex, Lck stabilizes its activity by phosphorylating it in a key residue.

The second temporal cluster of signaling events involves the mobilization of linker-adapter molecules that form a scaffold that supports the formation of complexes composed of signaling intermediates. This process couples proximal signaling to more distal downstream events. Linker-adapter molecules represent a general feature of signaling cascades in multiple immune and nonimmune cell types. In T cells, two molecules, LAT (for linker of activation T cells) and SLP-76 (SH2-containing leukocyte protein of 76 KDa), serve as substrates of ZAP-70 and form the linker/adapter bridge coupling ZAP-70 activation to downstream events such as MAP (mitogen-activated protein) kinase activation and Ca^{++} release. LAT and SLP-76 are linked to each other via the cellular adaptor GADS, and both also complex with PLC (phospholipase C)-γ, which promotes the release of intracellular calcium stores via hydrolysis of inositol phosphates. LAT and SLP-76 also serve distinct roles in signaling. LAT is coupled to the ras signaling pathway, and SLP-76 is involved in pathways related to cytoskeletal reorganization, integrin activation, and additional kinases that promote downstream events. Thus, LAT and SLP76 play central roles in the overall coordination of TCR-mediated signaling events. Their critical roles have been further established *in vivo*, as mice deficient

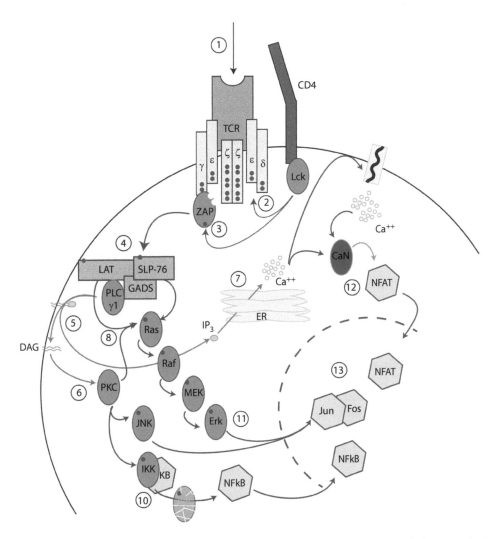

Figure 11.2 T-cell receptor signaling. TCR signaling is divided into three temporal clusters: *A. Proximal events*: (1) Antigen recognition in the context of MHC induces molecular changes in the CD3 molecules and approximates the Lck kinase (bound to CD4 or CD8). (2) Lck phosphorylates the ITAMs in the CD3 subunits. CD3-γ, δ, and ε possess one ITAM per molecule, but CD3ζ contains three. (3) ITAM phosphorylation allows the docking of ZAP-70 and its phosphorylation by Lck. *B. Linker/adapter events*: (4) LAT phosphorylation, by ZAP-70, allows the formation of a signaling hub comprised by LAT, SLP-76, GADS, and other proteins. (5) PLC-γ1 becomes activated and splits PIP_2 into DAG (diacylglycerol) and IP_3 (inositol triphosphate). *C. Distal events*: (6) DAG activates PKC and (7) IP3 induces calcium release from the endoplasmic reticulum (ER). (8) MAP kinases become activated by LAT and PKC. (9) The rise in intracellular calcium induces the opening of calcium channels in the cell membrane. (10) PKC activates IκB kinase (IKK). This causes its degradation and release of NF-κB. (11) MAP kinases activate Jun and Fos that form the heterodimer AP-1. (12) Increased calcium concentration activates calcineurin, a phosphatase that activates NF-AT. (13) The activated transcription factors enter the cell nucleus, where they instruct gene transcription.

in either LAT or SLP-76 have profound defects in T-cell development.

The distal TCR signaling events are directly coupled to transcription factor mobilization in the nucleus. One important distal event is the activation of MAP kinases (e.g., p38, Erk1/2, Jnk) that activate the transcription factors that control the genes that encode effector molecules. Another important distal event is the release of Ca^{++} from intracellular stores via second messengers. One of these messengers is inositol 1,4,5 triphosphate (IP_3), responsible for the additional rise in Ca^{++} that depends on intracytoplasmic stores. The activation of the calcium and calmodulin-dependent serine/threonine phosphatase calcineurin follows this second cytosolic calcium peak. The second critical messenger is diacylglycerol (DAG), responsible for the activation of protein kinase C (PKC). Together, calcium flux and MAP kinase activation lead to mobilization of transcription factors such as NF-AT (nuclear factor of activated T cells), NF-κB, and AP-1 that control transcription of *IL2* and other important genes.

The sequence of signaling events described refers to those directly coupled to the TCR; however, full T-cell activation requires engagement of the CD28 costimulatory receptor. While less is known concerning the precise signaling pathways coupled to CD28, two important processes have been found to be coupled to CD28 ligation. The first process is activation of a PI (phosphoinositol)-3 kinase that leads to mobilization of intracellular Ca^{++} stores. The second CD28-mediated signal target is the serine/threonine kinase AKT that is associated with cell survival and metabolic control.

Transcription factors for T-cell activation

The signaling cascades emanating from TCR and CD28 ligation culminate in transcription factor activation. Transcription factors need to be activated in order to induce the expression of a large number of molecules that control T-cell proliferation and differentiation. These molecules are not expressed by resting T cells, and their genes must be transcribed *de novo*. Multiple genes are expressed in a defined sequence starting minutes after activation of a helper cell and continuing for the next several days. Those genes encode critical transcription factors, enzymes, and substrates involved in proliferation, differentiation, and effector function.

Among the well-characterized transcription factors involved in T-cell activation, nuclear factor κB (NF-κB), nuclear factor of activated T cells (NF-AT), and AP-1 are particularly important for *IL2* transcription and for coordinating the initial events during T-cell activation. NF-κB is a DNA-binding protein found complexed with a specific inhibitor (IκB) in the cytoplasm of resting T lymphocytes. After phosphorylation by IκB kinase (IKK), IκB is destroyed, and the untethered NF-κB is allowed to move into the nucleus where it can bind to promoters of many genes, including those that encode the high-affinity IL-2 receptor (CD25) and Myc. Additionally, NF-κB activation is essential for the prevention of apoptotic cell death. NF-AT1 is almost exclusively found in hematopoietic cells. NF-AT1, along with AP-1, binds specific DNA sequences, found in the 5′ region of cytokine genes. An inactive phosphorylated form of NF-AT is located in the cytoplasm of resting T cells. This form is activated by dephosphorylation catalyzed by calcineurin. AP-1 is a nuclear protein induced when T cells are stimulated via the TCR plus ancillary signals mediated by CD28 cross-linking. It is formed by the association of two proto-oncogene products, c-Fos and c-Jun, whose synthesis is activated by PKC. The full expression of cytokine and cytokine receptor genes is controlled by promoter sequences recognized by NF-κB and/or by the complex of NF-AT-1 and AP-1. Their occupancy by these transcription factors is essential for control of their expression during T-cell activation.

IL-2 synthesis and T-lymphocyte proliferation

Two critical early events in T-cell activation are the transcription of IL-2 and of the high-affinity IL-2 receptor (CD25, or IL-2Rα). The upregulation of *IL2*, an essential step for T-cell proliferation at the onset of the immune response, requires occupancy of its promoter region by NF-AT/AP-1/NF-κB complexes. The expression of the IL-2Rα, in contrast, seems to be primarily controlled by NF-κB. The release of IL-2 into the cellular environment of activated T cells expressing IL-2 receptors has significant biological consequences.

AUTOCRINE AND PARACRINE EFFECTS OF IL-2

IL-2 stimulates lymphocyte proliferation in autocrine and paracrine loops. Released IL-2 binds the IL-2 receptors expressed by the producing cell and by nearby cells. The targets of the paracrine effects of IL-2 are helper T lymphocytes, cytotoxic T lymphocytes, B lymphocytes, and natural killer (NK) cells, all of which express IL-2 receptors.

IL-2 RECEPTOR

The IL-2R expressed by T and B lymphocytes is composed of three chains:

- **IL-2Rα** (CD25) is a 55 KDa polypeptide expressed by regulatory T cells, but not by resting conventional CD4 and CD8 T cells. It is sharply upregulated a few hours after T-cell activation. CD25 greatly increases the affinity of the IL-2 receptor for IL-2. However, it has a short intracytoplasmic domain unable to transduce signals.
- **IL2Rβ** (CD122) is a 70–75 KDa polypeptide expressed by resting T lymphocytes. IL-2Rβ has a long intracytoplasmic tail capable of signal transduction. Engagement of αβ dimers results in the recruitment of γ chains, forming the high-affinity trimeric IL-2R.
- **IL-2Rγ** is the third polypeptide that comprises the trimeric IL-2 receptor expressed after T-cell activation. The γ chain has a long intracytoplasmic segment, for transmission of intracellular signals. This protein subunit is shared by a number of cytokine receptors in addition to the IL-2R, including those for IL-4, IL-7, IL-9, and IL-15. Therefore, it is also called the common γ chain (γc).

CONSEQUENCES OF IL-2 BINDING TO THE IL-2 RECEPTOR

The binding of IL-2 to the trimeric high-affinity IL-2 receptor induces its association to the tyrosine kinase Lck and to JAK family tyrosine kinases. These proximal events lead to phosphorylation of transcription factors of the STAT family, which then dimerize and translocate to the nucleus, where they upregulate the expression of genes that encode cytokine receptors and induce the appearance of cyclins that drive the cell into the cell cycle. In addition, signals transduced via CD28 stabilize IL-2 production by triggering the synthesis of proteins that prolong the half-life of *IL2* mRNA, and induce antiapoptotic members of the Bcl-2 family.

T-LYMPHOCYTE PROLIFERATION AND DIFFERENTIATION

The production of IL-2 and upregulation of the IL-2R promote entry of the T cell into the cell cycle to initiate its proliferation and expansion.

This represents an essential part of the immune response. Antigen-specific T cells are present in very low frequency. In order for them to mount an efficient response, the relatively few cells activated during antigen presentation must expand and become thousands of cells with effector capacities. It is estimated that the initial helper T-lymphocyte population is capable of expanding 100-fold in 6 days, reaching more than 1,000-fold its starting number by day 10, the time that it takes to elicit a detectable primary immune response to most infectious agents. During the expansion phase, T cells undergo dramatic phenotypic changes that result from changes in gene expression. This "effector differentiation" yields short-lived effector cells able to eliminate the pathogen that elicited the immune response and also long-lived memory cells. Pathogen clearance is followed by the elimination of the no longer needed effector cells through apoptosis. In this manner, the immune response dwindles, and the system returns to a steady state. However, a population of antigen-specific memory T cells will remain and will allow the host to rapidly and effectively mount subsequent responses against the same antigen.

T-cell differentiation and effector functions

Antigen recognition and T-cell activation are roughly analogous in CD4 and CD8 T cells.

However, their response to cellular activation differs greatly. Therefore, they are discussed separately.

CD4 T CELLS

T cells that express the coreceptor CD4 have the capacity to engage antigen presented by class II MHC molecules. Because expression of MHC-II is restricted to APCs, CD4 T cells become activated only by these cells (i.e., dendritic cells [DCs] macrophages, B cells). CD4 T cells exert their effector functions by migrating to specific sites, where they modify the function and behavior of other immune and nonimmune cells through direct cell contact and, most importantly, through the secretion of soluble factors known as cytokines (Table 11.2). Signals conveyed by the APC during the priming of naïve CD4 T cells (i.e., the first activation of a CD4 T cell) determine the functional

Table 11.2 Major interleukins and cytokines

Interleukin/cytokine	Predominant source	Main targets	Biological activity
IL-1α,β	Monocytes, macrophages, and other cell types	T and B lymphocytes, dendritic cells, granulocytes, monocytes; nonimmune cells	Highly pro-inflammatory; activates a variety of cell types through the NF-κB pathway
IL-2	Activated T lymphocytes	T and B lymphocytes, NK cells	Promotes T and NK cell proliferation; cofactor for the proliferation of activated B cells; activates NK cells
IL-3	Activated T lymphocytes; mast cells and other myeloid cells	Hematopoietic stem cells; basophils	Hematopoietic growth factor; chemotactic for eosinophils
IL-4	Th2 lymphocytes; mast cells, basophils, and macrophages	Th1 lymphocytes, macrophages, B lymphocytes	Growth and differentiation factor for B lymphocytes; causes the expansion of Th2 lymphocytes (autocrine loop); promotes IgE synthesis
IL-5	Th2 lymphocytes, mast cells, eosinophils	Eosinophils, B lymphocytes	Promotes the growth and differentiation of eosinophils; chemotactic for eosinophils; B-cell differentiation
IL-6	Monocytes, fibroblasts, endothelial cells; also B and Th2 lymphocytes, plasma cells, macrophages	B and T lymphocytes, myeloid cells, nonimmune cells	B-cell differentiation factor; polyclonal B-lymphocyte activator; cofactor for T-lymphocyte differentiation; pro-inflammatory mediator; pyrogen
IL-7	Bone marrow, thymic stromal cells	Pro-B lymphocytes; activated T lymphocytes, thymocytes	Stimulates proliferation of pro-B lymphocytes and activated T lymphocytes; promotes thymic differentiation of T lymphocytes
IL-8 (CXCL8)	Macrophages, activated monocytes, fibroblasts, endothelial cells	Neutrophils, monocytes, T lymphocytes	Neutrophil and T-lymphocyte chemotactic factor
IL-9	Thymocytes, CD4+ Th9 lymphocytes	Mast cells, B lymphocytes, thymocytes	Growth factor

(Continued)

Table 11.2 (*Continued*) Major interleukins and cytokines

Interleukin/ cytokine	Predominant source	Main targets	Biological activity
IL-10	Th2 lymphocytes, T_{reg}, CD8$^+$ T cells	B lymphocytes, Th1 lymphocytes, macrophages, granulocytes	Inhibits cytokine synthesis predominantly in Th1 T lymphocytes and activated APCs; thymocyte growth factor; cytotoxic T-cell and B-cell differentiation factor; chemotactic factor for CD8+ T lymphocytes; mast cell costimulator
IL-11	Bone marrow stromal cells and mesenchymal cells	Hematopoietic stem cells	B-cell differentiation factor; stimulates proliferation and differentiation of hematopoietic stem cells, particularly megakaryocytes
IL-12	Monocytes, macrophages, dendritic cells	Th1 lymphocytes, NK cells	NK cell stimulating factor; Th1 lymphocyte activation and proliferation; enhances the activity of cytotoxic cells; induces interferon-γ production
IL-13	Activated Th2 and CD8$^+$ T lymphocytes, NK cells	B lymphocytes, monocytes, macrophages	Promotes immunoglobulin synthesis; induces the release of mediators from basophils and mast cells; suppresses monocyte/ macrophage functions
IL-14	T lymphocytes	B lymphocytes	B-lymphocyte growth factor
IL-15	Monocytes/ macrophages, microglia	T lymphocytes, monocytes, NK cells	Lymphocyte, mast cell, and NK cell growth factor; maturation factor for NK cells; chemoattractant for T lymphocytes
IL-16	CD8$^+$ T lymphocytes, fibroblasts, eosinophils, mast cells	CD4$^+$ T lymphocytes	Chemotactic and activating factor for CD4$^+$ T lymphocytes, macrophages, and eosinophils
IL-17	Th17 cells, neutrophils	Multiple immune cells; endothelial and epithelial cells	Proinflammatory; promotes osteoclast activation; promotes angiogenesis; chemoattractant for PMN leukocytes; promotes neutrophil maturation

(*Continued*)

Table 11.2 (*Continued*) Major interleukins and cytokines

Interleukin/cytokine	Predominant source	Main targets	Biological activity
IL-18	Dendritic cells, monocytes, macrophages, etc.	T cells and others	Proinflammatory; induces interferon-γ; promotes angiogenesis
IL-21	CD4+ T lymphocytes, T_{FH} cells	NK, T, and B lymphocytes	B-lymphocyte proliferation; T and NK cell costimulation
IL-23	Activated macrophages	T lymphocytes	Induces IL-17 synthesis and maintenance of Th17 cells; induces T-lymphocyte proliferation
IL-27	Activated APCs and mature dendritic cells	Naive CD4+ T lymphocytes, NK cells	Promotes proliferation of naive CD4+ T lymphocytes; activates Th1 responses (induces T-bet and downregulates GATA-3); induces interferon-γ synthesis
IL-32	Activated T and NK lymphocytes	Macrophages	Proinflammatory; induces the production of TNF, IL-8, and MIP-2
GM-CSF	Activated Th17 lymphocytes, macrophages, and endothelial cells; malignant plasma cells	Hematopoietic stem cells	Promotes proliferation and maturation of granulocytes and monocytes; proinflammatory; chemoattractant for neutrophils and eosinophils; activates neutrophils and basophils
IFN α/β	Plasmacytoid dendritic cells, leukocytes, cells infected with virus	Multiple	NK activator, pro-inflammatory, promotes antiviral responses in nonimmune cells
IFNγ	Th1 lymphocytes	Multiple	Macrophage and NK activator
TGFβ	Macrophages, lymphocytes (T_{reg}), endothelial cells	Multiple	Inhibits T, B, and NK cell proliferation; deactivates macrophages; anti-inflammatory and immunosuppressive
TNF	Activated APCs, CD4+ T lymphocytes, NK cells	Multiple	Cytotoxic for tumor cells; induces cachexia; septic shock mediator; B-lymphocyte activator; pro-inflammatory
LT-α (lymphotoxin, TNFβ)	T and B lymphocytes, leukocytes in general	Multiple	Activates B lymphocytes, PMN leukocytes, and NK cells; promotes fibroblast proliferation

characteristics of the effector CD4 T cells that will result from the encounter between the CD4 and the APC. Thus, when a CD4 T cell recognizes an antigen presented by an APC, it will become activated and proliferate, and during that process its progeny will acquire capacities tailored to the antigen that elicited the response. According to those capabilities, in particular, to the cytokine secretion profile that distinguishes them and to the expression of the key transcription factors that define their phenotype, effector CD4 T cells have been classified in the following subsets (Figure 11.3 and Table 11.3):

- **Th1 cells** express the transcription factor T-bet and produce large quantities of interferon (IFN)-γ, tumor necrosis factor (TNF)-α, IL-2, and granulocyte-macrophage colony-stimulating factor (GM-CSF). CD4 T cells differentiate into Th1 cells when IL-12 is produced during their priming. Th1 cells are extremely important in the immune response against intracellular pathogens, for example, *Mycobacterium tuberculosis*. The cytokines they produce activate macrophages, NK cells, and CD8 T cells to boost their effector capacities. Th1 cells are

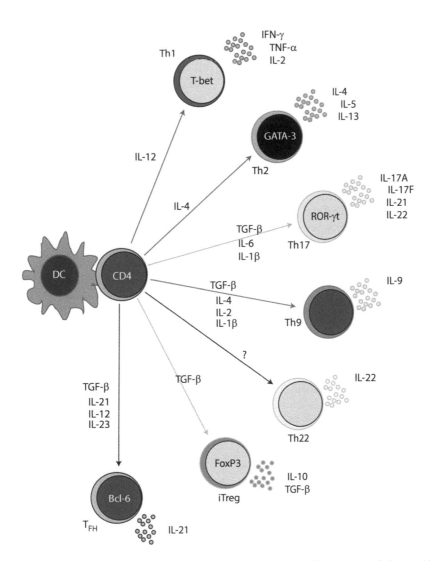

Figure 11.3 **CD4 T cell differentiation into effector subsets.** CD4 T cell priming is followed by the acquisition of different functional capacities that allow CD4 effector T cells to orchestrate immune responses tailored to the eliciting pathogen.

Table 11.3 Types of differentiated CD4 T cells and their properties

Effector cell type	Cytokines produced	Transcription factors	Cellular targets
Th1	IL-2, IFN-γ, TNF-α, IL-3, GM-CSF	T-bet	Macrophages, CD8 T cells
Th2	IL-4, IL-5, IL-13	GATA-3	B cells, mast cells, eosinophils
Th17	IL-17A, IL-17F, IL-22	ROR-γt	Endothelial and epithelial cells
Th9	IL-9	PU.1 (?)	
Th22	IL-22	?	Keratinocytes
Follicular helper T cells (TFH)	IL-21	Bcl-6	B cells
Cytotoxic T lymphocyte (CTL)	IFN-γ, TNF-α, perforin	T-bet, Eomes	MHC Class I+ Infected or tumor targets
Regulatory T cells (Treg)	IL-10, TGF-β	FoxP3	T cells, dendritic cells

highly inflammatory and have been associated with autoimmune diseases such as rheumatoid arthritis and type 1 diabetes and with type IV hypersensitivity reactions.

- **Th2 cells** are generated by the presence of IL-4 and produce IL-4, IL-5, and IL-13. These cells express the transcription factor GATA-3 and exert their function predominantly in the gut and airway epithelia, where they contribute to the maintenance of the mucosal barrier function, to the production of immunoglobulin, and to fight helminths and other extracellular parasitic infections. Th2 cells promote the production of IgE and are thought to participate in the pathogenesis of asthma and allergic diseases. Th2 cells, through the production of IL-4, inhibit Th1 differentiation and function. Analogously, Th1-derived IFN-γ inhibits Th2 cells.

- **Th17 cells** possess a potent pro-inflammatory capacity and are important in immune responses against fungi and extracellular bacteria. They produce IL-17A and IL-17F, as well as IL-21 and IL-22. They express the transcription factor ROR-γt that is elicited, during their activation, by the combination of TGF-β and pro-inflammatory cytokines such as IL-6 and IL-1β. The abundance of Th17 cells has been found to be abnormally high in patients with different autoimmune diseases such as psoriasis, multiple sclerosis, rheumatoid arthritis, and systemic lupus erythematosus. Moreover, Th17 cells have demonstrated to be pathogenic in murine models of autoimmune diseases.

- **Th9 and Th22 cells** represent recently defined CD4 effector subsets that produce, respectively,

IL-9 and IL-22. Th9 cells develop in the presence of IL-4, TGF-β, IL-2, and IL-1β. They participate in immune responses against nematodes by recruiting and activating mast cells. They potentiate Th2 responses and have also been linked to allergic diseases. Th22 cells produce IL-22 and TNF-α and have been found in the skin of patients with psoriasis. They are thought to contribute to immune responses in the skin and to promote wound healing through effects exerted on keratinocytes.

- **Induced regulatory T cells (iT$_{reg}$)** represent CD4 T cells that differentiate into suppressor cells in response to TGF-β and the absence of pro-inflammatory cytokines during priming. Similar to thymic-derived regulatory T cells, iT$_{reg}$ express the transcription factor FoxP3. Further, they produce the anti-inflammatory cytokines TGF-β and IL-10. iT$_{reg}$ that are thought to be important in the regulation of immune responses in the gut and have been shown to be responsible for oral tolerance.

- **Follicular helper T cells (T$_{FH}$)** are CD4 T cells that are specialized in providing help to B cells during the germinal center reaction. They differentiate from naïve CD4 T cells in the presence of IL-21, IL-12, IL-23, TGF-β, and signaling through the costimulatory molecule ICOS. Instead of exiting the secondary lymphoid organ and migrating to sites of inflammation, like the previously described subsets do, T$_{FH}$ cells upregulate a distinct chemokine receptor (CXCR5) that induces their migration to the B-cell follicle, where they interact with

B cells and promote their activation as well as their proliferation, somatic hypermutation, and isotype switching, through the production of cytokines (e.g., IL-21) and CD40 ligation.

As discussed before, antigen presentation to naïve CD4 T cells can produce immune responses that are highly variable. Moreover, these responses are not mutually exclusive and coexist. The DC, through differential expression of cell surface and soluble molecules, can skew the type of response that the CD4 T cells should mount. In this manner, different pathogens elicit different responses by inducing the differentiation of CD4 T cells that will produce specific cytokines, recruit specific immune cells, and promote the generation of a particular type of antibody response.

Effector CD4 T cells, large blast-like cells, are very different than the small metabolically quiescent naïve CD4 cells. They show increased expression of activation and differentiation markers, including adhesion molecules such as the integrin LFA-1, and the adhesion molecule CD44, reflecting their increased ability to interact with other cells. Effector CD4 T cells also lack the requirement for CD28/B7-derived costimulation to reactivate. Importantly, effector T cells also change their homing and recirculation patterns. While naïve lymphocytes primarily traffic through lymphoid tissue and blood, effector T cells have downregulated expression of the lymph node homing receptor CD62L (L-selectin) and are able to migrate to peripheral tissue sites. In this way, effector T cells can readily traffic to peripheral sites of antigen encounter for efficacious clearance.

In addition to profound changes in the cellular phenotype and function, effector T cells are relatively short-lived, lasting only days to weeks *in vivo*. The brief life span of effector T cells probably accounts for the lack of circulating effector T cells in healthy individuals. It is only in situations of chronic activation, such as chronic infection or autoimmunity, where effector T cells can be detected.

CYTOKINE RECEPTORS

The biological effects of cytokines are determined by the specific receptors expressed by different cell populations. The cytokine receptors can be grouped into several families depending on structural characteristics (Figure 11.4). Upregulation of a given subunit of these receptors is often a consequence of cellular activation and usually results in the expression of a high-affinity receptor able to transduce activation signals. The activation pathways triggered after receptor occupancy tend to be similar for receptors of the same family but differ for receptors of different families. The fact that several cytokines may share a given receptor explains why some biological properties are common to several interleukins.

The interleukin receptor family is the most common type of receptor. The receptors of this

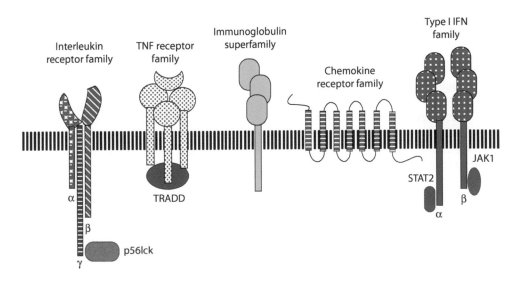

Figure 11.4 **The main families of cytokine receptors.**

family are heterodimers or heterotrimers and always include one α and one β chain, the latter with a longer intracytoplasmic segment and signaling functions. The receptors for IL-2, IL-3, IL-4, IL-5, IL-6, IL-7, IL-9, IL-15, and GM-CSF are included in this family. As mentioned previously, the receptors for IL-2, IL-4, IL-7, IL-9, and IL-15 share a common third chain (γ_c), which plays a significant role in signal transduction. One of the forms of severe combined immunodeficiency is secondary to abnormalities in the γ-chain gene (see Chapter 29).

Other receptor families include the **tumor necrosis factor receptor family**, including receptors for TNF, lymphotoxin-α (LT-α, TNFβ), CD40, and Fas. There are two types of TNF receptor, the TNFR-1 and TNFR-2. Activated TNFR-1 recruits a TNF receptor-associated death domain (TRADD), whose activation triggers a proapoptotic cascade that affects primarily tumor cells. Engagement of TRADD by TNFR-1 does not usually trigger cell death in immune cells, because an antiapoptotic pathway leading to NF-κB synthesis is simultaneously triggered and most often the T cells are activated and release pro-inflammatory cytokines. The binding of TNF to TNFR-2 does not engage TRADD and results in cell activation. Free TNFR-1 and TNFR-2 are detectable in serum and are commonly used biomarkers of inflammation.

The **immunoglobulin superfamily receptors** include the IL-1 (α and β) and IL-18 receptors, a receptor for colony-stimulating factor 1, and, as a special subfamily, the interferon receptors.

The **interferon receptors** signal the cells expressing them by pathways involving members of the JAK-STAT family, particularly STAT-1. STAT-1–deficient mice do not respond to interferons and are highly susceptible to bacterial and viral infections.

The **chemokine receptor family** includes receptors for IL-8, platelet factor-4 (PF-4), RANTES, and macrophage chemotactic and activating proteins. Two such receptors, CCR5 and CXCR4, are involved in the infection of memory T cells and macrophages (CCR5) and of naïve T lymphocytes (CXCR4) by the human immunodeficiency virus (HIV).

CD8 T CELLS

An essential function of cell-mediated immunity is the defense against intracellular infectious agents, particularly viruses. For example, circulating T lymphocytes isolated from individuals who are recovering from measles infection destroy MHC-identical fibroblasts infected with this virus in 2–3 hours. A number of experimental models have provided insights into the mechanisms of lymphocyte-mediated cytotoxicity against virus-infected cells.

Like CD4 effector cells, CD8 T cells undergo extensive rounds of proliferation following antigen presentation. During their proliferation, they acquire distinct functional characteristics (Table 11.3). They produce high levels of IFN-γ and TNF-α similar to Th1 effector cells. The transcription factors T-bet and eomesodermin control their effector capacities and cytokine production. Most effector CD8 T cells exhibit cytotoxic capability and lyse MHC class I–expressing target cells harboring their specific antigen. Their cytotoxicity is mediated by the presence of perforins and esterases in cytoplasmic granules and by increased expression of membrane-associated Fas ligand.

TARGET CELL KILLING

The cytotoxic reaction takes place in a series of successive steps (Figure 11.5). The first step involves the conjugation of cytotoxic T cells with their respective targets. For this to occur, the CD8 T cell must recognize a peptide-MHC-I complex on the target cell. In addition, other interactions are required to achieve a strong adhesion between the T cell and the target cell:

- The CD8+ molecule itself interacts with the nonpolymorphic domain of the MHC class I molecule, specifically with its α3 domain. The avidity of this interaction increases after TCR occupancy.
- The CD2 molecule interacts with the CD58 molecules expressed by the target cells. Any resting T cell can interact with CD58+ cells, but this interaction by itself is weak and does not lead to cell activation. The modification of the CD2 molecule after TCR engagement increases the affinity of the interaction between CD2 and CD58.
- The interaction between LFA-1 and ICAM-1 provides additional stabilizing bonds between the interacting cells. LFA-1 avidity for its ligand is also upregulated by T-cell activation.

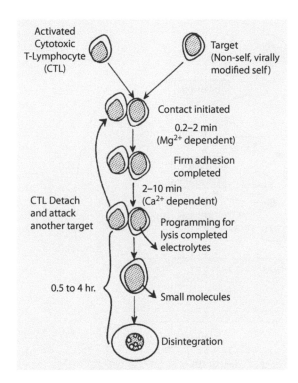

Figure 11.5 Sequence of events during a cytotoxic reaction. Notice that an activated cytotoxic (CD8+) T cell is able to kill several targets.

The conjugation of the CD8+ T cell to its target cell is firm but transient, and after about 30 minutes, the affinity of ICAM-1 for LFA-1 and of CD58 for CD2 reverts to resting levels. The cytotoxic T cell can then move on to another antigen-bearing target with which it will develop the same interaction. In this way, each CTL can kill several cells.

During the short period of intimate contact with its target, a series of reactions takes place, eventually resulting in the killing of the target cell. First, the cytoskeleton of the cytotoxic cell reorganizes. The microtubule-organizing center and the Golgi apparatus move in the direction of the area of contact with the target cell. This facilitates the transport of cytoplasmic granules toward the target. When the cytoplasmic granules reach the membrane, their contents are emptied into the virtual space that separates the cytotoxic T cells and target cells. These granules contain a mixture of proteins, including perforins and granzymes.

Perforins polymerize as soon as they are released, forming "polyperforins." These polyperforins insert into the membrane of the target cell and form transmembrane channels that allow the influx of water into the cell and may cause cell death in a manner analogous to the terminal components of complement. Additionally, the perforin channels facilitate the penetration of granzymes A and B into the target cell. These proteases activate proteolytic enzymes in the cytoplasm of the target cell, which initiate a cascade of events leading to apoptotic death.

Apoptosis or programmed cell death is characterized by nuclear and cytoplasmic changes. At the nuclear level, DNA is degraded and fragmented. The cytoplasm shows condensation, and there is an abnormal increase of membrane permeability, especially significant at the mitochondrial level. Caspases are a family of 13 cysteine proteases that cleave after aspartic acid residues. Some caspases (e.g., caspase 8 and 9) act as initiators of the sequence that leads to apoptosis, while others act as effector caspases, directly involved in the final steps of the cycle (e.g., caspase 3 and 7). Caspases exist as inactive proenzymes that need to be cleaved by proteases. CD8 T cell–derived granzymes can activate the effector caspases directly and through a pathway mediated by increased mitochondrial membrane permeability. Once activated, the effector caspases cleave an endonuclease-inactivating protein that forms an inactive complex with a cytoplasmic DNAse. As that protein is digested, the endonuclease becomes active and translocates to the nucleus, causing the DNA breakdown that is characteristic of apoptotic cell death (Figure 11.6).

A second pathway through which CD8 T cells can induce apoptosis in target cells is mediated by membrane-bound molecules such as FasL. FasL binds to Fas (CD95) and promotes the assembly of a death-inducing signaling complex in the Fas-bearing cell. The activation of this pathway is associated with activation of caspase 8, which in turn will trigger the cascade that leads to activation of effector caspases and apoptosis. These two pathways are not mutually exclusive. In fact, there is data that suggest that activation of both pathways is required *in vivo* for efficient cytotoxicity.

IMMUNE MEMORY

Immune memory refers to a long known phenomenon: that after infection with a pathogen, the host becomes resistant to a new infection with the same agent while remaining susceptible to other infectious agents. This phenomenon represents

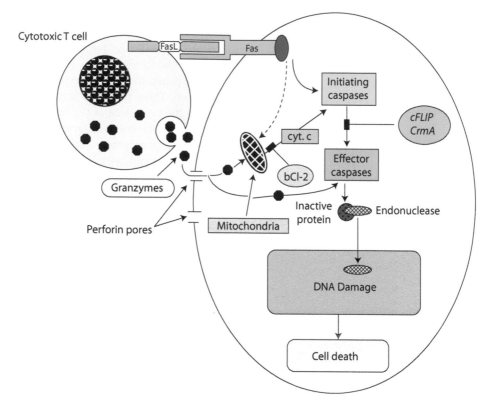

Figure 11.6 **Sequence of events leading to apoptosis of a target cell after interaction with an activated cytotoxic T cell.**

the raison d'être of the adaptive immune system. As mentioned earlier in the chapter, the adaptive immune system is composed of a large number of T and B cells, each bearing a unique antigen receptor. Within this vast antigen receptor repertoire, each receptor is present at a very low frequency. Because the anatomic organization of the immune system allows antigens to be sensed by a large number of cells, when low abundant specific T cells detect their antigen, they vigorously proliferate and differentiate into antigen-specific effector T cells. The expanded clones of T cells will orchestrate the immune response that will eventually clear the agent that elicited it. When the pathogen is eliminated, most of the T cells that were produced during the clonal expansion will be eliminated through apoptosis. However, a relatively small number of antigen-specific cells will remain. In contrast to the naïve T cells that were primed during the onset of the immune response, the antigen-specific T cells that remain will possess a number of characteristics that will allow them to confer protection if the host is invaded again by the

same pathogen. These characteristics represent the cellular basis of immune memory (Table 11.4):

a. *Life span*: Memory T cells are long lived and will survive in the host for the rest of its life. How much a memory T cell lives and how often it divides are still a matter of debate.

b. *Location*: Memory T cells will localize to strategic places within the host. Some of them will remain in secondary lymphoid organs, where they are exposed to a large amount of antigens. Others will migrate to epithelia where the pathogen is more likely to invade.

c. *Activation and effector capacities*: Memory T cells will become activated more easily than naïve T cells, and when they do, they will be able to exert their effector function more rapidly than their naïve counterparts.

These characteristics allow memory T cells to mount immune responses more rapidly and more effectively and thus to neutralize pathogens before they are able to cause disease.

Table 11.4 Distinguishing features of naïve and memory T cells

Property	Naïve T cell	Memory T cell
Phenotype	CD45RB^{hi} (Mo) CD45RA (Hu) CD44^{lo} CD11a^{lo} CD62L^{hi} CCR7^{hi} (Hu)	CD45RB^{lo} (Mo) CD45RO (Hu) CD44^{hi} CD11a^{hi}
Activation requirements		
Costimulation	Mandatory	Dispensable
APCs	Dendritic cell	Dendritic cell, B cells, macrophages, other cells
Responses to low antigen dose	Weak	Strong
Effector function	None	Effector cytokines, cytotoxicity
Kinetics	Slow (days)	Fast (hours)
Homing	Lymphoid organs	Lymphoid and nonlymphoid tissue

Abbreviations: Hu, human; Mo, mouse.

REGULATION OF THE IMMUNE RESPONSE

Immune responses are tightly regulated throughout their development. The activation of naïve T cells (i.e., T-cell priming) is restricted to DCs, which can deliver positive or negative signals, according to the costimulation molecules they express. DCs that have not been activated by pathogen-derived molecules (or by danger signals released from damaged cells) will present self antigens to self-reactive T cells and induce their functional inactivation or their deletion. In this manner, self-reactive T cells are constantly kept in check during steady state.

When a T cell is primed and begins its clonal expansion, the acquisition of specific functional characteristics represents a second regulatory level. The functional capacities that the clone acquires ensure that it migrates to the tissues where its functions are necessary and that it produces only the necessary cytokines. Immune responses that are skewed incorrectly will not be as efficient and may have pathological consequences.

Activated T cells also become susceptible to apoptosis. During clonal expansion, apoptosis induced by ligation of Fas and other related molecules curbs the magnitude of the immune response. For example, patients with X-linked lymphoproliferative disease can develop a lethal inflammatory response during viral infections due to failed restimulation–induced cell death. The length of the clonal expansion is also regulated by intrinsic and extrinsic factors that trigger apoptosis in the great majority of effector T cells generated during the response. When the antigen and cytokine levels dwindle, most activated effector cells undergo programmed cell death. These mechanisms illustrate how T-cell activation, expansion, and contraction are regulated by T-cell intrinsic and extrinsic processes. Another essential safeguard against immunopathology and inflammation is the presence of regulatory T cells (T$_{reg}$).

T$_{reg}$ limit the activation and effector function of other T cells and other immune cells (e.g., DCs and B cells) through several mechanisms. One mechanism is via the production of cytokines such as IL-10 and TGF-β. Another mechanism by which T$_{reg}$ have been shown to act is through modulation of APCs. For example, T$_{reg}$ can modulate certain types of DCs to render them tolerogenic rather than activating. Finally, another way T$_{reg}$ have been proposed to function is via direct effects on T cells, either by sequestration of IL-2, production of ADP, or even direct cytotoxicity.

During the T-cell ontogeny in the thymus, CD4 T cells that bear a self-reactive TCR can be deleted by negative selection, or selected to become a "thymic" or **natural T$_{reg}$ (nT$_{reg}$)**. The transcription factor FoxP3 is upregulated in nT$_{reg}$ that consequently acquire a distinct phenotype that grants them suppressive functions. The importance of T$_{reg}$ is exemplified by the dire consequences of mutations in

FOXP3. The absence of this transcriptional regulation causes a lethal autoimmune inflammatory syndrome that in humans is called IPEX (immunodysregulation polyendocrinopathy enteropathy X-linked). In children with this disease, the lack of T_{reg} causes uncontrolled activation of the immune system, indicating the importance of the regulatory function of T_{reg}.

As mentioned in earlier sections, naïve CD4 T cells can also acquire regulatory capacities during priming. These, "peripheral" or **induced T_{reg} (iT_{reg})**, also express the transcription factor FoxP3 and are, in many ways, similar to nT_{reg}. Perhaps the most important differences between nT_{reg} and iT_{reg} is the stability of the suppressive function. Whereas nT_{reg} stably express FoxP3, iT_{reg} have been shown to lose its expression and acquire pro-inflammatory capacities.

Other T_{reg} subpopulations have been described. These include suppressive CD8 T cells that home to the germinal center and regulate the germinal center response. Additionally, CD4 T cells share many features with follicular helper T cells but express FoxP3 and are also thought to home to the germinal center and exert local suppressive functions.

Finally, CD4 T cells primed in the presence of IL-10 can also become regulatory. These cells, called **Tr1 cells**, lack FoxP3 and express in their surface CD49b and lymphocyte activation gene (LAG)-3. Tr1 cells can regulate the function of dendritic cells by producing IL-10. Thus, a complex combination of intrinsic and extrinsic factors regulates the immune system to avoid inappropriate and prolonged responses.

CONCLUDING REMARKS

We discussed in this chapter how T cells become activated when they encounter antigen, including the molecular and cellular requirements and events involved in this process. We detailed how differentiation to effector T cells provides the key players for coordinating immune responses and removing foreign antigens. Finally, we discussed how immune memory is generated as a result of this process, and the different mechanisms the immune system uses to regulate immunity that could result in immunopathology. These cellular and molecular processes that form the basis of cellular immunity are important candidates for immunotherapies for modulating these responses in vaccines, autoimmunity, allergy, and transplantation.

BIBLIOGRAPHY

Chang JT, Wherry EJ, Goldrath AW. Molecular regulation of effector and memory T cell differentiation. *Nat Immunol.* 2014;15:1104–1115.

Chen L, Flies DB. Molecular mechanisms of T cell co-stimulation and co-inhibition. *Nat Rev Immunol.* 2013;13:227–242.

Courtney AH, Lo WL, Weiss A. TCR Signaling: Mechanisms of initiation and propagation. *Trends Biochem Sci.* 2018;43:108–123.

Crotty S. T Follicular helper cell differentiation, function, and roles in disease. *Immunity.* 2014;41:529–542.

Kaech SM, Cui W. Transcriptional control of effector and memory CD8+ T cell differentiation. *Nat Rev Immunol.* 2012;12:749–756.

Kaplan MH, Hufford MM, Olson MR. The development and *in vivo* function of T helper 9 cells. *Nat Rev Immunol.* 2015;15:295–307.

Ohkura N, Kitagawa Y, Sakaguchi S. Development and maintenance of regulatory T cells. *Immunity.* 2013;38:414–423.

Sallusto F. Heterogeneity of Human CD4+ T cells against microbes. *Annu Rev Immunol.* 2016;34:317–334.

Schildberg FA, Klein SR, Freeman GJ, Sharpe AH. Coinhibitory pathways in the B7-CD28 ligand-receptor family. *Immunity.* 2016;44:955–972.

Villarino AV, Kanno Y, Ferdinand JR, O'Shea JJ. Mechanisms of Jak/STAT signaling in immunity and disease. *J Immunol.* 2015;194:21–27.

Zhu J, Yamane H, Paul WE. Differentiation of effector CD4 T cell populations. *Annu Rev Immunol.* 2010;28:445–489.

12

Adaptive humoral immunity and immunoprophylaxis

GABRIEL VIRELLA

INTRODUCTION

The recognition of a foreign cell or substance triggers a complex set of events that result in the acquisition of specific immunity against the corresponding antigen(s). The elimination of "non-self" depends on effector mechanisms able to neutralize or eliminate the source of antigenic stimulation. While the inductive stages of most immune responses require T- and B-cell cooperation, the effector mechanisms can be clearly subdivided into cell dependent and antibody dependent (or humoral). The sequence of events that culminates in the production of antibodies specifically directed against exogenous antigen(s) constitutes the humoral immune response.

OVERVIEW OF INDUCTION OF HUMORAL IMMUNE RESPONSE

Exposure to natural immunogens

Infectious agents penetrate the organism generally via the skin, upper respiratory mucosa, and intestinal mucosa. In most cases, the immune system is stimulated in the absence of clinical symptoms suggestive of infection (subclinical infection). Constant exposure to immunogenic materials penetrating the organism through those routes is responsible for continuous stimulation of the immune system and explains why relatively large concentrations of immunoglobulins can be measured in the serum of normal animals. In contrast, animals reared in germ-free conditions synthesize very limited amounts of antibodies, and their sera have very low immunoglobulin concentrations.

B-cell activation

As discussed in greater detail in Chapters 4 and 11, B-cell activation requires multiple signals. The only specific signal is the one provided by the interaction between the antigen-binding site of surface immunoglobulins (sIg) located on the cell membrane with a given epitope of an immunogen. The additional signals, provided by Th2 helper cells and antigen-presenting cells (APCs), are nonspecific with regard to the antigen.

The recognition of an antigen by a resting B cell seems to be optimal when the immunogen is adsorbed to a follicular dendritic cell or to a macrophage. B lymphocytes recognize either unprocessed antigen or antigen fragments that conserve the configuration of the native antigen. All techniques used for measurement of specific antibodies use antigens in their original configuration as their basis, and succeed in detecting antibodies reacting with them. Whether or not some B cells may have membrane immunoglobulins reactive with immunogen-derived peptides associated with major histocompatibility complex II (MHC-II) molecules is not known.

Helper Th2 lymphocytes provide other signals essential for B-cell proliferation and differentiation. The activation of this CD4 subpopulation is favored by a low-affinity interaction between an immunogen-derived oligopeptide associated with an MHC-II molecule and the T-cell receptor, as well as by additional signals, some derived from cell-cell interactions, such as the CD28/CD86 interaction, and others from cytokines, such as interleukin (IL)-4. Activated Th2 cells, in turn, provide several costimulatory signals that promote B-cell proliferation and differentiation. Some of these signals derive from the interaction between cell membrane molecules upregulated during the early stages of Th2 and B-cell activation, e.g., CD40 L (CD154) on T cells and CD40 (on B cells), while others are mediated by cytokines, such as IL-4, IL-5, IL-6, and IL-10 (Figure 12.1).

When the proper sum of specific signals and costimulatory signals is received by the B cell, clonal proliferation and differentiation ensue. Since each immunogen presents a multitude of epitopes, a normal immune response is polyclonal, i.e., involves many different clones recognizing different epitopes of an immunogen. The induction of an immune response requires some time, for activation of all the relevant cells, and for proliferation and differentiation of B cells into plasma cells. Thus, there is always a lag phase between the time of immunization and the time when antibodies become detectable. It must be noted that while most activated B cells will become antibody-producing plasma cells, some will become memory cells (see discussion later in chapter).

Experimental animals immunized with a given immunogen (e.g., tobacco mosaic virus) often show marked postimmunization hypergammaglobulinemia, but only a very small fraction of the circulating immunoglobulins react with the

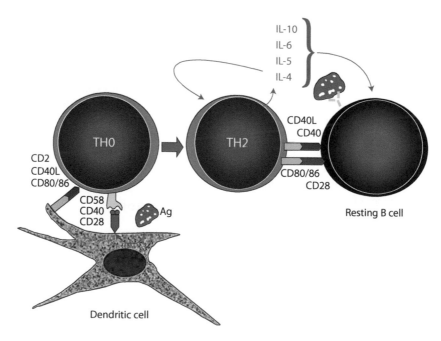

Figure 12.1 Induction of a humoral response. The activation of a resting B cell requires recognition of unprocessed antigen and costimulatory signals provided by activated Th2 cells through the release of cytokines and the increased expression of membrane proteins able to deliver activating signals to B cells expressing the corresponding ligand molecules.

immunogen. In humans, the initial burst of IgE production, after first exposure to an allergen, seems to be mainly constituted by nonspecific antibodies. This apparent lack of specificity of the immune response is more obvious in the primary immune response, after the first exposure to an immunogen. Most likely this is a consequence of the fact that the antibodies produced early in the immune response are of low affinity and may not be detectable in assays that favor the detection of high-affinity antibodies. It is also possible that the costimulatory signals provided by Th2 cells may enhance the immune response of neighboring B cells engaged in unrelated immune responses. This may result in the enhanced synthesis of antibodies reacting with other immunogens that the immune system is simultaneously recognizing. While the synthesis of unrelated antibodies is usually beneficial or inconsequential, it can also be the basis for at least some autoimmune reactions if strong help is provided to autoreactive B cells that otherwise would remain quiescent.

PRIMARY IMMUNE RESPONSE

The first contact with an antigen evokes a primary response, which has the following characteristics:

- A relatively long lag between the stimulus and the detection of antibodies by current methods (varying between 3 and 4 days after the injection of heterologous erythrocytes and 10 and 14 days after the injection of killed bacterial cells). Part of this variation depends on the sensitivity of antibody detection methods, but it is also a reflection of the potency of the immunogen.
- The first antibody class to be synthesized is usually IgM. Later in the response, IgG antibodies will predominate over IgM antibodies. This phenomenon, known as **IgM-IgG switch**, is controlled by different interleukins released by activated helper T lymphocytes and by specific costimulatory signals mediated by CD28/CD80, CD40/CD40L, and CD21/CD23.
- After rising exponentially for some time, antibody levels reach a steady state and then decline (Figure 12.2).
- Adjuvant administration will keep the antibody levels high for months.

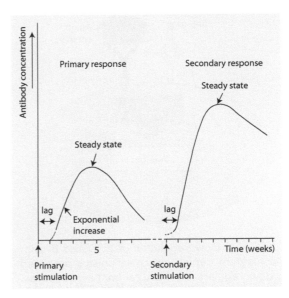

Figure 12.2 The sequence of events during a primary and a secondary immune response. (Modified from Eisen, H.N., *Immunology*, 2nd ed., Harper and Row, New York, NY, 1980.)

Downregulation of the humoral immune response

Several regulatory mechanisms will operate in order to turn off antibody production after the infectious agent (or any other type of immunogen) has been eliminated.

Antigen elimination. The most obvious downregulatory mechanism is the elimination of the antigen, which was the primary stimulus of the immune response.

Treg activation. As immune response progresses, the activity of T cells with suppressor activity, such as Treg, starts to predominate. IL-10, the major immunosuppressive cytokine released by activated CD4$^+$, CD25$^+$, FoxP3$^+$ Tregs, downregulates both Th1 and Th2 cells, thus reducing the delivery of costimulatory signals to B cells. T cells with suppressor activity persist after the antigen is eliminated, either as a consequence of their late activation or of a longer life span.

Immunoregulatory effects of soluble antigen-antibody complexes and anti-idiotypic antibodies. As the immune response proceeds and IgG antibodies are synthesized, IgG-containing antigen-antibody complexes are formed in circulation and in the extravascular compartments. The appearance of soluble antigen-antibody complexes is apparently

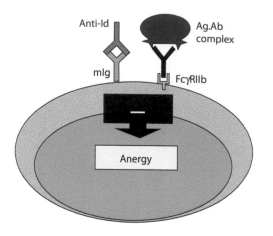

Figure 12.3 Downregulation of activated B cells. The diagram depicts two mechanisms proposed to downregulate the humoral immune response. Anti-idiotypic antibodies specific for the binding site of a given antibody emerge during the humoral response. The anti-idiotypic antibodies bind to the binding site of the surface immunoglobulins from the clone producing the antibody that triggered the anti-idiotype. In doing so, the anti-idiotype delivers an incomplete signal and prevents further interactions with unprocessed antigen. On the other hand, immune complexes formed by soluble, unprocessed, antigen and antibody, interact with the downregulatory FcγRIIb expressed by B cells. Both mechanisms can turn off activated B cells and are not mutually exclusive.

perceived by the immune system as evidence for having reached the main goal—elimination of the antigen. B cells express the FcγRIIb on their membranes, and experimental evidence shows that the ligation of B cell FcγRIIb with antigen-antibody complexes has a downregulating effect, similar to that attributed to anti-idiotypic antibodies (Figure 12.3).

Also during the immune response, as levels of antibodies keep increasing, antibodies reacting with variable region epitopes (idiotypes, see chapter 7) of those antibodies start being synthesized. The easiest way to understand this response is to accept that the normal state of tolerance to the millions of different idiotypes presented by antigen receptors is broken when one or a few specific antibodies are produced in large concentrations, suddenly exposing the immune system to large concentrations of molecules with identical idiotypes.

Anti-idiotypic antibodies are believed to participate in negative regulation of the immune response by binding to membrane immunoglobulins from antigen-specific B cells expressing variable regions of the same specificity as the antibody molecules that triggered the anti-idiotypic antibody. The binding of an antibody to a surface immunoglobulin induces B-lymphocyte proliferation, but the proliferating B cells fail to differentiate into antibody-producing cells for lack of costimulatory signals. At the same time, the occupancy of the sIg binding sites by the anti-idiotypic antibodies prevents the proper antigenic stimulation of the B lymphocyte.

SECONDARY OR ANAMNESTIC RESPONSE

Reexposure of an animal or human being to an immunizing antigen to which they have been previously exposed induces a secondary recall, or anamnestic response. The capacity to mount a secondary immune response can persist for many years, providing long-lasting protection against reinfection.

The secondary response has some important characteristics, some dependent on the existence of an expanded population of memory cells, ready to be stimulated, and others dependent on the prolonged retention of antigen in the lymph nodes with continuous stimulation of B cells over long periods of time.

Differentiation of B memory cells

During the peak of a primary response, there is a duality in the fate of activated B cells: while most will evolve into antibody-producing plasma cells, others will differentiate into memory B cells.

The differentiation of memory cells is believed to take place in the germinal centers of secondary lymphoid tissues. As a pre-memory B cell enters a follicle, it migrates into the germinal center where it undergoes active proliferation. At this stage, the "switch" from IgM to IgG or other isotype synthesis is taking place, and the V region genes undergo somatic hypermutation. After completing this round of proliferation, the resulting memory B cells need additional signals for full differentiation.

1. Clones with high-affinity sIg in the membrane will be able to interact with antigen molecules

immobilized by follicular dendritic cells. As a consequence, these clones will receive strong activation and differentiation signals. In contrast, clones with low-affinity sIg will not be able to compete with preformed antibody for binding to the immobilized antigen epitopes, will not receive adequate signals, and will undergo apoptosis.

2. The evolution of this antigen-stimulated memory B-cell precursor into a memory B cell requires a second signal provided by a helper T cell, in the form of the CD40/CD40 ligand interaction. Other signals, such as the one delivered by the CD21/CD23 interaction, may result in direct evolution of the prememory B cell into an antibody-producing plasma cell.

As discussed in Chapter 4, immunological memory is largely a T-cell function, but the expansion of the responding population of T cells will certainly contribute to the ability of B cells to respond more rapidly and effectively to a second exposure to the same antigen.

Consequences of the existence of expanded populations of memory cells. Three major features of a secondary immune response (Figure 12.2) result from the existence of expanded populations of memory cells, both T and B:

- **Lower threshold dose of immunogen**, i.e., the dose of antigen necessary to induce a secondary response is lower than the dose required to induce a primary response.
- **Shorter lag phase**, i.e., it takes a shorter time for the antibody to be detected in circulation after immunization.
- **Faster increase in antibody concentrations** and **higher titers of antibody** at the peak of the response.
- **Predominance of IgG antibody** is characteristic of the secondary immune response, probably a consequence of the fact that memory B cells express IgG on their membranes and will produce IgG after stimulation.

Consequences of prolonged retention of antigen and persistent B-cell stimulation. We previously discussed the downregulating effects of the interaction of soluble antigen-antibody complexes with B cells. However, antigen-antibody complexes formed early in a secondary immune response have a totally opposite effect when taken up by follicular dendritic cells that express Fcγ receptors on their membrane. They remain associated to these cells for a long period of time, with the following consequences:

- **Longer persistence of antibody synthesis**, slowing down the decay of antibody levels caused by the downregulatory mechanisms discussed previously.
- **Affinity maturation**. It is known that the affinity of antibodies increases during the primary immune response and even more so in the secondary and subsequent responses. This maturation is a result of the selection of memory B cells with progressively higher-affinity sIg antibodies during a persistent immune response. This selection is a direct consequence of the retention of antigen-antibody complexes by the follicular dendritic cells. The antigen moieties of the retained immune complexes are effectively presented to the immune system for as long as the complexes remain associated to the dendritic cells. As free antibodies and sIg compete for binding to the immobilized antigen, only B cells with sIg of higher affinity than the previously synthesized antibodies will be able to compete effectively and receive activation signals. Consequently, the affinity of the synthesized antibodies will show a steady increase.
- **Increased avidity and increased cross-reactivity**. During a long-lasting secondary response to a complex immunogen, clones responding to minor determinants emerge. Cryptic epitopes that are not recognized in the primary immune response may also be recognized as a consequence of repeated stimulation. Therefore, a wider range of antibodies is produced in the secondary immune response. This results in increased avidity (as discussed in Chapter 8, avidity is the sum of binding forces mediated by different antibody molecules binding simultaneously to the same antigen). But, as the repertoire of antibodies recognizing different epitopes of a given immunogen increases, so do the probabilities for the emergence of cross-reactive antibodies recognizing antigenic determinants common to other immunogens.

FATE OF ANTIGENS ON PRIMARY AND SECONDARY RESPONSES

Following intravenous injection of a soluble antigen, its concentration in serum tends to decrease in three phases (Figure 12.4):

- *Equilibration phase.* This phase is characterized by a sharp decrease of brief duration corresponding to the equilibration of the antigen between intra- and extravascular spaces.
- *Metabolic decay.* During this phase, the antigen slowly decays, due to its catabolic processing by the host.
- *Immune elimination.* When antibodies start to be formed, there will be a phase of rapid immune elimination, in which soluble antigen-antibody complexes will be formed and taken up by macrophages. The onset of this phase of immune elimination is shorter in the secondary immune response, virtually immediate if circulating

antibody exists previous to the introduction of the antigen, and nonexistent if the antigen is introduced in an immune-incompetent animal (Figure 12.5).

A similar sequence of events, with less distinct equilibration and metabolic decay phases, occurs in the case of particulate antigens. If the antigen is a live, multiplying organism, there might be an initial increase in the number of circulating or

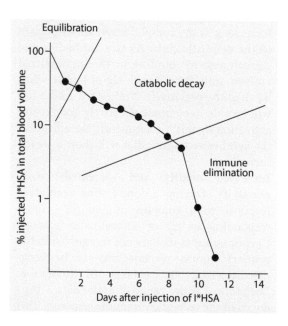

Figure 12.4 The immune elimination phenomenon. A few days following antigen administration, antibodies appear in the circulation and eliminate the antigen at a much more rapid rate than the rate in nonimmune individuals. Accelerated removal of an antigen from the blood circulation is a consequence of its interaction with specific antibody and elimination of antigen-antibody complexes through the mononuclear phagocyte system.

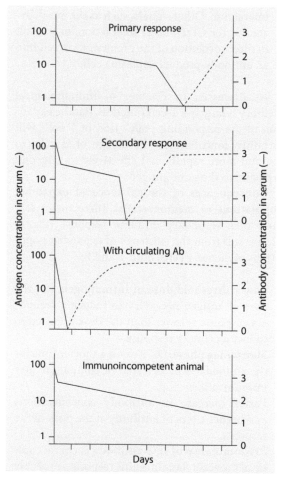

Figure 12.5 The fate of injected antigen in a nonimmune animal, which will undergo primary immune response; an immune animal that will show an accelerated, secondary response; an animal with circulating antibodies, which will very rapidly eliminate the corresponding antigen from circulation; and an immunoincompetent animal, which will slowly metabolize the antigen. (Modified from Talmage, D.F. et al., *J. Immunol.*, 67, 243–255, 1951.)

tissue-colonizing organisms, until the immune response promotes the elimination of the antigen by a variety of mechanisms discussed in later chapters.

MUCOSAL HUMORAL IMMUNE RESPONSE

The gastrointestinal and respiratory mucosae are among the most common portals of entry used by infectious agents. Since this constant exposure only rarely results in clinical disease, it seems obvious that strongly protective mechanisms must exist at the mucosal level. Some of those protective mechanisms are nonspecific and of a physicochemical nature, including the integrity of mucosal surfaces, gastric pH, gastrointestinal traffic, proteases and bile present in the intestinal lumen, as well as the flow of bronchial secretions, glucosidases, and bactericidal enzymes (e.g., lysozyme) found in respiratory secretions. At the same time, cell-mediated and humoral immune mechanisms are also operative in mucosal membranes.

Cell-mediated immune mechanisms at mucosal levels

Most evidence suggests that innate cell-mediated mechanisms predominate, including phagocytic cells and γ/δ T lymphocytes.

- Phagocytic cells (particularly macrophages) abound in the submucosa and represent an important mechanism for nonspecific elimination of particulate matter and microbial agents of limited virulence.
- γ/δ T lymphocytes are also present in large numbers in the submucosal tissues. It has been proposed that these cells seem able to cause the lysis of infected cells by MHC-independent recognition of altered glycosylation patterns of cell membrane glycoproteins or by recognition of cell-associated microbial superantigens.

Humoral immunity at mucosal level

A large volume of data has been compiled concerning the induction and physiological significance of humoral immunity at the mucosal level. A major established fact, supported by several lines of experimental work, is that the induction of

secretory antibodies requires direct mucosal stimulation. Seminal human studies showed that systemic administration of the attenuated poliovirus vaccine results in a systemic humoral response, while no secretory antibodies are detected. In contrast, oral administration of the same attenuated poliovirus results in both a secretory IgA response and a systemic IgM-IgG response (Figure 12.6).

In addition, it has been demonstrated that the stimulation of a given sector of the mucosal system (gastrointestinal [GI] tract) may result in detectable responses on nonstimulated areas (upper respiratory tract). This protection of distant areas is compatible with the unitarian concept of a mucosal immunological network with constant traffic of immune cells from one sector to another (Figure 12.7). For example, antigen-sensitized cells from the gut-associated lymphoid tissue (GALT), or from the peribronchial lymphoid tissues, enter the general circulation via the draining lymphatic vessels. Their systemic recirculation results in their migration toward the remaining secretory-associated lymphoid tissues, including the gastrointestinal tract, the airways, the urinary tract, and the mammary, salivary, and cervical glands of the uterus.

Passive transfer of mucosal immunity. In some mammalian species, milk-secreted antibodies are actively absorbed in the newborn's gut and constitute the main source of adoptive immunity in the neonate. This usually is observed in species in which there is limited or no placental transfer of antibodies. In humans, in which placental transfer of immunoglobulins is very effective, the antibodies ingested with maternal milk are not absorbed. However, milk antibodies seem to provide passive immunity at the GI level, which may be a very important factor in preventing infectious gastroenteritis in the newborn, whose mucosal immune system is not fully developed.

Physiological significance of mucosal immunity. The main immunological function of secretory IgA is believed to be to prevent microbial adherence to the mucosal epithelia, which usually precedes colonization and systemic invasion. However, in several experimental models, it has been demonstrated that disease can be prevented without interference with infection, so there are unresolved questions concerning the anti-infectious mechanism(s) of secretory antibodies.

The relative importance of cellular versus humoral mucosal defense mechanism has not been

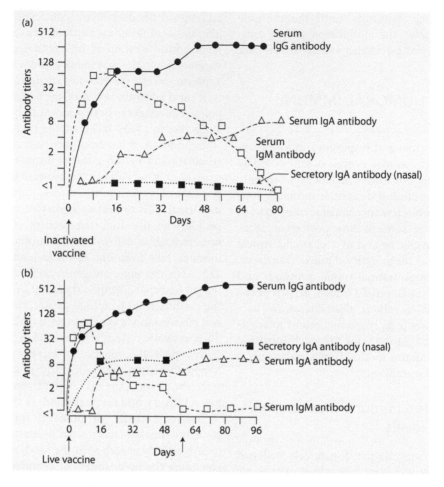

Figure 12.6 Comparison of the systemic and mucosal immune responses in human volunteers given killed polio vaccine (a) and live, attenuated polio vaccine (b). Note that secretory antibody was only detected in children immunized with live, attenuated vaccine. (Modified from Ogra, P.L. et al., *Engl. J. Med.*, 279, 893–900, 1968.)

properly established. However, many IgA-deficient individuals, with very low or absent circulating and secretory IgA, are totally asymptomatic, suggesting that cell-mediated mechanisms may play a significant protective role.

PASSIVE IMMUNIZATION

The parallel development of microbiology and immunology resulted in the discovery of the protective role of antibodies against a variety of infectious agents. This led Ehrlich, Roux and other eminent bacteriologists to develop serotherapy, i.e., the use of antibodies raised in horses to treat infectious diseases caused by bacteria they had just identified as the causative agents. The approach was successful, particularly for diseases caused by

exotoxins, such as diphtheria and tetanus, but it was also verified that the administration of horse serum was not without problems, leading to serum sickness as a consequence of the deposition of complexes made of horse proteins and antibodies produced by the patient who received them in different tissues and organs.

However, the advantages of immediate protection for the treatment and prevention of diseases in exposed patients remained obvious, and eventually human immunoglobulins, purified from patients with high antibody titers, were used for passive immunization, without the risk of developing serum sickness. Other than anti–snake venom antibodies, still produced in horses, passive immunization is currently carried out with human antibodies.

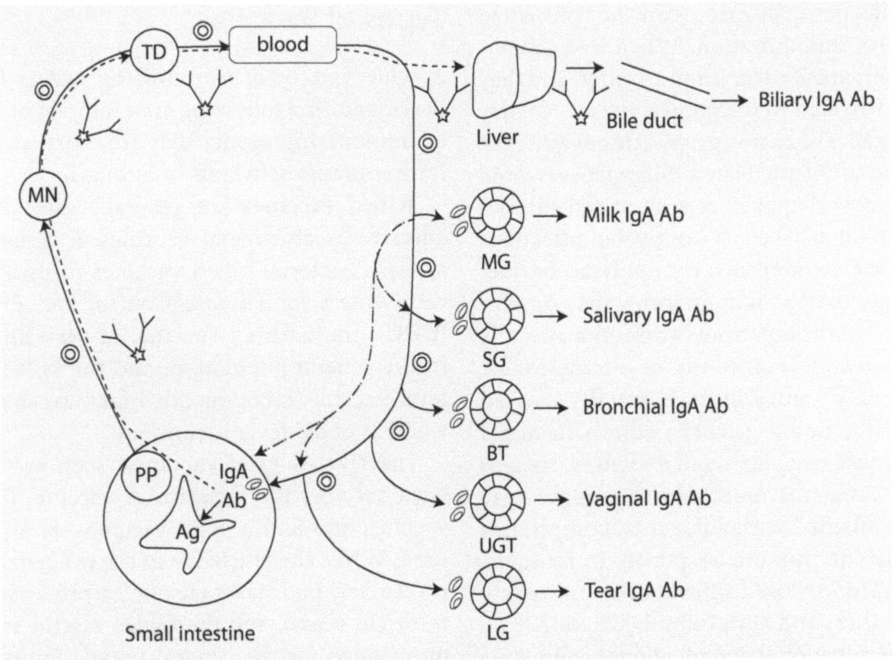

Figure 12.7 Pathways leading to the expression of IgA antibodies after antigenic stimulation of the GALT. IgA immunocytes (o) originating in Peyer's patches (PP) migrate to mesenteric lymph nodes (MN). Cells leave MN via the thoracic duct (TD) and enter circulation with subsequent homing to the mammary gland (MG), salivary gland (SG), lacrimal gland (LG), and lamina propria of the bronchial tree (BT), intestinal or urogenital tract (UGT) (o). The IgA antibodies are then expressed in milk, saliva, tears, and other secretions. IgA antibodies (⋆) entering circulation (---) are selectively removed by the liver and subsequently expressed in bile. Cell traffic between peripheral mucosal sites (- o - MG to SG, LG and small intestine) is included in this scheme. (Reproduced with permission from Montgomery, P.C. et al., In: Peeters, H., ed., *Protides of the Biological Fluids*, Pergamon Press, New York, NY, 1985, p. 43.)

IMMUNOPROPHYLAXIS

The concept of active immunization (immunoprophylaxis) as a way to prevent infectious diseases is more than two centuries old, if we consider the introduction of the cowpox vaccination by Jenner in 1796 as the starting point, or even older if we consider the much earlier practice of variolation in the Orient. Variolation, consisting of exposure of healthy humans to material collected from the pustules of patients with mild forms of smallpox, was introduced in Europe in 1721 following reports of its use in Turkey by Lady Montagu, but the critical step in the development of effective and safe vaccines arose from Jenner's acquaintance with Benjamin Jesty, a farmer who had immunized his wife and two children with pustular material from cows with cowpox, and with reports that milkmaids who had contracted cowpox were protected from smallpox. He then developed an immunization procedure based on the intradermal scarification of material from cowpox lesions. Empirically, he had discovered the principle of vaccine with live, attenuated microbes, which was later picked up by Louis Pasteur when he developed several of his vaccines. As infectious agents became better characterized, new vaccines were developed, some prepared with inactivated organisms, others with microbial components, and others still with attenuated infectious agents. Mass vaccination resulted in significant decreases of morbidity and mortality caused by infectious agents, particularly the most serious infectious diseases of childhood, such as diphtheria, measles, meningitis, and poliomyelitis. A major success was the virtual eradication of smallpox and poliomyelitis. However, at the global scale, infectious diseases are still a major cause of mortality, and the development of new and more effective vaccines remains a high priority.

Many infectious diseases can be prevented through active immunization. When live, attenuated organisms are used for immunization and they are usually delivered to the natural portal of entry of the organism. For example, a vaccine against the common cold using attenuated rhinoviruses would be most effective if applied as a nasal aerosol. But if inert compounds (such as inactivated infectious agents or their components, e.g., polysaccharides or toxoids) are used as immunogens, they have to be introduced in the organism by injection, usually intramuscularly, subcutaneously, or intradermally.

In humans, immunization is usually carried out by injecting the antigen or by administering it by the oral route (e.g., attenuated viruses, such as poliovirus). As a rule, injected immunogens are mixed or emulsified with adjuvants, compounds that enhance the immune response. In humans, the most commonly used adjuvants are inorganic gels such as alum and aluminum hydroxide.

The mechanism of action of adjuvants involves two important factors:

1. Adjuvants slow down the diffusion of the immunogen from the injected spot, so that antigenic stimulation will persist over a longer period of time.
2. Adjuvants induce the activation of macrophages and other antigen-presenting cells at the site of inoculation, thus enhancing the recruitment and activation of Th2 cells and B cells, and as such boosting the immune response. The adjuvants used in human vaccines are not the most potent enhancers of the immune response, but the more potent adjuvants cause severe inflammatory reactions.

Traditionally, vaccines are administered with the ultimate goal of inducing the synthesis of protective antibodies. However, most induce cell-mediated immunity as well. In some cases (tetanus toxoid, for example), the cell-mediated immune reaction is inconsequential. But in the case of viral vaccines, it may be as important or more important than humoral immunity. This could be particularly the case in HIV vaccines, because the antibodies elicited with several types of vaccines do not confer lasting protection. However, the evaluation of protective cell-mediated immunity is technically difficult, and this has hampered progress in the development of HIV vaccine targeting the activation of T cells.

Types of vaccines

A wide variety of immunizing agents has been developed. The following are examples of the types of immunizing agents that are most widely used for immunoprophylaxis in humans.

Killed vaccines are generally safe but not as effective as attenuated vaccines. Currently, there are two bacterial killed vaccines in use, listed by the Centers for Disease Control and Prevention (CDC): the anthrax vaccine, of very limited use in the general population, and the killed typhoid fever vaccine, recommended for travelers to areas where typhoid fever is common.

Inactivated viral vaccines, such as the influenza vaccine, the hepatitis A vaccine, the rabies vaccine, and Salk's polio vaccine, are still widely used. While the efficiency of the influenza vaccine is relatively poor (average of 60% protection, lower in recent years), and the rabies vaccine is not recommended for the general population, the hepatitis A and polio vaccines are very efficient. The currently used polio vaccine in the United States contains a mixture of the three known types of poliovirus, after inactivation with formalin. This vaccine has been as successful in the eradication of poliomyelitis as Sabin's attenuated oral vaccine. Its main advantage is safety, but it is not as effective or amenable to mass immunizations as the oral vaccine (see discussion later in chapter). However, the safety concerns have resulted in its adoption in the United States and other countries where poliomyelitis has been virtually eradicated and there is a greater risk of contracting polio from the attenuated vaccine (about once in every 2.4 million doses) than from a wild virus strain.

Component vaccines are safe, and their use has increased in the last decade. The original component vaccines were mostly made of bacterial toxoids and polysaccharides. Other modalities, such as conjugate vaccines and recombinant component vaccines, have been introduced with considerable success.

- Bacterial polysaccharide vaccines are widely used for *Streptococcus pneumoniae* and *Neisseria meningitidis*. A typhoid fever vaccine made of the Vi capsular polysaccharide is also available. Because of their T-independent nature, polysaccharide vaccines are not very potent (especially in young children) and do not elicit long-lasting memory. While conjugate vaccines (see later discussion) have replaced some polysaccharide vaccines, such as the old *Haemophilus influenzae* type B vaccine, the *Streptococcus pneumoniae* 23 serotype vaccine (Pneumovax 23) continues to be widely and successfully used in the adult population.

- Inactivated toxins (toxoids), such as tetanus and diphtheria toxoids, are prepared with formalin-inactivated toxins that have lost their active site but maintained their immunogenic determinants. Toxoids are strongly immunogenic proteins, induce high titers of antibodies able to neutralize the toxins, and induce long-lasting memory. Chemically inactivated pertussis toxin is also a key component of the acellular pertussis vaccine currently used.

- Viral component vaccines are based on the immunogenicity of isolated viral constituents. The best example is the hepatitis B vaccine, produced by recombinant yeast cells. The gene coding for the hepatitis B surface antigen (HBsAg) was isolated from the hepatitis B virus and inserted into a vector, flanked by promoter and terminator sequences. That vector was used to transform yeast cells, from which HBsAg was purified. All of the available hepatitis B vaccines are obtained by this procedure.

Mixed-component vaccines. The interest in developing safer vaccines for whooping cough led to the introduction of mixed-component acellular vaccines. The acellular pertussis vaccine is constituted by a mixture of inactivated pertussis toxin, a major determinant of the clinical disease, and one or several additional bacterial proteins, including adhesins (filamentous hemagglutinin) and outer membrane proteins (pertactin). These vaccines have replaced the old vaccine prepared with killed *Bordetella pertussis*.

Two vaccines have been developed by reverse vaccinology for group B meningococcus, using nonpolysaccharide components because group B polysaccharides are not immunogenic in humans. One is a quadrivalent vaccine for group B meningococcus (Bexsero) and contains an outer membrane component and recombinant subcapsular proteins (factor H binding protein, Neisserial adhesin A, and Neisserial heparin-binding antigen). This vaccine is moderately effective in young children (≥ 2 months of age) and more effective in adolescents and young adults. However, the levels of protective antibody are short-lasting, so repeated boosters are required to maintain protective immunity. The other is a bivalent vaccine (Trumenba) containing two recombinant variants of the factor H binding protein that include a lipid tail that enhances their immunogenicity. Protective titers were determined in over 80% of immunized adolescents and the antibody titers remained high 4 years after immunization in 50% of the subjects.

Conjugate vaccines. As previously mentioned, most polysaccharide vaccines have shown poor immunogenicity, particularly in infants. This lack of effectiveness is a consequence of the fact that polysaccharides induce mostly T-independent responses with little immunological memory. This problem appears to be eliminated if the polysaccharide is conjugated to an immunogenic protein, very much like a hapten-carrier conjugate.

- *Hib conjugate vaccine*. The first conjugate vaccines to be developed involved the polyribosyl-ribitol-phosphate (PRP) of *Haemophilus influenzae* type b (Hib). Four conjugate vaccines are available, based on Hib-polysaccharide conjugated to different protein carriers, such as diphtheria toxoid (PRP-D), a diphtheria toxoid-like protein (PRP-HbOC), tetanus toxoid (PRP-T), or meningococcal outer membrane protein (PRP-OMP). All are equally efficient, but to secure the carrier effect, critical for the boosting effect of repeated immunizations, the same vaccine should be used for the primary immunization and boosters.

  The introduction of these vaccines was followed by a 95% decrease in the incidence of *Haemophilus influenzae* type b infections affecting children of less than 5 years of age.

- *Pneumococcal polysaccharide vaccine (Prevnar 13)*. This vaccine contains the capsular polysaccharides of 13 *Streptococcus pneumoniae* serotypes that cause 80%–90% of cases of severe pneumococcal disease in the United States, conjugated to an inactive recombinant version of the diphtheria toxin. This vaccine has markedly reduced the incidence of severe pneumococcal infections and is the vaccine of choice for infants under 2 years of age, but there are no definite advantages for its use in older children and adults. On one hand, Prevnar does not require as many boosters as Pneumovax 23 to maintain protection, but on the other hand Pneumovax covers 10 additional serotypes. The effectiveness of Prevnar vaccination in the prevention of otitis media is considerably lower than the protection against invasive pneumococcal disease, but as noted before, infants under 2 years of age respond very poorly to Pneumovax, so there is not a more effective vaccine at that age group.

- *Quadrivalent meningococcal conjugate vaccine (MCV4 or MenactraT).* This vaccine can prevent four types of meningococcal disease (serogroups A, C, Y, and W-135) that include two of the three types most common in the United States. However, serogroup B polysaccharide is nonimmunogenic and is not included in the conjugate vaccine. As mentioned previously, new formulations including serogroup B outer membrane protein are being evaluated.

DNA vaccines. The observation that intramuscular injection of nonreplicating plasmid DNA encoding the hemagglutinin (HA) or nucleoprotein (NP) of influenza virus elicited humoral and cellular protective reactions attracted enormous interest from the scientific community. The recombinant DNA is taken up by APCs at the site of injection and is presented to T helper cells in a way that both humoral and cell-mediated immune responses are elicited. The safety and easy storage of candidate DNA vaccines are extremely appealing, and several different trials are ongoing. However, the initial impression from human trials is that DNA vaccines are far less potent in humans than they appear to be in experimental animals.

Attenuated vaccines. Attenuated vaccines are generally very efficient, but in rare cases they can cause the very disease they are designed to prevent, particularly in immunocompromised individuals.

- *Attenuated viral vaccines.* Most antiviral vaccines are made of viral strains attenuated in the laboratory, including the classical smallpox vaccine, the yellow fever vaccine, the oral polio vaccine (a mixture of attenuated strains of the three known types of poliovirus), the mumps-rubella-measles vaccine, the attenuated influenza vaccine (FluMist, applied intranasally), one of the two approved *Rotavirus* vaccines, and the varicella-zoster vaccine.

  Attenuated viral vaccines tend to be very potent, probably because of the infective nature of the immunizing agent. In the case of polio

vaccines, the attenuated virus can be transmitted by the fecal-oral route to nonimmunized individuals, thus increasing the proportion of immunized individuals in any given population. Another advantage of attenuated vaccines administered topically (by mouth or aerosol) is the simplicity of the immunization procedure. However, there are also drawbacks, such as the need for refrigeration.

- *Attenuated bacterial vaccines.* The bacillus of Calmette-Guérin (BCG), an attenuated strain of *Mycobacterium bovis*, has been used for decades as a vaccine for tuberculosis. Unfortunately, the rates of protection obtained with this vaccine are rather variable, from 80% to 0%. The trials conducted in the United States were particularly disappointing and resulted in the lack of interest in BCG as an immunoprophylactic agent. Current research with this agent is centered on creating recombinant strains of increased immunogenicity.

  Recently, an oral attenuated bacterial vaccine for cholera has been introduced with 90% efficacy at 10 days after administration and 79.5% efficacy 3 months after administration.

Recombinant vaccines. Recombinant attenuated bacteria have been approved for immunoprophylaxis. The best example is the oral vaccine prepared with the attenuated Ty21a strain of *Salmonella typhi* that grows poorly and is virtually nonpathogenic but induces protective immunity in 90% of the individuals. While the vaccine protects for an average of 5 years, it requires four doses prior to travel to a risk area, while the inactivated vaccine requires a single infection but only protects for about 1 year.

- *Recombinant viral vaccines.* A major success of vaccinology was the development of human papilloma virus (HPV) vaccines. The HPV vaccines are based on hollow virus-like particles (VLPs) assembled from recombinant HPV coat proteins. The quadrivalent vaccine (Gardasil) contains coat proteins from four different HPV strains: 6, 11, 16, and 18. Strains 16 and 18 currently cause about 70% of all cervical cancer, while strains 6 and 11 currently cause about 90% of all cases of genital warts. Recent observations suggest that the papilloma virus vaccines not only prevent cervical carcinoma but may cause regression of early lesions. The use of vaccines for tumor treatment is discussed in greater detail in Chapter 26.

A recombinant shingles vaccine has been recently approved by the U.S. Food and Drug Administration, consisting of a lyophilized recombinant varicella-zoster virus (VZV) glycoprotein E antigen that is reconstituted at the time of use with AS01B adjuvant suspension composed of lipid A from *Salmonella minnesota* and a saponin molecule, combined in a liposomal formulation consisting of dioleoyl phosphatidylcholine and cholesterol in phosphate-buffered saline solution. This vaccine requires two administrations and is about 90% effective, and it has been recommended to replace the older attenuated shingles vaccine.

A recombinant vaccine for influenza (Flublok) is also available, composed of purified recombinant hemagglutinin antigens derived from four influenza virus strains (two influenza A strains and two influenza B strains) selected for inclusion in the annual influenza vaccine by the World Health Organization and updated on an annual basis. The efficiency of this vaccine does not seem very different from that of the classical inactivated vaccine, but it does not contain egg proteins so it is safe for individuals allergic to those proteins.

Recommended immunizations

At the present time, a wide variety of vaccines is available for protection of the general population or of individuals at risk for a specific disease due to their occupation or to other factors (https://www.cdc.gov/vaccines/terms/usvaccines.html). Particularly important is the vaccination of children, which has resulted in significant decreases in infant and toddler mortality. In many cases, several vaccines are combined in a single preparation to reduce the number of injections in children. Additional details about the vaccination schedules in children and adults can be obtained from the CDC (https://www.cdc.gov/vaccines/acip/index.html). Additional information concerning recommended immunizations for adults, travelers, special professions, etc., can be obtained in a variety of specialized publications, including the *Report of the Committee on Infectious Diseases*, published annually by the American Academy of Pediatrics, the booklet *Health Information for International Travel*, published annually by the CDC, and the *Morbidity and Mortality Weekly Report* published by the CDC.

BIBLIOGRAPHY

Ahmed R, Gray D. Immunological memory and protective immunity: Understanding their relation. *Science*. 1996;272:54–60.

Biss E. *On Immunity: An Inoculation*, London, UK: Fitzcarraldo Editions; 2014.

Cui Z. DNA vaccine. *Adv Genet*. 2005;54:257–289.

Dennehy M, Williamson AL. Factors influencing the immune response to foreign antigen expressed in recombinant BCG vaccines. *Vaccine*. 2005;26:1209–1223.

Dunman PM, Nesin M. Passive immunization as prophylaxis: When and where will this work? *Curr Opin Pharmacol*. 2003;35:486–496.

Hammarlund E, Lewis MW, Hansen SG et al. Duration of antiviral immunity after smallpox vaccination. *Nat Med*. 2003;9:1131–1137.

Hanson LA, Korotkova M. The role of breastfeeding in prevention of neonatal infection. *Semin Neonatol*. 2002;7:275–281.

Källberg E, Jainandunsing S, Gray D, Leanderson, T. Somatic mutation of immunoglobulin V genes *in vitro*. *Science*. 1996;271:1285–1289.

Klaus GG, Humphrey JH, Kunkl A, Dongworth DW. The follicular dendritic cell: Its role in antigen presentation in the generation of immunological memory. *Immunol Rev*. 1980;53:3–28.

Kniskern PJ, Marburg S, Ellis RW. *Haemophilus influenzae* type b conjugate vaccines. *Pharm Biotechnol*. 1995;6:673–694.

McCullough KC, Summerfield A. Basic concepts of immune response and defense development. *ILAR J*. 2005;46:230–240.

Mestecky J, Lue C, Russell MW. Selective transport of IgA. Cellular and molecular aspects. *Gastroenterol Clin North Am*. 1991:20:441–471.

Noelle RJ, Erickson LD. Determinations of B cell fate in immunity and autoimmunity. *Curr Dir Autoimmun*. 2005;8:1–24.

Serruto D, Bottomley MJ, Ram S, Giuliani MM. The new multicomponent vaccine against meningococcal serogroup B, 4CMenB: Immunological, functional and structural characterization of the antigens. *Vaccine*. 2012;305:887–897.

Sette A, Rappuoli R. Reverse vaccinology: Developing vaccines in the era of genomics. *Immunity*. 2010;33:530–541.

Wilkins AL, Snape MD. Emerging clinical experience with vaccines against group B meningococcal disease. *Vaccine*. 2018;36:5470–5476.

13

Phagocytic cells and their functions

GABRIEL VIRELLA AND JOHN W. SLEASMAN

INTRODUCTION

The failure or success of an antibody response directed against an infectious agent depends entirely on the ability to trigger the complement system and/or to induce phagocytosis. Most mammals, including man, have developed two well-defined systems of phagocytic cells: the polymorphonuclear leukocyte system (particularly the neutrophil population) and the monocyte/macrophage system. Both types of cells can engulf microorganisms and cause their intracellular death through a variety of enzymatic systems, but the two systems differ considerably in their biological characteristics.

PHYSIOLOGY OF POLYMORPHONUCLEAR LEUKOCYTES

Neutrophils and other polymorphonuclear (PMN) leukocytes are "wandering" cells, constantly circulating around the vascular network, able to recognize foreign matter by a wide variety of immunological and nonimmunological mechanisms. Their main biological characteristics are summarized in Table 13.1. Their effective participation in an anti-infectious response depends on the ability to respond to chemotactic signals, ingest the pathogenic agent, and kill the ingested microbes.

Chemotaxis and migration to extravascular compartment

In normal conditions, the interaction between leukocytes and endothelial cells is rather loose and involves a family of molecules known as selectins, which are constitutively expressed on endothelial cells and glycoproteins expressed on the leukocyte cell membrane. These interactions cause the slowing down ("rolling") of leukocytes along the vessel wall but do not lead to firm adhesion of leukocytes to endothelial cells.

A variety of chemotactic stimuli can be involved in the recruitment of leukocytes to the extravascular space. In most cases, those chemotactic factors are of bacterial origin, but they can also be released as a consequence of tissue necrosis, as a result of monocyte and lymphocyte activation, or as a by-product of complement activation.

Among bacterial products, formyl-methionyl peptides, such as f-methionine-leucine-phenylalanine (f-met-leu-phe), are extremely potent chemotactic agents.

Complement-derived chemotactic factors (such as C5a) can be generated in several ways. Tissue damage may result in the activation of the plasmin system that may in turn initiate complement activation with generation of C5a. After the inflammatory process has been established, proteases released by activated neutrophils and macrophages

Table 13.1 Comparison of the characteristics of polymorphonuclear (PMN) leukocytes and monocytes/macrophages

Characteristic	PMN leukocytes	Monocyte/macrophage
Numbers in peripheral blood	$3-6 \times 10^3/\mu L$	$285-500/\mu L$
Resident forms in tissues	−	+ (macrophage)
Nonimmunological phagocytosis	++	+
Fc receptors	FcγRII,III	FcγRI,II,III
C3b receptors	++	++
Enzymatic granules	++	++
Bactericidal enzymes	++	++
Ability to generate superoxide and H_2O_2	+++	++
Synthesis and release of leukotrienes	+ (B4)	++ (B4, C4, D4)
Synthesis and release of prostaglandins	−	++
PAF release/response	++	±
Response to nonimmunologic chemotactic factors	+	−
Response to C5a/C3a	+	−
Response to cytokines	+ (IL-8)	++ (IFN-γ)
Release of cytokines	+	++
Antigen processing	−	++
Expression of HLA class II antigens	−	++
Phagocytosis-independent enzyme release	++	−

can also split C5, and the same cells may release leukotriene B4, another potent chemotactic factor, attracting more neutrophils to the site. Many microorganisms can generate C5a by activation of the complement system through the alternative pathway.

Finally, activated T cells and monocytes can also release chemokines such as interleukin (IL)-8, monocyte chemotactic protein-1, and RANTES that attract neutrophils and/or monocytes.

After receiving a chemotactic stimulus, the neutrophil undergoes changes in the cell membrane, which is smooth in the resting cell, and becomes "ruffled" after the cell receives the chemotactic signal. The activated PMN has a marked increase in cell adhesiveness, associated with increased expression of adherence molecules, namely, integrins of the CD11/CD18 complex, which include the following:

- CD11a (the α chain of LFA [leukocyte function antigen]-1)
- CD11b (the C3bi receptor or CR3, also known as Mac-1) molecule
- CD11c (also known as protein p150,95)
- CD18 (the β chain of LFA-1)

These cell adhesion molecules are common to the majority of leukocytes, but their individual density and frequency may vary in the two main groups of phagocytic cells. While CD11a and CD18 are expressed virtually by all monocytes and granulocytes, CD11b is more prevalent among granulocytes and CD11c is more frequent among monocytes.

The expression of these cell-adhesion molecules (CAMs) mediates a variety of cell-cell interactions such as those that lead to neutrophil aggregation, and, most importantly, those that mediate firm adhesion of neutrophils to endothelial cells. For example, CD11a (LFA-1) and CD11b interact with molecules of the immunoglobulin gene family, such as intercellular adhesion molecule (ICAM)-1, ICAM-2, and vascular cell adhesion molecule (VCAM)-1, expressed on the endothelial cell membrane. The expression of VCAM-1, and to a lesser degree, of ICAM-1 and -2, is also upregulated by cytokines released by activated monocytes and lymphocytes, such as IL-1 and tumor necrosis factor (TNF). Consequently, the adhesion of leukocytes to endothelial cells is further enhanced.

After adhering to endothelial cells, leukocytes migrate to the extravascular compartment. The transmigration involves interaction with a fourth member of the immunoglobulin gene family—platelet endothelial cell adhesion molecule-1 (PECAM-1)—which is expressed at the intercellular junctions between endothelial cells. The interaction of leukocytes with PECAM-1 mediates the process of diapedesis, by which leukocytes squeeze through the endothelial cell junctions into the extravascular compartment.

The diapedesis process involves the locomotor apparatus of the neutrophils, a contractile actin-myosin system stabilized by polymerized microtubules. Its activation is essential for the neutrophil to move to the extravascular space, and an intact CD11b protein seems essential for the proper modulation of microtubule assembly, which will not take place in CD11b-deficient patients.

Phagocytosis

At the area of infection, PMN leukocytes recognize the infectious agents, which are ingested and killed intracellularly. The sequence of events leading to opsonization and intracellular killing is summarized in Figure 13.1.

Several recognition systems appear to be involved in the phagocytosis step. The most important recognition systems are those that mediate the

ingestion of opsonized particles. Two major types of receptors expressed by phagocytic cells are involved in this process:

- **Fcγ receptors** are predominantly involved in promoting ingestion of antibody-coated particles. Neutrophils express two types of Fcγ receptors, FcγRII and FcγRIII, both of which are involved in phagocytosis. In experimental conditions, Fcα receptors may also be involved in phagocytosis, but their efficiency seems to be much lower than that of Fcγ receptors.
- **CR1 (C3b) receptor** is also able to mediate phagocytosis with high efficiency. This receptor is expressed by all phagocytic cells, including polymorphonuclear leukocytes, monocytes, and macrophages. The binding and ingestion of microorganisms through this receptor have been well established.

Opsonization with both IgG antibodies and C3b seems associated with maximal efficiency in ingestion. However, opsonization is not an absolute requirement for ingestion by phagocytic cells. A variety of receptors may be involved in nonimmune phagocytosis, as described in greater detail in Chapter 14. These nonimmune mechanisms are particularly effective in promoting the ingestion

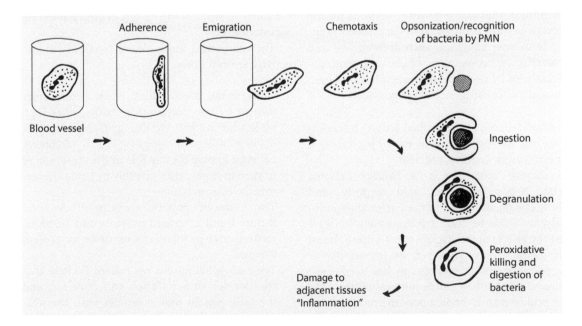

Figure 13.1 Sequence of events that takes place during PMN leukocyte phagocytosis. (Reproduced with permission from Wolach, B. et al., *Israel J. Med. Sci.*, 18, 897–916, 1982.)

of microorganisms with polysaccharide-rich outer layers. In addition, neutrophils are also able to ingest a variety of particulate matter, such as latex beads, silicone, asbestos fibers, etc., in the absence of opsonizing antibodies or complement.

Intracellular killing

Irrespectively of the nature of the receptors that may mediate it, ingestion is achieved through formation of pseudopodia that surround the particle or bacteria, and eventually fuse at the distal pole forming a phagosome. The cytoplasmic granules of the neutrophil (lysosomes) then fuse with the phagosomes, and their contents empty inside the phagosomes (degranulation). This degranulation process is very rapid and delivers a variety of antimicrobial substances to the phagosome:

- The azurophilic or primary granules contain, among other substances, myeloperoxidase, lysozyme, acid hydrolases (such as β-glucuronidase), cationic proteins, defensins, metalloproteinases (including proteases and collagenases), elastase, and cathepsin C2.
- The secondary granules or lysosomes contain lysozyme and lactoferrin.

Killing of ingested organisms depends on the effects of cationic proteins from the primary granules, lysosomal enzymes, such as lysozyme and lactoferrin, defensins, nitric oxide, and, most significantly, of by-products of the respiratory burst, activated as a consequence of phagocytosis.

- Lactoferrin has antimicrobial activity by chelating iron and preventing its use by bacteria that need it as an essential nutrient.
- Lysozyme splits the β-1,4 linkage between the N-acetylmuramic acid peptide and N-acetylglucosamine on the bacterial peptidoglycan. Some bacteria are exquisitely sensitive to the effects of this enzyme that causes almost immediate lysis. However, its importance as a primary killing mechanism has been questioned due to the relative inaccessibility of the peptidoglycan layer in many microorganisms, which may be surrounded by capsules or by the lipopolysaccharide-rich outer membrane (Gram-negative bacteria).

- Defensins are antimicrobial peptides released by almost all eukaryotic species, including plants, invertebrate animals, and vertebrate animals. Structurally, defensins are cationic molecules with spatially separated hydrophobic and charged regions which insert themselves into phospholipid membranes, causing their disruption. In mammalians, defensins are produced by specialized mucosal cells (i.e., the Paneth cells in the gut) and by phagocytic cells. The mucosal defensins are believed to play an important role in protecting mucosal cells from pathogenic bacteria. The neutrophil defensins are packaged on the azurophilic granules and are delivered to the phagosomes and also spilled into the extracellular environment.

RESPIRATORY BURST

From the bactericidal point of view, the activation of the superoxide generating system (respiratory burst) is the most significant killing mechanism of phagocytic cells. This system is activated primarily by opsonization but also by a variety of PMN activating stimuli, ranging from f-met-leu-phe to C5a. The activating stimuli are responsible for the induction of a key enzymatic activity (**NADPH oxidase**), a molecular complex located on the cell membrane, responsible for the transfer of a single electron from NADPH to oxygen, generating superoxide (O_2^-).

The component molecules of NADPH oxidase activity are as follows:

- Cytochrome b588, which is an heterodimer formed by two polypeptide chains, α, of high molecular weight (91 Kd, gp91phox) and β, of low molecular weight (22 Kd, p22phox), believed to play the key role in the reduction of oxygen to superoxide, possibly by being the terminal electron donor.
- Two cytosolic proteins (neutrophil cytosolic factors 1 and 2, termed p47phox and p67phox, respectively). p47phox is a substrate for protein kinase C.
- The rac2, a ubiquitous ras-related GTPase that translocates with p47phox and p67phox, and the rap1 protein that associates with the p22-phox component in the membrane, contribute to stabilize the enzymatic complex and regulate its biological activity.

In a resting cell, the complex is inactive and its components are not associated. After the cell is activated, p47phox is phosphorylated and becomes associated with p67phox and with rac2. The phosphorylated complex binds to cytochrome b588 in the lysosomal membranes, forming what is considered to be the active oxidase.

The electron transfer from NAPDH to oxygen is believed to involve at least three steps:

- Reduction of a flavin adenine dinucleotide (FAD), bound to the α chain of cytochrome b.
- Transfer of an electron from FADH2 to ferric iron in a heme molecule associated to the β chain of cytochrome b.
- Transfer of an electron from reduced iron to oxygen, generating superoxide.

The formation of the active molecular complex with oxidase activity coincides with phagolysosome fusion. Thus, the brunt of the active oxygen radicals generated by this system is delivered to the phagolysosome (Figure 13.2).

The respiratory burst generates two toxic compounds, essential for intracellular killing of bacteria: superoxide and H_2O_2. Through myeloperoxidase, H_2O_2 can be peroxided and led to form hypochlorite and other halide ion derivatives, which are also potent bactericidal agents. These compounds are also toxic to the cell, particularly superoxide, which can diffuse into the cytoplasm. The cell has several detoxifying systems, including superoxide dismutase, which converts superoxide into H_2O_2, and in turn, H_2O_2 is detoxified by catalase and by the oxidation of reduced glutathione, which requires activation of the hexose monophosphate shunt.

Activated phagocytic cells also express an inducible form on nitric oxide synthase (iNOS) that generates nitric oxide from arginine and molecular oxygen, using a variety of cofactors, including NADPH. Nitric oxide (NO) is a short-lived, highly cytotoxic free radical gas, which is believed to contribute significantly to intracellular killing. It can also participate in the induction of inflammatory reactions when spilled to the extracellular space.

PHYSIOLOGY OF MONOCYTE/ MACROPHAGE

Comparison of PMN leukocytes and monocytes/macrophages

The two populations of phagocytic cells share many common characteristics, such as the following:

- Presence of Fcγ and C3b receptors on their membranes.
- Ability to engulf bacteria and particles.
- Metabolic and enzymatic killing mechanisms and pathways.

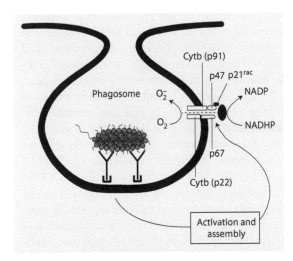

Figure 13.2 Major events involved in the respiratory burst of phagocytic cells. The occupancy of Fc and/or CR1 receptors triggers the activation sequence, which involves protein kinase activation, enzyme activation, and phosphorylation of at least one cytosolic protein (p47). As a result, a molecular complex, constituted by cytochrome B (Cyt b), p47, and p67, is assembled on the cell membrane, which is folding to constitute a phagosome. This complex has NADPH oxidase activity, oxidizes NADPH, and transfers the resulting electron to an oxygen molecule, resulting in the formation of superoxide (O_2^-).

In contrast, other functions and metabolic pathways differ considerably between these two types of cells (see Table 13.1). One important distinguishing feature is the involvement of the monocyte/macrophage series of cells in the inductive stages of the immune response, due to their ability to process antigens and present antigen-derived peptides to the immune system. Monocytes and macrophages are also involved in immunoregulatory signals, providing both activating signals (in the form of IL-1, IL-6, and IL-12) and downregulating signals (mainly in the form of PGE$_2$) to T lymphocytes.

PMN leukocytes and monocytes/macrophages have different preferences as far as phagocytosis. For example, PMN leukocytes are able to ingest inert particles such as latex but have very little ability to engulf antibody-coded homologous erythrocytes, while the reverse is true for the monocyte/macrophage. While neutrophils seem to be constitutively ready to ingest particulate matter, the circulating monocytes and the tissue-fixed (resident) macrophages are usually resting cells that need to be activated by several types of stimuli before they can fully express their phagocytic and killing potential. The activating factors include microorganisms or their products and cytokines. The main activating cytokine is interferon-γ, released by activated Th1 cells.

The **activated macrophage** has unique morphologic and functional characteristics. Morphologically, the activated macrophage is larger, and its cytoplasm tends to spread and attach to surfaces. The composition of the plasma membrane is changed, and the rates of pinocytosis and engulfment are increased (phagocytosis through C3b receptors is only seen after activation). Intracellularly, there is a marked increase in enzymatic contents, particularly of plasminogen activator, collagenase, and elastase. The oxidative metabolism (leading to generation of superoxide and H_2O_2) as well as the activity of iNOS are greatly enhanced.

MACROPHAGE HETEROGENEITY

Macrophages can be separated into three populations: M0, M1, and M2. M0 macrophages are resting cells, able to ingest by phagocytosis or endocytosis, while M1 and M2 are activated macrophage populations. In humans, M1 macrophages, also known as classically activated macrophages, do not endocytose. Two main activation stimuli have been used: LPS and interferon γ (IFNγ). Once activated, they express CD64, and when LPS is added to IFNγ or used by itself, the M1 macrophages also express CD80. M1 macrophages are proinflammatory and express CCL17 and CCL18, but they release different cytokines depending on how they are activated. IFNγ activation induces the release of additional IFNγ, while LPS-activated M1 release very small amounts of IFNγ and predominantly release TNF, IL-1β, RANTES, IL-8, and other proinflammatory

cytokines, closer to what is observed when human macrophages are activated via the Fcγ receptors. Activation with IFNγ suppresses the expression of cell recruitment genes activated by LPS, thus suggesting that it can also contribute to the resolution of an inflammatory reaction.

Differentiation of M2 macrophages requires activation by IL-4, IL-3, or a combination of IL-4 and IL-13, and this population expresses CD209, CD200R, CD1a, and CD1b. While M1 macrophages are actively involved in phagocytosis, M2 macrophages are predominantly involved in endocytosis, involving alternative receptors, such as the mannose receptor (MR, CD206). M2 macrophages secrete IL-10 and TGF-β. They also contribute on production of extracellular matrix components and tissue remodeling.

ROLE OF MACROPHAGES IN PHAGOCYTOSIS OF DEAD CELLS

As cells die, either by apoptosis or by necrosis, they express cell membrane markers that allow ingestion by macrophages, dendritic cells, and related cells. This results in the presentation of peptides derived from the dead cells on MHC-I molecules. In physiological conditions, the ingestion of dead cells by tissue macrophages is associated with the release of anti-inflammatory cytokines such as TGFβ1 (which is linked to the differentiation of Treg cells) and IL-10, and the immune system remains ignorant of the presented self peptides. However, presentation of peptides derived from ingested dead cells cross-loaded to MHC-I molecules by dendritic cells may elicit a CD8+ immune response against those peptides. It can be theorized that if the dead cells are ingested in nonphysiological conditions, e.g., as a consequence of the reaction against an infective agent, the likelihood for uptake and presentation in conditions favorable to the induction of an immune response increases. Such immune responses have been postulated to play a significant role in the emergence of autoimmune diseases. Also, the inflammatory complications of chronic granulomatous disease (CGD) result, in part at least, from defective phagocytosis of apoptotic neutrophils, resulting in the release of intracellular components such as DNA, proteases, and cationic proteins that are proinflammatory.

PHAGOCYTIC CELL ACTIVATION AND INFLAMMATION

One of the most biologically important consequences of phagocytosis is the release of pro-inflammatory cytokines. In the case of ingestion of opsonized particles, the engagement of Fcγ receptors and C3b receptors triggers the activation cascade that leads to the release of cytokines, proteases, oxygen radicals, and other proinflammatory compounds. However, such activation can also be induced as a consequence of innate immunity reactions involving the recognition of pathogen-associated molecular patterns (PAMPs) or endogenous danger-associated molecular patterns (DAMPs) by pattern-recognition receptors (PRRs). The activation of PPRs results in a cascade of events including the assembly of multimolecular complexes known as inflammasomes, which recruit inactive pro-caspase-1 proteins that oligomerize and are auto-proteolytically cleaved into caspase-1. Activated caspase-1 cleaves the inactive precursors of IL-1 and IL-18 that are consequently released in their active forms. One of the main components of the inflammasome are nod-like receptor proteins (NLRPs), particularly NLRP3 and NLRC4. Functionally, NLRs are sensors required for the formation of the inflammasome and recognize a variety of cellular damage or cellular infection products including DAMPs and PAMPs. Structurally, NLRPs contain a pyrin domain, while NLRC contain a caspase activation and recruitment domain (CARD). There is a major difference between those inflammasomes. NLRP3, after priming as a consequence of the binding of LPS to TLR4, can be activated by a wide variety of stimuli, such as reactive oxygen species, mitochondrial DNA, cardiolipin, or the release of cathepsins. NLRC4 (NLR family CARD domain-containing protein 4) needs to oligomerize with NAIP (NLR family apoptosis inhibitory protein) forming a NAIP/NLCR4 inflammasome that contains ASC (Adaptor Protein Apoptosis-Associated Speck-Like Protein Containing CARD) required for maximal inflammasome activation. Dying cells release ASC that can be taken up by other cells, propagating its proinflammatory activity from cell to cell. Probably a consequence of these properties, the NAIP/NLCR4 inflammasome has been identified as a cause of spontaneous autoinflammatory disorders.

Auto-inflammatory disorders

Auto-inflammatory disorders are a collection of diseases that result from exaggerated inflammasome activation usually associated with mutations in different inflammasomes, particularly those with pyrin domains, leading to uncontrolled inflammation. They range in severity from chronic inflammation and recurrent fever to severe life-threatening systemic inflammation and death.

Familial Mediterranean fever (FMF) is associated with recurrent fevers, polyserositis, chronic abdominal pain, arthritis, cutaneous erythema, inflammatory bowel disease, and amyloidosis leading to multiple organ failure. There are both autosomal dominant and recessive forms, and as the disease name implies, people of Mediterranean origin—including Sephardic and Mizrahi Jews, Armenians, Azerbaijanis, Arabs, Greeks, Turks, and Italians—are most commonly affected. The mutations in MEFV result in abnormal pyrin-mediated inflammasome assembly, and secretion of the pro-inflammatory cytokines (such as IL-18 and IL-1β) is a response to enterotoxins from bacteria.

Mevalonate kinase deficiency, also known as **hyper IgD syndrome**, causes a less severe form of periodic fever syndrome associated with chronic adenopathy, oral aphthosis ulcers, chronic diarrhea, and mevalonate acidosis during attacks. Laboratory findings include leukocytosis and elevated IgD levels.

TNF receptor–associated periodic fever syndrome (TRAPS) leads to fever, serositis, erythematous rash, periorbital edema, conjunctivitis, and amyloidosis, as is seen in FMF. Treatment is targeted at the TNF pathway using TNF inhibitors or the use of colchicine, particularly for FMF.

Cold autoinflammatory syndromes (cryopyrin-associated periodic syndromes [CAPS]) are hereditary autosomic-dominant diseases characterized by nonpruritic urticarial, arthritis, fever, and leukocytosis after cold exposure. The predominant genetic defect is within the *NLRP3* gene, resulting in gain of function and constitutional hyperactivity of the inflammasome. This results in abnormally high production of IL-1β due to alterations of cryopyrin inflammasomes by abnormal *NLRP3* signaling. Treatment consists of drugs that prevent IL1-β signaling, such as anakinra, rilonacept, and canakinumab.

Familial cold autoinflammatory syndrome (FCAS), also known as familial cold urticaria, is a mild form of CAPS typically triggered by cold exposure and characterized by febrile urticarial rash with headache, arthralgia, and occasionally conjunctivitis, but no central nervous system symptoms.

Muckle–Wells syndrome usually is a disease of later onset. The affected patients have similar symptoms as those seen in CAPS, but conjunctivitis and uveitis are more frequent, and sensorineural deafness and potentially life-threatening amyloidosis may also develop.

Neonatal-onset multisystem inflammatory disease (NOMID) is a severe form of these diseases characterized by neonatal-onset rash, continuous fevers, inflammation, aseptic meningitis, deforming arthropathy, sensineuronal hearing loss, and visual loss.

LABORATORY EVALUATION OF PHAGOCYTIC FUNCTION

The evaluation of phagocytic function is usually centered on the study of neutrophils that are considerably easier to isolate than monocytes or macrophages. Phagocytosis by neutrophils can be depressed as a result of reduction in cell numbers or as a result of a functional defect. Functional defects affecting every stage of the phagocytic response have been reported and have to be evaluated by different tests. The following is a summary of the most important tests used to evaluate phagocytic function.

Neutrophil count

This is the simplest and one of the most important tests to perform since phagocytic defects due to neutropenia are, by far, more common than the primary congenital defects of phagocytic function. As a rule, it is believed that a neutrophil count below $1000/\mu L$ represents an increased risk of infection, and when neutrophil counts are lower than $200/\mu L$, the patient will invariably be infected.

Adherence

The increased adherence of activated phagocytic cells to endothelial cells is critical for the migration of these cells to infectious foci. Although there are specialized tests available to measure aggregation

and adherence of neutrophils in response to stimuli such as $C5a_{desarg}$ (a nonchemotactic derivative of C5a), presently this property is evaluated indirectly, by determining by flow cytometry the expression of the different components of CD11/CD18 complex that mediate adhesion.

Chemotaxis and migration

The migration of phagocytes in response to chemotactic stimuli can be studied *in vitro*, using the Boyden chamber. The basic principle of all versions of the Boyden chamber is to have two compartments separated by a membrane whose pores are too tight to allow PMN leukocytes to passively diffuse from one chamber to the other but large enough to allow the active movement of these cells from the upper chamber where they are placed, to the lower chamber.

The movement of the cells is stimulated by adding to the lower chamber a chemotactic factor such as C5a, the bacterial tetrapeptide f-met-leu-phe, IL-8, leukotriene B4, or platelet-activating factor (PAF). The results are usually based on either counting the number of cells that reached the bottom side of the membrane, or by determining the number of ^{51}Cr-labeled PMN trapped in the filter separating the two chambers (as illustrated in Figure 13.3).

It must be noted that all versions of this technique are difficult to reproduce and standardize and are not used in routine laboratory diagnosis.

Ingestion

Ingestion tests are relatively simple to perform and reproduce. They are usually based on incubating PMN with opsonized particles, and after an adequate incubation, determining either the number of ingested particles or a phagocytic index:

$$\text{Phagocytic index} = \frac{\text{Number of cells with ingested particles}}{\text{Total number of cells}} \times 100$$

Several types of particles have been used, including latex, zymosan (fragments of fungal capsular polysaccharidic material), killed *Candida albicans*, and IgG-coated beads (Immunobeads). All of these particles will activate complement by either one of the pathways and become coated with C3, although opsonization with complement is not the major

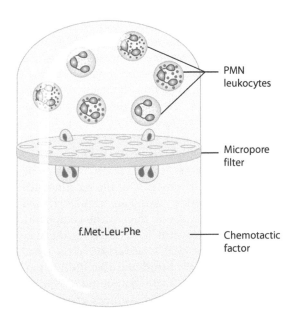

PMN
leukocytes

Micropore
filter

f.Met-Leu-Phe

Chemotactic
factor

Figure 13.3 **Principle of chemotaxis assays using the Boyden chamber and ⁵¹Cr-labeled PMN leukocytes. A chemotactic factor (N-formyl-methionyl-leucyl-phenylalanine, f-Met-Leu-Phe) is added to one of the compartments of the chamber, and leukocytes are added to the opposite compartment. The number of cells trapped in the filter separating the two chambers reflects the chemotactic response to f-Met-Leu-Phe.**

determinant of phagocytosis. The easiest particles to visualize once ingested are fluorescent latex beads; their use considerably simplifies the assay (Figure 13.4), particularly if performed in a flow cytometer. Fluorescein-labeled killed *C. albicans* and killed *Staphylococcus aureus* can also be used in flow cytometry–based ingestion assays.

Ingestion tests are also not used routinely because other tests are available that test both for ingestion and for the ability to mount a respiratory burst (see later discussion in chapter).

Degranulation

When the contents of cytoplasmic granules are released into a phagosome, there is always some leakage of their contents into the extracellular fluid. The tests to study degranulation involve ingestion of particulate matter as previously mentioned, but in this case, the supernatants are analyzed for their contents of substances released by the PMN granules such as myeloperoxidase, lysozyme, β-glucuronidase, and lactoferrin.

Oxidative burst

Most diagnostic laboratories that test for neutrophil function run a variant or another of a test

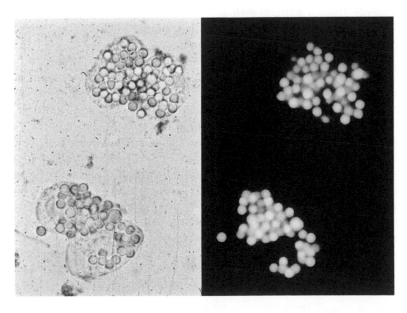

Figure 13.4 **Use of fluorescent latex beads for evaluation of phagocytosis. The panel on the left reproduces a photograph of a microscopic field showing the phagocytic cells that have ingested latex beads under visible light. The panel on the right shows the same field under UV light.**

to measure the oxidative burst. Several different assays are available, using different parameters and methodologies. Tests based on the reduction of nitroblue tetrazolium (**NBT reduction tests**) were the first successfully used for evaluation of the oxidative burst but have been largely replaced by flow cytometry tests based on the reduction of fluorescent substrates.

The principle of the NBT assays is relatively simple. Oxidized NBT, colorless to pale yellow in solution, is transformed by reduction into blue formazan. The test usually involves incubation of purified neutrophils, NBT, and a stimulus known to activate the respiratory burst. Two types of stimuli can be used:

- **Opsonized particles**, which need to be ingested to stimulate the burst. In this way the test examines both the ability to ingest and the ability to produce a respiratory burst.
- **Diffusible activators**, such as PMA (phorbol-12-myristate-13-acetate) or f-met-leu-phe. These compounds diffuse into the cell, activate the NADPH-cytochrome B system, and induce the respiratory burst directly, bypassing the ingestion step. A patient whose neutrophils respond to stimulation with phorbol ester but not to stimulation with opsonized beads is likely to have an ingestion defect. In contrast, neutrophils from a patient with a primary defect in the ability to generate the respiratory burst will not respond to any kind of stimulus.

The oxidative burst can be measured by colorimetric assays. Classical tests involved the simultaneous exposure of opsonized particles and NBT, and the change of color of the supernatant from pale yellow to gray or purple (as a result of the spillage of oxidizing products during phagocytosis) was measured. This assay was rendered practical and convenient by the introduction of kinetic colorimeters. Using this type of equipment, the color change of NBT can be measured without the need to extract the dye from the cells or to separate the cells from the supernatant.

The techniques more widely used in diagnostic laboratories utilize fluorescent dyes, which allow the use of flow cytometry to measure the oxidative burst activated by phorbol myristate acetate (PMA). A widely used flow cytometry test uses dihydrorhodamine (DHR), the nonfluorescent derivative of rhodamine. DHR is taken up by leukocytes following *ex vivo* incubation. When the cells are subsequently activated by PMA, the NAD/NADPH electron transport system is activated, DHR is reduced by products of the nicotinamide adenine dinucleotide phosphate (NADPH) and transforms into a green fluorescent compound, and a fluorescence shift is detected by the flow cytometer (Figure 13.5). Comparison of the mean fluorescence intensity before and after PMA stimulation is measured as a stimulation index. Normal neutrophils have a stimulation index greater than 150, while patients with different forms of CGD have stimulation indexes between 1 and 3. Female carriers of CGD have two populations of neutrophils, one with normal oxidative burst activity because they activate the normal X chromosome, and the other with abnormal respiratory burst activity because the abnormal X chromosome is activated.

It must be noted that the flow cytometry test measures the activation of the oxidative burst by PMA but will not detect defects in ingestion of opsonized particles.

Killing assays

The main protective function of the neutrophil is the ingestion and killing of microorganisms. This ability can be tested using a variety of bacteria and fungi that are mixed with PMN in the presence of normal human plasma (a source of opsonins), and after a given time, the cells are harvested, lysed, and the number of intracytoplasmic viable bacteria is determined.

Killing assays are difficult and cumbersome and require close support from a microbiology laboratory, and for this reason they have been less used than the indirect killing assays based on detection of the oxidative burst of the PMN mentioned in the previous section.

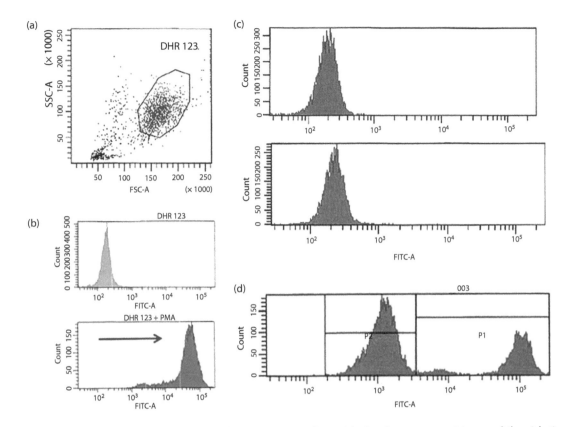

Figure 13.5 Assessment of neutrophil function using the oxidative burst assay. Neutrophil oxidative burst activity through the NAD/NADPH pathway can be measured by flow cytometry. (a) Neutrophils can be identified by their unique forward (FSC) and side scatter (SSC) characteristics. (b) Resting neutrophils when incubated with dihydrorhodamine (upper panel). Following stimulation with phorbol myristate acetate (PMA), normal neutrophils oxidize the dihydrorhodamine to cause a fluorescence shift (lower panel). The degree of oxidative burst activity is measured as the mean fluorescence intensity (MFI) of the PMA-stimulated cells divided by the MFI of unstimulated cells. (c) Lack of the oxidative burst pattern in a child with chronic granulomatous disease (CGD) in which there is no shift in MFI after PMA stimulation. (d) Respiratory burst pattern of a female carrier for X-linked CGD in which two peaks are seen for neutrophils expressing either the normal or an abnormal X chromosome.

BIBLIOGRAPHY

Aderem A, Unerhill DM. Mechanisms of phagocytosis in macrophages. *Annu Rev Immunol.* 1999;17:593–623.

Arandjelovic S, Ravichandran KS. Phagocytosis of apoptotic cells in homeostasis. *Nature Immunology.* 2015;16:907–917.

Boxer LA, Blackwood RA. Leukocyte disorders: Quantitative and qualitative disorders of the neutrophil. *Pediatr Rev.* 1996;17:19–28. (part 1) and 47–50 (part 2).

De Torre-Minguela C, Mesa del Castillo P, Pelegrín P. The NLRP3 and pyrin inflammasomes: Implications in the pathophysiology of autoinflammatory diseases. *Front Immunol.* 2017;8:43.

Errante P, Frazão JB, Condino-Neto A. The use of interferon-γ therapy in chronic granulomatous disease. *Recent Pat Antiinfect Drug Discov.* 2008;3:225–230.

Gu BJ, Sun C Fuller S et al. A quantitative method for measuring innate phagocytosis by human monocytes using real-time flow cytometry. *Cytometry Part A.* 2014;85:313–321.

Guo H, Callaway JB, Ting JP. Inflammasomes: Mechanism of action, role in disease, and therapeutics. *Nat Med.* 2015;21:677–687.

Hoeksema MA, Brendon P, Scicluna MC et al. IFN-γ priming of macrophages represses a part of the inflammatory program and attenuates neutrophil recruitment. *J Immunol.* 2015;194:3909–3916.

Ottonello L, Dapino P, Pastorino G et al. Neutrophil dysfunction and increased susceptibility to infection. *Eur J Clin Invest.* 1995;25:687–692.

Pallister CJ, Hancock JT. Phagocytic NADPH oxidase and its role in chronic granulomatous disease. *Brit J Biomed Sci.* 1995;52:149–156.

Robinson JP, Carter WO, Narayanan P. Functional assays by flow cytometry. In: Rose NR, de Macario EC, Folds JD, Lane HC, Nakamura RM, eds. *Manual of Clinical Laboratory Immunology,* 5th ed. Washington, DC: American Society for Microbiology; 1997: 245–254.

Tarique AA, Logan J, Thomas E et al. Phenotypic, functional, and plasticity features of classical and alternatively activated human macrophages. *Am J Respir Cell Mol Biol.* 2015;53:676–688.

Umeki S. Mechanisms for the activation/electron transfer of neutrophil NADPH-oxidase complex and molecular pathology of chronic granulomatous disease. *Ann Hematol.* 1994;68:267–277.

Virella G. Diagnostic evaluation of neutrophil function. In: Gabrilovich DI, ed., *The Neutrophils: New Outlook for Old Cells,* London, UK: Imperial College Press; 1999:275–297.

Vuorte J, Jansson SE, Repo H. Standardization of a flow cytometric assay for phagocyte respiratory burst activity. *Scand J Immunol.* 1996;43:329–334.

14

Anti-infectious innate and adaptive immune responses

CARL ATKINSON AND GABRIEL VIRELLA

INTRODUCTION

During evolution, an extremely complex system of anti-infectious defenses has emerged. However, as vertebrates and mammals developed their defenses, so microbes continued to evolve, and many became adept at avoiding the consequences of anti-infectious defense mechanisms. The interplay between host defenses, microbial virulence, and microbial evasion mechanisms determines the outcome of the constant encounters between humans and pathogenic organisms.

INNATE IMMUNITY

The term *innate immunity* defines a variety of anti-infectious defenses that preexist before contact with an infectious agent. This term was designed to contrast with adaptive immunity that is triggered by the recognition of non-self components, is specific for the inducing agent, and takes several days to develop. A summary of the characteristics that differentiate some of the best-defined components

of innate immunity from adaptive immunity is presented in Table 14.1.

As with other domains of immunity, innate immune defenses may play other roles in addition to protection against infectious agents, but in this chapter, we focus our attention on the protective mechanisms.

Constitutive nonspecific defense mechanisms

Constitutive nonspecific defense mechanisms play an important role as a first line of defense by preventing penetration of microorganisms beyond the outer exposed surfaces of the body. As summarized in Table 14.2, some of these nonspecific defense mechanisms are local, while others are systemic. The local mechanisms consist of physical and chemical barriers that protect the organism from infectious agents, and their importance is apparent from the prevalence of infections when their integrity is compromised. The systemic

Table 14.1 Nonspecific anti-infectious defense mechanisms

Local	Systemic
Physical integrity of skin and mucosae	Fever
Lysozyme in tears, saliva, sweat, and other secretions	Defensins
Gastric acidity	Production of interferons
Flow of mucosal secretions in the respiratory tract	Nonimmune opsonization; phagocytosis
Intestinal transit	Nonimmune killing; natural killer cells
Urinary flow	

mechanisms can be activated directly and immediately by infectious agents.

INNATE IMMUNE MECHANISMS

Several anti-infectious defenses can be included in the broad category of innate immunity, ranging from antibacterial compounds to phagocytic cells.

Antimicrobial peptides: Defensins and cathelicidins

Defensins are antimicrobial peptides released by specialized mucosal cells (i.e., the Paneth cells in the gut) and by phagocytic cells. The mucosal defensins are believed to play an important role in protecting mucosal cells from pathogenic bacteria. The neutrophil defensins are packaged in the azurophilic granules and are delivered to the phagosomes as well as being spilled into the extracellular environment. Mammalian defensins are grouped into two families: α and β.

β defensins have been shown to have chemotactic properties for immature dendritic cells and T lymphocytes, and because of this activity may play a significant role in promoting the onset of the adaptive immune response.

Lymphocytes, phagocytic cells, and epithelial cells of the gastrointestinal and respiratory tracts express cathelicidins. Their antibacterial activity affects both Gram-positive and Gram-negative bacteria. In addition, engagement of toll-like receptors 1 and 2 (see later discussion in this chapter) by mycobacterial lipopeptides triggers a vitamin D–dependent anti-mycobacterial response mediated by increased synthesis of cathelicidin.

Activation of complement system via alternative pathway

A variety of microorganisms (bacteria, fungi, viruses, and parasites, see Table 14.3) can activate complement directly in the nonimmune host via all three activation pathways. Certain microbial structures can directly bind C1q (initiates classical pathway), mannose-binding protein (lectin pathway), and can accept spontaneously deposited C3 (alternative pathway). The subsequent generation of chemotactic complement activation products

Table 14.2 Features of innate and adaptive immunity

Innate immunity	Adaptive immunity
Pathogen recognized by receptors encoded in the germline	Pathogen recognized by receptors generated randomly during differentiation
Receptors have broad specificity, i.e., recognize many related molecular structures called PAMPs (pathogen-associated molecular patterns)	Receptors have very narrow specificity, i.e., recognize a unique epitope
PAMPs are essential polysaccharides and polynucleotides that differ little from one pathogen to another but are not found in the host	Most epitopes are derived from polypeptides (proteins) or polysaccharides and reflect the individuality of the pathogen
Receptors are PRRs (pattern recognition receptors)	Receptors are B-cell (BCR) and T-cell (TCR) receptors for antigen
Immediate response	Slow (3–8 days) response (because of the need for clones of responding cells to develop)
No memory of prior exposure	Memory of prior exposure

Table 14.3 Examples of infectious agents able to activate the alternative pathway of complement without apparent participation of specific antibody

a. Bacteria
   Haemophilus influenzae type b
   Streptococcus pneumoniae
   Staphylococcus aureus
   S. epidermidis
b. Fungi
   Candida albicans
c. Parasites
   Trypanosoma cyclops
   Schistosoma mansoni
   Babesia rodhaini
d. Viruses
   Vesicular stomatitis virus

(C3a and C5a) and the opsonization of microbes by C3b and iC3b promote leukocyte recruitment and microbe phagocytosis, as discussed in more detail in Chapter 9.

γ/δ T lymphocytes

This T-cell subpopulation is predominantly localized to epithelia and appears to recognize and eliminate infected epithelial cells. In humans, there are two major subsets of γ/δ T cells identified by their γ/δ chain. γ/δ1 T cells are predominant in the thymus and epithelial tissues and recognize various stress-related antigens. γ/δ2 T cells constitute the majority of blood γ/δ T cells. Both subsets share a common Vγ9 chain. Human Vγ9/Vδ2$^+$ T cells can be activated by microbial products (e.g., phosphorylated metabolites) as well as by markers of cellular stress released by infected or transformed cells. The activation of γ/δ T cells can be mediated by their T-cell receptors (TCRs) assisted by costimulatory signals from natural killer (NK)-type receptors but do not involve major histocompatibility complex (MHC)–associated presentation of the activating compounds. The γ/δ TCRs also recognize lipid antigens presented by CD1 molecules, in particular CD1d. Once activated, γ/δ T cells show a great degree of plasticity. They can release proinflammatory cytokines, cause cytolysis of infected or transformed cells by the same mechanisms as classical cytotoxic CD8 T cells, and become professional antigen-presenting cells. Thus, γ/δ T cells appear to be one of the bridges between innate and adaptive immunity.

Phagocytic cells

As a microbe penetrates beyond the skin or mucosal surface, it will encounter cells able to ingest it. Two types of cells are particularly adept at non-immune phagocytosis: granulocytes (particularly neutrophils) and tissue macrophages. This nonimmune phagocytosis involves a variety of recognition systems (Figure 14.1):

- CR1 and CR3 receptors, able to interact with complement opsonins C3b and iC3b on the microbial surface that are deposited as a consequence of complement activation.
- C-type lectins, such as mannose receptors, able to mediate ingestion of organisms with mannose-rich polysaccharides, such as *Candida albicans*. A mannose-binding protein that promotes phagocytosis through complement activation amplifies mannose-mediated phagocytosis.
- C-reactive protein binds to certain bacterial polysaccharides and has very similar effects to the mannose-binding protein, activating complement and promoting phagocytosis, both through CR1 and CR3, as well as by other receptors, including the FcγRI and C1q receptors.
- TLRs, structurally similar to the Toll receptors of insects, recognize pathogen-associated molecular patterns (PAMPS) or, in other words, are pattern-recognition receptors (PPRs). There are 10 types of TLRs, most of them present in phagocytic cells and antigen-presenting cells (APCs) and six of which recognize microbial products. Some (TLR-1, -2, -4, and -5) are expressed on the cell membranes, while TLR-3, -7, and -9 are expressed in endosomes. The specificities of these receptors are as follows:
  - TLR-1 and -2 recognize glucan, peptidoglycan, lipopeptides, and some lipopolysaccharides.
  - TLR-3 recognizes viral dsRNA.
  - TLR-4 recognizes most types of lipopolysaccharide.
  - TLR-5 recognizes flagellin.
  - TLR-7 recognizes viral ssRNA.
  - TLR-9 recognizes bacterial DNA.

The binding of these products to TLRs induces phagocytosis, activation of signaling cascades involving NFkB, and, in some cases (TLR-1/2), synthesis of antimicrobial peptides, such as cathelicidins. It is now clear that these processes are

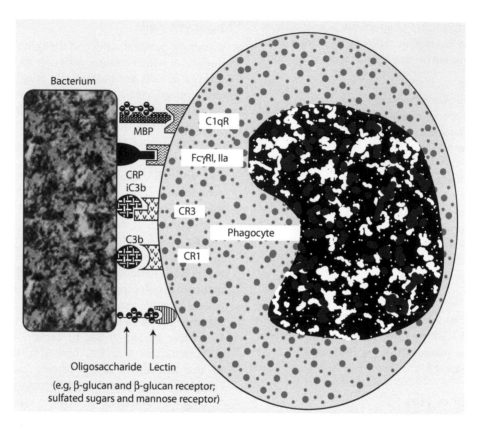

Figure 14.1 Different receptors that may mediate nonimmune phagocytosis. (CRP, C-reactive protein; MBP, mannose-binding protein.)

also of significance in bridging innate and adaptive immune responses, such as by activating APCs. A special case seems to be that of TLR-7, expressed in endosomal vesicles, where they can interact with viral ssRNA released as engulfed viral particles are denatured. The stimulation of TLR-7 by viral ssRNA induces the release of interferon-α and pro-inflammatory cytokines, which may play an important role in the innate response to viruses. Similarly, TLR-9 is expressed intracellularly, within the endosomal compartment, and functions to alert the cell to bacterial or viral infections by binding to unmethylated CpG sequences in DNA. Thus, in keeping with the other TLRs, activation of TLR-9 induces cytokines such as type-1 interferon, interleukin (IL)-6, IL-12, and tumor necrosis factor (TNF)-α as a means to tune the inflammatory response to invading pathogens.

These initial antimicrobial steps are not specific and of limited amplitude. However, they assist in antigen presentation in association with MHC-I and MHC-II, which will be critical for the initiation

of the adaptive immune response. In turn, the activation of the adaptive immune response results in targeted phagocytosis and elimination of the engulfed microbe, and the inflammatory response is considerably more intense when antigen-antibody complexes (immune complexes [ICs]) interact with the phagocytic cells Fcγ receptors (FcγR). The nature and role of pro-inflammatory cytokines and chemokines released by activated T cells and phagocytic cells are discussed later in this chapter.

NATURAL KILLER CELLS

NK cells represent another bridge between innate and acquired immunity, where the two systems become closely related. NK cells were recognized for their ability to kill certain tumor cell lines and viral infected cells. They are also one of the main cell populations involved in antibody-dependent cellular cytotoxicity (ADCC). The physiological significance of NK cells results from the fact that these cells seem to fulfill the need for a rapid response to a viral infection. The mobilization of a T lymphocyte–mediated cytotoxic response is a relatively slow process. In a resting immune system, the cytotoxic T-cell precursors exist in relatively low numbers ($<1/10^5$). Proliferation and differentiation are required to generate a sufficient number of fully activated effector $CD8^+$ T cells. Even the response of a primed individual takes a few days. Thus, an effective primary antiviral cytotoxic T-cell primary response is seldom deployed in less than 5–6 days and may take as long as 2 weeks. During this time, the host depends on defenses that can be deployed much more rapidly, such as the production of type I interferons (α and β), initiated as soon as the virus starts replicating, and the activity of NK cells.

NK cell activation

NK cells receive autocrine and paracrine activation signals from NK cells, T lymphocytes, and monocytes/macrophages. Those signals are mediated by cytokines released from those cells, particularly type I interferons (α and β), IL-2, and IL-12. The activating effect of IL-2 is mediated by the interaction of this cytokine with a functional IL-2 receptor, predominantly constituted by the β chain (p75 subunit) expressed by NK cells. Because the α chain is not expressed, NK cells are, for the most part, $CD25^-$. However, this variant of the IL-2 receptor enables NK cells to be effectively activated by IL-2, without the need for any additional costimulating factors or signals.

Type I interferons enhance the cytotoxic activity of NK cells. Thus, the release of these interferons from infected cells mobilizes nonspecific defenses before the differentiation of MHC-restricted cytotoxic T lymphocytes is completed. IL-12, produced at the same time as interferons α and β, is believed to play a crucial role in the early activation of NK cells.

The mechanism of recognition of target cells by NK cells is totally different from the antigen recognition mechanisms of B and T lymphocytes (Figure 14.2). A major difference is that NK cells can recognize virus-infected cells without clonal restriction. Normal cells deliver both activating and downregulating signals that neutralize each other. Viral infections are associated with changes in the constitution of membrane glycoproteins and often interfere with the interaction of MHC-I molecules (HLA-C) with the inhibitory receptor, either by replacing a self peptide on HLA-C by a non-self

peptide, or from the reduced expression of MHC-I molecules on the cell membrane. In either case, the end result will be that the activating receptor will deliver a strong signal that is not counteracted by an equivalent signal from the inhibitory receptor. In all of these circumstances, the activated NK cell will be able to cause the death of the target cell by mechanisms similar to those involved in T lymphocyte–mediated cytotoxicity (see Chapter 11).

NATURAL ANTIBODIES

Preexisting antibodies may play a very important anti-infectious protecting role. Their origin and nature are somewhere in between natural and adaptive immunity. The term *natural* is misleading, implying that those antibodies emerged in the absence of specific antigen stimulation. However, the origin of natural antibodies, in most cases, appears to be unsuspected cross reactions. The classical example is experimental production of agglutinins recognizing the human AB alloantigens by chickens. Interestingly, the isoagglutinins are only produced by chicks fed conventional diets; chicks fed sterile diets do not develop them. Furthermore, anti-A and anti-B agglutinins develop as soon as chicks fed sterile diets after birth are placed on conventional diets later in life. These observations pointed to some dietary component as a source of immunization. It was eventually demonstrated that the cell-wall polysaccharides of several strains of Enterobacteriaceae and the AB oligosaccharides of human erythrocytes are structurally similar. Thus, cross-reactive antibodies to Enterobacteriaceae are responsible for the "spontaneous" development of antibodies to human red cell antigens in chickens.

Newborn babies of blood groups A, B, or O do not have anti-A or anti-B isoagglutinins in their cord blood but develop them during the first months of life, as they get exposed to common bacteria with polysaccharide capsules. However, newborns are tolerant to their own blood group substance, so they will only make antibodies against the blood group substance that they do not express. Blood group AB individuals never produce AB isoagglutinins. Other mechanisms, such as the mitogenic effects of T-independent antigens and the nonspecific activation of B cells by lymphokines released by antigen-stimulated T lymphocytes could explain the rise of "nonspecific" immunoglobulins that is observed in the early

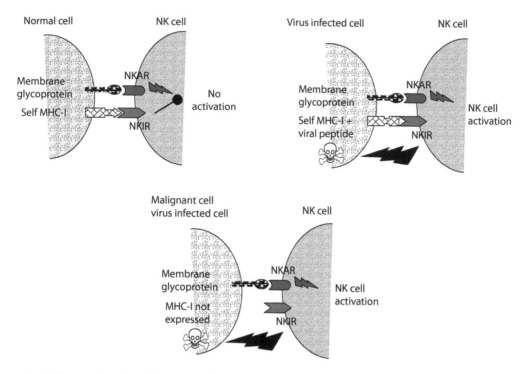

Figure 14.2 The mechanism of target cell recognition by NK cells. The activation or lack of activation of cytotoxic pathways depends on the balance between activating receptors (NKAR, such as NKR-P1, which interacts with cellular glycoproteins) and inhibitory receptors (NKIR, such as KIR, which interacts with self MHC-I molecules). If the inhibitory receptor is not triggered (due to either lack of interaction of the inhibitory receptor with MHC-I–peptide complex, or to downregulation of expression of MHC-I molecules on the cell membrane), stimulatory activity prevails, and the target cell is killed. Overexpression of modified cellular glycoproteins (in malignant cells of viral-infected cells) can cause a very strong activating signal, able to override the downregulating signal mediated by MHC-I recognition.

stages of the humoral response to many different antigens. It is only a matter of random probability that some of these nonspecific immunoglobulins may play the role of "natural antibodies" relative to an unrelated antigen. Finally, there is experimental evidence for the existence of polyspecific or promiscuous antibodies, able to react with different antigens. These promiscuous antibodies are believed to be germline encoded, usually of the IgM isotype, structurally flexible and able to bind with low affinity a large number of unrelated antigens. The cinical relevance of these promiscuous antibodies has not been definitely established.

Irrespective of their origin, "natural" antibodies may play an important protective role, as shown by the experiments summarized in Figure 14.3. Antibodies elicited to *Escherichia coli* K100 cross-react with the polyribophosphate of *Haemophilus influenzae* and can protect experimental animals against infection with the latter

organism. It is logical to assume that such cross-immunizations may be rather common and play an important protective role against a variety of infectious agents.

ADAPTIVE IMMUNITY

Humoral immune response

If a pathogen is not eliminated by nonimmunological means and continues to replicate, it will eventually spread through the blood and lymph, and will usually be trapped by macrophages and dendritic cells in the lymph nodes and spleen. These cells are able to internalize antigens interacting with receptors such as the mannose receptor process the antigen in the endosomic compartment, and express MHC-II-associated antigen-derived peptides. This creates ideal conditions for the onset of a specific immune response: B lymphocytes can

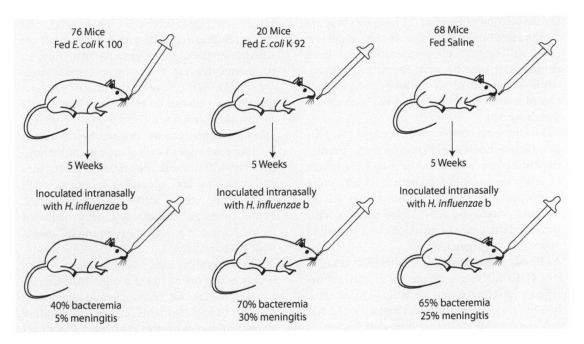

Figure 14.3 An experiment proving the anti-infectious protective role of cross-reactive "natural" antibodies. Three groups of mice were orally immunized with *Escherichia coli* K100, *E. coli* K92, and saline, as a control. Five weeks later all animals were challenged with *Haemophilus influenzae* type b by the intranasal route. *E. coli* K100 has cross-reactivity with *H. influenzae* type b, but the same is not true for *E. coli* K92. The animals immunized with *E. coli* K100 showed significantly lower rates of bacteremia and meningeal infection than the animals immunized with *E. coli* K92 or controls fed with saline. (Based on Moxon R, Anderson P, *J. Infect. Dis.* 1979; 140: 471–478.)

interact with membrane-bound antigen, while helper T cells recognize MHC-II with antigen-derived peptides presented by the same APC. The antigen-recognizing cells will interact and costimulate each other and after a time lag necessary for proliferation and differentiation of B cells into antibody-producing cells, circulating antibody will become detectable.

As described in Chapter 12, a primary immune response will take 5–7 days (sometimes as long as 2–3 weeks) to be detected. The predominating isotype of the antibodies made early in a primary immune response is IgM, and these antibodies are of relatively low affinity. In contrast, a secondary immune response has a shorter lag phase (as short as 3–4 days), and the predominant isotype of the antibodies is IgG, which have higher affinity. These different characteristics can be exploited for diagnostic purposes. The predominance of IgM or of low-affinity antibodies indicates that a given immune response has been elicited recently and that the infection is recent or ongoing.

ANTIBODY-DEPENDENT ANTI-INFECTIOUS EFFECTOR MECHANISMS

As soon as specific antibodies become available, they can protect the organism against infection by several different mechanisms:

- **Complement-mediated lysis** can result from activation of the complete sequence of complement. However, as discussed later, both mammalian cells and most pathogenic microorganisms have developed mechanisms that allow them to resist complement-mediated lysis.
- **Opsonization and phagocytosis** are critically important. Several proteins can opsonize and promote phagocytosis, as discussed previously, but IgG antibodies are the most efficient opsonins among the immunoglobulins. Opsonization is potentiated when complement is activated as a consequence of the antigen-antibody reaction occurring on the surface of the infectious agent and C3b, and iC3b joins IgG on the microbial cell membrane. This synergism is explained by

the association of Fcγ and C3 receptors that are coexpressed on the membranes of all phagocytic cells. Killing through opsonization has been demonstrated for bacteria, fungi, and viruses, while phagocytosis of antibody/complement-coated unicellular parasites has not been clearly demonstrated.

The biological significance of phagocytic cells as ultimate mediators of the effects of opsonizing antibodies is obvious; the protective effects of antibodies are lost in patients with severe neutropenia or with severe functional defects of their phagocytic cells. Those patients have increased incidence of infections by a variety of opportunistic organisms:

- **Antibody-dependent cell mediated cytotoxicity (ADCC)**: NK cells express the FcγRIII, a low-affinity Fc receptor that binds IgG-coated cells. IgG binding results in the activation of the NK cell and lysis of the target, a process known as ADCC. ADCC-dependent activation and killing are not inhibited by the NKIR (p58,70) inhibitory receptor.

Other cell populations with Fc receptors may be able to participate in killing reactions that target antibody-coated cells. IgG1, IgG3, and IgE antibodies and cells with FcγR or FcεR are usually involved. Large granular lymphocytes or monocytes are the most common effector cells in ADCC, but in the case of parasitic infections, eosinophils play the principal role in cytotoxic reactions (Figure 14.4). Different effector mechanisms are responsible for killing by different types of cells. Large granular lymphocytes kill through the release of granzymes and signaling for apoptosis; monocytes kill by releasing oxygen active radicals and nitric oxide; eosinophil killing is mostly mediated by the release of a "major basic protein" that is toxic for parasites:

- **Toxin neutralization**: Many bacteria release toxins, which are often the major virulence factors responsible for severe clinical symptoms. Antibodies to these toxins prevent their binding to cellular receptors and promote toxin elimination by phagocytosis.
- **Virus neutralization**: Most viruses spread from an initial focus of infection to a target tissue via the bloodstream. Antibodies binding to the circulating virus can change its external configuration

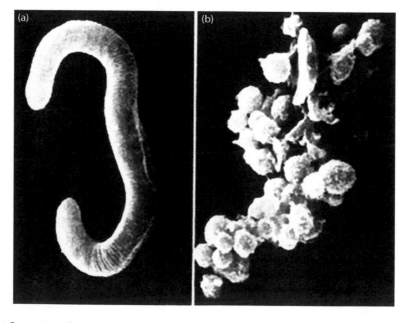

Figure 14.4 (a) Scanning electron microphotograph of a *Trichinella spiralis* larva incubated with eosinophils and complement-depleted normal (nonimmune) mouse serum for 4 hours. (b) Scanning electron microphotograph of a *T. spiralis* larva incubated with eosinophils and complement-depleted immune serum for 4 hours. Notice that the attachment of eosinophils happened only when eosinophils were added to *T. spiralis* larvae in the presence of immune sera containing antibodies directed against the parasite. (Reproduced with permission from Kazura, J.W., Aikawa, M., *J. Immunol.*, 124, 355–361, 1980.)

and prevent either its binding to cell receptors or its ability to release nucleic acid into the cell.

- **Mucosal protection**: Secretory antibodies seem to confer their protective role by preventing the attachment and subsequent penetration of microbial agents through mucosal surfaces.

FACTORS INFLUENCING EFFECTIVENESS OF ANTI-INFECTIOUS HUMORAL RESPONSE

The effectiveness of the humoral immune response in preventing an infectious disease depends on the time differential between the incubation period of the disease and the time needed to mount the immune response. If antibodies can be synthesized before the organism proliferates or before it secretes its exotoxins, then the humoral response will prevent the infection's clinical manifestations.

If relevant antibodies are present in the circulation, as a result of vaccination, previous infection, or cross-reaction between different microorganisms, then protection is most effective since the microorganism or its toxin(s) will be almost immediately neutralized, and the infection will remain subclinical.

If preformed antibodies are not present, protection will depend on whether antibody synthesis can take place before the "incubation period" (period of time during which the infectious agent is multiplying but has not yet reached sufficient mass to cause clinical disease) is over. Some infectious agents, such as the influenza virus, have very short incubation periods (about 2–3 days), and in such cases, not even a secondary immune response is protective. In most infections, however, the duration of the incubation period is sufficiently long as to allow a secondary immune response to provide protective antibodies. Thus, for many infections, particularly the common viral diseases of childhood, previous exposure and acquisition of memory ensure that antibody will be produced in time to contain infection upon subsequent exposures. Thus, reinfection plays the role of natural "booster" doses, explaining the "immunity for life" associated with some of the most common childhood diseases. However, this effect appears to be lost when the spread of the infectious agent is limited as a consequence of vaccination, but not totally eliminated. Two examples of this situation are measles and whooping cough, rarely seen in childhood when most children were immunized, but still causing disease among young adults who had lost their immunity.

The goal of prophylactic immunization may vary from case to case. In diseases with very short incubation periods, it is essential to maintain the levels of neutralizing antibody in the circulation necessary to immediately abort infection. In most other diseases, it may be sufficient to induce immunological memory, since once memory has been induced, the immune system will be able to respond in time to prevent the development of clinical infection.

Finally, it must be noted that protection by humoral immunity is only possible if the infectious agent is easily available to the antibodies produced against it. Thus, intracellular pathogens are not easy to eliminate by antibodies. In addition, as discussed in detail later in this chapter, there are organisms able to change their antigenic makeup during the course of an infection and that can persist in spite of a vigorous humoral response.

Cell-mediated immunity

Many organisms have the ability to grow and replicate intracellularly. For some it is an absolute requirement, whereas for others it is an option that allows them to survive after phagocytosis. Antibodies are largely ineffective against intracellular organisms, and T lymphocytes play a major role in their elimination. A cell-mediated immune response is indicated by the finding of lymphocytic infiltrates in tissues infected by intracellular infectious agents, such as viruses. The immune system has two basic options to eliminate intracellular organisms: to kill the infected cell or to enhance the infected cell's ability to kill intracellular organisms.

Lymphocyte-mediated cytotoxicity seems particularly significant for the elimination of viral-infected cells. It can be easily demonstrated that viral-infected cells are lysed as a consequence of their incubation with "immune" lymphocytes that are obtained from an animal previously exposed to the same virus. The sequence of events involves recognition of viral-derived peptides expressed in association with MHC-I molecules by CD8$^+$ lymphocytes, followed by differentiation into cytotoxic T cells specific for the same MHC-I–peptide complex that they recognized when initially activated. The differentiation requires Th1 help.

The activation of Th1 cells is triggered by the recognition of MHC-II–peptide complexes. Considering that macrophages are common targets for most viral infections, they are likely to present viral peptides associated both with MHC-I and MHC-II molecules. This duality should allow the simultaneous activation of CD4$^+$ and CD8$^+$ T cells in close proximity, an ideal setup for delivery of "help" to activated precursors of cytotoxic T cells.

Lymphocyte-mediated activation of macrophages and other inflammatory cells. Most intracellular bacteria and parasites infect tissue macrophages but fail to induce efficient cytotoxic reactivity. The persistence of the infection depends on a delicate balance between a state of relative inactivity by the macrophage and mechanisms that allow the infectious agent to escape proteolytic digestion once inside the cytoplasm. The immune system can react through a largely ineffective humoral response, or through a Th1-mediated inflammatory response, which may actually induce the elimination of the pathogen.

The effective response involves activation of CD4$^+$ Th1 lymphocytes and, particularly, the release of IL-12. The role of IL-12 appears to be critical, because IL-12 receptor deficiency is associated with the predisposition to develop tuberculosis, a classical example of intracellular infection. When properly activated by IL-12, Th1 lymphocytes release a variety of lymphokines, particularly interferon-γ, which activates macrophages and enhances their ability to kill intracellular organisms, and GM-CSF, which promotes differentiation and release of granulocytes and monocytes from the bone marrow. As a consequence of the delivery of activation signals, macrophages and lymphocytes enter into a complex cycle of self and mutual activation involving a variety of cytokines.

PRO-INFLAMMATORY CYTOKINES

One of the most remarkable consequences of the activation of the populations of leukocytes involved in the immune response is the synthesis of cytokines, soluble molecules that have a variety of biological effects, including inflammation and modulation of the activity of other leukocyte populations. A special subset of cytokines is the interleukins, of which 40 different ones have been well characterized. Although activated CD8$^+$ cells may produce some cytokines, and macrophages and other APCs produce others, CD4$^+$ Th cells are their major source. The biological effects of cytokines and chemokines are extremely diverse; they influence not only the immune response but also inflammatory processes and hematopoiesis.

Inflammation is always present when the immune system is trying to eliminate an infectious agent. In the acute phase of the disease, this is part and parcel of the effort to eliminate the infection and heal the damage caused by it. But if the inflammatory reaction persists, it may become the source of adverse effects and it will need to be treated to avoid unnecessary tissue damage.

The group of soluble factors, which influence inflammatory reactions, includes IL-1, IL-6, IL-15, IL-18, TNF (also known as cachectin), and interferon-γ (Table 14.4). IL-1 and TNF have membrane-associated and secreted forms and seem to be directly or indirectly responsible (in conjunction with IL-6) for the acute-phase reaction associated with acute inflammatory processes, as well as for the systemic metabolic abnormalities and circulatory collapse characteristic of shock associated with severe infections.

Interleukin-1. IL-1 exists in two molecular forms, IL-1α and IL-1β, encoded by two separate genes and displaying only 20% homology to one another. In spite of this structural difference, both forms of IL-1 bind to the same receptor and share identical biological properties. IL-1α tends to remain associated to cell membranes, while IL-1β, synthesized as an inactive precursor, is released from the cell after being processed post-translationally by a cysteine-asparagin protease (caspase-1 or interleukin-converting enzyme, ICE). Il-1β is the predominant form in humans.

Tumor necrosis factor. TNF is produced by a variety of cells, including activated T lymphocytes and activated macrophages, and has multiple targets. Its original designation was derived from its cytotoxic effects on malignant cells.

Biological properties of IL-1 and TNF. These interleukins have effects at three different levels (Table 14.5). At the metabolic level, IL-1 and TNF induce the synthesis of many proteins, such as α-1 antitrypsin, fibrinogen, and C-reactive protein in the liver. These proteins are known generically as acute-phase reactants, because of their increase in situations associated with inflammatory reactions. In cases of prolonged and severe infections, protracted TNF production may result in negative protein balance, loss of muscle mass, and progressive wasting (cachexia).

Table 14.4 Major pro-inflammatory cytokines

Cytokine	Predominant source	Main targets	Biological activity
IL-1	Macrophages, monocytes, and other cell types	T and B lymphocytes; many other cells	Stimulates T cells; activates several types of cells; pro-inflammatory mediator; pyrogen
IL-6	B and T lymphocytes, macrophages	B and T lymphocytes, others	B-cell differentiation factor; polyclonal B-cell activator; pro-inflammatory mediator; pyrogen
IL-15	Macrophages, APC	NK cells, T lymphocytes, macrophages, synovial cells	NK cell differentiation; increases and sustains TNF and interferon-γ synthesis by macrophages and NK cells; chemotactic for T cells
IL-18	Macrophages, APC	Macrophages, neutrophils, NK cells, endothelial cells	Stimulates interferon-γ synthesis; enhances Th1 and NK cell maturation
TNF (cachectin)	APCs, CD4$^+$ T cells	Multiple	Cytotoxic for some cells; cachexia; septic shock mediator; B-lymphocyte activator; pyrogen
Inteferon-γ	Activated T cells (especially CD4$^+$ Th1 cells) and NK cells	T cells, phagocytic cells, endothelial cells	Downregulates Th2 and B cells; Activates macrophages; induces ICAM-1 in endothelial cells

Table 14.5 Cellular sources and biological effects of IL-1 and TNF

	IL-1	TNF
Cellular source	Monocytes, macrophages, and related cells	Monocytes, macrophages, and related cells; CD4$^+$ T lymphocytes
Biologic property		
Pyrogen	+	+
Sleep inducer	+	+
Shock	+	+
Synthesis of reactive proteins	+	+
T-cell activation	+	+
B-cell activation	+	+
Stem cell proliferation and differentiation	+	−

At the vascular level, IL-1β and TNF cause the upregulation of cell adhesion molecules, particularly P-selectin and E-selectin in vascular endothelial cells. This upregulation associated with the release of chemokines promotes the adherence and egress to the extravascular space of inflammatory cells, where they form tissue inflammatory infiltrates. One of the possible consequences of the adherence of activated endothelial cells and inflammatory cells is endothelial cell damage.

This is a major component of Gram-negative septic shock and of toxic shock syndrome, both dramatic examples of the adverse effects of massive stimulation of cells capable of releasing excessive amounts of interleukins.

At the central nervous system level, IL-1 and TNF do not cross the blood-brain barrier but act on the periventricular organs where the blood-brain barrier is interrupted. They interact with a group of nuclei in the anterior hypothalamus, causing fever (secondarily to stimulation of prostaglandin synthesis) and sleep, and increase the production of ACTH.

Interleukin-6. IL-6 is synthesized primarily by monocytes, macrophages, and other antigen-presenting cells, and has pro-inflammatory and hematopoietic activities. Its role as a pro-inflammatory cytokine is similar to those of IL-1 and TNF, particularly in the induction of the synthesis of acute-phase response proteins by the liver.

Interferon-γ. IFNγ is released by activated Th1 lymphocytes, and its main targets are macrophages that are activated by IFNγ, enhancing their ability to destroy intracellular bacteria and parasites. Also, IFNγ, in concert with IL-1β, induces an increase in the expression of adhesion molecules involved in the transmigration of lymphocytes across the endothelial barrier (ICAM-1, LFA-1, VLA-4). At the same time, IFNγ inhibits the expression of E and P-selectins, critical for the transmigration of neutrophils, and induces the release of several α-chemokines, such as CXCL9, CXCL10, and CXCL11, that attract activated Th1 cells, NK cells, monocytes, and dendritic cells. Therefore, because of the combined effects of IFN-γ and CXC chemokines, large numbers of T lymphocytes and monocytes will exit the vascular bed in areas near the tissues where activated Th1 cells are releasing interleukins and will form perivascular mononuclear cell infiltrates, characteristic of delayed hypersensitivity reactions. It must be noted that excessive and protracted production of IFN-γ may have adverse effects. Hyperstimulated monocytes and macrophages may become exceedingly cytotoxic and may mediate tissue damage in inflammatory reactions and autoimmune diseases.

Interleukin-12. In conjunction with nitric oxide, IL-12 stimulates the cytotoxic activity of NK cells, enhancing their release of interferon-γ. Interferon-γ and IL-12 also have an important role in promoting Th1 lymphocyte differentiation.

Interleukin-15. IL-15 has similar properties to IL-2, including the ability to activate T cells through the IL-2 receptor. However, it has other unique properties, such as inducing the development and differentiation of NK cells. IL-15, in concert with IL-12, induces the release of interferon-γ, TNF, and macrophage inflammatory proteins (MIP)1α and 1β by NK cells.

Interleukin-18. IL-18, produced primarily by macrophages and related cells, was initially named "interferon-γ inducing factor," reflecting its major biological role. In many respects, it is similar to IL-1 and IL-12. IL-18 is produced and released by APCs, and its main targets are Th0/Th1 CD4$^+$ T cells and NK cells. However, in combination with other cytokines and cell-cell interactions, it can also induce Th2 lymphocyte activation.

Macrophage migration inhibitory factor. MIF, one of the first cytokines discovered and one of the last to be characterized, bridges the gap between innate and adaptive immunity. It is expressed by a variety of cells, including monocytes, macrophages, neutrophils, activated T cells, and anterior pituitary cells. Its release by leukocytes is triggered by the exposure to microbial products, such as LPS, Gram-positive exotoxins, or other pro-inflammatory cytokines (TNF, IFNγ). Several receptors of MIF have been identified, including CD74, CXCR2 and CXCR4. MIF appears to be involved in the recruitment of leukocytes in conjunction with other proinflammatory cytokines, whose release is also stimulated by MIF. It also increases the expression of TLR-4, thus playing a significant role in anti-infectious defense against Gram-negative bacteria. However, experimental data suggest that excessively high levels of MIF may actually exacerbate the effects of endotoxin. This may result from immunoregulatory properties of MIF, which can inhibit the immunosuppressive effects of glucocorticoids on immune cells and p53-dependent macrophage apoptosis, both effects leading to enhanced adverse inflammatory responses.

CHEMOKINES

This designation is given to a group of cytokines with chemotactic properties. They are divided into two major groups, α and β, depending on their tertiary structure. In the α chemokines, one amino acid separates the first two cysteine residues (Cys-aminoacid-Cys) and for that reason they are also known as CXC chemokines, the preferred term in modern literature. In β chemokines the first two cysteine residues are adjacent to each other and for that reason are also known as CC chemokines.

CXC chemokines

Interleukin-8 (neutrophil-activating factor) is the most important of the CXC chemokines. It is released by T lymphocytes and monocytes stimulated with TNF or IL-1. It functions as a chemotactic and activating factor for granulocytes, the cell population with the highest level of IL-8 receptor expression. IL-8 recruits granulocytes to areas of inflammation and increases their phagocytic and pro-inflammatory abilities. It has also been demonstrated to be chemotactic for T lymphocytes. In addition to IL-8, the CXC chemokines include the previously mentioned interferon-γ–inducible chemokines (CXCL9, CXCL10, and CXCL11).

CC Chemokines

CC Chemokines include four major cytokines, which act predominantly on mononuclear cells, the cells that predominantly express the receptors for this group of cytokines:

- **CCL5 (RANTES, regulated on activation, normal T-cell expressed and secreted)** is released by T cells and attracts T cells with memory phenotype, NK cells, eosinophils, and mast cells.
- **Macrophage inflammatory proteins (MIPs)** are released by monocytes and macrophages and attract eosinophils, lymphocytes, and NK and LAK cells.
- **Macrophage chemotactic proteins (MCPs)** are produced by monocytes, macrophages, and related cells and attract monocytes, eosinophils, NK, and LAK cells.
- **Eotaxin** is a chemokine induced by IL-4 that recruits eosinophils and Th2 CD4$^+$ T cells to the sites of allergic inflammation.
- **β-Defensins** are released primarily by granulocytes and have also been characterized as chemotactic for T lymphocytes.

IMMUNE DEFICIENCY SYNDROMES FOR STUDY OF IMMUNE DEFENSES AGAINST HUMAN INFECTIONS

Most of our information about the immune system in humans has been learned from the study of immunocompromised patients and patients with immunodeficiency diseases. The most characteristic clinical features of immunocompromised patients are repeated or chronic infections, often caused by opportunistic agents. There are some characteristic associations between specific types of infections and generic types of immune deficiency which illustrate the physiological roles of the different components of the immune system:

- Patients with antibody deficiencies and conserved cell-mediated immunity suffer from repeated and chronic infections with pyogenic bacteria.
- Patients with primary deficiencies of cell-mediated immunity usually suffer from chronic or recurrent fungal, parasitic, and viral infections.
- Neutrophil deficiencies are usually associated with bacterial infections caused by common organisms of low virulence that would normally be kept in check through nonimmune phagocytosis.
- Isolated deficiencies of terminal complement components (C6-C9) are also associated with bacterial infections, most frequently involving *Neisseria* sp., whose elimination appears to require formation of the cytolytic membrane attack complex.

ESCAPE FROM IMMUNE RESPONSE

Many infectious agents have developed the capacity to avoid the immune response. Several mechanisms are involved:

- **Complement inhibitory activity** has been characterized for bacterial capsules and membrane proteins of some bacteria, parasites, and enveloped viruses. Some pathogens can also acquire host complement inhibitory proteins from serum or cell membranes. Complement inhibitory activity on the pathogen surface results in a decreased level of opsonization by C3b, and other complement fragments, reducing the efficacy of complement-mediated phagocytosis.
- **Resistance to phagocytosis**, either mediated by polysaccharide capsules that repel and inhibit the function of phagocytic cells or provide the ability to survive after ingestion. Resistance to phagocytosis is characteristic of the group of bacteria known as facultative intracellular (*Mycobacteria*, *Brucella*, *Listeria*, and

Salmonella, among others), as well as of some fungi and protozoa (*Toxoplasma, Trypanosoma cruzi,* and *Leishmania* sp.). Infectious agents have developed many different strategies to survive intracellularly. Some infectious agents secrete molecules that prevent the formation of phagolysosomes allowing the infectious agent to survive inside phagosomes, relatively devoid of toxic compounds (e.g., *Mycobacterium tuberculosis, Legionella pneumophila,* and *Toxoplasma gondii*). Others have outer coats that protect the bacteria against proteolytic enzymes and free toxic radicals (such as the superoxide radical) or have developed mechanisms that allow them to exit the phagosome and survived unharmed in the cytoplasm (e.g., *Trypanosoma cruzi*). Finally, others depress the response of the infected phagocytic cells to activating cytokines, such as interferon-γ.

Some organisms combine several different mechanisms to survive intracellularly. For example, *Mycobacterium leprae* is coated with a phenolic glycolipid layer that scavenges free radicals and releases a compound that inhibits the effects of interferon-γ. In addition, the release of IL-4 and IL-10 by infected macrophages is enhanced, contributing to the downregulation of Th1 lymphocytes.

- **Ineffective immune responses**: Some infectious agents appear to have acquired evolutionary advantage by not inducing effective immune responses. For example, polysaccharide capsules protect many bacteria and fungi against phagocytosis through physicochemical effects and also by the fact that their immunogenicity is not as strong as that of proteins. Polysaccharides are not presented to helper CD4 T cells, and in the absence of adequate T cell help, the response to polysaccharides involves predominantly IgM and IgG2 antibodies, which are inefficient as opsonins (the FcγR of phagocytic cells recognize preferentially IgG1 and IgG3 antibodies). Another example is *Neisseria meningitidis,* which often induces the synthesis of IgA antibodies. *In vitro* data suggest that IgA can act as a weak opsonin or induce ADCC (monocytes/macrophages and other leukocytes express Fcα receptors on their membranes), but the physiological protective role of IgA antibodies is questionable. Patient sera with high titers of IgA antibodies to *N. meningitidis* fail to show

bactericidal activity until IgA-specific anti-*Neisseria meningitidis* antibodies are removed. This observation suggests that IgA antibodies may act as "blocking factors," preventing opsonizing IgG antibodies from binding to the same epitopes.

- **Release of soluble antigens** from infected cells that are able to bind and block antibodies before they can reach the cells have been demonstrated in the case of the hepatitis B virus. The circulating surface antigens act as a "deflector shield," which protects the infected tissues from "antibody aggression."

- **Loss and masking of antigens with absorbed host proteins** have been demonstrated with several worms, particularly schistosomula (the larval forms of schistosome). The ability of parasitic worms to survive in the host is well known and is certainly derived from the ability to evade the immune system.

- **Antigenic variation** has been characterized in bacteria (*Borrelia recurrentis*), protozoan parasites (trypanosomes, *Giardia lamblia*), and viruses (human immunodeficiency virus, HIV).

One of the best-studied examples of antigenic variaion is the African trypanosomes. These protozoa have a surface coat constituted of a single glycoprotein (variant-specific surface glycoprotein or VSG), for which there are about 10^3 genes in the chromosome. At any given time, only one of those genes is expressed, the others remaining silent. For every 10^6 or 10^7 trypanosome divisions, a mutation occurs that replaces the active VSG gene on the expression site by a previously silent VSG gene. The previously expressed gene is destroyed, and a new VSG protein is coded, which is antigenically different. The emergence of a new antigenic coat allows the parasite to multiply unchecked. As antibodies emerge to the newly expressed VSG protein, parasitemia will decline, only to increase as soon as a new mutation occurs, and a different VSG protein is synthesized. *Giardia lamblia* has a similar mechanism of variation, but the rate of surface antigen replacement is even faster (once every 10^3 divisions).

Borrelia recurrentis, the agent of relapsing fever, carries genes for at least 26 different variable major proteins (VMPs) that are sequentially activated by duplicative transposition to an expression site. The successive waves of bacteremia and fever correspond to the emergence of new mutants, which, for a while, can proliferate unchecked until antibodies are formed.

HIV exhibits a high degree of antigenic variation that results from errors introduced by the reverse transcriptase when synthesizing viral DNA from the RNA template. The mutation rate is relatively high (one in every 10^3 progeny particles), and the immune response selects the mutant strains that present new configurations in the outer envelope proteins, allowing the mutant to proliferate unchecked by preexisting neutralizing antibodies.

- **Cell-to-cell spread**: This allows infectious agents to propagate without being exposed to specific antibodies or phagocytic cells. This strategy is commonplace for viruses, especially for herpesviruses, retroviruses, and paramyxoviruses, and allows the fusion of infected cells with noninfected cells allowing viral particles to pass from cell to cell without exposure to the extracellular environment.

  Some intracellular bacteria have also developed the ability to spread from cell to cell, with the best-known example being *Listeria monocytogenes*. After becoming intracellular, *L. monocytogenes* can travel along the cytoskeleton and promote the fusion of the membrane of an infected cell with the membrane of a neighboring noninfected cell, which is subsequently invaded.

- **Immunosuppressive effects of infection**: Although immunosuppressive effects have been described in association with bacteria and parasitic infections, the best-documented examples of infection-associated immunosuppression are those described in viral infections. The effects of HIV on the immune system are described in detail in Chapter 30, but many other viruses have the ability to depress immune functions. For example, patients in the acute phase of measles are more susceptible to bacterial infections, such as pneumonia. The patients have lymphopenia caused by arrest of differentiation affecting predominantly dendritic cells and T cells. As a consequence, both delayed hypersensitivity responses and *in vitro* lymphocyte proliferation in response to mitogens and antigens are significantly depressed during the acute phase of measles and the immediate convalescence period, usually returning to normal after 4 weeks.

Mothers and infants infected with cytomegalovirus (CMV) show depressed responses to CMV virus but normal responses to T-cell mitogens, suggesting that in some cases the immunosuppression may be antigen specific, while in measles it is obviously nonspecific.

Influenza virus has been found to depress cell-mediated immunity in mice, apparently due to an increase in the suppressor activity of T lymphocytes.

Epstein-Barr virus releases a specific protein that has extensive sequence homology with IL-10. The biological properties of this viral protein are also analogous to those of IL-10; both are able to inhibit lymphokine synthesis by T-cell clones.

ABNORMAL CONSEQUENCES OF THE IMMUNE RESPONSE

In the vast majority of situations, the immune response has a protective effect that allows the organism to recover from infection without major illness and without long-term sequelae. However, there are well-known examples of deleterious effects triggered by an exaggerated or misdirected immune response.

Activation of T lymphocytes by bacterial "superantigens"

A variety of bacterial exotoxins, such as staphylococcal enterotoxins-A and -B (SE-A and SE-B), staphylococcal toxic shock syndrome toxin-1 (TSST-1), exfoliating toxin, and streptococcal exotoxin A, as well as other unrelated bacterial proteins (such as streptococcal M proteins) have been characterized as "superantigens."

Superantigens are defined by their ability to stimulate T cells without being processed. The stimulation of T cells is polyclonal; thus, the designation "superantigen" is a misnomer, but it has gained popularity and is widely used in the literature. The best-studied "superantigens" are the staphylococcal enterotoxins, which are potent polyclonal activators of murine and human T lymphocytes, inducing T-cell proliferation and cytokine release. TSST-1 also appears to activate monocytes and is a potent B-cell mitogen, inducing B-cell proliferation and differentiation.

The stimulatory effects of "superantigens" are a consequence of the direct and simultaneous binding to the nonpolymorphic area of class II MHC on professional accessory cells (macrophages and related cells) and to the Vβ chain of the α/β TCR (Figure 14.5). For example, staphylococcal enterotoxins bind exclusively to specific subfamilies of Vβ chains that are expressed only by certain individuals. When expressed, these Vβ chain regions can be found on 2%–20% of a positive individual's T cells, and the cross-linking of the TCR2 and of the APC by the enterotoxin activates all T cells (both CD4 and CD8+) expressing the specific Vβ region recognized by the enterotoxin. The massive T-cell activation induced by superantigens results in the release of large amounts of IL-2, interferon-γ, lymphotoxin-α (LTα), and TNF. After the initial burst of cytokine release, the stimulated T cells either undergo apoptosis or become anergic. This effect could severely disturb the ability of the immune system to adequately respond to bacteria releasing superantigens.

Patients infected by bacteria able to release large amounts of superantigens (e.g., *Staphylococcus aureus* releasing enterotoxins or TSST-1 and Group A *Streptococcus* releasing exotoxin A) may develop septic shock as a consequence of the systemic effects of these cytokines. These systemic effects include fever, endothelial damage, profound hypotension, disseminated intravascular coagulation, multiorgan failure, and death.

Infection as consequence of uptake of antigen-antibody complexes

The immune response, in some cases, facilitates the access of infectious agents to cells in which they will be able to proliferate. For example, intracellular organisms that are ingested as a consequence of opsonization often infect macrophages.

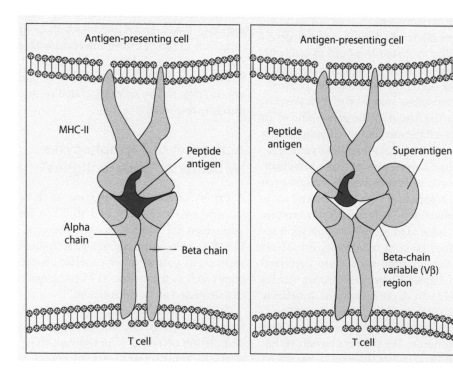

Figure 14.5 Comparison of the mechanisms of T-cell stimulation by conventional antigens and staphylococcal enterotoxins. While conventional antigens are processed into oligopeptides, which bind to MHC-II molecules, and then bind specifically to a TCR binding site (left panel), bacterial "superantigens" interact with nonpolymorphic areas of the Vβ chain of the TCR and of the MHC-II molecule on an APC (right panel). Notice that "superantigen" binding overrides the need for TCR recognition of the MHC-II–associated oligopeptide, and thus T cells of many different specificities can be activated. It is also important to note that both APC and T cells can be stimulated as a consequence of the extensive cross-linking of membrane proteins. (Modified from Johnson, H.M. et al., *Sci. Am.*, 266, 92–95, 1992.)

Leishmania organisms are intracellular parasites that penetrate the host's cells after reacting with complement, particularly C3. Epstein–Barr virus (EBV) normally infects B cells through CR2, a complement receptor. However, if dimeric IgA reactive with the virus is produced and released into the mucosal secretions, the resulting IgA-EBV complex is able to infect mucosal cells through the poly-Ig receptor that binds dimeric IgA (see Chapter 6). Mucosal infection in the nasopharynx can eventually acquire malignant characteristics.

Postinfectious tissue damage

Several examples of the pathogenic role of an anti-infectious immune response have been characterized. The following are some of the best-known examples:

- **Immune-complex induced inflammation**: Antigen-antibody complexes, if formed in large amounts, can cause disease by becoming trapped in different capillary networks and leading to inflammation. The clinical expression of immune complex-related inflammation depends on the localization of the trapped complexes: vasculitis and purpura occur when the skin is predominantly affected, glomerulonephritis if trapping takes place on the glomerular capillaries, and arthritis when the joints are affected. Viruses (particularly Hepatitis C virus) are often involved in the formation of circulating antigen-antibody complexes.
- **Immune destruction of infected cells and tissues**: An immune response directed against an infectious agent may be the main cause of damage to the infected tissue. For example, in **subacute sclerosing panencephalitis**, a degenerative disease of the nervous system associated with persistent infection with the measles virus, the response against viral epitopes expressed in infected neurons is believed to be the primary mechanisms of disease. Also, in some forms of **chronic active hepatitis** (see Chapter 17), the immune response directed against viral epitopes expressed by infected hepatocytes seems to cause more tissue damage than the infection itself.
- **Cross-reactions with tissue antigens**: have been proposed as the basis for the association of streptococcal infections with rheumatic carditis and glomerulonephritis. Antibodies to type 1 streptococcal M protein cross-react with epitopes of myocardium and kidney mesangial cells and cause inflammatory changes in the heart and glomeruli, respectively.
- **Autoimmunity**. The role of infectious agents as triggers of autoimmune reactions is discussed in detail in Chapter 16.

EPILOGUE

The outcome of an infectious process depends on a very complex set of interactions with the immune system. A successful pathogen is usually one that has developed mechanisms that avoid fast elimination by an immunocompetent host. These mechanisms allow the infectious agent to replicate, cause disease, and spread to other individuals before the immune response is induced. The immune response, on the other hand, is a powerful weapon that, once set in motion, may destroy friendly targets. Thus, a therapeutic strategy for infectious disease has to consider such questions as the particular survival strategy of the infectious agents, the effects of the infection on the immune system, and the possibility that the immune response may be more of a problem than the infection itself.

BIBLIOGRAPHY

Avota E, Gassert E, Schneider-Schaulies S. Measles virus-induced immunosuppression: From effectors to mechanisms. *Medical Microbiol Immunol.* 2010;199:227–237.

Borst P, Graves DR. Programmed gene rearrangements altering gene expression. *Science.* 1987;235:658–667.

Calandra T, Roger T. Macrophage migration inhibitory factor: A regulator of innate immunity. *Nat Rev Immunol.* 2003;3:791–800.

De Smet K, Contreras R. Human antimicrobial peptides: Defensins, cathelicidins and histatins. *Biotechnol Lett.* 2005;27:1337–1347.

Ferri C, Giuggioli D, Cazzato M et al. HCV-related cryoglobulinemic vasculitis: An update on its etiopathogenesis and therapeutic strategies. *Clin Exp Rheumatol.* 2003;21(6 Suppl 32):S78–S84.

Gleeson PA. The role of endosomes in innate and adaptive immunity. *Semin Cell Dev Biol.* 2014;31:64–72.

Gracie JA, Robertson SE, McInnes IB. Interleukin-18. *J Leukoc Biol.* 2003;73:213–224.

Griffith JW. Chemokines and chemokine receptors: Positioning cells for host defense and immunity. *Ann Rev Immunol.* 2014;32:659–702.

Hamerman JA, Ogasawara K, Lanier LL. NK cells in innate immunity. *Curr Opin Immunol.* 2005;17:29–35.

Hazlett L, Wu M. Defensins in innate immunity. *Cell Tissue Res.* 2011;343:175–188.

Justiz Vaillant AA, Qurie A. Interleukin. In: StatPearls [Internet]. Treasure Island (FL): StatPearls Publishing; 2019 Jan. Available from: https://www.ncbi.nlm.nih.gov/books/NBK499840/.

Kawai T, Akira S. The role of pattern-recognition receptors in innate immunity: Update on toll-like receptors. *Nature Immunol.* 2010;11: 373–384.

Kraus W, Dale JB, Beachey EH. Identification of an epitope of type 1 streptococcal M protein that is shared with a 43-kDa protein of human myocardium and renal glomeruli. *J Immunol.* 1990;145:4089.

Laffy JML, Dodev T, Macpherson JA et al. Promiscuous antibodies characterised by their physicochemical properties: From sequence to structure and back. *Prog Biophys Mol Biol.* 2017;128:47–56.

Lanier LL. NK cell recognition. *Annu Rev Immunol.* 2005;23:225–274.

Lawand M, Déchanet-Merville J, Dieu-Nosjean M-C. Key features of $\gamma\delta$ T-cell subsets in human diseases and their immunotherapeutic implications. *Front Immunol.* 2017;8:761.

Li H, Llera A, Malchiodi EL, Mariuzza, RA. The structural basis of T cell activation by superantigens. *Annu Rev Immunol.* 1999;17:435–466.

Mauel J. Macrophage-parasite interactions in Leishmania infections. *J Leukoc Biol.* 1990;47: 187–193.

Tosi MF. Innate immune responses to infection. *J. Allergy Clin Immunol.* 2005;116:241–249.

15

Diagnostic applications of immunology

AJAY GROVER, VIRGINIA LITWIN, AND GABRIEL VIRELLA

INTRODUCTION

Scientists have made use of the exquisite sensitivity and specificity of antibody recognition for use in assays for both diagnostic and basic research applications. Technological advances in methods to generate antibodies and to detect antibody-antigen binding have transformed laboratory medicine and basic research in many fields. A variety of platforms make use of a variety of tags (fluorescence, electrochemiluminescence, heavy metals) to detect antibody-antigen interactions. These technologies are sensitive, specific, quantitative, and relatively rapid. Immunoassays and flow cytometry have replaced more laborious, less-sensitive methods that relied on the detection of antibody-antigen aggregates in gel-based systems (immunodiffusion). Applications of these serologic and molecular methods are quite broad. They have been applied to the diagnosis of infectious diseases, the detection of previous infection, the monitoring of neoplasms and vaccine efficacy, the assay of hormones and drugs, and pregnancy diagnosis. In some cases, the antigen being measured is itself an antibody. Measurement of specific antibodies has found wide application in the diagnosis of infectious, allergic, autoimmune, and immunodeficiency diseases.

SEROLOGICAL ASSAYS

Immunoserologic assays can be developed for antigen or antibody detection or quantitative assay. For antibody detection or measurement, a purified preparation of antigen must be available. For example, when human serum is tested for antibody to diphtheria toxoid, a purified preparation of the toxoid must be available. Next, a method for detecting the specific antigen-antibody reaction must be developed. Conversely, to detect antigens in biological fluids, specific antibodies must be available. In both types of assays, positive and negative controls are mandatory for proper interpretation of the results.

CLASSICAL ASSAYS

Precipitation assays, such as **radial immunodiffusion** (RID) (Figure 15.1) are still used for certain

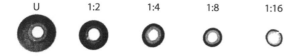

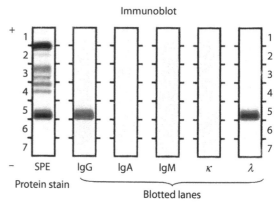

Figure 15.1 The principle of radial immunodiffusion. Five wells carved into antibody-containing agar were filled with serial dilutions of the corresponding antigen. The antigen diffused, reacted with antibody in the agar, and eventually precipitated in a circular pattern. The diameters or areas of these circular precipitates are directly proportional to the concentration of antigen in each well.

Figure 15.2 Use of the immunoblotting technique for typing a monoclonal protein. From right to left, the pictures show a reference lane in which the serum proteins were electrophoresed and stained, showing an homogeneous protein of γ mobility, near the bottom of the separation. The next five lanes were blotted with the indicated antisera, washed, and then stained to reveal which antisera reacted with the homogeneous protein visualized in the reference lane. The results indicate that the homogeneous protein is a monoclonal protein of the IgG heavy-chain isotype, with λ light chains.

applications, but these tend to be low-volume assays, available only in highly specialized reference laboratories. In precipitation assays, the presence of antibody (or antigen) in the sample causes the formation of a precipitate in agar containing the specific antigen (or antibody). RID plates are prepared with agarose gel containing polyclonal antibodies to the protein antigen at an optimized concentration. After incubation, a precipitin ring forms because of the antibody-antigen reaction, the diameter of which is dependent on the analyte concentration. The concentration of the protein in the sample is determined by comparison to standard calibrators of known levels of antigen.

Immunonephelometry is a preferred alternative for gel-based precipitation assays, as this technique is more sensitive and can be automated. Immunonephelometry is also based on the formation of antigen-antibody complexes and makes use of antibody and/or antigen calibrators. The analyte of interest is measured by light dispersion (nephelometry).

Immunofixation (immunoblotting) is a multistep process (Figure 15.2). In the first step, several aliquots of the patient's serum are simultaneously separated by electrophoresis. One of the separation lanes is stained as reference for the position of the different serum proteins (extreme right lane in the figure), while paper strips embedded with different antibodies are laid over the remaining separation lanes. The antibodies diffuse into the agar and react with the corresponding immunoglobulins. After washing off unbound immunoglobulins and antibodies, the lanes where immunofixation take place are stained, revealing whether the antisera did or did not recognize the proteins they are directed against. In this example, a monoclonal protein reacting with anti-IgG and anti-λ antisera

was revealed. This test is useful in diagnosing myeloma, macroglobulinemia of Waldenström, and other plasma cell dyscrasias where the detection and characterization of a monoclonal gammopathy are essential for the diagnosis.

Western blot

Western blotting (Figure 15.3) is a technique that identifies specific proteins in a given sample after their separation using polyacrylamide gel electrophoresis. The polyacrylamide gel is placed adjacent to a membrane, which is typically nitrocellulose or PVDF (polyvinylidene fluoride), and the application of an electrical current induces the proteins to migrate from the gel and immobilize on the membrane. The membrane is subsequently stained with an antibody. The confirmatory HIV test employs a Western blot to detect anti-HIV antibody in a human serum sample. Proteins from known HIV-infected cells are separated and blotted on a membrane as discussed previously. Then, the serum to be tested is applied in the primary antibody incubation step; free antibody is washed away, and a secondary antihuman antibody linked

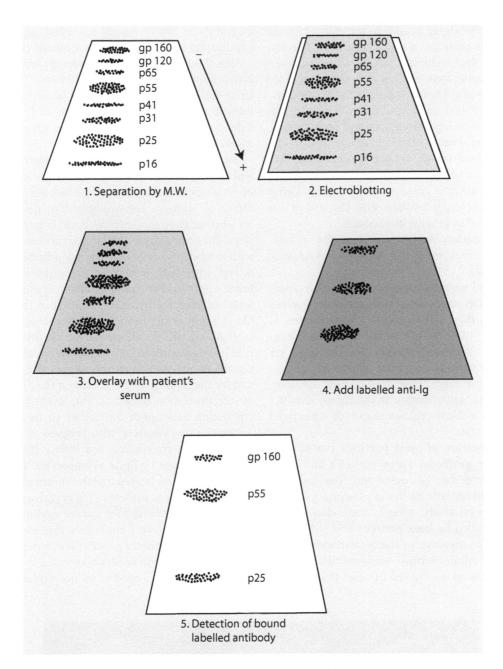

Figure 15.3 A Western blot study to confirm the existence of anti-HIV antibodies. In the first step, a mixture of HIV antigens is separated by size (large antigens remain close to the origin where the sample is applied, smaller antigens move deep into the acrylamide gel used for the separation). In the second step, the separated antigens are electrophoresed into a permeable nitrocellulose membrane (electroblotting). Next, the patient's serum is spread over the cellulose membrane to which the antigens have been transferred. If antibodies to any of these antigens are present in the serum, a precipitate will be formed at the site where the antigen has been transferred. After washing excess of unreacted antigens and serum proteins, a labeled second antibody is overlaid on the membrane; if human antibodies precipitate by reacting with blotted antigens, the second antibody (labeled anti-human immunoglobulin) will react with the immunoglobulins contained in the precipitate. After washing off the excess of unreacted second antibody, labeled antibody bound to human antibody-viral protein complexes is revealed. Its binding to an antigen-antibody precipitate can be detected either by adding a color-developing substrate or by measuring chemiluminescence, depending on the label.

to an enzyme signal is added. The stained bands indicate the proteins to which the patient's serum is specific. This technique has the advantage over other screening assays of not only detecting antibodies, but also identifying their target antigens, resulting in increased specificity. However, the procedure is of low throughput and requires specialized personnel in certified laboratories. To circumvent these issues, antigen-specific blots that need only be probed with the patient serum and developed, are now commercially available. Using these commercially available kits, the testing can be conducted in general laboratories.

Agglutination assays are used for a variety of purposes in bacteriology and diagnostic immunology.

Bacterial agglutination is observed when a bacterial suspension is mixed with antibody directed to their surface determinants. Agglutination is rapid and visible by eye, without special instrumentation. Its disadvantages are the need for isolated organisms and poor sensitivity, requiring relatively large concentrations of antibody. Nonetheless, agglutination is commonly used for serotyping isolated organisms and for some rapid diagnostic tests.

Agglutination of inert particles coated with antigen or antibody. Latex particles and other inert particles can be coated with purified antigen and will agglutinate in the presence of specific antibody. Conversely, specific antibodies can be easily adsorbed by latex particles and will agglutinate in the presence of the corresponding antigen. The method becomes semiquantitative when serum dilutions are created in order to determine

an end point. The reciprocal of the last agglutinating dilution is designated as the antibody titer.

The flexibility of this methodology allows for broad applications in clinical diagnosis ranging from the detection of rheumatoid factor for rheumatoid arthritis diagnosis (Figure 15.4) to the detection of bacterial and/or fungi in the cerebrospinal fluid for meningitis diagnosis.

Red cell agglutination (hemagglutination). Red cell agglutination is the basis of a wide array of serological tests that can be subclassified as direct or indirect hemagglutination, depending on whether the assay involves a single step or two steps. Direct hemagglutination tests are carried out with washed red cells that are agglutinated when mixed with IgM antibodies recognizing membrane epitopes. For example, direct agglutination tests are used for the determination of the ABO blood group and titration of isohemagglutinins (anti-A and anti-B antibodies), for the titration of cold hemagglutinins (IgM antibodies which agglutinate RBC at temperatures below that of the body), and for the monospot test, useful for the diagnosis of infectious mononucleosis. This last test detects circulating heterophile antibodies (cross-reactive antibodies that combine with antigens of an animal of a different species) and induce the agglutination of sheep or horse erythrocytes. Indirect hemagglutination is used to detect antibodies that react with antigens present in the erythrocytes but that by themselves cannot induce agglutination. Usually, these are IgG antibodies that are not as efficient agglutinators of red cells as polymeric IgM antibodies. A second antibody directed to human immunoglobulins is used to induce agglutination

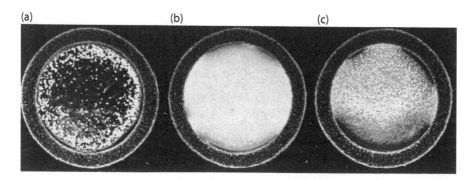

(a)   (b)   (c)

Figure 15.4 Detection of rheumatoid factor by the latex agglutination technique. A suspension of IgG-coated latex particles is mixed with a 1:20 dilution of three sera. Obvious clumping is seen in (a), corresponding to a strongly positive serum; no clumping is seen in (b), corresponding to a negative serum; very fine clumping is seen in (c), corresponding to a weakly positive serum.

by reacting with the red-cell bound IgG molecules, and consequently, cross-linking the red cells. The best known example of indirect agglutination is the antiglobulin or Coombs' test that is used in the diagnosis of autoimmune hemolytic anemia.

TESTS BASED ON IMMUNOFLUORESCENCE

Immunofluorescence relies on the use of antibodies chemically conjugated to fluorescent dyes (also called fluorophores) such as fluorescein

isothiocyanate (FITC). The fluorophore allows visualization of cell- or tissue-fixed antigens in the sample under a fluorescent microscope. There are several variations of immunofluorescence that can be used to detect the presence of antigens in cells or tissues and the presence of antibodies in patient's serum (Figure 15.5).

Direct immunofluorescence

Direct immunofluorescence uses a single antibody that is chemically linked to a fluorophore. The

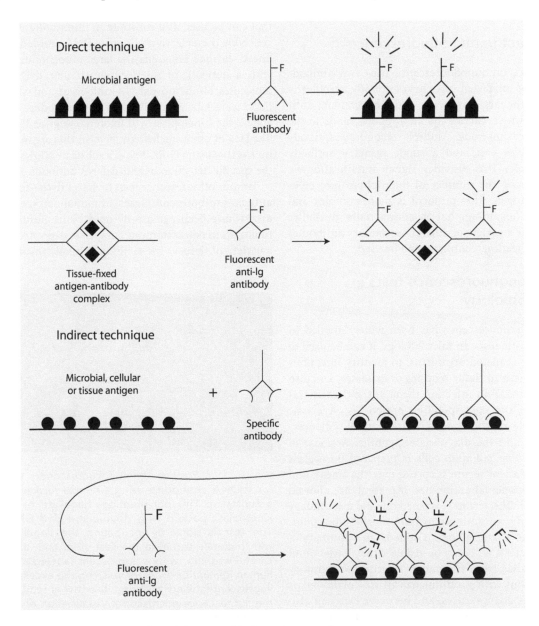

Figure 15.5 General principles of direct and indirect immunofluorescence.

antibody recognizes the target molecule and binds to it, and the fluorophore it carries can be detected via microscopy. This technique has several advantages over the secondary (or indirect) protocol discussed later because of the direct conjugation of the antibody to the fluorophore. This reduces the number of steps in the staining procedure, making the process faster, and can reduce background signal by avoiding some issues with antibody cross-reactivity or nonspecificity. However, since the number of fluorescent molecules that can be bound to the primary antibody is limited, direct immunofluorescence is less sensitive than indirect immunofluorescence.

Indirect immunofluorescence

Indirect immunofluorescence uses two antibodies: the unlabeled (primary) antibody specifically binds the target molecule, and the secondary antibody, which carries the fluorophore, binds to the primary antibody. Multiple secondary antibody molecules can bind a single primary antibody molecule. This provides signal amplification by increasing the number of fluorophore molecules per antigen. This protocol is more complex and time consuming, but it allows more flexibility because a variety of different secondary antibodies and detection techniques can be used.

Immunofluorescence tests in microbiology

Immunofluorescence has been widely applied in diagnostic tests. In microbiology, it can be used to identify isolated organisms, to identify infectious organisms in tissue biopsies or exudates, and also to diagnose an infection through the demonstration of the corresponding antibodies. A classic example of the use of indirect immunofluorescence is in the diagnosis of syphilis. A smear of *Treponema pallidum* cells is prepared on a glass slide. Patient serum is spread over the smear, and antitreponemal antibodies, if present, are allowed to bind. The serum is washed off, and a secondary antibody, an antihuman immunoglobulin conjugated to a fluorophore, is added. On examination, the bacteria will only be visible if they have bound antibodies from the patient's serum. Respiratory infections with parainfluenza viruses, orthomyxoviruses, adenoviruses, and herpesviruses can also be diagnosed using immunofluorescence staining.

Immunofluorescence tests for detection of autoantibodies

The presence of antinuclear antibodies (ANAs) may be a marker of an autoimmune process and is associated with several autoimmune disorders such as systemic lupus erythematosus (SLE). The indirect immunofluorescence technique on monolayers of cultured epithelial cells is the current recommended method. Samples are classified as positive or negative on the basis of specific staining patterns.

Crithidia luciliae is a single-cell hemoflagellate that can be used as a substrate in immunofluorescence for the detection of anti-dsDNA antibodies. The *C. luciliae* kinetoplast, a large mitochondrion with a network of interlocking circular dsDNA molecules, binds anti-dsDNA antibodies, and when fluorescent-labeled antihuman Ig antibodies are added, the kinetoplast will fluoresce (Figure 15.6). The lack of other nuclear antigens in this organelle means that using *C. luciliae* as a substrate allows for the specific detection of anti-dsDNA antibodies.

Immunofluorescence tests to detect tissue-fixed antigen-antibody complexes. Immunofluorescence assays have been extensively used by immunopathologists to detect immune complexes deposited in a variety of tissues. The technique usually involves

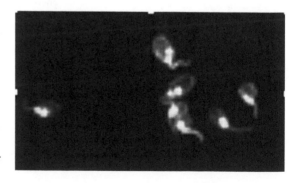

Figure 15.6 Positive immunofluorescence test for dsDNA antibodies using *Crithidia luciliae* as a substrate. This noninfectious flagellate has a kinetoplast packed with double-stranded DNA. The test is done by incubating the flagellate with patient's serum in the first step, and, after careful washing, with a fluorescent labeled antihuman IgG antibody. After washing the excess of fluorescent-labeled antibody, the test is read on the fluorescence microscope. Visualization of the kinetoplast reflects the binding of anti-dsDNA.

a biopsy that is frozen and sectioned. The sections are incubated with fluorescent-labeled antibodies specific for immunoglobulins, C3, and fibrinogen (which is usually deposited in inflamed lesions).

The principles of **quantitative immunofluorescence** are similar to those described for indirect fluorescence assays: antigen is bound to a solid phase, exposed to a serum sample containing specific antibody, unbound immunoglobulins are rinsed off, and a fluorescein-labeled antibody is added to reveal specific antibody. A fluorometer is used to measure the amount of fluorescence emitted by the second antibody. Since the amount of fluorescent antibody added to the system is fixed, the amount that remains bound is directly proportional to the concentration of antibody present in the sample. Thus, a quantitative correlation can be drawn between the intensity of fluorescence and the concentration of antibody. These quantitative tests have been adapted to microbiological assays and can identify IgG and IgM antibodies.

MONOCLONAL ANTIBODY-BASED ASSAYS

The methodology for production of monoclonal antibodies was first reported by Kohler and Milstein in the 1970s, and the Nobel Prize was awarded to these investigators in recognition of the significance of the technology.

The production of monoclonal antibodies involves two cell populations and three major steps: fusion, selection, and screening. Most commonly, spleen cells from a mouse immunized with the antigen of interest are fused with transformed murine plasma cells. This fusion results in the formation of hybrid cells (hybridomas) that will proliferate like transformed cells. The B-cell hybridomas will produce the same antibody as the parental B cell (Figure 15.7). The hybridomas are grown and selected in culture conditions that will support their growth but not that of the fusion partner or the nonfused splenocytes.

A lengthy screening process follows, the aim of which is to select from the large number of hybridomas produced by fusion those that produce antibody against antigens of interest. Single cells are seeded (by manual limiting dilution or cell sorting by flow cytometry) into individual receptacles containing tissue culture medium and allowed to grow

into clones producing antibody of a single specificity (monoclonal antibody [mAb]).

Hundreds of monoclonal antibodies identifying different membrane and intracellular markers on lymphocytes and other cell types have been generated. These cellular antigens are complex molecules expressing many different epitopes. Accordingly, monoclonal antibodies raised in different laboratories potentially recognized slightly different parts of the same molecule. Historically, each laboratory would identify a molecule by a unique name, and the field became rather complicated; as each cellular antigen might be known by several different names. As a consequence, workshops sponsored by the World Health Organization were developed in order to establish a standardized nomenclature. During the workshops, newly developed monoclonal antibodies were evaluated, the cellular antigen they recognize verified, and a designation given to the newly defined antigen. A given cellular antigen recognized by novel monoclonal antibodies is designated by the initials CD, for clusters of differentiation (a designation that recognizes the fact that each marker has multiple antigenic determinants), followed by a number. The numerical designations are assigned based partly on the order of discovery, and partly on the ontogenic order of appearance. For instance, the monoclonal antibody recognizing what, at the time, was considered ontogenetically as the most primitive T-lymphocyte membrane marker, was designated as CD1, and the T lymphocytes expressing it are known as CD1$^+$. Some of the most common CD markers are described in Chapter 10.

FLOW CYTOMETRY

Flow cytometry has become one of the most important and powerful technologies for clinical immunology, basic research, and drug development. A flow cytometer is an instrument that measures cells (cytometry) in a fluid stream (flow) (Figure 15.8). Within the flow cell, cells pass in a fluid stream in front of a laser light source, which allows for the measurement of multiple properties from individual cells. When the individual cells are intercepted by the laser light source, the light will be dispersed (or scattered). When the cells are labeled with fluorescent dyes, the laser light will excite the fluorescent dyes, and fluorescent energy will be emitted. The flow cytometer is equipped

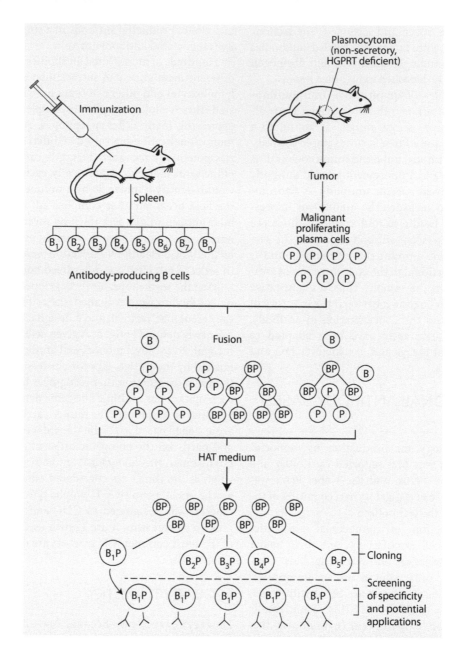

Figure 15.7 **Major steps involved in hybridoma production. First, antibody-producing lymphocytes are fused with nonsecretory malignant plasma cells, deficient in hypoxanthine guanine phosphoribosyl transferase (HGPRT). Nonfused lymphocytes will not proliferate, and nonfused plasma cells will die in a hypoxanthine-rich medium (HAT). The HGPRT-deficient plasma cells cannot detoxify hypoxanthine, while the hybrid cells have HGPRT provided by the antibody-producing B lymphocytes. The surviving hybrids are cloned by limiting dilution, and the resulting clones are tested for the specificity and potential value of the antibodies produced.**

with multiple detectors to capture the light scatter and fluorescence emission signals, which allows for the simultaneous measurement of multiple characteristics of a single cell. Therein lies the true power of flow cytometry—multiparameter data acquisition/analysis from individual cells. Data collected from the light scatter provides information about the size and complexity of the individual cells. Larger cells will disperse more light in the forward direction (forward scatter), and cells with

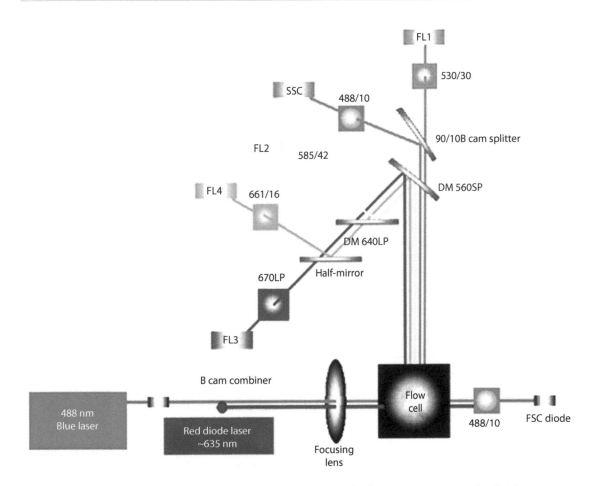

Figure 15.8 A typical flow cytometer. The key components of a flow cytometer are the fluidics system, the optical system, and the electronics system. The purpose of the fluidics is to focus the cells, single file, in the center of a fluid stream that is intercepted by the laser light source. This occurs within the flow cell. The optical components include the laser light source and a series of photomultiplier tubes (PMTs) and a photodiode for collecting the light signals. In this figure, there is a photodiode for forward scatter light (FSC), a PMT for side scatter light (SSC), and four PMTs detect separate fluorescence signals (FL1, FL2, FL3, FL4). A series of mirrors and filters directs fluorescence emission of the appropriate wavelength to the designated detector. The most commonly used fluorescent dyes are fluorescein isothiocyanate (FITC), phycoerythrin (PE), peridinin chlorophyll protein (PerCP), and allophycocyanin (APC), which are detected in FL1, FL2, FL3, and FL4, respectively. An electronic system converts optical signals into electronic impulses, which are in turn converted to digital values and sent to a computer.

greater internal complexity such as granulocytes will disperse more light in the 90° angle (side scatter). The most common clinical instruments are equipped with three lasers and 8–10 detectors for fluorescence emission. This allows for the collection of 10–12 parameters (two light scatter measurements and 8–10 fluorescence measurements) for each individual cell.

Data acquisition is rapid, routinely thousands of cells can be analyzed in a few seconds. The collection of such a large number of events eliminates the need for replicate analysis. Because multiple measurements are collected on each individual cell, mixed populations of cells can be assayed without prior physical separation. Later, during data analysis, cells with specific properties can be "electronically" separated or "gated," as described later.

Using a combination of membrane and intracellular probes, countless assays can be performed. Flow cytometry allows the gathering of information about the stage of development and the activation state of a cell, if a cell is dividing, if a cell is undergoing cell death by apoptosis or necrosis, or if a cell is normal or leukemic.

The most common clinical applications of flow cytometry are the diagnosis and monitoring of leukemia and HIV infection, the quantitation of CD34+ peripheral blood stem cells, and the diagnosis of paroxysmal nocturnal hemoglobinuria. Furthermore, flow cytometry has become an important tool for the counting of leukocytes in blood components after leukocyte depletion. Whole blood can be stained directly; following incubation with a cocktail containing fluorochrome-conjugated monoclonal antibodies, the RBC are lysed and the samples are ready for acquisition. Using a CD45 versus side-scatter gating technique, lymphocytes are selected, and percentages of the various cell surface markers (CD3, CD4, CD8, CD19, CD16/CD56) are determined (Figure 15.9). When fluorescent quantitation beads are added to the sample, the absolute cell count of each marker can be determined directly. Both the absolute cell count and the percentage are reported for each marker.

In patients with HIV infection, the CD4+ T-cell level and the CD4+/CD8+ ratio typically decline shortly after seroconversion. CD4+ levels above 500 cells/mm³ are usually associated with asymptomatic infection, whereas levels <200 cells/mm³ are consistent with a transition to AIDS. CD4+ levels rise in response to effective antiretroviral therapy.

Identifying deficiency in T, B, or natural killer (NK) cells allows classification of severe combined immunodeficiency (SCID) and other immunodeficiencies into one of the following types: T+B+NK+, T+B+NK−, T+B−NK+, T−B+NK+, T+B−NK−, T−B+NK−, T−B−NK+, and T−B−NK−. Such classification facilitates appropriate genetic counseling and clinical management (see Chapter 29).

Immunophenotyping is also critical in the diagnosis of leukemias and lymphomas, and to monitor therapy. Samples are analyzed using various panels of antibodies that have been established for various types of leukemia or lymphoma. The markers that are present on the cells as detected by immunophenotyping will help characterize the abnormal cells present.

It must be kept in mind that while findings represent comparisons to "normal" results and to known antigen associations with leukemias and lymphomas, abnormal immunophenotype profiles can be present in a variety of hematological malignancies. The EuroFlow Consortium has developed and standardized flow cytometric assays for diagnosis and prognostic (sub)classification of hematological malignancies as well as for evaluation of treatment effectiveness during follow-up.

Other clinical applications of flow cytometry

The applications of flow cytometry in the clinical and research laboratory are numerous. Monoclonal antibodies to cell surface antigens can be combined with mAb to intracellular proteins and nucleic binding dyes. For intracellular protein and nucleic acid staining, cells are fixed and then permeabilized with detergent or alcohol solutions. For example, intracellular cytokine staining of CD4 lymphocytes can provide information about the nature of an immune response, given that Th1 cells produce IFNγ, Th2 cells produce IL-4, Th17 cells produce IL-17, and Th21 cells preferentially produce IL-21.

CELL ISOLATION

Some flow cytometers have the ability to collect populations of cells or individual cells expressing a given phenotype. The sorted cells are used for a variety of downstream applications that include functional analysis and molecular profiling. Cell sorting is common in a research setting but is not used in clinical laboratories for patient care and treatment.

Another method for cell isolation uses immunomagnetic beads, used mostly in research laboratories. This technique is more rapid and less expensive than sorting on a flow cytometer. The limitation is that single-cell cloning is not possible. A mixed population of cells is incubated with monoclonal antibodies directed against the cell of interest. The antibodies can be directly conjugated to magnetic beads, or a secondary antibody directly conjugated to the magnetic bead can be used. Next, the cells bound to the immunomagnetic beads are isolated by placing the mixture near a magnetic field that attracts the labeled cells. Cells not recognized by the monoclonal antibody remain in the flow-through and can be collected for further fractionation or discarded. When the magnetic field is removed, the positively selected cells can be used in functional assays.

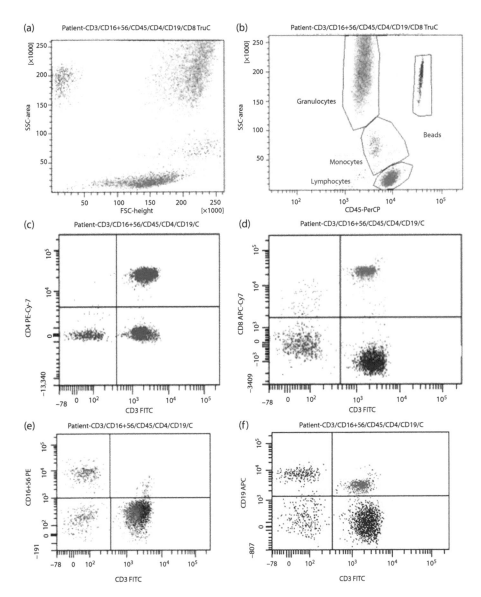

Figure 15.9 Lymphocyte immunophenotyping. Whole blood is stained with two antibody cocktails each containing monoclonal antibodies directly conjugated to one of six fluorochromes: FITC, PE, PerCP, PE-Cy7, APC-Cy7 or APC (see Figure 15.8). During data analysis, lymphocytes are selected or gated from the other leukocytes based on their light scatter properties or a combination of light scatter and CD45 (common leukocyte antigen) expression (a, b). Next, lymphocyte subsets are characterized. T cells that express CD3+ and CD4+ are part of the T-helper cell subset, while those that express CD3+ and CD8+ are part of the T cytotoxic cell subset (c, d). NK cells are identified as CD3−, and CD16+/ CD56+ (e), and B cells are identified as CD19+ (f).

IMMUNOHISTOCHEMISTRY

Immunohistochemistry is the result of the application of monoclonal antibodies to the detection of antigens in tissues, and has replaced immunofluorescence in many applications due to the specificity of mAbs. What distinguishes this technique from flow cytometry is that the cells are evaluated within their physiological context because the tissue remains in its original microenvironment. Consequently, it is possible to observe the localization of the antigens of interest with regard to the neighboring cells and the cellular compartments (i.e., cytoplasm, nucleus, or membrane). In addition to the gross histology (changes in the cells), the pathologist can now also observe changes in specific proteins within the cells. This was the first proven method to deliver the promise of "personalized medicine." For example, Her2/neu+ staining is an indication for the use of Herceptin, a monoclonal antibody therapy that specifically targets the Her2 receptor, in Her2/neu+ breast cancer patients. Clinically, it has been demonstrated that patients with high levels of this receptor benefit from the use of Herceptin, and, as a consequence, several immunohistochemistry tests have been developed that allow pathologists to measure Her2 expression levels.

HIGHLY SENSITIVE IMMUNOASSAYS

The use of monoclonal antibodies and specialized readout systems (enzymatic, fluorescent, chemiluminescent) have led to the generation of highly sensitive immunoassays that replaced older platforms such as radioimmunoassay.

ENZYME IMMUNOASSAY

The enzyme-linked immunosorbent assay (ELISA), currently known as enzyme immunoassay (EIA), is a flexible platform for the detection of an unlimited number of antigens in a variety of matrices. EIA is most often performed in a 96-well plate format and can be highly specific and sensitive in the nanomolar and picomolar ranges, when the correct configuration of high-quality, highly specific, serological reagents (monoclonal or polyclonal) is incorporated into the assay. The assay can be quantitative if an appropriate standard curve is incorporated into it. With the use of the 96-well plate format and automated pipetting devices, EIA can be high throughput and can be performed in different configurations:

In a **sandwich EIA capture assay** (Figure 15.10a), an antibody (the capture antibody) is adsorbed to the wells of a 96-well plate. The sample, in liquid format (i.e., plasma, serum, tissue culture media, cell lysate), containing the analyte of interest is then added to the well, and the antigen is allowed to bind the immobilized antibody. After washing away unbound proteins, the bound antigen can be detected with a second antibody coupled to an enzyme, usually peroxidase or alkaline phosphatase. Usually the second antibody recognizes a different epitope than the capture antibody, to avoid mutual interference between the capture antibody and the detection antibody. After unbound detection antibody is removed, a chromogenic, fluorogenic, or chemiluminescent substrate is added to the well. The enzyme-coupled detection antibody hydrolyzes the substrate generating a colored, fluorescent, or chemiluminescent product, which can easily be detected in the appropriate plate reader.

In a **direct antibody assay**, the antigen is immobilized in the 96-well plate, incubated with controls with known concentrations of antibody and samples to be tested for the presence of the antibody, and after incubation and washing off unbound proteins, a labeled anti-Ig antibody is used to detect the bound antibody (Figure 15.10b).

In a **competitive EIA**, a mixture of enzyme-labeled antigen and unlabeled antigen is added to a well coated with the capture antibody. The concentrations of labeled antigen and antibody are kept constant, and the concentration of unlabeled antigen is variable. After incubation and washing, the substrate is added. If the substrate develops color, the color intensity is directly proportional to the amount of bound labeled antigen, which, in turn, is inversely proportional to the concentration of unlabeled antigen added to the mixture.

Clinical applications of EIA

As a result of its relative simplicity and versatility, enzyme immunoassays are very widely used. Commercially available EIA kits have been developed for antimicrobial antibodies, antigen detection, hormone detection, and drug assay. In infectious diseases, immunoassays are used to distinguish disease-specific IgG versus IgM responses. IgG antibodies can be present in circulation for extended periods of time; whereas, IgM antibodies are characteristic of the early stages of the primary immune response. Thus, assays specifically designed to detect IgM antibodies are particularly useful for the diagnosis of ongoing infections.

Rapid EIA tests

One of the more innovative approaches to the immunoassay has been the development of the rapid diagnostic EIA kits, which can be performed

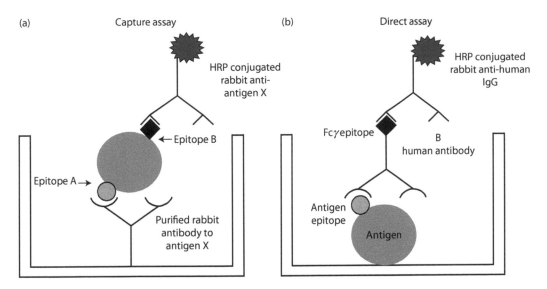

Figure 15.10 The principles of different types of enzyme immunoassays. In a competitive assay (a), a capture antibody is immobilized, reacts with the corresponding antigen, and a second enzyme-labeled antibody to a different epitope of the antigen is used to reveal its presence in the plate through a colorimetric reaction that takes place after adding a color-generating substrate to the enzyme coupled to the second antibody. The diagram illustrated the use of a horseradish peroxidase (HRP)–conjugated second antibody. In the direct assay (b), the antigen is adsorbed to the solid phase, antibodies to that antigen will become immobilized as a consequence of binding, and an enzyme-conjugated rabbit antibody to human IgG (or other immunoglobulin isotypes) is used to detect bound antibody. The intensity of color generated after adding a color-generating substrate will be proportional to the concentration of human antibody bound to the antigen and labeled antibody reacting with the human antibody.

with minimal training and instrumentation at a physician's office and even at home by patients themselves. Rapid tests have been developed for pregnancy, for a variety of infections including streptococcal sore throat, respiratory syncytial virus infections, viral influenza, and HIV infection, and for detection of occult blood in feces.

The original rapid tests for pregnancy were sandwich assays that used two monoclonal antibodies recognizing two different, noncompeting epitopes in human chorionic gonadotrophin. One antibody was immobilized onto a solid phase, and its function is to capture the antigen (hCG). The second was labeled with an enzyme and would be retained on the solid surface only if antigen had been captured by the first antibody. The retention of labeled antibody was detected by a color reaction secondary to the breakdown of an adequate substrate. These tests usually involved two or more steps. One-step tests were later developed, but the manufacturers have not divulged their exact design.

ELISpot

The enzyme-linked immunospot (ELISpot) assay (Figure 15.11) is a highly sensitive immunoassay that measures the frequency of cytokine-secreting cells at the single-cell level. In this assay, cells are cultured on a surface coated with a specific capture antibody in the presence or absence of stimuli. Cytokine secreted by the cells are captured. After an appropriate incubation time, cells are removed, and the secreted molecule is detected using a detection antibody in a similar procedure to that employed by the EIA. A variety of detection systems such as enzymatic or fluorescent can be used. Since the cytokines are retained by the antibody immobilized on the test surface, the end result is visible spots on the surface where the cytokine has been captured, and if an adequate dilution is used, each spot corresponding to an individual cytokine-secreting cell. T-SPOT is a type of ELISpot assay used for tuberculosis diagnosis, which belongs to the group of interferon-γ release assays. This assay

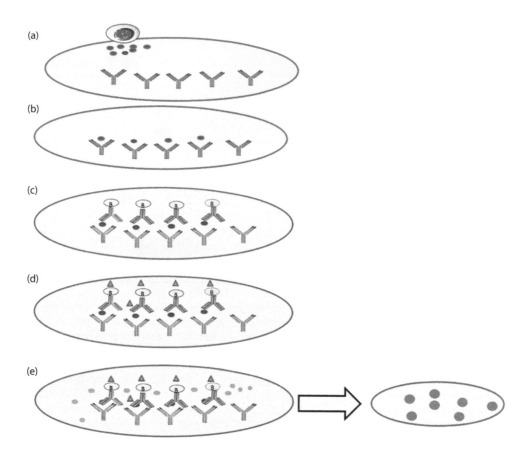

Figure 15.11 ELISpot assay. ELISpot employs the sandwich enzyme-linked immunosorbent assay (ELISA) technique. (a) Either a monoclonal or a polyclonal antibody specific for the chosen analyte is precoated onto a PVDF (polyvinylidene difluoride)–backed microplate. Appropriately stimulated cells are pipetted into the wells, and the microplate is placed into a humidified 37°C CO_2 incubator for a specified period of time. (b) During this incubation period, the immobilized antibody, in the immediate vicinity of the secreting cells, binds secreted analyte. (c) After washing away any cells and unbound substances, a biotinylated polyclonal antibody specific for the chosen analyte is added to the wells. (d) Following a wash to remove any unbound biotinylated antibody, alkaline-phosphatase conjugated to streptavidin is added. (e) Unbound enzyme is subsequently removed by washing, and a substrate solution (BCIP/NBT) is added. A blue-black colored precipitate forms and appears as spots at the sites of cytokine localization, with each individual spot representing an individual analyte-secreting cell. The spots can be counted with an automated ELISpot reader system.

counts the number of effector T cells that produce interferon-γ in a sample of blood. This gives an overall measurement of the host immune response against mycobacteria, including *Mycobacterium tuberculosis*.

Multiplex immunoassays

Immunoassays can be adapted to formats that allow multiple simultaneous readings, known as multiplex assays. Two basic formats exist, a plate format and a microsphere format. The bead technology can be compared to an "ELISA-on-a-bead," the marriage of the ELISA and the flow cytometer. The capture antibody is conjugated to a fluorescent microsphere, and all incubations are performed in solution. The bound antigen is detected with a fluorescent-conjugate detection antibody. The innovation of this method comes from the use of microspheres with varying levels of fluorescence and detection antibodies conjugated to different fluorochromes. This allows for multiplexing so that multiple antigens can be detected from the same sample in the same assay. While it is theoretically possible to measure 100 analytes from a single 50 μL plasma sample, in reality robust assays have been developed for about 5–10 analytes at a time. Challenges of this technology are to find the appropriate buffer conditions for multiple analytes. Furthermore, the assays are not as sensitive or reproducible as some immunoassays for the detection of low levels of antigen. This technology has had great impact in the field of transplantation where it is now routinely used to test for circulating anti-HLA antibodies in the recipients.

In plate-based multiplex assays, antibodies of different specificities are chemically bound to 96-well assay plates (with round or square wells), and the bound analyte is revealed with an enzyme-labeled antibody. Although the maximum number of antibodies that can be spotted on each well has not been definitively set, 9–12 analytes/well formats are commonly used. The antibodies are spotted precisely in the same positions in each well, and the detection unit is able to measure the signal intensity of each spot without interference from nearby spots. These assays have been of special interest to clinical investigators interested in measuring cytokine profiles in their patients.

EVALUATION OF CELLULAR IMMUNE RESPONSES

Lymphocyte functional assays can be performed directly in whole blood samples or in peripheral blood mononuclear cell (PBMC) preparations, which include monocytes and lymphocytes. PBMCs are prepared by density gradient centrifugation using a separation medium that has a specific gravity, which lies between the density of erythrocytes, granulocytes, and lymphocytes. Whole blood is layered over the separation medium and centrifuged. After centrifugation, the erythrocytes and granulocytes are below the separation medium, while the PBMCs will rest on top of the separation medium but underneath the platelet-rich plasma (Figure 15.12). About 80% of the PBMCs are lymphocytes and 20% are monocytes.

LABORATORY TESTS FOR ASSESSMENT OF LYMPHOCYTE FUNCTION *EX VIVO*

The evaluation of cell-mediated immunity presents considerably more difficulties than the evaluation of the humoral immune responses. *In vivo* tests, such as skin tests with common antigens known to induce delayed hypersensitive reactions, are difficult to standardize. *Ex vivo* functional tests are

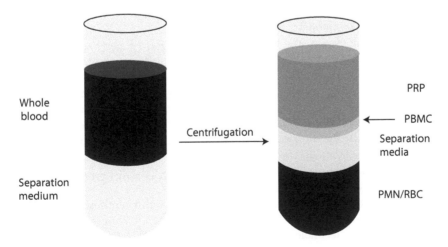

Figure 15.12 Peripheral blood mononuclear cell (PBMC) isolation by density gradient centrifugation. Whole blood is carefully layered atop a dextran sucrose-based separation medium of approximately the same density as PBMC. After centrifugation, the cells with higher density (RBC and polymorphonuclear cells [PMN]) will sediment below the separation medium. PBMC will rest directly on top of the medium beneath the platelet-rich plasma (PRP).

difficult to execute, time consuming, and require specialized personnel and sophisticated equipment.

Ex vivo stimulation

Lymphocytes in whole blood samples or in purified PBMCs can be stimulated *ex vivo* by specific antigens or by mitogenic substances. Ideally, specific antigens would be used to study lymphocyte function; however, given the fact that very few peripheral lymphocytes are specific for a given antigen, this approach is difficult. Alternatively, mitogens, which stimulate lymphocytes by antigen-independent mechanisms, are commonly used for *ex vivo* stimulation. Typical end points used to assess *ex vivo* lymphocyte activation are proliferation, cytokine production, changes in membrane expression of activation markers, and immunoglobulin production by B cells. Technically, the assays to assess *ex vivo* are relatively simple to perform; however, the data can be difficult to interpret, given that reference values for the responses in healthy individuals have not been established and individual variability in responses is high.

The common mitogens are lectins, such as phytohemagglutinin (PHA) and pokeweed mitogen (PWM). PWM stimulates both B cells and T cells, while PHA stimulates T cells only. A more physiologically relevant method is to stimulate the T cell receptor (TCR) directly with immobilized anti-CD3 monoclonal antibodies. The antigens most commonly used for *ex vivo* stimulation are purified protein derivative (PPD), *Candida albicans* antigens, keyhole limpet hemocyanin, and tetanus toxoid (which stimulates both T and B cells).

Proliferation assays

Incorporation of tritiated thymidine [^{3}H-Tdr] into dividing cells was traditionally the most common end point used to measure lymphocyte proliferation. When [^{3}H-Tdr] is added after 72 hours of stimulation, it is incorporated into the newly synthesized DNA. The amount of ^{3}H-Tdr incorporated into the cells can be correlated to proliferation.

Using newer, innovative technologies, the same information about immune function can be obtained in a simpler assay, without the use of radioactive isotopes. Cylex has developed a streamlined method to measure cell stimulation that requires only 18 hours of incubation and measures an early response to stimulation by detecting intracellular

ATP synthesis, which increases within the cells responding to the stimulant and thus correlates to cellular activation. When this assay is performed on isolated CD4 lymphocytes, the results are thought to be an indicator of a patient's overall immune cell function. As the response to immunosuppressive therapy varies among individuals, assessment of a patient's immune cell function may provide useful information to the clinician in the course of individual patient management.

Cytokine production assays

Cytokine production from *ex vivo* stimulation assays can be measured by a variety of methods, ELISA, ELISpot, multiplex bead assays, and intracellular cytokine staining by flow cytometry of the measurement of cytokine mRNA by qRT-PCR. IL-2 production is probably the cytokine of choice for the evaluation of the initial stages of activation of the T-helper cell population. Low or absent release of IL-2 has been observed in a variety of immunodeficiency states, particularly in patients with AIDS. Measurement of other cytokines such as IL-4, IL-5, IL-6, IL-10, IL-12, GM-CSF, TNF, LTα, and IFN-γ can provide a more complete picture of the functional response of T lymphocytes. For example, predominant release of IL-4, IL-5, or IL-10 is characteristic of Th2 responses, while predominant release of IFN-γ, IL-2, or GM-CSF is characteristic of Th1 responses.

Expression of activation markers

Changes in membrane expression of activation markers by flow cytometry can also be used to evaluate *ex vivo* stimulation. Upregulation of CD25 and CD69, or downregulation of CD62L is typical in activated lymphocytes.

Immunoglobulin production

Immunoglobulin synthesis is the best indicator of B-cell function. Changes in the levels of IgG and IgM after PWM stimulation can be easily measured in immunoassays.

Tetramer assays

One of the developments with greater potential significance has been the development of

MHC-peptide multimers. MHC-I and MHC-II multimers able to bind specific peptides have been constructed, and those tetramers, once loaded with a peptide, interact specifically with CD8$^+$ or CD4$^+$ T cells with TCR able to recognize the peptide-MHC combination in question. For example, MHC-I–peptide complexes loaded with peptides derived from melanoma-associated antigens have been shown to be able to bind specifically to CD8$^+$ lymphocytes from melanoma patients that can then be purified and shown to be able to lyse melanoma tumor cells *in vitro*. In contrast, MHC-II tetramers loaded with an influenza hemagglutinin (HA) peptide have been shown to bind and activate HA-specific CD4$^+$ T cells. The potential for application of this technique to characterize normal and abnormal aspects of cell-mediated immune responses appears almost unlimited.

Assays for cytotoxic effector cells

Traditionally, the functional evaluation of cytolytic activity in cytotoxic T lymphocytes (CTL) and NK cells was based on chromium (^{51}Cr) release cytotoxicity assays. Target cells prelabeled with ^{51}Cr were incubated with effector cells. Upon target cell lysis, ^{51}Cr is released into the culture media. The amount of ^{51}Cr release correlates with the cytotoxic effector cell function. More recently, a flow cytometric assay for cytolytic potential has been developed. This assay measures the level of CD107 on the plasma membrane. In resting CTL or NK cells, CD107 is expressed intracellularly on the membrane of the cytotoxic granules. Upon activation-induced degranulation, CD107 can be detected on the cellular membrane, reflecting degranulation and loss of intracellular perforin. Thus, the CD107-positive CTL or NK cells represent the subset with lytic potential. This innovative assay is more rapid than a traditional cytotoxicity assay and does not require the use of radiolabeled materials.

The cellular targets for cytotoxic cells vary according to cytotoxic cell population to be evaluated. The evaluation of CTL requires mixing sensitized cytotoxic T cells with targets expressing the sensitizing antigen. NK cell activity is usually measured with tumor cell lines known to be susceptible to NK cell killing. Antibody-dependent cellular cytotoxicity is measured using antibody-coated target cells.

LABORATORY TESTS FOR ASSESSMENT OF LYMPHOCYTE FUNCTION *IN VIVO*

While antigenic and mitogenic stimulation assays test lymphocyte reactions under more or less physiological conditions, the target cells are those present in circulation, and it can be argued that the sampling does not adequately reflect the state of activation of their tissue counterparts. This is particularly problematic when the objective is to assess the role of the T-cell system in a patient with a hypersensitivity disease. Several groups have proposed that the assay of circulating cytokines or cytokine receptors (shed as a consequence of cell activation) is more reflective of the state of activation of T cells *in vivo*. It must be noted that these assays have not proven to be as useful as expected. A major limiting factor is their lack of disease specificity, which makes their correlation with specific clinical conditions rather difficult.

Plasma IL-2 levels have been measured as a way to evaluate the state of T-lymphocyte activation *in vivo*. Increased levels of circulating IL-2 have been reported in patients with multiple sclerosis, patients with rheumatoid arthritis, and patients undergoing graft rejection, situations in which T-cell hyperactivity would fit with the clinical picture. However, a significant problem with these assays is the existence of factors that interfere with the assay of IL-2 by ELISA, and the results may be inaccurate. Activated T cells shed many of their membrane receptors, including the IL-2 receptor (IL-2R). Elevated levels of circulating soluble receptors (shed by activated T lymphocytes) can be demonstrated in patients with hairy cell leukemia, AIDS, rheumatoid arthritis, graft rejection, etc. In general, the results of assays for IL-2R show parallelism with the results of assays for IL-2.

Urinary levels of IL-2 can also be measured in an immunoassay. Urine is a good matrix as it contains fewer interfering substances than plasma. Increased urinary levels of IL-2 have been reported in association with kidney allograft rejection and proposed as a parameter that may help differentiate acute rejection from cyclosporine A toxicity.

Serum levels of IL-6, TNF, soluble TNF receptors 1 and 2, MCP-1, and MIF correlate with chronic inflammatory diseases such as systemic lupus erythematosus and atherosclerosis.

LABORATORY TESTS FOR ASSESSMENT OF PHAGOCYTIC CELL FUNCTION

Phagocytic cell function tests can be performed with isolated peripheral blood neutrophils or directly in whole blood. Killing defects are the most frequent primary abnormalities of these cells, and can be tested in a variety of ways. Bacterial killing tests are not routinely available in diagnostic laboratories. Instead, tests based on the induction and measurement of the oxidative burst are used to investigate those defects. These tests are discussed in detail in Chapter 13.

BIBLIOGRAPHY

Burska A, Boissinot M, Ponchel F. Cytokines as biomarkers in rheumatoid arthritis. *Mediators Inflamm*. 2014;2014:545493.

Denny T, Alexander T, Litwin V, eds. *Immunology Section, Clinical Microbiology Procedures Handbook*, 4th ed. Washington, DC: ASM Press; 2016.

Detrick B, Schmitz JL, Hamilton RG, eds. *Manual of Molecular and Clinical Laboratory Immunology*, 8th ed. Washington, DC: ASM Press; 2016.

Hunt KJ, Baker NL, Cleary PA, Klein R, Virella G, Lopes-Virella MF; and the DCCT/EDIC Group of Investigators. Longitudinal association between endothelial dysfunction, inflammation, and clotting biomarkers with subclinical atherosclerosis in type 1 diabetes: An evaluation of the DCCT/EDIC Cohort. *Diabetes Care*. 2015;38:1281–1289.

Litwin V, Marder P, eds. *Flow Cytometry in Drug Discovery and Development*. New York, NY: Wiley-Blackwell; 2010.

McKinnon KM. Multiparameter conventional flow cytometry. In: Hawley T, Hawley R, eds. *Flow Cytometry Protocols. Methods in Molecular Biology*. vol. 1678. New York, NY: Humana Press; 2018.

Oldaker T, Whitby L, Saber M, Holden J, Wallace PK, Litwin V. ICCS/ESCCA consensus guidelines to detect GPI-deficient cells in paroxysmal nocturnal hemoglobinuria (PNH) and related disorders part 4—Assay validation and quality assurance. *Cytometry B Clin Cytom* 2018;94:67–81.

16

Tolerance and autoimmunity

GEORGE C. TSOKOS AND GABRIEL VIRELLA

DEFINITION AND GENERAL CHARACTERISTICS OF TOLERANCE

Tolerance is best defined as a state of antigen-specific immunological unresponsiveness. This definition has two important corollaries:

- When tolerance is experimentally induced, it does not affect the immune response to antigens other than the one used to induce tolerance. This is a very important feature that differentiates tolerance from generalized immunosuppression, in which there is a depression of the immune response to a wide array of different antigens. Tolerance may be transient or permanent, while immunosuppression is usually transient.
- Given the antigen specificity that characterizes it, tolerance must be established at the clonal level. In other words, if tolerance is antigen specific, it must involve the T- and/or B-lymphocyte clone(s) specific for the antigen in question and not affect any other clones.

MECHANISMS OF TOLERANCE: CLONAL DELETION

At the cellular level, tolerance can result from clonal deletion or clonal anergy. Clonal deletion involves different processes for T and B lymphocytes. T lymphocytes are massively produced in the thymus and once generated will not rearrange their receptors. Memory T cells are long lived, and there is no clear evidence that new ones are generated after the thymus ceases to function in early adulthood. Therefore, elimination of autoreactive T cells has been postulated to occur at the production site (thymus) at the time the cells are differentiating their T-cell receptor (TCR) repertoire. Clonal deletion of T lymphocytes in the thymus is not a completely efficient process. The clones most likely to be eliminated are those that express T-cell receptors that interact with high affinity with self peptides associated with major histocompatibility complex (MHC) molecules. This process assumes that autoantigens are expressed in the thymus. Truly, mutation of the gene *AIRE* (autoimmune regulator) in both humans and mice results in the "autoimmune polyendocrinopathy syndrome." AIRE protein is responsible for the expression in the thymus of proteins typically seen in peripheral organs. T cells that are specific for antigens not expressed in the thymus escape negative selection (central tolerance) and move to the periphery where they may attack tissues and organs.

The fate of the T cells that encounter autoantigen in the thymus depends on their affinity for the TCR. If the affinity is high, the cells will die. This process is known as **negative selection**, and it occurs in the stage of double-positive T cells in the thymic cortex and in early single-positive cells in the medulla. This explains why most T cells in the periphery do not recognize self-antigen. Some T cells that recognize self-antigen in the thymus are not deleted and differentiate into regulatory T cells specific for this antigen (referred to as tTregs), and they control the immune response after they exit the thymus. Other self-reactive cells escape into the periphery where they are subject to control by regulatory cells.

In contrast, B lymphocytes are continuously produced by the bone marrow throughout life and initially express low-affinity IgM on their membranes. In most instances, the interaction of these resting B cells with circulating self molecules neither activates them nor causes their elimination. Selection and deletion of autoreactive clones seem to take place in the peripheral lymphoid organs during the onset of the immune response. At that time, activated B cells can modify the structure of their membrane immunoglobulin as a consequence of somatic mutations in their germ-line immunoglobulin genes. B cells expressing self-reactive immunoglobulins of high affinity can emerge from this process, and their elimination takes place in the germinal centers.

Both T- and B-cell clonal deletion fail to eliminate all autoreactive cells. In the case of T cells, clonal deletion is very effective to eliminate autoreactive cells with high-affinity receptors for autoantigens, but autoreactive cells with moderate- to low-affinity receptors will be spared. Other critical factors that determine how effective clonal deletion is include the affinity and stability of the interaction of self-reactive peptides with MHC molecules and the level of expression of the MHC-peptide complexes. In other words, any condition that interferes with the effective presentation of a self-reactive peptide in association with an MHC molecule decreases the efficiency of clonal deletion. Clonal deletion will also not affect clones that recognize self-antigens not expressed in the thymus. Furthermore, as the thymic function declines with age, alternative mechanisms have to be in place to ensure the inactivation of autoreactive clones emerging from the differentiation of lymphoid stem cells.

The causes of B-cell escape from clonal deletion are not as well defined, but they exist nonetheless. Thus, peripheral tolerance mechanisms must exist to ensure that autoreactive clones of T and B cells are neutralized after their migration to the peripheral lymphoid tissues.

MECHANISMS OF TOLERANCE: CLONAL ANERGY

One of the postulated peripheral tolerance mechanisms is known as clonal anergy, a process that incapacitates or disables autoreactive clones that escape selection by clonal deletion. Thus, anergy can be experimentally induced after the ontogenic differentiation of immunocompetent cells has reached a stage in which clonal deletion is no longer possible.

By definition, anergic clones lack the ability to respond to stimulation with the corresponding antigen. Thus, the most obvious manifestation of clonal anergy is the inability to respond to proper stimulation. Anergic B cells carry IgM autoreactive antibody in their membrane but are not activated when they encounter antigen. Anergic T cells express TCR for the tolerizing antigen but fail to properly express the IL-2 and IL-2 receptor genes and to proliferate in response to antigenic stimulation.

In a simplistic way, it can be stated that anergy results from an internal block of the intracellular signaling pathways caused by increased expression of molecules that suppress the signaling process, or from downregulating effects exerted by other (regulatory) cells. One major mechanism that is involved in anergy is the incomplete signaling of an immunocompetent cell. This may result in either a block of the intracellular activation pathways or the developmental arrest of autoreactive clones, which fail to fully differentiate into mature clones of effector cells. Both mechanisms are discussed in detail later in this chapter.

As is often the case, when several mechanisms leading to a similar end result are defined, they end up not being mutually exclusive. Indeed, there is ample evidence suggesting that tolerance results from a combination of clonal deletion and clonal anergy. Both processes must coexist and complement each other under normal conditions so that autoreactive clones, which escape deletion during embryonic development, may be downregulated and become anergic. The failure of either one of these mechanisms may result in the development of an autoimmune disease. The contribution of regulatory T cells to the maintenance of peripheral tolerance is of paramount importance, and it is discussed later in this chapter.

ACQUIRED TOLERANCE

Acquired tolerance can be induced in experimental animals under the right conditions, known as tolerogenic conditions, and in clinical practice using a number of drugs or biologics that enhance mechanisms responsible for immune tolerance (Table 16.1). Several factors influence the development of tolerance. The clinical significance of understanding acquired tolerance is reflected in the need to reestablish tolerance in autoimmune diseases. Reestablishing tolerance limited only to antigens that lead to autoimmune pathology represents the only hope for specific treatment. Certain approaches that have claimed possible clinical effect include the following:

- Modulation of antigen receptors off the surface of B cells results in an inability to bind autoantigen and therefore to respond to it. Example: A tetramer of small DNA fragments binds to anti-DNA immunoglobulin expressing B cells, forces the disappearance of surface antigen receptor, and subsequently, the B cell does not recognize autoantigen.

Table 16.1 Factors influencing the development of tolerance

- Host
- Genetic predisposition
- Soluble, small-sized antigen
- Antigen structurally similar to self protein
- Intravenous administration of antigen
- High or low dose of antigen

- Engagement of the inhibitory FcRIIb limits the responsiveness of B cells to antigen.
- Altering the route of administration may suppress the response to the autoantigen. Oral administration of basic myelin or collagen, the suspected autoantigens in multiple sclerosis and arthritis, may lead to disease suppression.
- Immunosuppressive drugs, if given at proper doses, may suppress autoreactive clones in autoimmune diseases although nonautoreactive immune cells are eliminated.
- Development of T- or B-cell receptor ligands that have altered (lower) avidity and through binding to the corresponding receptor induce anergy rather than a productive response.
- Blockade of costimulation results in T-cell anergy. CTLA4-Ig (in a soluble form fused to the Fc portion of IgG) or CTLA4 antibodies block the delivery of costimulation through CD28 provided by CD80/86. Direct engagement of the inhibitor receptor known as programmed cell death protein 1 (PD-1) may cause unresponsiveness.

EXPERIMENTAL APPROACHES TO DEFINITION OF MECHANISMS OF LYMPHOCYTE TOLERANCE

The understanding of the mechanisms involved in tolerance has received a significant boost through the use of transgenic mice. These mice are obtained by introducing a gene in the genome of a fertilized egg that is subsequently implanted in a pseudo-pregnant female in which it develops. The new gene introduced in the germ line is passed on, allowing the study of the acquisition of tolerance to a defined antigen under physiological conditions. Double-transgenic mice expressing a given antigen and an antibody with predetermined specificity have been constructed by breeding transgenic mice. The tissue expression of the transgene can be manipulated by coupling a tissue-specific promoter to the gene in question.

B-lymphocyte tolerance models

The main characteristics of B-cell tolerance are summarized in Table 16.2. Experimental evidence supporting both anergy and clonal deletion as mechanisms leading to B-cell tolerance has been

Table 16.2 B-cell tolerance

B-cell anergy	Antigen is soluble
	Reactivation may occur
	Direct proof:
	A. Double-transgenic animals (soluble egg lysozyme and anti-egg lysozyme Ab genes): B cells synthesize egg lysozyme but do not secrete anti-lysozyme Ab
	B. Transgenic animals (anti-DNA Ab gene on B cells): B cells do not secrete anti-DNA Ab
B-cell deletion	Antigen is surface bound
	Direct proof:
	A. Double-transgenic mice (genes coding for surface bound lysozyme and anti-lysozyme Ab): B cells do not produce lysozyme or anti-lysozyme Ab
	B. Transgenic mice with B cells with genes coding for anti-H2-K^k antibody mated with H2-K^k mice produce offspring that lack H2-K^k antibody-positive B cells

obtained in transgenic mouse models. One of the most informative models for the understanding of B-cell tolerance was obtained by breeding double-transgenic mice from animals transgenic for hen egg lysozyme, which develop tolerance to this protein during development, and animals of the same strain carrying the gene coding for IgM egg lysozyme antibody. The double-transgenic F1 hybrids express the gene coding for egg lysozyme in nonlymphoid cells, and B lymphocytes of these mice also express IgM anti-egg lysozyme antibody. These antibody-positive B lymphocytes are present in large numbers in the spleen. The predominance of B cells with membrane IgM specific for lysozyme is a consequence of allelic exclusion: The insertion of a completely rearranged immunoglobulin transgene blocks rearrangement of the normal immunoglobulin genes.

The relevance of this model to the understanding of tolerance lies in the fact that the double-transgenic F1 hybrids failed to produce anti-egg lysozyme antibodies after repeated immunization with egg lysozyme. Thus, these animals have B lymphocytes carrying and expressing a gene that codes for a self-reactive antibody but cannot respond to the antigen. Experiments on these cells suggest that one or several of the kinases activated during the response of a normal B cell to antigenic stimulation remain in an inactive state, interrupting the activation cascade.

Reversibility of B-cell anergy

By definition, a state of anergy should be reversible. Reversibility was experimentally proven by transferring lymphocytes from double-transgenic F1 hybrids expressing the gene coding for anti-egg lysozyme antibody to irradiated nontransgenic recipients of the same strain. In this new environment, from which egg lysozyme was absent, the transferred B lymphocytes produced anti-egg lysozyme antibodies upon immunization. These experiments suggest that continuous exposure to the circulating self-antigen is necessary to maintain B-cell anergy.

Another approach to activate anergic cells is to separate peripheral blood B lymphocytes from an anergic animal and stimulate them *in vitro* with lipopolysaccharide, which is a polyclonal mitogen for murine B lymphocytes. As a consequence of this stimulation, the signaling block that characterizes anergy is overridden, and autoreactive B cells secreting antilysozyme antibody can be detected.

In the bone marrow, upon encounter with certain autoantigens, B cells undergo "receptor editing," which results in the inability to respond.

Models for B-lymphocyte clonal deletion

Evidence supporting clonal deletion in B-cell tolerance has also been recently obtained in transgenic animal models. Experiments were carried out in F1 double-transgenic mice that were raised by mating animals that expressed egg lysozyme not as a soluble protein, but as an integral membrane protein, with transgenic mice of the same strain carrying the gene for IgM anti-egg lysozyme antibody. In the resulting double-transgenic F1 hybrids, B lymphocytes carrying IgM anti-egg lysozyme antibody could not be detected.

Additional experiments have proven that stimulation of an immature IgM/IgD autoreactive B-cell clone by a self-antigen abundantly expressed on a cell membrane leads to clonal deletion by apoptosis. The elimination of autoreactive clones seems to take place in the lymph node germinal centers.

Thus, the sum of experimental data suggests that B-cell tolerance can result both from clonal anergy and clonal deletion, and the choice of mechanism depends on whether the antigen is soluble or membrane bound. Clonal deletion involves apoptosis of the self-reactive cells, but we do not know why only membrane-bound antigens appear to trigger apoptosis. B-cell anergy, conversely, is associated with a block in the transduction of the activating signal resulting from the binding of antigen to the membrane immunoglobulin, probably consequent to the lack of costimulatory signals usually delivered by activated Th2 cells. Experimental data suggest that the signal delivered to CD40+ B cells by interacting with the CD40 ligand expressed by T cells is critically important for B-cell differentiation. In the absence of CD40 signaling, B cells are easy to tolerize.

T-LYMPHOCYTE TOLERANCE MODELS

The main characteristics of T-cell tolerance are summarized in Table 16.3. As in the case of B-cell anergy, experimental evidence supporting both anergy and clonal deletion as mechanisms leading to T-cell tolerance has been obtained in transgenic mouse models.

There is solid experimental evidence supporting clonal deletion as a mechanism involved in T-cell tolerance. Of seminal importance were the experiments in which transgenic mice were transfected with the gene coding for a TCR cloned from an MHC-I–restricted CD8+ cytotoxic T-cell clone specific for the male HY antigen (Figure 16.1). This TCR was able to mediate a cytotoxic reaction against any cell expressing the HY antigen. While female transgenic mice (HY−) were found to have mature CD8+ cells expressing the TCR specific for HY, none of the transgenic male animals (HY+) had detectable mature CD8+ cells expressing the anti-HY TCR. However, functionally harmless CD4+ cells with the autoreactive TCR could be detected in male animals.

These observations were interpreted as meaning that those lymphocytes expressing the autoreactive TCR and the CD8+ antigen interacted effectively with a cell presenting an immunogenic HY-derived peptide in association with a MHC-I molecule, and those cells were deleted. CD4+ lymphocytes, even if carrying the same TCR, cannot interact effectively with MHC-I–associated HY-derived peptides and were spared. Similar experiments using mice transfected with genes coding for MHC class-II–restricted TCRs showed that the CD4+ lymphocytes were selectively deleted, as expected from the fact that the reaction between a TCR and an MHC-II–associated peptide is stabilized by CD4 molecules. In other words, the role of CD4 and CD8, as stabilizers of the reaction between T lymphocytes and antigen-presenting cells (APCs), is not only important for antigenic stimulation but is also critical for clonal deletion.

Mechanisms of T-cell clonal deletion

A common point to all types of clonal deletion is that cell death is due to apoptosis, involving interaction of the Fas molecule with its ligand. However, many details concerning the control of T-cell apoptosis remain unexplained, and, as discussed previously, it is clear that clonal deletion is an imperfect mechanism that needs to be complemented by mechanisms ensuring that persisting autoreactive clones remain inactive.

T-cell anergy

Experimental models addressing the question of how T cells become tolerant to tissue-specific determinants that are not expressed in the thymus have

Table 16.3 T-cell tolerance

Clonal deletion	Ag presented in the thymus
	T cells die by apoptosis
	TCR repertoire bias
	Never absolute (residual autoreactive cells seem to persist)
Clonal anergy	Occurs in periphery
	Stimulation of T cells in the absence of proper costimulation leads to anergy

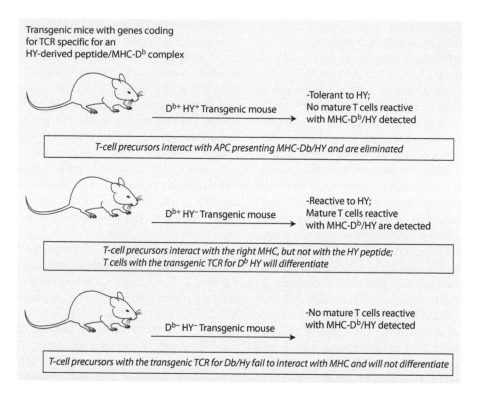

Figure 16.1 An experiment in which transgenic animals expressing a TCR specific for an HY-derived peptide–MHC-D^b complex were shown to become tolerant to the HY peptide, but only in D^{b+} animals. The tolerance in this model was apparently due to clonal deletion, since mature T cells reactive with MHC-D^b/HY could not be detected in the tolerant animals.

provided evidence for the role of clonal anergy. Transgenic mice were constructed in which the transgene was coupled to a tissue-specific promoter that directed their expression to an extra-thymic tissue. For example, heterologous MHC class-II (I-E) genes were coupled to the insulin promoter prior to their injection into fertilized eggs. Consequently, the MHC class-II antigens coded by the transfected genes were expressed only in the pancreatic islet β cells. Class-II (I-E) specific helper T cells were detectable in the transgenic animals, but they could not be stimulated by exposure to lymphoid cells expressing the transfected MHC-II genes. Thus, tolerance to a peripherally expressed MHC-II self-antigen can be due to clonal anergy.

Mechanisms of T-cell anergy

Proper stimulation of mature CD4$^+$ T lymphocytes requires at least two signals: one delivered by the interaction of the TCR with the MHC-II-Ag complex, and the other delivered by the accessory cell. Both signals require cell-cell contact, involving a variety of surface molecules, and the release of soluble cytokines. When all these signals are properly transmitted to the T lymphocyte, a state of activation ensues. Several experiments suggest that the state of anergy develops when TCR-mediated signaling is not followed by costimulatory signals. For example, a state of anergy is induced when T lymphocytes are stimulated with chemically fixed accessory cells (which cannot release cytokines or upregulate membrane molecules involved in the delivery of costimulatory signals) or with purified MHC-II–antigen complexes (which also cannot provide costimulatory signals).

From the multitude of costimulatory pairs of molecules that have been described, the CD28/CTLA4-B7 family is the most significant in the physiology of T-cell anergy. CD28-mediated signals are necessary to induce the production of IL-2, which seems to be critical for the initial proliferation of Th0 cells and eventual differentiation of Th1 cells. CD28 engagement also results in a lower threshold for effective TCR activation and therefore may enhance the lower avidity interactions between TCR and autoantigens. If the interaction between CD28 and its ligand is prevented at the onset of the immune response, anergy and tolerance ensue. Also, if CD80/86 molecules interact with CTLA4 rather than CD28, a downregulating signal is delivered to the T lymphocyte (see Chapter 11). CTLA4 has a 10- to 20-fold higher avidity for CD80 than CD28. In contrast to the interactions involving CD28, those that involve CTLA4 may increase the threshold of T-cell activation and inhibit T-cell responses to low-affinity autoantigens.

Another inhibitory receptor is PD-1 (programmed death 1, called so because it was originally thought to be involved in apoptosis). It recognizes two ligands, PD-L1 and PD-L2. Its cytoplasmic region recognizes phosphatases that inhibit T-cell function. Mice deficient in PD-1, like those deficient in CTLA4, develop autoimmunity. Tumors that express PD-L1 and L2 inhibit T-cell cytotoxic function. PD-1, PD-L1 or CTLA4 antibodies (checkpoint inhibitors) have met success in the treatment of certain tumors.

In conclusion, clonal deletion seems extremely efficient during embryonic differentiation, but a large number of potentially autoreactive clones seem to escape deletion. Whether those autoreactive clones remain anergic or are activated may just depend on whether the autoantigens against which they are directed are ever presented in a context able to induce an active immune response, i.e., by activated APCs able to deliver costimulatory signals to the autoreactive T and/or B cells. Under normal physiologic conditions, the recognition of autoantigens is more likely to take place in the absence of costimulatory signals by helper T cells, conditions that are likely to contribute to the perpetuation of a state of T-cell anergy. The perpetuation of the anergic state by incomplete signaling of autoreactive clones is believed to be significant in the maintenance of tolerance in adult life.

Regulatory T cells

The immune system uses a multitude of mechanisms to regulate T cell–dependent immune responses. Suppression of the immune response following infection obviates the continuous expansion and exhaustion of the immune system. Failure to control the immune response will result in autoimmunity and organ damage.

The most important cells in the suppression of self-reactive T cells are the CD4+ T cells that express forkhead box P3 (FOXP3; regulatory T cells [Treg]). Humans and mice that lack FOXP3 develop multiorgan autoinflammatory syndrome (Scurfy mice; immune dysregulation, polyendocrinopathy, enteropathy, X-linked (IPEX) syndrome in humans).

Treg heterogeneity: FOXP3+ T cells constitute 5%–10% of peripheral blood cells in mice and humans. FOXP3 stabilizes the Treg lineage by reinforcing a specific gene program. The differentiation of Treg cells depends on IL-2. Tregs express increased amounts of the low-avidity IL-2 receptor α chain (CD25) and low amounts of the α chain of the IL-7 receptor (CD127). Some activated T cells express FOXP3, and some FOXP3+ cells may display a pro-inflammatory phenotype).

Treg cells are classified into **two major groups**: those originating in the thymus (tTreg) and those developing in the periphery (pTreg). Stimulation through CD3/TCR and CD28 leads to the expression of transcription factors that bind to conserved noncoding region (CNS)2 and CNS3 of the FOXP3 gene to drive FOXP3 expression. Subsequently, IL-2 receptor signaling leads to the generation of pSTAT5 that keeps the FOXP3 locus open, hence the dependence of Tregs on IL-2. In addition, pTregs, but not tTregs, depend on TGFβ signaling to complete their differentiation, and protocols to induce Tregs *in vitro* require TGFβ. pTregs, unlike tTregs display significant plasticity. A well-established scenario has been shown with Tregs in the gut. Gut Tregs are pTregs and suppress responses to microbiota, yet during infection, these Tregs convert to Th1 and Th2 pro-inflammatory cells.

Functional heterogeneity of Tregs: Multiple mechanisms have been ascribed to mouse and human Treg cells that suppress autoreactive T cells:

- Secretion of immunomodulatory proteins by Treg cells, such as IL-10 and TGFβ, which suppress pro-inflammatory responses. A functional group of Tregs is known as effector (e) Tregs, which produce IL-10, are found in sites of inflammation and are probably responsible for the control of inflammation.

- Expression of CD80 and CD86 and increased release of the immunosuppressive enzyme, indoleamine-2,3-dioxygenase (IDO) can result in the conversion of dendritic cells to tolerogenic cells.
- High expression of the ectoenzymes CD39 and CD73 converts ATP to AMP (CD39) and AMP to adenosine (CD73), which is a strong suppressor molecule after it binds to cells expressing adenosine receptors.

More subsets of Tregs have been recognized as responsible for the control of specific effector T-cell subsets. Treg cells expressing Tbet, GATA, STAT3, and Bcl6 suppress Th1, Th2, Th17, and T-follicular helper (Tfh) cells, respectively.

Another recognized feature of Treg heterogeneity is that the Tregs that reside in various tissues express unique characteristics. Tregs in the gut express the retinoic acid receptor-related orphan nuclear receptor gamma (RORγt), and they can produce IL-17. Tregs in visceral adipose tissue express PPARγ that regulates insulin sensitivity. Skin Tregs express a different type of ROR, RORα, which downregulates the proliferation of type 2 innate lymphoid cells (ILC2) and Th2 cells, suppresses IL-4 expression, and enhances the expression of the death receptor 3 (DR3). These combined effects protect against the development of skin allergic reactions.

Another novel feature of Tregs is their involvement in tissue regeneration. Tregs that express amphiregulin (an epithelial cell growth factor) accumulate in sites of muscle or skin injury and promote tissue repair.

Molecular requirements of Treg cells: As mentioned, the differentiation and expansion of Treg cells depends on IL-2 signaling, and they were first recognized when it was noticed that mice and humans defective on IL-2 or IL-2 receptor develop inflammation. Delivery of Il-2 to Treg cells in low doses has been shown in a number of diseases to expand Treg cells and result in clinical improvement.

Certain levels of the mechanistic or mammalian target of rapamycin (mTOR) factor are needed for the proper function of Tregs. The phosphatases PTEN (phosphatase and tensin homolog) and PP2A (protein phosphatase 2A) contribute to the good function of Tregs through distinct mechanisms. In contrast, Notch signaling is detrimental to the function of Tregs.

Besides FOXP3, additional transcription factors are needed for the proper function and sustenance of Tregs. These include STAT5, the transcription regulator Bach2, and the chromatin remodeler special AT-rich sequence binding protein (SATB1).

As already mentioned, lack of FOXP3, IL-2, IL-2 receptor, CTLA4, and PD-1 in humans results in autoimmunity and represents monogenic autoinflammatory diseases due to Treg deficiency. Functional and/or numerical Treg abnormalities have been reported in systemic and organ-specific autoimmune diseases.

MUCOSAL TOLERANCE

Ingested antigens seldom cause an immune response. If we consider the immensity of potentially immunogenic proteins to which the digestive mucosae are exposed over a lifetime, the incidence of food allergies is miniscule, proof of the general lack of immunogenicity of ingested non-self material. It is also well documented that ingestion of proteins or nonreplicating organisms is not an efficient approach to immunization. At the same time, reports of the therapeutic benefit of oral administration of collagen to patients with rheumatoid arthritis raised considerable interest in the concept of oral tolerance.

The sum of experimental data collected so far suggests that the administration of large doses of oral antigen causes Th1 anergy-driven tolerance. However, this seems to be a rather exceptional mechanism with little clinical application. In contrast, the administration of low doses of antigen is believed to stimulate Th2 responses and cause bystander suppression of autoreactive Th1 cells. A proposed framework for this type of suppression is as follows:

1. The ingested antigen (usually a protein) is transported to submucosal accessory cells in the Peyer's patches where it is processed and presented to regulatory T cells (both of CD4+ and CD8+ phenotypes, including special subpopulations of γδ CD4+ and CD8+ T cells), which after proliferation and differentiation become functional suppressors. The suppressor effect is mediated by secretion of TGF-β, IL-10, and IL-4 after reexposure to the tolerizing antigen.
2. When the antigen is introduced in small doses as a nasal aerosol, the main effect seems to be

the stimulation of immunoregulatory $\gamma\delta$ CD8$^+$ cells that cause a shift from a predominant and pathogenic Th1 response to a less harmful Th2 response.

3. The activated regulatory T cells enter the circulation and are attracted to areas of ongoing reactivity. In the peripheral lymphoid tissues, they may downregulate immune responses to the tolerizing antigen. In tissues where effector cells are causing inflammatory changes, the recruitment of activated regulatory T cells releasing TGF-β and IL-10 may suppress the activity of Th1 assisting the local immune response process, resulting in a downregulation of the inflammatory response. As indicated, regulatory T cells in the mucosa display plasticity and may convert to Th17 cells, particularly under inflammatory conditions.

The antigen used to induce oral tolerance does not need to be identical to that recognized by the autoreactive T cells *in vivo*, since the suppressor effects of IL-10 and TGF-β are nonspecific and can affect T cells reacting with other antigens (bystander suppression). However, the best results with oral tolerization protocols are obtained when antigens structurally related to the autoantigens are given orally. Thus, cross-reactivity between the two antigens may be important in localizing the activated suppressor CD8$^+$ cells to the right tissue.

TERMINATION OF TOLERANCE

A state of tolerance dependent on the downregulation of self-reactive clones can be terminated if those clones are adequately activated. Several possible scenarios can be envisaged and, in some cases, experimentally proven to explain the activation of anergic clones:

- Exposure of anergic cells to an antigen that cross-reacts with a tolerogen may induce the activation of T-helper lymphocytes specific for the cross-reacting antigen (molecular mimicry). As a consequence, the activated T$_H$ cells will provide autoreactive pro-inflammatory Th1 or B lymphocytes with the necessary costimulatory signals necessary to initiate a response against the tolerogen.
- Proper stimulation of anergic T lymphocytes may reestablish the costimulatory pathways,

terminate anergy, and initiate the autoreactive process. Experimental evidence supporting this concept was obtained in studies of transgenic mice expressing a lymphocytic choriomeningitis viral glycoprotein on the pancreatic cells. These transgenic mice have T lymphocytes that recognize the glycoprotein but remain anergic. However, the state of anergy in these transgenic mice can be terminated by an infection with the lymphocytic choriomeningitis virus. The infection stimulates the immune system and induces the overexpression of MHC-II–self-peptide complexes and costimulatory signals, and previously unresponsive T cells are activated. Consequently, the previously tolerant animals develop inflammatory changes in the Langerhans islets (insulitis) caused by lymphocytes reacting with the viral antigen expressed on the pancreatic cells. Those changes precede the development of diabetes. Infections involving superantigen-producing organisms may be for termination of tolerance. Those superantigens react with most MHC-II molecules and with the TCR of specific variable region families. Those TCR families are expressed by as much as one-third of the total T-cell population. The cross-linking of TCRs on large numbers of T lymphocytes in close apposition with activated APCs delivers strong activating signals to T lymphocytes. The consequence is that previously anergic self-reactive T cells will be activated, and a previously downregulated autoimmune response becomes active.

AUTOIMMUNITY

Failure of the immune system to "tolerate" self-antigens may result in the development of pathological processes known as **autoimmune diseases**. At the clinical level, autoimmunity is thought to be involved in a variety of apparently unrelated diseases such as systemic lupus erythematosus (SLE), insulin-dependent diabetes mellitus, myasthenia gravis, rheumatoid arthritis, multiple sclerosis, and hemolytic anemia. There are at least 40 diseases known or considered to be autoimmune in nature, affecting about 5% of the general population. Their distribution by gender and age is not uniform. As a rule, autoimmune diseases predominate in women and have a bimodal age distribution. A first peak of incidence is around puberty, whereas the second peak is in the forties and fifties.

CLASSIFICATION OF AUTOIMMUNE DISEASES

There are several different ways to classify autoimmune diseases. Because several autoimmune diseases are strongly linked with MHC antigens, one of the proposed classifications, shown in Table 16.4, groups autoimmune diseases according to their association with class-I or class-II MHC markers. It is interesting to notice that although autoimmune diseases may afflict both sexes, there is a female preponderance for the class II–associated diseases and a definite increase in the prevalence of class I–associated diseases among males.

PATHOPHYSIOLOGY OF AUTOIMMUNE DISEASES

The autoimmune pathologic process may be initiated and/or perpetuated by autoantibodies, immune complexes containing autoantigens, and autoreactive T lymphocytes. Each of these immune processes plays a preponderant role in certain diseases or may be synergistically associated, particularly in multiorgan, systemic autoimmune diseases.

Table 16.4 **Classification of autoimmune diseases**

I. MHC Class II–Associated

  A. Organ specific
    (autoantibody directed against a single organ or closely related organs)

  B. Systemic
    (Systemic lupus erythematosus—variety of autoantibodies to DNA, cytoplasmic antigens, etc.)

II. MHC Class I–Associated

  A. HLA-B27–related spondyloarthropathies (ankylosing spondylitis, Reiter's syndrome, etc.)

  B. Psoriasis vulgaris (which is associated with HLA-B13, B16, and B17)

Pathogenic role of autoantibodies

B lymphocytes with autoreactive specificities remain nondeleted in the adult individuals of many species. In mice, polyclonal activation with lipopolysaccharide leads to production of autoantibodies. In humans, bacterial and viral infections (particularly chronic) may lead to the production of anti-immunoglobulin and antinuclear antibodies. In general, it is accepted that polyclonal B-cell activation may be associated with the activation of autoreactive B lymphocytes.

Autoantibody-associated diseases are characterized by the presence of autoantibodies in the individual's serum and by the deposition of autoantibodies in tissues. Antibodies with high affinity for the antigen are considered to be more pathogenic because they form stable immune complexes (ICs) that can activate complement more effectively. Other characteristics of the antibodies and corresponding agents may play a determinant pathogenic role. For example, DNA antibodies, very prevalent in SLE, have a weak positive charge at physiological pH and bind to the negatively charged glomerular basement membrane, which also binds DNA. Such affinity of antigens and antibodies for the glomerular basement membrane creates the ideal conditions for *in situ* IC formation and deposition, which is usually followed by glomerular inflammation. Some DNA antibodies cross-react with NMDA receptors in the brain and cause pathology. Finally, autoantibodies may bind only to cells and tissues that have been exposed to a stressor such as ischemia, activate complement, and cause tissue injury. This may explain why titers of autoantibodies almost never correlate with autoimmune disease severity.

Autoantibodies may be directly involved in the pathogenesis of some diseases, while in others, they may serve simply as disease markers without a known pathogenic role. For example, the anti-Sm antibodies that are found exclusively in patients with SLE are not known to play a pathogenic role. However, in many other situations, autoantibodies may be able to trigger various pathogenic mechanisms leading to cell or tissue destruction (Table 16.5). This is particularly true of complement-fixing antibodies (IgG and IgM). Finally, other autoantibodies may have a pathogenic role dependent not on causing cell or tissue damage, but on the interference with cell functions resulting from their binding to physiologically important cell receptors.

Table 16.5 Pathogenic mechanisms triggered by autoantibodies

Mechanism	Disease	Comments
C'-mediated cell lysis	Autoimmune cytopenias	C'-activating immunoglobulin binds to cell-membrane antigen; C' is activated; membrane attack complex is formed; cell is lysed
Tissue destruction by inflammatory cells	SLE	Antinuclear antibodies bind to tissue-fixed antigens; C' is activated; C3a and C5a are produced; polymorphonuclear cells are attracted; inflammation develops
Blockage of receptor	Insulin-resistant diabetes mellitus (acanthosis nigricans)	Anti-insulin receptor antibodies bind to insulin receptor and compete with insulin
Charge facilitated	Lupus nephritis	Cationic anti-DNA tissue deposition; antibodies bind to glomerular basement membrane
Activation of C'	Membranoproliferative glomerulonephritis	Anti-C3bBb antibodies (nephritic factors) bind to and stabilize the C3 convertase (C3bBb) that cleaves C3
Phagocytosis and intracellular lysis	Autoimmune cytopenias	Antibody binds to cell; may or may not activate C'; cell-antibody (C3b, C3d) complexes are phagocytosed by Fc receptor and/or complement receptor-bearing cells

Table 16.6 Antibody-mediated autoimmune diseases

Disease	Antigen
Autoimmune cytopenias (anemia, thrombocytopenia, neutropenia)	Erythrocyte, platelet or neutrophil cell surface determinant
Goodpasture's syndrome	Type IV collagen
Pemphigus vulgaris	Cadherin on epidermal keratinocytes
Myasthenia gravis	Acetylcholine receptor
Hyperthyroidism	Thyroid-stimulating hormone receptor (Graves' disease)
Insulin-resistant diabetes (acanthosis nigricans)	Insulin receptor
Pernicious anemia	Intrinsic factor, parietal cells

Representative human autoimmune diseases in which autoantibodies are believed to play a major pathogenic role are listed in Table 16.6. It must be noted that in some of these diseases there is also a cell-mediated immunity component. For example, in myasthenia gravis, autoreactive T lymphocytes have been described, and both autoreactive cell lines and clones have been successfully established from patients' lymphocytes.

Pathogenic role of immune complexes in autoimmune diseases

In autoimmune diseases, there is ample opportunity for the formation of IC involving autoantibodies and self-antigens. Several factors determine the pathogenicity of IC, as discussed in greater detail in Chapter 23. They include the size of the IC (intermediate-size IC are the most pathogenic), the ability of the host to clear IC (individuals with low complement levels or deficient Fc receptor and/or complement receptor function have delayed IC clearance rates and are prone to develop autoimmune diseases), and physicochemical properties of IC (which determine the ability to activate complement and/or the deposition in specific tissues). In many occasions, ICs are formed *in situ*, activate the complement system, complement split products are formed, and neutrophils are attracted to the area of IC deposition where they will mediate the IC-mediated tissue destruction. SLE and polyarteritis nodosa are two classic examples of autoimmune diseases in which ICs play a major pathogenic role. In SLE, DNA and other nuclear antigens are predominantly involved in the formation of IC, while in polyarteritis nodosa, the most frequently identified antigens are related to hepatitis B.

Role of activated T lymphocytes in pathogenesis of autoimmune diseases

Typical T cell–mediated autoimmune diseases are summarized in Table 16.7. T lymphocytes that are involved in the pathogenesis of such autoimmune diseases may be autoreactive and recognize self-antigens, recognize foreign antigen associated with self determinants (modified self), or respond to foreign antigens but still induce self tissue destruction by nonspecific mechanisms.

Cytotoxic CD8+ lymphocytes play a pathogenic role in some autoimmune diseases, usually involving the recognition of non-self peptides expressed in the context of self MHC and destroying the cell expressing such "modified" self. For example, coxsackie B virus–defined antigens expressed on the surface of myocardial cells may induce CD8+-mediated tissue destruction, causing a viral-induced autoimmune myocarditis.

Activated CD4+ helper cells, particularly those of the Th1 phenotype, appear to be more frequently involved in cell-mediated autoimmune reactions than their CD8+ counterparts. Their pathogenic effects are mediated by the release of pro-inflammatory cytokines and chemokines. Th2 cells can also be involved, promoting the activation of autoreactive B lymphocytes.

Th17 cells have been shown to contribute significantly to autoimmune pathology including the skin (e.g., psoriasis), the joint (rheumatoid and psoriatic arthritis), and the kidney (lupus nephritis).

PATHOGENIC FACTORS INVOLVED IN ONSET OF AUTOIMMUNE DISEASES

Multiple factors have been proposed as participating in the pathogenesis of autoimmune diseases. These factors can be classified as immunologic, genetic, environmental, and hormonal. Each group of factors is believed to contribute in different ways to the pathogenesis of different diseases.

Abnormal immunoregulation. Multiple lymphocyte abnormalities have been described in patients with autoimmune diseases. Prominent among them are B-lymphocyte overactivity, the presence of spontaneously activated T and B lymphocytes, and decreased T regulatory cell function. These abnormalities are typified in SLE and are discussed in Chapter 18.

Genetic factors. Clinical observations have documented increased frequency of autoimmune diseases in families, and increased rates of clinical concordance in monozygotic twins. The basis for these associations seems to be complex, involving multiple sets of genes, only some of which have been identified. The same seems to be true in experimental animals. The study of congenic mice has shed some light onto how different loci contribute, through positive and negative epistatic interactions, to loss of tolerance to autoantigens and the progressive establishment of a lupus-like disease. The number of genes involved in human lupus must be significantly higher. A similarly high number of loci have been proposed for diabetes, inflammatory bowel disease, and arthritis in humans and laboratory animals.

Single genetic traits have been shown to lead to autoimmunity in mice and humans through distinct pathophysiologic processes. Following is a partial list that expands continuously as whole DNA sequencing becomes more available to clinical investigators:

Table 16.7 Examples of T cell–mediated autoimmune diseases

Disease	Specificity of T-cell clone/line[a]	T cell involved
Experimental allergic encephalomyelitis	Myelin basic protein	CD4+
Autoimmune thyroiditis	Thyroid follicular epithelial cells	?
Insulin-dependent diabetes mellitus	Pancreatic islet β cells	CD8+ (CD4+)
Viral myocarditis	Coxsackie B virus	CD8+

[a] Derived from cells isolated from tissue lesions or peripheral blood of patients and animals affected by the experimental disease. Some of these T-cell lines have been used for adoptive transfer of the disease. In experimental animals, treatment with anti–T cell antibodies may improve the clinical manifestations of the disease.

- Lack of AIRE (autoimmune regulator) leads to autoimmune polyendocrinopathy syndrome because peripheral autoantigens are not expressed in the thymus to execute negative selection of T cells.
- Lack of Fas and Fas ligand leads to autoimmune lymphoproliferative syndrome because T and B cells are not eliminated through apoptosis.
- Lack of C4 and C1q leads to lupus-like syndromes because of defective clearance of immune complexes.
- Lack of FOXP3 causes IPEX because of failure to generate T regulatory cells.
- CTLA-4 mutations associate with Graves' disease, type 1 diabetes, and SLE because of failure in T-cell anergy and reduced activation threshold of self-reactive T cells.

MHC markers. Several studies have also documented associations between HLA antigens and various diseases.

The classic example of linkage with MHC-I markers is the association between HLA-B27 and inflammatory spondyloarthropathies (ankylosing spondylitis, reactive arthritis, etc.). The pathogenic relevance of HLA-B27 is strongly supported by experiments with transgenic mice carrying the gene for HLA-B27. Those transgenic animals spontaneously develop inflammatory disease involving the gastrointestinal tract, peripheral and vertebral joints, skin, nails, and heart. It has been postulated that the autoimmune reaction is triggered by an infectious peptide presented by HLA-B27 and followed by cross-reactive lymphocyte activation by an endogenous collagen-derived peptide, equally associated with HLA-B27.

The linkage of autoimmunity with MHC-II markers is better understood. With the expanded definition of MHC-II alleles due to the development of antisera and DNA probes and because of the successful sequencing of the genes coding for the constitutive polypeptide chains of MHC-II molecules, the significance of MHC-II alelles has become clear. For example, insulin-dependent diabetes mellitus (IDDM) is strongly associated with serologically defined MHC-II markers (HLA-DR3 and HLA-DR4) but is even more strongly correlated with the presence of uncharged amino acids at position 57 of the β chain of DQ (DQβ).

Molecular mimicry, i.e., cross-reactivity between peptides derived from infectious agents and peptides derived from autologous proteins that are expressed by most normal resting cells in the organism. Anergic autoreactive T-cell clones would be activated by an immune response against an infectious agent due to this type of cross-reactivity.

Lack of expression of major histocompatibility complex alleles able to bind critical endogenous peptides

This possibility has been documented in animal models of type 1 diabetes and multiple sclerosis. The MHC molecules associated with autoimmunity either are expressed in very low levels in differentiating cells and resting cells of adult animals, or are associated with unstable peptides that are easily degraded and not efficiently presented. Under those circumstances, potentially autoreactive T-lymphocyte clones would not be eliminated and would remain available for later activation due to an unrelated immune response or the presentation of a cross-reactive peptide.

T-cell receptor variable region types

The TCR repertoire of a given individual seems to be another important determinant of autoimmunity. Several autoimmune diseases show associations with specific TCR variable region types. This is not surprising because the specific recognition of different oligopeptides by different T lymphocytes depends on the diversity of the TCR. Therefore, the development of an autoimmune response should require that the genome of an individual includes genes encoding a particular array of V-region genes whose transcription resulted in the expression of TCR able to combine with a specific autologous peptide. In addition, the clones expressing such receptors must not be deleted during embryonic differentiation.

These postulates are supported by immunogenetic studies in different animals and humans with different manifestations of autoimmunity. Those studies suggest that linkages between specific TCR V-region genes and specific autoimmune diseases may actually exist (for example, insulin-dependent diabetes mellitus, multiple sclerosis, and SLE). Even in identical twins, however, concordance for a particular autoimmune disease never exceeds 40%, suggesting that the presence of autoimmunity-associated TCR V-region genes is not sufficient to cause disease by itself. Indeed, with certain exceptions, human autoimmune diseases are multigenic, and the number of the involved genes has not been determined.

ENVIRONMENTAL FACTORS

Molecular mimicry

The most important environmental factors are believed to be foreign antigens sharing structural similarity with self determinants. Exposure to these epitopes can trigger autoimmune reactions. The term *molecular mimicry* is used to describe identity or similarity of either amino acid sequences or structural epitopes between foreign and self-antigens.

One of the best-known examples of autoimmunity resulting from the exposure to cross-reactive antigens is the cardiomyopathy that complicates many cases of acute rheumatic fever. Group A β-hemolytic streptococci have several epitopes cross-reactive with tissue antigens. One of them cross-reacts with an antigen found in cardiac myosin. The normal immune response to such a cross-reactive strain of *Streptococcus* will generate lymphocyte clones that will react with myosin and induce myocardial damage long after the infection has been eliminated.

Several other examples of molecular mimicry have been described, as summarized in Table 16.8, and additional ones await better definition. For example, molecular mimicry between the envelope glycolipids of Gram-negative bacteria and the myelin of the peripheral nerves may explain the association of Guillain-Barré syndrome with *Campylobacter jejuni* infections. Mimicry between LFA-1 and the *Borrelia burgdorferi* outer surface protein A is considered responsible for the rheumatic manifestations of Lyme disease. Mimicry between glutamate decarboxylase, an enzyme concentrated in pancreatic β cells, and coxsackievirus P2-C, an enzyme involved in the replication of coxsackievirus B, has been considered responsible for the development of insulin-dependent diabetes in humans and in murine models of this disease.

Infectious agents, particularly viruses, can precipitate autoimmunity by inducing the release of sequestered antigens. In autoimmune myocarditis associated with coxsackie B3 virus, the apparent role of the virus is to cause the release of normally sequestered intracellular antigens as a consequence of virus-induced myocardial cell necrosis. Autoantibodies and T lymphocytes reactive with sarcolemma and myofibril antigens or peptides derived from these antigens emerge, and the auto-reactive T lymphocytes are believed to be responsible for the development of persistent myocarditis.

Table 16.8 Human proteins with structural homology to human pathogens

Disease	Human protein	Pathogen
Ankylosing spondylitis, Reiter's syndrome	HLA-B27	*Klebsiella pneumoniae*
Rheumatoid arthritis	HLA-DR4	Epstein–Barr virus
IDDM	Insulin receptor	Papillomavirus
	HLA-DR	Cytomegalovirus
	Glutamate decarboxylase	Coxsackievirus P2-C enzyme
Myasthenia gravis	Acetylcholine receptor	Poliovirus
Ro-associated clinical syndromes	Ro/SSA antigen	Vesicular stomatitis virus
Rheumatic heart disease	Cardiac myosin	Group A streptococci
Celiac disease	A-gliadin or wheat gluten	Adenovirus type 12
Acute proliferative glomerulonephritis	Vimentin	*Streptococcus pyogenes* type 1
Lyme disease (rheumatic manifestations)	LFA-1	*Borrelia burgdorferi* outer surface protein-A

Latent viral infections are believed to be responsible for the development of many autoimmune disorders. Latent infection is commonly associated with integration of the viral genome into the host chromosomes. While integrated viruses very seldom enter a full replicative cycle and do not cause cytotoxicity, they can interfere, directly or indirectly, with several functions of the infected cells. T-cell activation secondary to an inapparent viral infection has the potential to induce autoimmunity secondary to the release of interferon-γ and TNF, both known to be potent inducers of MHC-II antigen expression. The increased expression of class-II MHC antigens would then create optimal conditions for the onset of an autoimmune response directed against MHC-II–self peptide complexes. Such a mechanism has been proposed to explain the onset of autoimmune thyroiditis. An unknown nonlytic virus would cause T-lymphocyte activation in the thyroid gland, followed by increased expression of MHC-II and thyroid-derived peptides, and finally, an antithyroid immune reaction would develop.

Finally, physical trauma can also lead to immune responses to sequestered antigens. The classic example is sympathetic ophthalmia, an inflammatory process of apparent autoimmune etiology affecting the normal eye after a penetrating injury of the other. This process may not be limited to trauma; tissue injury induced by any cause may result in the generation of autoreactive T cells that recognize previously cryptic epitopes. Over time, this process will lead to expansion of the immune response by facilitating the onset of immune responses to additional epitopes. This process is known as *epitope spreading*.

Unresolved issues in molecular mimicry

There are still difficulties in proving that infections are the cause of autoimmune diseases. The infection may have resolved long before the appearance of disease or the infection may be inapparent, thus obscuring the temporal association between infection and autoimmunity. Alternatively, molecular mimicry may be the result rather than the cause of autoimmunity. The infectious process may result in the alteration of nonimmunogenic antigenic determinants as a consequence of tissue injury. The autoantibodies that appear when the disease is diagnosed may then result from tissue injury rather than be the cause of it.

The increased frequency of autoimmune diseases in countries where infections have either been eradicated or are being effectively treated has advanced the argument that infections may also suppress autoimmunity. This is known as the "sterile" hypothesis of autoimmunity, and there is experimental, besides epidemiologic, evidence to support it.

ANIMAL MODELS OF AUTOIMMUNITY

Our understanding of autoimmune disease has been facilitated by studies in animal models. Several animal models have been developed, each sharing some characteristics of a human disease of autoimmune etiology. These animal models often provide the only experimental approaches to the study of the pathogenesis of autoimmune diseases.

In some experimental models, injecting normal animals with antigens extracted from the human target tissues induces autoimmune diseases. A rapid onset and an acute course characterize the resulting diseases. These models have been particularly useful in the study of autoimmune thyroiditis and arthritis (collagen-induced arthritis). Most useful for the study of autoimmunity are animals that spontaneously develop autoimmune disease of protracted course, which parallels closely the disease as seen in humans. Representative animal models of different autoimmune diseases are listed in Table 16.9.

Experimental allergic encephalomyelitis (EAE) in mice and rats is the best-characterized experimental model of multiple sclerosis. Immunizing animals with myelin basic protein and adjuvant induces the disease. One to two weeks later, the animals develop encephalomyelitis characterized by perivascular mononuclear cell infiltrates and demyelination. The mononuclear cell infiltrates show a predominance of CD4$^+$ T lymphocytes, which upon activation release cytokines that attract phagocytic cells to the area of immunological reaction; those cells are, in turn, activated and release enzymes that are responsible for the demyelination. CD4$^+$ T lymphocyte clones from animals with EAE disease can transfer the disease to normal animals of the same strain. Genetic manipulations leading to deletion of the genes coding for two specific variable regions of the TCR β chain (Vβ8 and Vβ13) prevent the expression of disease. These two Vβ regions must obviously be involved in the recognition of a dominant epitope of human myelin.

Table 16.9 Representative autoimmune disease models and their human analogs

	Animal model	Human disease analog
A. Antigen induced		
Myelin basic protein	Experimental allergic encephalomyelitis	Multiple sclerosis
Collagen type II	Collagen-induced arthritis	Rheumatoid arthritis
B. Induced by injecting mycobacterial extract	Adjuvant arthritis	Rheumatoid arthritis
C. Chemically induced		
$HgCl_2$	Nephritis in rats	Nephritis
D. Spontaneous models		
NZB, (NZB × NZW)F$_1$ MRL lpr/lpr BXSB murine strains	Murine lupus	Systemic lupus erythematosus
Nonobese diabetic mice and rats Inbred BB rats	Diabetes	Type 1 (autoimmune) diabetes
E. Transgenic animals		
HLA-B27 transgenic rats	Spondyloarthropathy	Inflammatory spondyloarthropathies

Diabetes develops spontaneously in inbred BB rats, as well as in nonobese diabetic (NOD) mice. In both strains the onset of the disease is characterized by T cell–mediated insulitis, which evolves into diabetes. This disease demonstrates H-2 linkage remarkably similar to that observed between human insulin-dependent diabetes mellitus and HLA-DR3, DR4, and other MHC-II alleles. In NOD mice, a decreased expression of MHC-I genes, secondary to a TAP-1 gene deficiency, has also been characterized. Such deficiency would prevent these animals from deleting autoreactive cytotoxic T-cell clones during lymphocyte differentiation.

A number of murine strains spontaneously develop autoimmune disease that resembles human **systemic lupus erythematosus** (SLE):

- (NZB X NZW)F$_1$ female mice develop glomerulonephritis, hemolytic anemia, and anti-DNA antibodies. Numerous alterations in T- and B-lymphocyte function, cytokine release, and macrophage functions have been described in these animals. It has also been demonstrated that this and other SLE and autoimmune-prone mouse strains, such as MRL/lpr, BXSB, and NOD, express reduced levels of the inhibitory FcγRIIB receptor on activated B cells. The low expression of this receptor removes an important downregulating control for autoantibody-producing cells.
- MRL-lpr/lpr mice that lack Fas antigen and *gld* mice that lack Fas ligand produce autoantibodies and develop arthritis and kidney disease, but they also develop massive lymphadenopathy, which is not seen in human disease.
- BXSB mice develop anti-DNA antibodies, nephritis, and vasculitis. In this strain, in contrast to the others, disease susceptibility is linked to the Y chromosome and is caused by a duplication of the TLR7 locus.

IMMUNOMODULATION IN TREATMENT OF AUTOIMMUNE DISEASES

Standard therapeutic approaches to autoimmune disease usually involve symptomatic palliation with anti-inflammatory drugs and attempts to downregulate the immune response. Glucocorticoids, which have both anti-inflammatory and immunosuppressive effects, have been widely used, as well as immunosuppressive and cytotoxic drugs. However, the use of these drugs is often associated with severe side effects and is not always efficient. Other therapeutic approaches that have been tried have had as their objective to downregulate the autoimmune response by disrupting costimulation (Table 16.10) and, if possible, to induce tolerance.

Induction of tolerance to the responsible antigen is the most logical approach to the treatment of autoimmune disorders. This approach is hampered by the fact that the identity of the antigen is not known with certainty in many diseases and because of the individual variations to tolerization that will

Table 16.10 Summary of interventions aimed at disrupting costimulation of T cells in animal models of autoimmune diseases

Model	Anti-CD80 Ab	Anti-CD86 Ab	CTLA4-Ig
SLE-like disease in (NZBXNZW) F1 mice			Benefit
Insulin-dependent diabetes in NOD mice	Worsening	Prevention	
Experimental allergic encephalomyelitis	Benefit (↑Th2)	Worsening	

be encountered in humans, due to their high degree of genetic diversity. The need for well-defined tolerogens may not be an insurmountable obstacle due to the phenomenon recently described as "bystander tolerance." For example, when a cross-reactive antigen is used to induce oral tolerance, immunoregulatory cells secreting IL-10 and TGF-β differentiate in the submucosa and migrate to lymphoid organs and inflamed sites, where they suppress the activity of pro-inflammatory Th1 cells. The effects of regulatory cells are not antigen specific, so they may extend to autoreactive T cells interacting with a peptide different from those generated by the orally administered tolerogen. Examples of the beneficial effects of oral tolerization have been described, both in animal models and humans. In experimental animals, oral administration of basic myelin protein has been shown to decrease the severity of experimental allergic encephalitis. In patients with rheumatoid arthritis, oral administration of collagen type II was followed by clinical improvement.

B-cell tolerization has been tried in patients with SLE. A reportedly successful protocol involved administration of a construct of four short DNA fragments conjugated to a dextran backbone that caused cessation of DNA antibody synthesis. Apparently, the construct bound to B-cell surface immunoglobulins in DNA-specific B cells and caused its internalization. The reason why this causes the interruption of antibody synthesis has not been clarified.

BIBLIOGRAPHY

Barturen G, Beretta L, Cervera R et al. Moving towards a molecular taxonomy of autoimmune rheumatic diseases. *Nat Rev Rheumatol.* 2018;14:75–93.

Christen U, von Herrath MG. Infections and autoimmunity—Good or bad? *J Immunol.* 2005;174:7481–7486.

Goodnow CC. Multistep pathogenesis of autoimmune disease. *Cell* 2007;130:25–35.

Goodnow CC, Sprent J, Fazekas de St Groth B et al. Cellular and genetic mechanisms of self-tolerance and autoimmunity. *Nature* 2005;435:590–597.

Malhotra N, Leyva-Castillo JM, Jadhav U et al. RORα-expressing T regulatory cells restrain allergic skin inflammation. *Sci Immunol.* 2018;3(21). doi: 10.1126/sciimmunol.aao6923

Moulton VR, Suarez-Fueyo A, Meidan E et al. Pathogenesis of human systemic lupus erythematosus: A cellular perspective. *Trends Mol Med.* 2017;23:615–635.

Ohkura N, Kitagawa Y, Sakaguchi S. Development and maintenance of regulatory T cells. *Immunity.* 2013;38:414–423.

Paterson AM, Sharpe AH. Taming tissue-specific T cells: CTLA-4 reins in self-reactive T cells. *Nat Immunol.* 2010;11:109–111.

Rezende RM, Weiner HL. History and mechanisms of oral tolerance. *Semin Immunol.* 2017;30:3–11.

Rioux JD, Abbas AK. Paths to understanding the genetic basis of autoimmune disease. *Nature* 2005;435:584–589.

Sakaguchi S, Vignali DA, Rudensky AY et al. The plasticity and stability of regulatory T cells. *Nat Rev Immunol.* 2013;13:461–467.

Schildberg FA, Klein SR, Freeman GJ et al. Coinhibitory pathways in the B7-CD28 ligand-receptor family. *Immunity.* 2016;44:955–972.

Theofilopoulos AN, Kono DH, Baccala R. The multiple pathways to autoimmunity. *Nat Immunol.* 2017;1:716–724.

Tsokos GC, Fleming SD. Autoimmunity, complement activation, tissue injury and back. *Curr Dir Autoimmun.* 2004;7:149–164.

Ueda H, Howson JM, Esposito L et al. Association of the T-cell regulatory gene CTLA4 with susceptibility to autoimmune disease. *Nature.* 2003;423:506–511.

Weiner HL, da Cunha AP, Quintana F et al. Oral tolerance. *Immunol Rev.* 2011;241:241–259.

17

Organ-specific autoimmune diseases

GABRIEL VIRELLA AND GEORGE C. TSOKOS

INTRODUCTION

Autoimmune diseases can be roughly divided into organ-specific and systemic diseases, based both on the extent of their involvement and the type of autoantibodies present in the patients. The systemic forms of autoimmune diseases, best exemplified by systemic lupus erythematosus (SLE) and rheumatoid arthritis, are discussed in Chapters 18 and 19. Less-generalized autoimmune processes may affect virtually every organ system (Table 17.1); in many instances, only certain cell types within an organ system will be affected in a particular disease, i.e., gastric parietal cells in pernicious anemia. In this chapter, we restrict our discussion to the major autoimmune diseases that affect specific organs and the associated autoantibodies with the understanding that in many cases these antibodies are not the cause of the disease, but just a secondary manifestation. Our understanding of the pathogenesis of most organ-specific autoimmune disorders is schematically illustrated in Figure 17.1. The key cells are autoreactive T cells, which under the wrong circumstances become activated. The activated T cells can be controlled by T-regulatory cells (Tregs). If they manage to overcome the downregulating effects of the Tregs, the activated T cells are able to cause the death of cells expressing the autoantigens that triggered the reaction both directly and through activated macrophages.

AUTOIMMUNE DISEASES OF THE THYROID GLAND

Autoimmune factors have been implicated in two major thyroid diseases, Graves' disease and Hashimoto's disease.

Autoantibodies

THYROID-STIMULATING HORMONE RECEPTOR ANTIBODIES

Graves' disease, also known as thyrotoxicosis, diffuse toxic goiter, and exophthalmic goiter, is the result of the production of antibodies against the thyroid-stimulating hormone receptor (TSHR), usually of the IgG1 isotype. Three functional types of TSHR antibodies can be detected in patients with Graves' disease. In 80%–90% of the patients with Graves' disease, the antibodies

Table 17.1 Representative examples of organ-specific and systemic autoimmune diseases

Disease	Target tissue	Antibodies mainly against
Organ-specific diseases		
Graves' disease	Thyroid	TSH receptor
Hashimoto's thyroiditis	Thyroid	Thyroglobulin
Myasthenia gravis	Muscle	Acetylcholine receptors
Pernicious anemia	Gastric parietal cells	Gastric parietal cells intrinsic factor (IF) B12-IF complex
Addison's disease	Adrenals	Adrenal cells microsomal antigen
Insulin-dependent diabetes mellitus	Pancreas	Pancreatic islet cells, insulin
Primary biliary cirrhosis	Liver	Mitochondrial antigens
Autoimmune chronic active hepatitis	Liver	Nuclear antigens, smooth muscle, liver-kidney, microsomal antigen, soluble liver antigen, etc.
Autoimmune hemolytic anemia	RBCs	RBCs
Idiopathic thrombocytopenic purpura	Platelets	Platelets
Systemic diseases		
Systemic lupus erythematosus	Kidney, skin, lung, brain	Nuclear antigens, microsomes, IgG, etc.
Rheumatoid arthritis	Joints	IgG, nuclear antigens
Sjögren's syndrome	Salivary and lachrymal glands	Nucleolar mitochondria
Goodpasture's syndrome	Lungs, kidneys	Basement membranes

stimulate the production of thyroid hormones by activating the adenylate cyclase system after binding to the TSH receptor the activity of the thyroid gland. For that reason they have been known by a variety of descriptive terms, including long-acting thyroid stimulator (LATS). A second type of TSHR antibodies induces apoptosis of the cells expressing it, contributing to the development of thyroid inflammation. Finally, a third type of TSHR antibodies blocks the receptor and does not stimulate the production of thyroid hormones. These antibodies are detected in about 4% of patients with Graves' disease, and when their activity predominates (in about 50% of the cases in which they are detected), cause hypothyroidism, while the remaining patients may be euthyroid or hyperthyroid depending on the ratio of blocking versus stimulating antibodies. These blocking antibodies can also be detected in about 10% of patients with Hashimoto's thyroiditis.

Thyroid peroxidase (TPO) antibodies are present in more than 80% of patients with Graves' disease and Hashimoto's thyroiditis. TPO is a membrane-bound enzyme responsible for iodine oxidation and iodination of tyrosyl residues of thyroglobulin. They can be of any class, but most of them are either IgG1 or IgG4. Their contribution to disease pathology is unclear.

Thyroglobulin antibodies do not appear to contribute to disease expression and reflect massive thyroid cell destruction. They are present in more than 50% of patients with Graves' disease and Hashimoto's thyroiditis. They are polyclonal and usually of the IgG1 and IgG4 classes. TPO and thyroglobulin antibodies are present in about 15% of normal subjects.

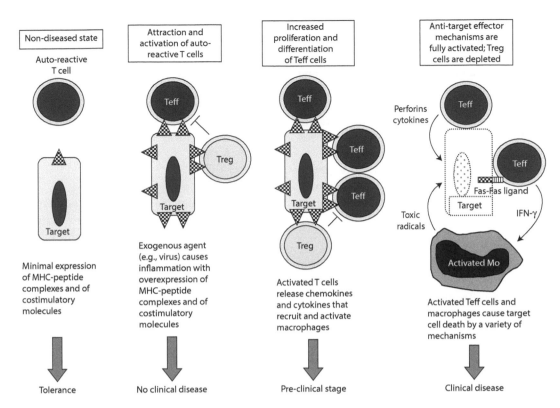

Figure 17.1 **Pathogenesis of organ-specific autoimmunity.** In normal, tolerant conditions, autoreactive clones remain inactive because the cells expressing the corresponding autoantigens express them in low density and do not provide costimulatory signals. A combination of genetic and environmental factors, such as a viral infection leading to inflammatory changes and activation of accessory cells, might lead to the breaking of self-tolerance and activation of autoreactive T cells designated in the figure as T effector cells (Teff). Further inflammation might attract more such cells, for example, if a virus persists or autoantigens are being presented in a chronic manner. The ultimate outcome is determined by the magnitude of the autoreactive response. Many aggressive T cells, such as CTL and Th1 lymphocytes will enhance progression, whereas the presence of (autoreactive) Tregs will dampen inflammation. Penetrance of clinical disease is directly correlated with the amount of target cell (organ) destruction and is determined by this balance of Tregs to pro-inflammatory (Th1) and cytotoxic T cells. The cytotoxic effects on target cells can be directly mediated by activated T-effector cells or by activated macrophages. (Modified from a figure contributed by Dr. Matthias von Herrath, La Jolla, CA.)

Pathogenesis

THYROID INFLAMMATION

Biopsy of the thyroid gland shows diffuse lymphoplasmacytic interstitial infiltration. Several factors may contribute to chronic inflammation of the thyroid gland. High intake of **iodine** increases the antigenicity of thyroglobulin because it exposes neoantigens and activates TPO. Oxidative stress may cause increased expression of ICAM1 on the surface of thyrocytes and the expression of death receptor (DR) 5 on thyroid cells, enhanced dendritic cell maturation, and increased accumulation of T and B cells able to produce autoantibody. Both Th1 and Th17 cells have been found in the thyroid tissues of patients with autoimmune thyroid disease, whereas the function of Tregs appears to be deficient. Autoreactive CD4 cells recruit cytotoxic CD8 cells that destroy thyrocytes by release of granzyme and perforin. Other cytokines including IFNγ, IL-2, and GM-CSF are also involved in the pathogenesis of the inflammatory reaction. This chronic inflammation is likely to contribute to the perpetuation of the disease both by activating antibody-producing cells and by depleting TSHR$^+$ cells.

Genetic factors contribute significantly to the expression of the disease. HLA class-II antigens have been linked to autoimmune thyroid disease. HLADR3 has been linked to Graves' disease and several other genetic markers (including CD3, DQ7) have been linked to Hashimoto's disease. Polymorphisms of the CTLA4, PTN22, vitamin D receptor, IL-4, and TNF genes have also been linked to autoimmune thyroid disease.

Autoimmune thyroid disease is more **prevalent in women**, and the role of both hormones and skewed X-chromosome inactivation has been studied.

INFECTIONS AND MICROBIOME

Several viruses, including hepatitis C virus, Epstein–Barr virus, herpes simplex virus, HTLV1, and others, as well as the gut microbiota have been proposed to be involved in the pathogenesis of thyroid disease.

Graves' disease

Graves' disease has its peak incidence in the third to fourth decade and has a female-to-male ratio of 4–8:1. Patients usually present with diffuse goiter, and 60%–70% of patients have ocular disturbances. Symptoms of hyperthyroidism include increased metabolic rate with weight loss, nervousness, weakness, sweating, heat intolerance, and loose stools. Abnormalities on physical examination include diffuse and nontender enlargement of the thyroid, tachycardia, warm and moist skin, tremor, exophthalmos, and pretibial edema.

GRAVES' OPHTHALMOPATHY

One of the clinical hallmarks of Graves' disease is exophthalmos (protrusion of the eyeball). Exophthalmos can be unilateral or bilateral and may be associated with proptosis, conjunctivitis, and/or periorbital edema. Exophthalmos is secondary to retro-orbital accumulation of fibroblasts, adipocytes, and muscle cells, all of which exhibit TSH receptor antigen to which TSI binds and alters their function.

Diagnosis

The diagnosis is usually investigated on patients with hyperthyroidism found to have increased levels of thyroid hormones (triiodothyronine, T3, and thyroxin, T4) and increased uptake of T3.

The diagnosis is confirmed by demonstration of antithyroid receptor antibodies that can be done with two types of assays. Some assays are based on the inhibition of TSH binding by TSI antibodies (TSH-binding inhibition assay), while others are based on the functional consequences of thyroid receptor antibody binding to TSH such as increased adenylate cyclase activity and increased levels of cAMP.

Therapy

The therapy is directed at reducing the thyroid's ability to respond to stimulation by antibodies. This can be achieved surgically, by subtotal thyroidectomy, or pharmacologically, either by administration of radioactive iodine (^{131}I) (which is difficult to dose) or by the use of antithyroid drugs such as propylthiouracil and methimazole, which are useful but slow in their effects.

Hashimoto's thyroiditis

Hashimoto's thyroiditis is the most common form of thyroiditis, and it usually has a chronic evolution. Its incidence peaks during the third to fifth decades, with a female-to-male ratio of 10:1. It is characterized by a slow progression to hypothyroidism, and symptoms develop insidiously.

Hashimoto's thyroiditis is pathologically characterized by severe lymphocytic infiltration of the thyroid parenchyma associated with destruction of the thyroid follicles and hypothyroidism. The inflammatory infiltrate of the thyroid gland shows predominance of activated, lymphokine-secreting T lymphocytes. Numerous plasma cells can also be seen.

Autoantibodies against thyroglobulin are detected in 60%–75% of patients with Hashimoto's thyroiditis, but whether they play a pathogenic role is unclear. Of note is the fact that increased ingestion of iodine is associated both with enhanced production of thyroglobulin antibodies and development of Hashimoto's thyroiditis. T lymphocytes reacting with thyroglobulin can be detected in the peripheral blood of normal controls and in patients with Hashimoto's thyroiditis, but the patients have greater numbers of these lymphocytes that also show an enhanced response to thyroglobulin.

In the early stages, glucocorticoids may be used as mild immunosuppressants, with the aim of reducing the autoimmune response and extending the asymptomatic phase. When patients develop hypothyroidism, thyroid hormone replacement is indicated.

ADDISON'S DISEASE (CHRONIC PRIMARY HYPOADRENALISM)

Addison's disease can either be caused by exogenous agents (e.g., infection of the adrenals by *Mycobacterium tuberculosis*) or be idiopathic. The idiopathic form is believed to have an autoimmune basis, since 50% of patients have been found to have antibodies to the microsomes of adrenal cells (as compared to 5% in the general population) by immunofluorescence. The autoantibodies directed against the adrenal react mainly in the zona glomerulosa, zona fasciculata, and zona reticularis and are believed to play the main pathogenic role in this disease, causing atrophy and loss of function of the adrenal cortex. Biopsy of the adrenal glands shows marked cortical atrophy with an unaltered medulla. Abundant inflammatory mononuclear cells are seen between the residual islands of epithelial cells.

The diagnosis is confirmed by demonstration of anti-adrenal antibodies by indirect immunofluorescence in the presence of clinical and laboratory hypoadrenalism.

AUTOIMMUNE POLYGLANDULAR SYNDROMES

Autoimmune polyglandular syndrome I (APS-I) is a rare childhood disease with Mendelian recessive inheritance mode. The three major components are chronic mucocutaneous candidiasis, hypoparathyroidism, and autoimmune Addison's disease. Other endocrine glands may be involved. The entity is also known as autoimmune polyendocrinopathy-candidiasis-ectodermal dystrophy (APECED). The molecular basis for this entity has been established. These patients lack autoimmune regulator (AIRE), a transcriptional regulator that is believed to control the expression of tissue-specific genes in the thymus. Therefore, autoreactive T cells do not see self-antigens in the thymus, and they are not deleted during the negative selection process in the thymus. The second variant of APS, APS-II, is more common than APS-I and afflicts young adults. Main features include diabetes and Addison's disease. Some patients may have vitiligo, pernicious anemia,

celiac disease, and other autoimmune diseases. It is proper, therefore, that patients presenting with diabetes or Addison's disease be screened for other autoimmune diseases.

AUTOIMMUNE DIABETES MELLITUS

The critical defect of type 1A diabetes mellitus (DM) is a decreased-to-absent production of insulin secondary to β-cell destruction. In type 1B DM, considerably less frequent than type 1A DM, the patients (usually of African, Hispanic, or Asian origin) have permanent insulin deficiency and suffer from episodic ketoacidosis, but lack immunological evidence for β-cell autoimmunity.

Pathogenesis

The original body of evidence on which the concept that the majority of cases of type 1 diabetes are the consequence of an autoimmune disease was based is the detection of many different types of autoantibodies in patients with this disease. These antibodies, however, do not seem to play a major pathogenic role, at least as initial pathogenic insults, but they seem to reflect the intensity of the underlying autoimmune reaction against the islet cell β cells. The autoantibodies can be detected before diabetes becomes clinically evident, and the number of different autoantibodies that are detected seems to be inversely correlated with the length of the disease-free interval in positive individuals.

Autoantibodies. The following are the major types of autoantibodies detected in patients with type 1 diabetes:

- **Anti-islet cell antibodies (ICA)** are classically detected by indirect immunofluorescence and react against membrane and cytoplasmic antigens of the islet cells. These antibodies are detected in as many as 90% of type 1 diabetic patients at the time of diagnosis, but they diminish in frequency to 5%–10% in patients with long-standing DM. Other interesting characteristics of ICA are their isotype distribution, with predominance of subclasses IgG2 and/or IgG4 (which have limited complement-activating properties), and their detection months or years before the appearance of clinical symptoms.
- **Antibodies to β-cell antigens**. The best characterized islet cell antigens against which

antibodies have been demonstrated in type 1 diabetics and individuals predisposed to develop the disease are **IA-2α** and **IA-2β** (**phogrin**), two closely related β cell–associated tyrosine phosphatases. About two-thirds of patients have antibodies to **IA-2α** and about 60% of patients have antibodies to **IA-2β**. Epitope mapping studies suggest that the immunogenic epitopes are located in the intracytoplasmic segment of these enzymes. Antibodies to glutamic acid decarboxylase (**GAD**) are also present in a large proportion of newly diagnosed diabetics (84%).

- **Insulin autoantibodies** are responsible for a rare form of diabetes known as insulin autoimmune syndrome (IAS), characterized by the combination of fasting hypoglycemia, high concentration of total serum immunoreactive insulin, and presence of autoantibodies to native human insulin in serum. The combination of insulin autoantibodies with insulin alters the pharmacokinetics and bioavailability of insulin, causing dissociation between the activity of insulin and blood glucose levels. This disease has been reported in Japan and has no relation with the common form of type 1 diabetes, characterized by permanent insulin deficiency.

Insulin autoantibodies are detected in as many as 92% of non-insulin-treated patients with type 1 diabetes at the time of diagnosis, but their pathogenic significance is not clear.

Induced anti-insulin antibodies can be found in all diabetic patients treated with insulin. The incidence of these antibodies was greater when bovine or porcine insulin was used. However, human anti-insulin antibodies can also be detected (less frequently) in patients treated with recombinant human insulin, whose tertiary configuration differs from that of the insulin released by the human pancreas. The antibodies directed against therapeutically administered insulin appear to be predominantly of the IgG2 and IgG4 isotypes and may cause insulin resistance, similar to what is observed in the IAS, but in a much milder form.

Cell-mediated immunity is believed to be the main pathogenic factor causing islet cell damage. The predominant cells in the islet cell infiltrates are T lymphocytes, including both activated CD4+ and CD8+ T lymphocytes. Activated macrophages are also present in the infiltrates. The major pathogenic role seems to be played by CD4+ T cells, with a Th0-Th1 cytokine-secreting pattern. Those cells secrete large amounts of IL-2 and interferon-γ (IFNγ).

The significance of increased IL-2 secretion may lie in the fact that it causes the upregulation of MHC-II in islet β cells, thus creating favorable conditions for the induction of autoreactive cells. In experimental animal models, this change precedes the development of insulitis. IFN-γ, in contrast, activates macrophages, causing the release of cytokines, such as IL-1 and IL-12, and toxic radicals. IL-1 has been shown to lead to β-cell damage by indirect mechanisms. IL-12 may promote the differentiation and activation of additional Th1 cells as well as the activation of cytotoxic T cells and NK cells. Toxic radicals, such as superoxide and nitric oxide, are known to damage islet cells *in vitro*. Recently it has been shown that IFN-γ can also activate the synthesis of oxygen-active radicals and nitric oxide in β cells. These compounds can react with each other forming peroxinitrate, which is highly toxic. Activated CD8+ cells may also be involved in monocyte activation through the secretion of IFNγ. The main question that remains unanswered is the nature of the epitopes that are recognized by these cells and trigger their activation.

Of crucial importance to our understanding of the pathogenesis of DM is the definition of the insult(s) that may activate autoreactive T lymphocytes and trigger the disease. It is generally accepted that an environmental insult, most likely a viral infection (rubella virus and coxsackievirus B4 have been repeatedly suggested as culprits), plays the initiating role, causing β-cell cytotoxicity. Experimental data suggest several possible pathways for the pathogenic effects of viral infections. Infected cells in the pancreas can present viral-derived peptides to the CD8+ cytotoxic T lymphocytes and in this way initiate the autoimmune response. However, experimental studies suggest that this is a rather ineffective pathway, and evidence suggesting the need for activation of accessory cells has been accumulating. One mechanism proposed for such activation would involve the interaction of viral particles with toll-like receptors, particularly TLR-3. Mononuclear cells activated in this way release interferon-α that can facilitate β-cell destruction either directly or indirectly, upregulating the expression of MHC-I in β cells, thus rendering them more susceptible to T cell–mediated cytotoxicity. Another possible mechanism of activation of accessory cells is the engulfment of dead cells, killed as a consequence of viral replication.

There is suggestive evidence supporting the pathogenic role of viral infections in some patient populations. For example, 12%–15% of patients with congenital rubella develop type I diabetes, particularly when they are DR3 or DR4 positive. But for the majority of diabetic patients, a link with any given viral infection remains elusive.

The nature of the epitopes recognized by autoreactive T cells is still being investigated, but published data suggest that proinsulin, insulin, GAD, and IA-2α and β are the source of peptides recognized by autoreactive T cells. The overall evidence suggests that the T-cell autoimmune response is polyclonal.

Using tetramer technology, autoreactive Th1 lymphocytes recognizing proinsulin and GAD-derived peptides have been found in the circulation of at-risk patients, who are also positive for ICA and insulin antibodies. Whether the identification of self-reactive T cells in this patient population has greater prognostic significance is not known.

Genetic factors

Type 1 DM is a polygenic disease. Eighteen to twenty different chromosomal regions possibly influencing the development of this form of diabetes have been identified. Of those, two have been better characterized.

1. The **IDDM1 region**, which includes the MHC genes determining resistance/susceptibly to diabetes, is considered to be the major genetic determinant of predisposition for the development of diabetes. Several DP and DQ alleles are associated with predisposition or resistance to diabetes (Table 17.2).
   - Ninety-five percent of diabetics express DR3 (HLA-DRB1*03) and/or DR4 (HLA-DRB1*04), compared to 42%–54% of nondiabetics. This corresponds to a relative disease risk of 2 to 5. It has been proposed that this association is due, at least in part, to linkage disequilibrium between DR and DQ.
   - Several haplotypes that include different DQ and DRB1 alleles are associated with susceptibility or resistance to diabetes. The nomenclature of these haplotypes is complex. Because both α and β chains are polymorphic, alleles have a dual nomenclature

Table 17.2 Insulin-dependent diabetes-related major histocompatibility complex markers

Markers associated with protection	Markers associated with predisposition
DR2	DR3 (DRB1*0301)[a]
DR5	DR4 (DRB1*0401, 0405)[a]
DQA1*0102-DQB1*0602[b,c]	DQA1*0301-DQB1*302[d,e]
	DQA1*0501-DQB1*0201[e]
	DQA1*0401-DQB1*0402[e]
	DQA1*0101-DQB1*0501[e]

[a] Association secondary to linkage disequilibrium between DR and DQ; maximal risk in DR3/DR4 heterozygous individuals.
[b] DQ3.1 heterodimer.
[c] Contains an aspartic acid residue on DQB57; maximal protection is associated with expression of two Asp 57+ DQB alleles.
[d] DQ8 heterodimer.
[e] Maximal predisposition is associated either with the expression of two Asp-57 alleles of DR3 or DR4 or with the expression of an Asp 57-, Arg52+ DQ3.1 heterodimer.

indicating to which A and B chains they correspond. For example, the haplotypes HLADRB1*0401-DQA1*0301-DQB1*0302 and HLADRB1*0301-DQA1*0501-DQB1*0201 are associated with a high risk for the development of diabetes. A heterozygous individual expressing both of these haplotypes has a risk of 25%–40% of developing type 1 diabetes. Other haplotypes seem to be associated with resistance to type 1 DM. In Caucasians, resistance is associated with a DQ 3.1 heterodimer (DQA1*0102-DQB1*0602), characterized by the presence of aspartate (a negatively charged amino acid) in position 57 of the β chain (DQB1*0602 allele). The presence of a neutral amino acid in that same position, as well as the presence of arginine in position 52 of DQα, are characteristic of susceptibility alleles. Individuals with two susceptibility-determining Asp-DQ3.1 alleles have the highest degree of predisposition to develop DM. It is also worth noting that the protection or susceptibility to develop diabetes associated with DQ8 haplotypes (DQB1*0302) is influenced by the

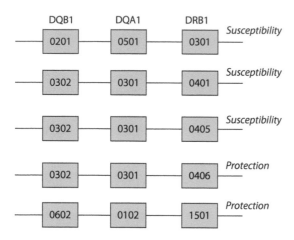

DQB1   DQA1   DRB1

0201	0501	0301	*Susceptibility*
0302	0301	0401	*Susceptibility*
0302	0301	0405	*Susceptibility*
0302	0301	0406	*Protection*
0602	0102	1501	*Protection*

Figure 17.2 Some MHC-II haplotypes associated with susceptibility or protection relative to type 1 diabetes mellitus. DR3 (DRB1*0301) and DR4 (DRB1*04) alleles are commonly associated with susceptibility while the DQ3.1 haplotype containing the DQB1*602 allele is associated with resistance. Note that the effect of the DQ8 haplotype DQA1*0301–DQB1*0302 is closely related to the DRB1 allele linked to it. While the association with DRB1*0405 determines susceptibility to type 1 diabetes, the association with DRB1*0406 determines resistance. (Modified from Undlien DE et al. *Trends Genet.*, 2001;17:93.)

DR4 alleles linked to them. In fact, the same DQ8 haplotype can be protective or not depending on its association with different DR4 alleles (see Figure 17.2).

2. **MHC-I genes associated with predisposition to develop diabetes** have also been identified. These MHC-I molecules are believed to be involved in the presentation of "diabetogenic" peptides to CD8+ cells, as supported by the finding of activated CD8+ T cells in the infiltrates surrounding the islets.
3. The **IDDM2 region** has been mapped to a variable number of tandem repeats (VNTRs) that flank the insulin gene and the insulin-growth factor II genes on chromosome 11. Those VNTR alleles that are associated with low expression of the insulin gene in the thymus would impair the ability to develop central tolerance to insulin-derived peptides.
4. Several other regions are linked to diabetes predisposition with variable consistency. These include regions where there are loci coding for insulin-growth factor-binding proteins (chromosome 2), which appear to be linked with

predisposition to develop diabetes, particularly in females, and the CTLA-4 gene (also in chromosome 2), which is believed to play a significant role in the induction of peripheral tolerance. Recent data suggest that a high level of CTLA-4 expression is associated with protection from diabetes, the reverse being also true.

How genetic factors influence the development of diabetes. Several hypotheses have been advanced to explain how MHC molecules, proteasomes, and TAP proteins influence the development of diabetes, all of them hinging on their ability to generate and present in association with MHC molecules β cell–derived peptides involved in the elicitation of the autoimmune response resulting in diabetes (diabetogenic peptides). One of the many interpretations that has been put forward is the basis for the MHC-II role in protection or predisposition for type 1 DM is related to the differential ability to bind diabetogenic peptides generated from the ingestion of β cells undergoing spontaneous apoptosis or viral-induced cell death and present them to the immune system. Protective MHC-II molecules would present diabetogenic peptides to the immune system, inducing central and/or peripheral tolerance (it is possible that the insulin gene is expressed in thymic cells during differentiation), while predisposing MHC-II molecules would not.

Sequence of pathogenic events leading to the development of insulin-dependent diabetes mellitus

Based on our current knowledge of the control of immunological responses and tolerance and on data accumulated from studies of IDDM patients and experimental animal models, the following hypothetical sequence of events leading to the development of IDDM can be proposed. First, one has to admit that autoreactive clones potentially able to be engaged in autoimmunity against pancreatic β cells persist in adult life. Even if the MHC-II molecules associated with predisposition and respective diabetogenic peptides were recognized by self-reactive T cell receptors (TCRs), their expression in resting antigen-presenting cells unable to deliver costimulatory signals would result in tolerogenic or apoptotic signaling of the autoreactive T cells.

A viral infection affecting the β cells or neighboring tissues has the potential to cause the activation of accessory cells and of Th cells involved in the antiviral response. Those cells will deliver costimulatory signals to the autoreactive Th cells, pushing them into a state of activation rather than anergy. Other cytokines will act on β cells, increasing their susceptibility to immune destruction. Thus, interferon-α released by activated accessory cells enhances the expression of MHC-I molecules, while IL-2 and other cytokines released by activated T cells induce the expression of MHC-II and CAMs.

The activated autoreactive T cells accumulate in the pancreatic islets and release chemotactic cytokines and interferon-γ, which will attract and activate monocytes/macrophages to the area, where interactions with islet cells overexpressing CAMs will contribute to their fixation in the islets. The activated monocytes/macrophages release cytokines such as IL-1, IL-12, and TNF, and toxic compounds such as oxygen active radicals and nitric oxide. The cytokines contribute to the damage by increasing the level of activation of Th1 cells (IL-12), monocytes, and macrophages (IL-1, TNF). In addition, IL-1 and interferon-γ (released by activated Th1 cells) induce the expression of Fas on islet cells. Islet cell death is a consequence of several mechanisms, including Fas-FasL apoptosis signaling and the release of toxic radicals that lead to oxidative changes of cell and organelle membrane lipids.

In addition to the immunological pathways involved in the pathogenesis of type 1 DM, dietary and nutritional factors appear to play also an important role. Cow's milk consumption, for example, has been linked to an increased risk for the development of type 1 DM, while breast milk feeding appears to have a protective effect. The ingestion of processed foods containing a variety of antioxidants and additives has also been suggested to favor the onset of type 1 DM. On the other hand, omega-3 fatty acids, vitamins D and E, and zinc have been proposed as having a protective effect.

Immunotherapy

Two main approaches to immunotherapy have been evaluated, one involving the use of immunosuppressants, and the other involving tolerization.

Among immunosuppressants, cyclosporin A received considerable attention in trials with the goal of preventing the full development of type 1A DM. To be effective, immunosuppressive therapy needs to be instituted to recently diagnosed patients with residual β-cell function, but the treatment is only effective while cyclosporin A is administered. In the vast majority of cases, progression to diabetes is seen soon after immunosuppressive therapy is discontinued.

Induction of tolerance by administration of insulin either by aerosol or by the oral route was investigated. Aerosol administration seems to result in the induction of γ/δ CD8+ T cells that secrete IL-10 and IL-4 and, in experimental animal models, are able to prevent the development of diabetes. Oral administration seems to generate a similar set of γ/δ CD4+ regulatory cells that secrete large amounts of TGF-β in addition to IL4 and IL-10. However, clinical trials have not shown any evidence of clinical effectiveness of these protocols on children identified at risk of developing type 1A DM.

A wide variety of interventions designed either to induce tolerance or depress the autoimmune response have been tested in clinical trials, but to date none has resulted in restoring normal insulin levels and clinical cure.

ACANTHOSIS NIGRICANS

Acanthosis nigricans is a rare syndrome that received its name because of thickening and hyperpigmentation of the skin in the flexural and intertriginous areas, in which patients develop a particularly labile form of diabetes associated with antibodies directed against the insulin receptor. These antibodies block the binding of insulin to the receptor. If the antibodies themselves are devoid of activating properties, they induce insulin-resistant diabetes. On the other side, the antibodies may stimulate the insulin receptor and cause hypoglycemia.

The clinical symptoms can be rather variable, depending on the biological properties of the predominant antibody population. Blocking antibodies to the insulin receptor cause hyperglycemia that does not respond to the administration of insulin (insulin-resistant diabetes). In contrast, insulin receptor antibodies with stimulating properties may induce the cellular metabolic effects usually triggered by insulin, albeit in an abnormal and unregulated fashion. The clinical picture is one of hyperinsulinism. The same patient may undergo cycles of predominance of hypo- and hyperinsulinism-like symptoms, mimicking an extremely brittle and difficult-to-control form of diabetes.

AUTOIMMUNE DISEASES OF THE GASTROINTESTINAL TRACT AND LIVER

Pernicious anemia

Pernicious or megaloblastic anemia is a severe form of anemia secondary to a special type of chronic atrophic gastritis associated with lack of absorption of vitamin B12. Pathologically, the disease is associated with chronic atrophic gastritis and defective production and/or function of intrinsic factor, which is required for the absorption of vitamin B12. Three types of autoantibodies have been described in patients with this disease:

- **Type I (blocking) antibodies**, present in 75% of patients, bind to intrinsic factor (IF) and prevent its binding to vitamin B12.
- **Type II (binding) antibodies** react with the IF-vitamin B12 complex and inhibit IF action. The type II antibody is found in 50% of patients, and it does not occur in the absence of antibody I.
- **Type III (parietal canalicular) antibodies**, present in the microvilli of the canalicular system of the gastric mucosa, are detected in 85%–90% of patients and react with the parietal cell, inhibiting the secretion of IF.

Animal models of pernicious anemia strongly implicate Th1 CD4$^+$ cells in the pathogenesis of the disease. Autoreactive CD4$^+$ T cells that have escaped thymic selection and recognize gastric epithelial cell antigens (in mice H/K ATPase) home the gastric mucosa, where they secrete cytokines such as IFNγ and IL-10. Macrophages are also present in the early mucosal infiltrates. The action of the effector CD4$^+$ T cells is under normal conditions under the control of CD4$^+$CD25$^+$ Treg cells. Experimental depletion of these cells allows the expression of the disease, whereas their presence blocks the expression of the disease.

In 10%–15% of patients with pernicious anemia, no antibody can be detected with currently available techniques. Other autoimmune diseases such as thyroiditis and Addison's disease are diagnosed with abnormally high frequency in patients with pernicious anemia.

Severe neuropathy and megaloblastic anemia dominate the clinical picture in patients with vitamin B12 deficiency. The development of neuropathy is a consequence of the fact that vitamin B12 is an essential coenzyme for the metabolism of homocysteine, the metabolic precursor of methionine and choline. Choline is required for the synthesis of choline-containing phospholipids, and methionine is also needed for the methylation of basic myelin.

Treatment involves intramuscular injection of vitamin B12 that will correct both hematological and neurological manifestations.

Chronic active hepatitis

Chronic active hepatitis (CAH) is a disease characterized by persistent hepatic inflammation, necrosis, and fibrosis, which often lead to hepatic insufficiency and cirrhosis. It can be subclassified by its etiology as viral induced, drug or chemically induced, autoimmune, and cryptogenic (cases that do not fit into any of the other groups).

Autoimmune chronic active hepatitis is characterized by the presence of autoantibodies and by lack of evidence of viral infection. Based on the pattern of autoantibodies detected in different patients, CAH can be subclassified into four types. The best characterized in the classic autoimmune chronic hepatitis (also known as "lupoid hepatitis") is defined by the detection of antinuclear antibodies. The term *lupoid* is used to stress the common feature (i.e., antinuclear antibodies) between this type of CAH and SLE. The antinuclear antibodies in autoimmune CAH are heterogeneous and are not directed against any specific nuclear antigen. In addition, autoantibodies to liver membrane antigens and smooth muscle are also detected in patients with this type of CAH. The other types of autoimmune CAH are characterized by different patterns of detection of autoantibodies to smooth muscle, liver-kidney microsomal antigens, and soluble liver antigens.

The autoimmune form of CAH affects predominantly young or postmenopausal women (80% of all patients) with an approximate incidence of 1 person per 100,000. The strong association with certain MHC-II antigens, particularly HLA-DRB1 alleles of DR3 and DR4, suggests a genetic predisposition. In addition, relatives may suffer from a variety of "autoimmune" diseases, such as thyroiditis, diabetes mellitus, autoimmune hemolytic anemia, and Sjögren's syndrome. Evidence suggesting a dysregulation of the immune system in these patients includes marked hypergammaglobulinemia, and detection of multiple autoantibodies.

Pathogenesis. Liver damage in all forms of CAH is believed to be the result of a cell-mediated immune response against altered hepatocyte membrane antigens. Both circulating and liver-derived lymphocytes from these patients have been shown to be cytotoxic for liver cells *in vitro*. Antibody-dependent cell-mediated cytotoxicity has also been suggested as playing a pathogenic role.

In the case of viral infections, the expression of viral proteins in the cell membrane of infected cells could be the initiating stimulus for the response. The trigger of most autoimmune forms of CAH remains unknown. In some cases, drugs, particularly α-methyldopa, may play the initiating role. α-methyldopa is believed to modify membrane proteins of a variety of cells and induce immune responses, which cross-react with native membrane proteins and perpetuate the damage, even after the drug has been removed.

The pathogenesis of cryptogenic CAH, in which there is no evidence of viral infection, exposure to drugs known to be associated with CAH, or autoimmune responses, remains unknown. Liver damage results from a series of events in which CD4T cells play a key role. Th1 lymphocytes secreting IL-2 and IFNγ activate cytotoxic CD8 T cells and stimulate hepatocytes to express HLA class-II antigens. The expression of self peptides by MHC-II will, in turn, activate monocytes/macrophages to release proinflammatory cytokines such as IL-1 and TNF; Th2 lymphocytes that produce IL-4 that assists autoreactive B cells to produce more autoantibody; and Th17 lymphocytes that exacerbate the inflammatory response.

Diagnosis of CAH is usually established by liver biopsy. Typically, the biopsy will reveal a picture of "piecemeal necrosis," characterized by marked mononuclear cell infiltration of the periportal spaces and/or paraseptal mesenchymal-parenchymal junctions, often expanding into the lobules. Plasma cells are often prominent in the infiltrate. There is also evidence of hepatocyte necrosis at the periphery of the lobules, with

evidence of regeneration and fibrosis. It is believed that this picture reflects an immune attack of the infiltrating lymphocytes directed against the periportal and paraseptal lymphocytes. In one-quarter to one-half of the patients (depending on the study), evidence of postnecrotic cirrhosis is detected; and in some patients, the evolution toward cirrhosis is progressive.

Treatment involves administration of glucocorticoids in the autoimmune forms and antiviral agents in cases associated with viral infection. α-Interferon administration seems beneficial for patients with viral CAH, who can complete several months of therapy without severe side effects. In some patients, interferon administration is associated with the emergence of antinuclear antibodies, which usually disappear after therapy is discontinued, but rarely may evolve toward a complete picture of autoimmune CAH requiring glucocorticoid therapy.

AUTOIMMUNE DISEASES OF THE NEUROMUSCULAR SYSTEMS

Myasthenia gravis

Myasthenia gravis is a chronic autoimmune disease caused by a disorder of neuromuscular transmission. Two main pathological findings are characteristic of myasthenia gravis: the production of anti-nicotinic-acetylcholine receptor antibodies, detected in 85%–90% of the patients, and a 70%–90% reduction in the number of acetylcholine receptors in the neuromuscular junctions.

The reduction in the number of acetylcholine receptors is believed to be due to their destruction by the immune system. This could be a consequence of complement activation by the nicotinic-acetylcholine receptor antibodies, opsonization, ADCC, activation of phagocytic cells, or T cell–mediated cytotoxicity. Cell-mediated immunity has been suggested as playing the major pathogenic role due to the lymphocytic infiltration that is often seen at the neuromuscular junction level, and because blast transformation can be achieved *in vitro* by stimulating T lymphocytes isolated from myasthenia gravis patients with acetylcholine receptor protein. These T lymphocytes may provide help to autoreactive B lymphocytes producing acetylcholine receptor antibodies. In such cases, autoreactive T lymphocytes could be more central in the pathogenesis of the disease than autoantibody-producing B lymphocytes. However, the pathogenic role of autoantibodies is evident from the fact that newborns to mothers with myasthenia gravis develop myasthenia-like symptoms for as long as they have maternal autoantibodies in circulation. It is important also to note that the lymphocytic infiltrates are not detected in a significant number of patients clinically indistinguishable from those with infiltrates.

Thymic abnormalities are frequent in myasthenia gravis. Seventy percent of patients have increased numbers of B-cell germinal centers within the thymus, which some authors have suggested to be the source of autoantibodies. About 10% of patients develop malignant tumors of the thymus (thymomas).

Symptoms of myasthenia gravis include increased muscular fatigue and weakness, especially becoming evident with exercise. The diagnosis is confirmed by the finding of acetylcholine receptor antibodies.

Treatment can involve the administration of acetylcholinesterase inhibitors, such as neostigmine and pyridostigmine (Mestinon), in combination with atropine. Virtually complete or partial relief of symptoms can be achieved with medical treatment in a significant number of patients. Another approach is thymectomy that is followed by improvement in 75% of patients and remission in the other 25%, although it may be several months after surgery when clinical improvement starts to be obvious.

Those patients who do not respond to either form of therapy may be treated with glucocorticoids, which can induce clinical improvement in 60%–100% of patients, depending on the series.

Multiple sclerosis

Multiple sclerosis (MS) is an autoimmune disease that results from the destruction of the myelin sheath in the central nervous system. MS lesions observed at autopsy are characterized by areas of myelin loss surrounding small veins in the deep white matter. A perivenous cuff of inflammatory cells is associated with acute lesions but is absent from old lesions where gliosis replaces myelin and the oligodendrocytes that produce and support it.

The inflammatory cells found in MS lesions are a mixture of T and B lymphocytes and macrophages (which are known as microglial cells in the central nervous system). The T lymphocytes are mostly CD4$^+$ and secrete IFN-γ, IL17, or both. One-fifth of the cells also produce GM-CSF. Peripheral blood CD4 T cells collected from patients with MS prior to treatment display increased propensity to differentiate to Th1 or Th17 cells. A few CD8$^+$ lymphocytes are also present in the lesions. Two main lines of evidence support the importance of T lymphocytes in the pathogenesis of MS. First, experimental allergic encephalomyelitis (EAE), the best animal model for MS, is transferred by CD4$^+$ T lymphocytes but not by serum. Injection of T-cell clones specific for the immunodominant epitope of myelin basic protein (MBP) derived from sick animals is the most efficient protocol to transmit the disease to healthy animals.

Second, MBP-specific CD4 clones can be established from lymphocytes isolated from the spinal fluid of MS patients. These clones generally recognize an epitope located at amino acids 87–99, but clones specific for other groups of 12 amino acids in the MBP molecule and to other myelin components, such as myelin proteolipid protein and myelin-associated glycoprotein, are also expanded. Therefore, many different T-cell clones with different TCRs appear to be involved in the autoimmune response.

The T cells present in MS lesions are clonally restricted, suggesting a role for autoantigen in the process. Autoreactive cells specific for MBP can be found in the peripheral blood of MS patients. The cell types involved are Th1 (secreting IFN γ, TNF, and lymphotoxin) and Th17 (secreting IL-17) that appear to migrate from the periphery to central nervous system (CNS). The MBP-reactive T cells express a number of chemokines and chemokine receptors, including MCP-1, RANTES, CCR5, and CXCR3, which apparently enable their migration to the CNS. They also express a series of adhesion molecules, such as ICAM-1 and LFA-1, which allow adhesion and inappropriate homing around microglial cells which in MS patients have been found to express adhesion molecules.

MS occurs mostly in young adults between the ages of 16 and 40 with a 3:1 female predominance. As in many other autoimmune diseases, the role of genetic factors was suggested by the finding that some HLA alleles are overrepresented among MS patients, particularly HLA-DR2 and HLA- DQ1, which are found in up to 70% of patients. These class-II MHC molecules are likely to be involved in peptide presentation to CD4+ lymphocytes. It has been demonstrated that normal individuals have myelin-specific T cells in their blood, suggesting that MBP-specific T lymphocytes are not deleted during differentiation, probably because myelin antigens are not expressed in the thymus. However, many of the normal individuals who have myelin-specific T cells in their blood do not develop MS, even when they are HLA-DR2. Thus, in normal individuals, these clones remain in a state of anergy or tolerance. Genome-wide association studies have revealed additional loci linked to MS. Most of those loci are linked to immune response rather than resident cell genes. The most important is the linkage with IL2-Rα (CD25) and IL7-Rα.

Very little is known about what activates previously tolerant MBP-specific clones and other autoreactive clones involved in MS. Viral infections have been proposed as the trigger for MS, perhaps as a consequence of molecular mimicry. In fact, many viral antigens from coronaviruses, Epstein–Barr virus, hepatitis B virus, herpes simplex virus, and others have sequences identical to MBP epitopes. Consequently, the immune response to the virus would activate a set of T cells whose TCR would cross-react with MBP peptides. Another possibility is that a viral superantigen could accidentally activate an MBP-specific T lymphocyte and cause its expansion.

In any case, autoreactive T lymphocytes by themselves are incapable of damaging the myelin sheath. However, autoreactive T lymphocytes secrete interferon-γ that activates the macrophages found in the lesions. Some of these activated macrophages are seen attached to the myelin sheath that they actively strip and phagocytize, becoming lipid laden. In addition, once they have engulfed myelin, they present myelin-derived antigens to T cells, contributing to the perpetuation of the immune reaction.

Clinical manifestations. Frequent symptoms at diagnosis include visual abnormalities, abnormal reflexes, and sensory and motor abnormalities. This variety of manifestations reflects the fact that lesions can occur anywhere in the white matter of the brain, cerebellum, pons, or spinal cord, at any time. The multiplicity and progression (both in number and extent) of MS lesions is the major clinical diagnostic criterion for this disease.

The course of MS is characterized by relapses and remissions in about 80% of patients, but each new attack may bring additional deficits when the myelin sheaths are incompletely or imperfectly replaced. Frequently, after 5–15 years of evolution, these patients enter a phase of relentless chronic progression and become wheelchair bound, bedridden, and totally dependent for all activities of daily living. In the remaining 20% of cases, MS is chronically progressive from onset.

The **diagnosis of MS** may be assisted by magnetic resonance imaging (MRI), which demonstrates breakdown of the blood-brain barrier that is always present at the beginning of a new attack, and spinal fluid electrophoresis, which may detect oligoclonal bands (multiple electrophoretically homogeneous bands) of IgG in the spinal fluid.

Treatment. The treatment of MS is not satisfactory. Glucocorticoids have been used extensively during the past 20 years. Usually high doses are required (to seal the blood-brain barrier), not suitable for long-term administration. In addition, glucocorticoid administration does not significantly affect disease progression.

Recombinant interferon β1b and the closely related interferon β1a are recommended for the treatment of relapsing-remitting MS. These interferons act by downregulating IFN-γ production and class-II expression on antigen-presenting cells. Interferon-β administration has been shown to slow down the progression of MS.

Glatiramer acetate (Copaxone, copolymer-1 [COP-1]), a synthetic basic copolymer of four amino acids designed to resemble MBP epitopes, without the ability to induce T-cell proliferation, has been used with some success. Administration of this product reduces the frequency of relapses of MS, lessens disease activity as measured by MRI, and can induce neurological improvement.

Two mechanisms of action have been proposed for glatiramer acetate. One is that this compound is a TCR antagonist of the immunodominant 82–100 epitope of MBP, thus turning off the immune response to MBP. The other is that glatiramer acetate administration may lead to a tolerant state by downregulating T-cell immune responses to MBP. This effect is supposed to be mediated by IL-10–secreting Treg lymphocytes.

In humans, administration of Copaxone is associated with an elevation of serum IL-10 levels and profound changes in T-lymphocyte activity, including suppression of TNF mRNA, and elevation of TGF-β and IL-4 mRNA. These results suggest that Copaxone may induce a shift from Th1 to a Treg cytokine profile, possibly associated with bystander suppression of the autoreactive immune response.

Recently, several new pharmacological agents have been found to be useful in the treatment of MS. Teriflunomide, a pyrimidine synthesis inhibitor, has been found in phase III trials to be equivalent to IFNβ. Dimethyl fumarate has a comparable clinical effect that correlates inversely with lymphocyte counts and has been approved by the U.S. Food and Drug Administration (FDA). Fingolimod, a sphingosine-1-phosphate-1 receptor antagonist, inhibits the egress of lymphocytes from lymph nodes to the bloodstream. It has been shown to have a good clinical effect and has also been approved by the FDA. Natalizumab is a humanized monoclonal antibody that recognizes the adhesion molecule α4 integrin and blocks its interaction with the vascular cell adhesion molecule 1. Natalizumab has great clinical efficacy. A downside is there is a substantial risk for the development of progressive multifocal leukoencephalopathy caused by activation of the JC virus. Other monoclonal antibodies shown to be clinically valuable and used to treat MS are the B cell–depleting antibodies (rituximab and ocrelizumab).

BIBLIOGRAPHY

Ajjan RA, Weetman AP. The pathogenesis of Hashimoto's thyroiditis: Further developments in our understanding. *Horm Metab Res*. 2015; 47:702–710.

Axisa PP, Hafler DA. Multiple sclerosis: Genetics, biomarkers, treatments. *Curr Opin Neurol*. 2016;29:345–353.

Baecher-Allan C, Kaskow BJ, Weiner HL. Multiple sclerosis: Mechanisms and immunotherapy. *Neuron* 2018;97:742–768.

Baeten DL, Kuchroo VK. How cytokine networks fuel inflammation: Interleukin-17 and a tale of two autoimmune diseases. *Nat Med*. 2013;19:824–825.

Bone RN, Evans-Molina C. Combination immunotherapy for type 1 diabetes. *Curr Diab Rep*. 2017;17(7):50. doi: 10.1007/s11892-017-0878-z.

Caturegli P, Kimura H, Rocchi R, Rose NR. Autoimmune thyroid diseases. *Curr Opin Rheumatol*. 2007;19:44–48.

Diana T, Krause J, Olivo PD et al. Prevalence and clinical relevance of thyroid stimulating hormone receptor-blocking antibodies in autoimmune thyroid disease. *Clin Exp Immunol*. 2017;189:304–309.

Eisenbarth GS. Type 1 diabetes: Molecular, cellular and clinical immunology. *Adv Exp Med Biol*. 2004;552:306–310.

Fröhlich E, Wahl R. Thyroid autoimmunity: Role of anti-thyroid antibodies in thyroid and extrathyroidal diseases. *Front Immunol*. 2017;8:521. doi: 10.3389/fimmu.2017.00521.

Green EA, Flavell RA. The initiation of autoimmune diabetes. *Curr Opin Immunol*. 1999;11:663–669.

Koeleman BPC, Lie BA, Undlien DE et al. Genotype effects and epistasis in type 1 diabetes and HLA-DQ trans dimer associations with disease. *Genes Immun*. 2004;5:381–388.

Kolb H, von Herrath M. Immunotherapy for type 1 diabetes: Why do current protocols not halt the underlying disease process? *Cell Metab*. 2017;25:233–241.

Lindstrom J, Shelton D, Fujii Y. Myasthenia gravis. *Adv Immunol*. 1988;42:233–284.

Morshed SA, Davies TF. Graves' disease mechanisms: The role of stimulating, blocking, and cleavage region TSH receptor antibodies. *Horm Metab Res*. 2015;47:727–734.

Patel DD, Kuchroo VK. Th17 cell pathway in human immunity: Lessons from genetics and therapeutic interventions. *Immunity* 2015;43:1040–1051.

Rekers NV, von Herrath MG, Wesley JD. Immunotherapies and immune biomarkers in type 1 diabetes: A partnership for success. *Clin Immunol*. 2015;161:37–43.

Virtanen SM. Dietary factors in the development of type 1 diabetes. *Pediatr Diabetes*. 2016;17(Suppl 22):49–55.

Wong FS, Karttunen J, Dumont C et al. Identification of an MHC class-I restricted autoantigen in type 1 diabetes by screening an organ-specific cDNA library. *Nat Med*. 1999; 5:1026–1031.

18

Systemic lupus erythematosus

GEORGE C. TSOKOS

INTRODUCTION

Systemic lupus erythematosus (SLE) is a generalized autoimmune disorder associated with multiple cellular and humoral immune abnormalities and protean clinical manifestations. It is most common in women of childbearing age.

CLINICAL MANIFESTATIONS

The clinical expression of SLE varies among different patients. The kind of organ (vital versus nonvital) that becomes involved determines the seriousness and the overall prognosis of the disease. The average frequency of some main clinical manifestations of SLE that may be observed during the entire course of SLE is shown in Table 18.1.

Diagnosis

The diagnosis is based on the verification that any four of the clinical and/or laboratory manifestations that are listed in Table 18.2 are present simultaneously or serially during a period of observation.

Course

Flares and remissions, heralded by the appearance of new manifestations and reappearance or worsening of preexisting symptoms, give the disease its fluctuating natural history. Over time, damage of the involved organs accumulates. Although high levels of autoantibodies and low levels of serum complement (C3, C4) may accompany clinical disease activity, there is no laboratory marker as of yet that can reliably predict an upcoming flare.

Overlap syndromes

Occasionally, physicians observe clinical situations in which the differentiation between SLE and another connective tissue disease is difficult. In some patients, the distinction may be impossible, and they are classified as having an overlap syndrome. This syndrome represents the association of SLE with another disorder such as scleroderma or rheumatoid arthritis. There are also some patients who have symptoms and laboratory findings that are reminiscent of lupus, yet a formal diagnosis (defined by the criteria listed in Table 18.2) cannot be made. Patients who take certain drugs (hydralazine, procainamide, etc.) may present with an incomplete picture of lupus known as drug-induced lupus. Other patients may present with an incomplete picture of lupus that may remain stable over a period of years or evolve with the appearance of additional manifestations.

Table 18.1 Main clinical manifestations of systemic lupus erythematosus

Manifestation	Percentage (%) of patients
Musculoarticular	95
Renal disease	60
Pulmonary disease (pleurisy, pneumonitis)	60
Cutaneous disease (photosensitivity, alopecia, etc.)	80
Cardiac disease (pericarditis, endocarditis)	20
Fever of unknown origin	80
Gastrointestinal disease (hepatomegaly, ascites, etc.)	45
Hematologic/reticuloendothelial (anemia, leukopenia, splenomegaly)	85
Neuropsychiatric (organic brain syndrome, seizures, peripheral neuropathy, etc.)	20

Table 18.2 Diagnostic features of systemic lupus erythematosus[a]

Facial erythema (butterfly rash)
Discoid lupus
Photosensitivity
Oral or nasopharyngeal ulcers
Arthritis without deformity
Pleuritis, or pericarditis
Psychosis, or seizures
Hemolytic anemia, leukopenia, lymphopenia, or thrombocytopenia
Heavy proteinuria, or cellular casts in the urinary sediment
Positive lupus erythematosus cell preparation, positive anti-dsDNA, anti-Sm antibodies, false-positive syphilis serology, positive anti-cardiolipin antibodies
Antinuclear antibody

[a] Established by the American College of Rheumatology.

IMMUNOLOGICAL ABNORMALITIES IN SYSTEMIC LUPUS ERYTHEMATOSUS

Autoantibodies

The **LE cell** is a peculiar-looking polymorphonuclear leukocyte that has ingested nuclear material. It is possible to reproduce this phenomenon *in vitro* by incubating normal neutrophils with damaged leukocytes preincubated with sera obtained from SLE patients. Investigations concerning the nature of this phenomenon led to the discovery that antibodies directed against nuclear antigens can promote the formation of LE cells, and subsequently, to the definition of a heterogeneous group of antinuclear antibodies.

Antinuclear antibodies (ANAs) are detected by indirect immunofluorescence using a variety of tissues and cell lines as substrates. A positive result is indicated by the observation of nuclear fluorescence after incubating the cells with the serum of the patient and subsequently with an anti-human immunoglobulin serum labeled with fluorochrome. Four patterns of fluorescence can be seen, indicating different types of antinuclear antibodies (see Table 18.3). The test for ANAs is not very specific but is very sensitive. A negative result virtually excludes the diagnosis of SLE (more than 95% of patients with SLE are ANA positive), while high titers are strongly suggestive of SLE but not confirmatory. ANAs can be detected in other conditions including other systemic autoimmune/collagen diseases and chronic

Table 18.3 Immunofluorescence patterns of antinuclear antibodies

Pattern	Antigen	Disease association(s)
Peripheral	Double-stranded DNA	SLE
Homogeneous	DNA-histone complexes	SLE and other connective tissue diseases
Speckled	Non-DNA nuclear antigens	
	Sm	SLE
	Ribonucleoprotein	Mixed connective tissue disease, SLE, scleroderma, etc.
	SS-A, SS-B	Sjögren's disease
Nucleolar	Nucleolus-specific RNA	Scleroderma

infections, as well as in normal individuals, albeit in low titers.

DNA antibodies are the most important in SLE. They can react with single-stranded DNA (ssDNA) or double-stranded DNA (dsDNA). Two-thirds of patients with SLE have circulating DNA antibodies. Although ssDNA antibodies may be found in many diseases besides SLE, dsDNA antibodies are found almost exclusively in SLE (40%–60% of the patients). They can be detected by immunofluorescence using as a substrate a noninfectious flagellate, *Crithidia luciliae*, which has a kinetoplast packed with double-stranded DNA. Using this test, the antibodies can be semiquantitated by titrating the serum, determining the highest serum dilution associated with visible fluorescence of the kinetoplast after addition of a fluorescent-labeled IgG antibody.

Antibodies to the DNA-histone complex are present in over 65% of patients with SLE. The use of enzyme-linked immunosorbent assay (ELISA) has permitted the identification of antibodies to all histone proteins including H1, H2A, H2B, H3, and H4. Histone antibodies are also present in patients with drug-induced SLE, most frequently associated with hydralazine and procainamide treatment.

Antibodies to nonhistone proteins that have been characterized best include the following:

- *Anti-Sm*: Antibodies to the Sm (Smith) antigen are present in one-third of patients with SLE but not in other conditions. The antigenic determinant is on a protein that is conjugated to one of six different small nuclear RNAs (snRNA).
- *Anti-U1-RNP*: The antigenic epitope is on a protein conjugated to U1-RNA. Antibodies to this antigen are present in the majority of patients

with SLE and mixed connective tissue disease—which represents an overlap syndrome.
- *Anti-SS-A/Ro*: These antibodies are present in one-third of patients with SLE and two-thirds of patients with Sjögren's syndrome (SS). Antibodies to the Ro antigen are frequently found in patients with SLE who are ANA-negative. Babies born to mothers with Ro antibodies may have heart block, leukopenia, and/or skin rash.
- *Anti-SS-B/La*: The antigenic epitope recognized by this antibody is on a 43 Kd protein conjugated to RNA. Antibodies to La antigen are present in about one-third of patients with SLE and in approximately one-half of patients with Sjögren's syndrome.

Cardiolipin and phospholipid antibodies are frequently found in patients with SLE. The cardiolipin antibodies recognize a cryptic epitope on β2-glycoprotein I that is exposed after it binds to anionic phospholipids. A related group of antibodies includes the phospholipid antibodies that react with phospholipids and are apparently implicated as one of the causes of clotting disorders in SLE.

Lupus anticoagulant is detected by prolongation of *in vitro* clotting assays. It represents a major form of phospholipid antibodies with some overlap with the ELISA-detected antiphospholipid antibodies.

Pathogenic role of autoantibodies in SLE

There are three groups of autoantibodies: those that have not been assigned a role in pathogenesis and are not helpful in diagnosis; those that are helpful in diagnosis or are associated with a particular clinical manifestation but have not been shown to cause certain pathology (Sm antibody); and those that cause, or at least initiate, a pathologic process (anti-erythrocytic antibodies bind to red blood cell membranes, activate complement, and cause red cell hemolysis). Increasingly, SLE autoantibodies are assigned new roles such as entering live cells and altering cell biochemistry, binding cell surface membranes and altering cell function, binding to cells that have already been stressed or injured, and activating complement.

T-cell antibodies are believed to bind and eliminate certain subsets of T cells and disturb homeostasis that may result in decreased effector T-cell function and increased antibody production by B cells. Also, T-cell antibodies may alter the function of T cells; for example, they cause decreased production of IL-2.

Antibodies against CR1 (complement receptor 1) and against the **C3 convertase** are occasionally detected. CR1 antibodies may block the receptor and interfere with the clearance of immune complexes. Antibodies to the C3 convertase prolong its half-life and contribute to increased C3 consumption.

Anti–red cell antibodies and **antiplatelet antibodies** are the cause, respectively, of hemolytic anemia and thrombocytopenia.

Autoantibodies directed against central nervous system (CNS) molecules such as the NR2 subunit of the N-methyl-d-aspartate glutamate (NMDA) receptor contribute to neuronal malfunction and loss of cognition.

DNA antibodies form immune complexes by reacting with DNA and are implicated in the pathogenesis of glomerulonephritis (see discussion later in this chapter).

Cardiolipin antibodies, phospholipid antibodies, and **lupus anticoagulant** are detected frequently in SLE patients. The cardiolipin antibodies cause false positivity in serological tests for syphilis. Cardiolipin and phospholipid antibodies are also associated with miscarriages, thrombophlebitis and thrombocytopenia, and various central nervous system manifestations, secondary to vascular thrombosis. The constellation of these symptoms is known as antiphospholipid antibody syndrome, and although it was first recognized in lupus patients, the majority of the cases do not fulfill the diagnostic criteria for SLE.

Ro antibodies, when present in mothers with SLE, seem associated with the development of heart block in their babies. Ro antibodies may interfere with the electrophysiology of the cells involved with the conductance within the heart.

Diagnostic value of autoantibodies

Some autoantibodies may not be linked with any specific clinical manifestations but are very useful as disease markers. For example, dsDNA and Sm antibodies are diagnostic of SLE. Most other autoantibodies are present in more than one clinical disease or syndrome.

PATHOGENESIS OF SLE

Multiple environmental, hormonal, genetic, and immunoregulatory factors are involved in the expression of the disease. In any given patient, different factors contribute variably to the expression of the disease.

Genetic factors

The understanding of the pathogenic mechanisms underlying the progression of SLE has been facilitated by the discovery of spontaneously occurring disease in mice that resembles SLE in many respects. During the inbreeding of mice, it was observed that the F1 (first-generation) hybrids obtained by mating white and black mice from New Zealand [(NZB × NZW)F1] spontaneously developed a systemic autoimmune disease involving a variety of organs and systems. Throughout the course of their disease, the mice develop hypergammaglobulinemia, reflecting a state of hyperactivation of the humoral immune system. The animals have a variety of autoantibodies and manifestations of autoimmune disease and immune complex disease similar to those seen in humans with SLE. As the disease progresses, they develop nephritis and lymphoproliferative disorders and die.

The importance of genetic factors in the development of disease in NZB mice is underlined by the observation that the parental NZB mice have a mild form of the disease manifested by autoimmune hemolytic anemia, but that the introduction of the NZW genetic background causes the disease to appear earlier and in severe form. Genetic linkage studies indicate that many of the immunologic abnormalities are under multigenic control, one gene(s) controlling the animal's ability to produce anti-DNA antibodies, another gene the presence of anti-erythrocyte antibodies, and still other genes controlling high levels of IgM production and lymphocytic proliferation.

Two other mouse strains that develop an SLE-like disease spontaneously have been identified: MRL *lpr/lpr* and MRL *gld*. The first strain has a defect in the FAS gene, whereas the second has a defect in the FAS ligand gene. The products of these two genes are responsible for the programmed cell death of cells also known as apoptosis, which is critical for the control of undesirable immune responses. Patients with Fas deficiency develop an autoimmune lymphoproliferative syndrome with lymph node enlargement and autoimmune elements.

Several pieces of evidence indicate that genetic factors also play a role in the pathogenesis of human SLE. Serum DNA and T-cell antibodies as well as cellular abnormalities are present in healthy relatives of lupus patients. There is a moderate degree of clinical disease concordance among monozygotic twins. The fact that the clinical concordance between twins is only moderate strongly indicates that genetic factors alone may not lead to the expression of the disease and that other factors are needed. The genes which could play a role, probably in synergy with environmental factors, have not been identified. Current evidence indicates that in humans, as in mice, these genes are probably linked to the major histocompatibility complex (MHC). For example, the HLA-DR2 haplotype is overrepresented in patients with SLE. As mentioned before, an SLE-like disease develops frequently in individuals with C4 and C2 deficiencies (C4 and C2 genes are located in chromosome 6, in close proximity to the MHC genes). Also, individuals lacking C1q are also prone to developing lupus. Recently, genome-wide searches for "lupus" genes have been undertaken. These studies have reported more than 50 genomic loci to be associated with lupus. Interestingly, many of these areas are found in 6p and 1q.

Immune response abnormalities

SLE is a disease associated with profound immunoregulatory abnormalities, affecting both humoral and cellular responses.

B-CELL ABNORMALITIES

Increased numbers of B cells and plasma cells are detected in the bone marrow and peripheral lymphoid tissues secreting immunoglobulins spontaneously. The hyperactive status of B cells and plasma cells in SLE seems to result from several factors (summarized in Figure 18.1).

Signals derived from the occupation of B-cell receptors (BCRs), surface IgM (sIgM) or sIgD lead to significantly enhanced production of tyrosine-phosphorylated cellular proteins and increased formation of inositol triphosphate when compared to B-cell responses from either normal or disease-control individuals. These events are followed by a significantly increased free Ca^{2+} flux in the cytoplasm, which is contributed primarily by the intracellular calcium stores (Figure 18.2). Thus, the responses are more vigorous than normal. In addition, the modulation of B-cell responses by costimulatory molecules is also abnormal. The coactivation signals derive from the occupation of complement receptor type 2 (CR2, a complex of CD21, CD19, CD81) and the lowering of the threshold of B-cell activation secondary to the cross-linking of CR2 and BCR (which co-cross-linking is enhanced in SLE, as a consequence of the abundance of circulating CR2 ligands [C3d, C3dg, and iC3d]). In contrast, feedback mechanisms believed to assist in the downregulation of B-cell responses appear to be deficient in SLE. Normally, the B-cell FcγRIIB1 coreceptor causes an early termination of B-cell receptor-initiated signals when co-cross-linked with sIg (i.e., when Ag is presented to B cells in the form of immune complexes). In SLE, the function of Fc receptors is defective, and this downregulating effect is depressed.

The number of activated B cells and plasma cells correlates with disease activity. Only a limited number of light- and heavy-chain genes are used by autoantibodies, demonstrating that the autoantibody response involves only a few of all B-cell clones available. Furthermore, the changes appearing in their sequence over time strongly suggest that they undergo affinity maturation, a process that requires T-cell help. It also suggests that a few antigens drive the response.

Immunosuppressive drug treatment of both murine and human lupus causes clinical improvement associated with decreased B-cell activity. Any infection that induces B-cell activation is

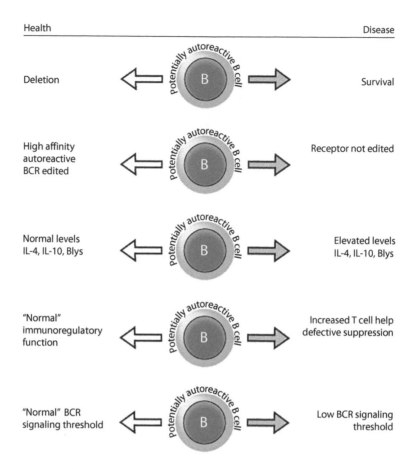

Figure 18.1 Summary of the immunoregulatory abnormalities associated with systemic lupus erythematosus.

likely to cause a clinical relapse in patients with inactive SLE.

T-CELL ABNORMALITIES

They are numerous and contribute invariably to disease pathogenesis:

- The numbers and function of CD4 T cells expressing FoxP3 (regulatory T cells) are low, allowing uncontrolled function of B cells.
- A subset of $CD3^+$ cells that express neither CD4 nor CD8 has been found to provide help to autologous B cells synthesizing DNA antibodies and to produce the proinflammatory cytokine IL17.
- A recently defined subpopulation of T cells known as T-follicular helper T cells are expanded in patients with SLE and provide help to B cells.
- Cytotoxic responses to viral or other nominal antigens are decreased and contribute to increased rates of infection.
- Production of the central cytokine IL-2 is decreased, and this accounts for decreased regulatory and cytotoxic cell function.
- In humans, restriction fragment length polymorphism studies of the constant region of the T-cell receptor (TCR) demonstrated an association between TcRα chain polymorphism and SLE and TcRβ chain polymorphism and production of anti-Ro antibodies. More recently, sequence information of the TCR chains of pathogenic human T-cell clones demonstrated bias in the T-cell repertoire selection process.

DENDRITIC CELL ABNORMALITIES

Plasmacytoid dendritic cells may present autoantigen to T and B cells at increased rates in patients with SLE. Interferon-α and circulating immune complexes (acting through Fc receptors and toll-like receptor 9) stimulate dendritic cell function in SLE.

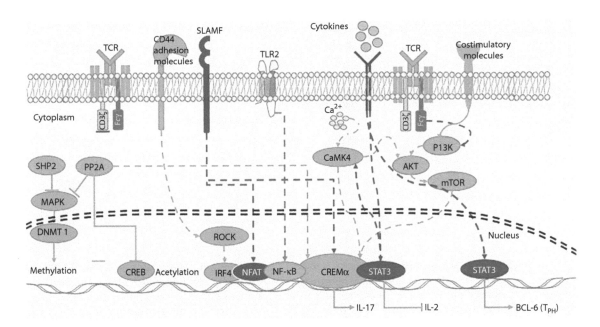

Figure 18.2 Molecular defects that lead to T-cell abnormalities in systemic lupus erythematosus. T cells initiate the activation process after the engagement of the T-cell receptor (TCR) by antigen or circulating anti-CD3/TCR antibodies. The CD3 complex is rewired in SLE T cells with the CDζ chain being replaced by FcRIγ (Fcγ) that results in increased calcium flux, activation of the calcium/calmodulin kinase 4 (CaMK4), which in turn increases the binding of transcription factors such as cyclic AMP response element modulator α (CREM)α to the promoters of the IL-2 and IL17 genes suppressing the first and enhancing the second. Engagement of the cytokine receptors is also altered in SLE T cells. IL-2 signaling is compromised with decreased levels of the signal transducers of activation and transcription 5 (STAT5), which translate to decreased Treg activity, whereas IL-6 signaling results in increased STAT3 activity, which translates in increased IL-17 production. Costimulatory receptor signaling is also altered, resulting in increased mTOR activity. Engagement of adhesion molecules (CD44) results in increased Rho-associated protein kinase (ROCK) activity that translates to increased adhesion and also increased IL-17 production. T cells from SLE patients express increased levels of the serine/threonine phosphatase 2 (PP2A), which contributes to increased demethylation of certain genes and decreased activity of the transcriptional enhancer cyclic AMP-responsive element-binding protein 1 (CREB). Altered levels of signaling lymphocytic activation molecule family (SLAMF) on the surface of T cells account for decreased Treg and cytolytic T-cell function in SLE patients.

Immune complexes in SLE

The pathogenic role of immune complexes (ICs) in SLE has been well established. As summarized in Figure 18.3, this pathogenic role is a result of a variety of abnormal circumstances.

First, marked elevations in the levels of circulating immune complexes can be detected in the sera of patients with SLE during acute episodes of the disease by a variety of techniques. Since patients with active SLE have high levels of free circulating DNA and most have also DNA antibodies, DNA-anti-DNA ICs are likely to be formed either in circulation or in collagen-rich tissues and structures, such as the glomerular basement membrane, which have avidity for DNA.

Besides the fact that immune complexes are formed at increased rates in patients with SLE, the clearance rate of circulating immune complexes is decreased as a consequence of several factors:

- Immune complexes are cleared by the Fc-receptor-bearing cells of the reticuloendothelial system. Many patients with lupus nephritis have alleles of Fc receptors that bind IgG with less avidity. This results in slower immune complex clearance.
- Immune complexes often have adsorbed complement components and split products, including C3b, which reacts with CR1. Consequently, ICs are transported to the reticuloendothelial system by red blood cells which bind them

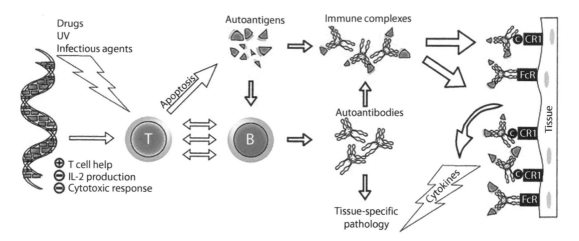

Figure 18.3 Overview of the pathogenesis of systemic lupus erythematosus: Multiple genetic, environmental, and hormonal factors influence the function of T and B lymphocytes. T cells display a wide spectrum of abnormalities including decreased cytotoxic responses and increased ability to help B cells to produce antibodies. Lupus B cells, with the help of T cells, produce autoantibodies that bind to autoantigens found on cells and tissues and others released in the circulation by apoptotic cells. The resulting immune complexes are not cleared effectively because, besides the fact that they are produced at increased rates, the receptors that are responsible for their clearance, i.e., Fc and complement receptors, are deficient either in numbers or in function. Once deposited in tissues, immune complexes initiate a cascade that eventually results in tissue injury.

through their CR1. Patients with SLE have decreased numbers of CR1, a fact that may compromise the clearance of ICs and contribute to the development of IC-induced inflammatory reactions.

- ICs are partially solubilized as a consequence of complement activation, a process that contributes to their inactivation and clearance. Individuals with C4 deficiency develop a disease with clinical features resembling those of SLE. This observation can be explained by the fact that immune complexes are cleared at slower rates in C4-deficient individuals, perhaps due to the role of C4 fragments in the solubilization and clearance of circulating immune complexes.

The pro-inflammatory properties of immune complexes in SLE are suggested by a variety of observations. First, rising levels of DNA antibodies in conjunction with falling serum C3 levels (reflecting consumption by antigen-antibody complexes) are associated with disease flares. Second, patients with IgG1 and IgG3 (complement-fixing) DNA antibodies develop lupus nephritis more frequently than those patients in whom DNA antibodies are of other isotypes. Glomerulonephritis,

cutaneous vasculitis, arthritis, and some of the neurologic manifestations of SLE are fully explainable by the development of local inflammatory lesions secondary to the formation or deposition of ICs. What remains unclear is whether tissue-fixed ICs are circulating ICs that eventually become deposited in tissues or if they result from the formation of antigen-antibody complexes *in situ*.

In SLE patients, immune complex deposits have also been noted on the dermoepidermal junction of both inflamed skin and normal skin, appearing as a fluorescent "band" when a skin biopsy is studied by immunofluorescence with antisera to immunoglobulins and complement components (band test).

Glomerulonephritis

Immunofluorescence studies indicate that the capillary tufts of renal glomeruli in patients with lupus nephritis contain deposits of immunoglobulins and complement. Several lines of evidence support the conclusion that those deposits represent immune complexes and that these ICs are likely to play a primary pathogenic role. DNA and DNA antibodies can be eluted from the kidneys of lupus patients, confirming that they correspond to antigen-antibody complexes. The deposition of IC in the glomerular basement membrane can be explained in five different ways:

- Deposition of soluble, circulating ICs.
- Formation of ICs *in situ*. DNA has affinity to glomerular basement membranes and, once immobilized, may react with circulating DNA antibodies to form antigen-antibody complexes.
- Cross-reaction of DNA antibodies with collagen and cytoskeleton proteins.
- Anti-C1q antibodies, highly associated with nephritis, cause renal damage if ICs have already been deposited. This experimental fact suggests a cascade of events that involves the deposition of ICs, complement, and anti-C1q antibodies leading to renal injury.
- IgG from patients with SLE enters podocytes using the neonatal Fc receptor (FcRn) and compromises their structure and function.

The pathogenic role of ICs deposited in the kidney is supported by ample evidence for complement activation via the classic and alternative pathways in patients with active nephritis. Circulating levels of C3 and C4 are usually decreased, whereas plasma levels of complement breakdown products such as C3a, C3d, and Bb are increased. C1q, C3b, and complement split products such as C3d, C3bi, and C3c can be detected attached to circulating ICs.

Nonimmune factors influencing the course of SLE

In addition, and in close interplay with genetic and immunological factors, a variety of other factors have an apparent effect on the evolution of the disease.

Hormonal effects. The expression of the genetic and immunologic abnormalities characteristic of murine lupus-like disease is influenced by female sex hormones. For example, in (NZB × NZW) F1 mice, the disease is more severe in females. Administration of estrogens aggravates the evolution of the disease, which is only seen in castrated male mice and not in complete males.

The extent of the hormonal involvement in human SLE cannot be proven directly, but the large female predominance (9:1 female-to-male ratio) as well as the influence of puberty and pregnancies at the onset of the disease, or the severity of the disease's manifestations, indicate that sex hormones play a role in the modulation of the disease. Estrogens and prolactin administered to animals promote anti-DNA antibody selection in animals.

Environmental factors. Several environmental insults have been related to the onset or relapse of SLE.

Sunlight exposure was the first environmental factor influencing the clinical evolution of human SLE to be identified. Exposure to sunlight may precede the clinical expression of the disease or disease relapse. This could be related to the fact that the Langerhans cells of the skin and keratinocytes release significant amounts of interleukin-1 upon exposure to ultraviolet (UV) light, and could thus represent the initial stimulus tipping off a precarious balance of the immune system.

Infections also seem to play a role. The normal immune response to bacterial and viral infections may spin off into a state of B-cell hyperactivity, triggering a relapse. Infection through the "molecular mimicry" can initiate an autoimmune response. Also, various infections may suppress the autoimmune response, and in their absence, autoimmune manifestations may occur at increased rates.

Drugs, particularly those with DNA-binding ability, such as hydantoin, isoniazid, and hydralazine, can cause a drug-induced lupus-like syndrome. These drugs are known to cause DNA hypomethylation. Because hypomethylated genes are transcribed at higher rates, it is theoretically possible that they cause SLE by increasing the transcription rate of genes that are involved in the expression of the disease. ANAs appear in 15%–70% of patients treated with any of these drugs for several weeks. These ANAs belong, in most cases, to the IgM class and react with histones. Only when the antibodies switch from IgM to IgG does the patient become symptomatic. ANAs usually disappear after termination of the treatment. Patients with drug-induced SLE usually have a milder disease without significant vital organ involvement.

TREATMENT

Improvement of our understanding of the pathogenesis of SLE has led to reasonable therapeutic strategies that have dramatically improved the well-being and life expectancy of patients with SLE, whose survival rate at 10 years is now 80%. The therapeutic approach to each patient is determined by the extent of the disease and, most importantly, by the nature and extent of organ involvement. Careful avoidance of factors implicated in the induction of relapses, such as high-risk medications, exposure to sunlight, infections, etc., is always indicated, but in most cases, administration of anti-inflammatory and immunosuppressive drugs is essential.

Glucocorticoids combine anti-inflammatory effects with a weak immunosuppressive capacity. The anti-inflammatory effect is probably beneficial in disease manifestations secondary to immune complex deposition, while the immunosuppressive effect may help to curtail the activity of the B-cell system.

Nonsteroidal anti-inflammatory drugs are frequently used in order to control arthritis and serositis.

Immunosuppressive drugs are often used in the treatment of patients with vital organ involvement (i.e., glomerulonephritis, CNS involvement). **Cyclophosphamide**, given intravenously, has been successfully used to prolong adequate renal function with only few side effects. Maximal benefit is achieved when long-term treatment is started early, with relatively good renal function. In some patients, clinical effects require the administration of high (nonablative) doses of cyclophosphamide. Infections, sterility, and malignancies are frequent side effects.

Mycophenolate is being used extensively to treat patients with more severe disease and lupus nephritis. It has fewer side effects than cyclophosphamide and it appears (not proven) equally effective.

A monoclonal antibody against BLyS (B-lymphocyte stimulator) has been approved by the U.S. Food and Drug Administration for the treatment of patients with SLE, but it takes 6–7 months to notice any effect, usually limited to minor manifestations.

Experimental therapeutic approaches are under study in patients with SLE. These new approaches capitalize on information that has been generated from the study of the pathogenesis of the disease.

As discussed earlier, much of the produced autoantibody is the result of cognate interaction between helper T cells and B lymphocytes. Therefore, the interruption of this interaction by either humanized antibodies (see Chapter 24) or fusion proteins (recombinant molecules constituted by the binding site of a receptor or ligand and the Fc portion of IgG to prolong serum half-life) is expected to have therapeutic value. Such reagents include anti-CD40 ligand antibody and the CTLA4-Ig.

Complement activation mediates significant pathology in human lupus. An anti-C5 antibody that disrupts complement activation is currently in clinical trials to determine its role in the treatment of lupus.

Anti-CD20 antibody, able to deplete B cells, although helpful in some patients has not been evaluated by qualified clinical trials.

Numerous trials carried out in patients with SLE have failed for a number of reasons, including clinical and pathogenic heterogeneity of the disease.

Additional trials will determine the possibility of curing, or setting back the lupus clock, by ablating (by means of administration of large doses of cytotoxic drugs or total body irradiation) the patient's own immune system and reinfusing autologous hematopoietic stem cells.

BIBLIOGRAPHY

Agmon-Levin N, Damoiseaux J, Kallenberg C et al. International recommendations for the assessment of autoantibodies to cellular antigens referred to as anti-nuclear antibodies. *Ann Rheum Dis.* 2014;73:17–23.

Boumpas DT, Fessler BJ, Austin HA 3rd et al. Systemic lupus erythematosus: Emerging concepts. Part 1: Renal, neuropsychiatric, cardiovascular, pulmonary, and hematologic disease. *Ann Intern Med.* 1995;21:940–950.

Boumpas DT, Fessler BJ, Austin HA 3rd et al. Systemic lupus erythematosus: Emerging concepts. Part 2: Dermatologic and joint disease, the antiphospholipid antibody syndrome, pregnancy and hormonal therapy, morbidity and mortality, and pathogenesis. *Ann Intern Med.* 1995;123:42–53.

Deng Y, Tsao BP. Updates in lupus genetics. *Curr Rheumatol Rep.* 2017;19:68. doi: 10.1007/s11926-017-0695-z.

Giannakopoulos B, Krilis SA. The pathogenesis of the antiphospholipid syndrome. *N Engl J Med.* 2013;368:1033–1044.

Liu Z, Davidson A. Taming lupus—A new understanding of pathogenesis is leading to clinical advances. *Nat Med.* 2012;18:871–882.

Mader S, Brimberg L, Diamond B. The role of brain-reactive autoantibodies in brain pathology and cognitive impairment. *Front Immunol.* 2017;8:1101. doi: 10.3389/fimmu.2017.01101.

McClain MT, Heinlen LD, Dennis GJ et al. Early events in lupus humoral autoimmunity suggest initiation through molecular mimicry. *Nat Med.* 2005;11:85–89.

Moulton VR, Suarez-Fueyo A, Meidan E et al. Pathogenesis of human systemic lupus erythematosus: A cellular perspective. *Trends Mol Med.* 2017;23:615–635.

Presumey J, Bialas AR, Carroll MC. Complement system in neural synapse elimination in development and disease. *Adv Immunol.* 2017;135: 53–79.

Tsokos GC. Systemic lupus erythematosus. *N Engl J Med.* 2011;365:2110–2121.

19

Rheumatoid arthritis

GEORGE C. TSOKOS AND GABRIEL VIRELLA

INTRODUCTION

Rheumatoid arthritis (RA) is a chronic autoimmune disease characterized by inflammatory and degenerative lesions of the distal joints, frequently associated with multiorgan involvement. This disease affects just under 1% of the population, and its etiology is complex; immunologic, genetic, and hormonal factors are thought to determine its development. RA progresses variably in different individuals and, if not treated early and aggressively, will eventually cause joint destruction and incapacitating deformities.

CLINICAL AND PATHOLOGICAL ASPECTS OF RHEUMATOID ARTHRITIS

Localized disease: Clinical presentation

A chronic inflammatory process of the joints that progresses through different stages of increasing severity (Table 19.1) characterizes RA. The damage is reversible until cartilage and bones become involved (stages 4 and 5). At that time, the changes become irreversible and result in severe functional impairment.

The most common clinical presentation of RA is the association of pain, swelling, and stiffness of the metacarpophalangeal and wrist joints, often associated with pain in the sole of the foot, indicating metatarsophalangeal involvement. The disease is initially limited to small distal joints. With time, RA progresses from the distal to the proximal joints so that in the late stages, joints such as the ankles, knees, and elbows may become affected.

PATHOLOGICAL MANIFESTATIONS OF LOCALIZED DISEASE

In the early stages, the inflammatory lesion is limited to the lining of the normal diarthrodial joint. A thin membrane composed of two types of synoviocytes, the type A synoviocyte, which is a phagocytic cell of the monocyte-macrophage series with a rapid turnover, and the type B synoviocyte, which is believed to be a specialized fibroblast, constitutes the normal synovial lining. This cellular lining sits on top of a loose acellular stroma that contains many capillaries.

The earliest pathological changes, seen at the time of the initial symptoms, affect the endothelium

Table 19.1 The stages of rheumatoid arthritis

Stage	Pathologic process	Symptoms	Physical signs
1	Antigen presentation to T lymphocytes	None	None
2	Proliferation of T and B lymphocytes	Malaise, mild joint stiffness	Swelling of small joints
3	Neutrophils in synovial fluid; synovial cell proliferation	Joint pain and morning stiffness, malaise	Swelling of small joints
4	Invasive pannus; degradation of cartilage	Joint pain and morning stiffness, malaise	Swelling of small joints
5	Invasive pannus; degradation of cartilage; bone erosion	Joint pain and morning stiffness, malaise	Swelling of small joints; deformities

of the microvasculature, whose permeability is increased, as judged by the development of edema and of a sparse inflammatory infiltrate of the edematous subsynovial space, in which polymorphonuclear leukocytes predominate. Several weeks later, hyperplasia of the synovial lining cells and perivascular lymphocytic infiltrates can be detected, some of which may appear as lymphoid follicles.

In the chronic stage, the size and number of the synovial lining cells increase, and the synovial membrane takes a villous appearance. There is also subintimal hypertrophy with massive infiltration by lymphocytes, plasmablasts, and granulation tissue (forming what is known as pannus). This thick pannus behaves like a tumor and in the ensuing months and years continues to grow, protruding into the joint. The synovial space becomes filled with exudative fluid, and this progressive inflammation causes pain and limits motion. With time, the cartilage is eroded, and there is progressive destruction of bones and tendons, leading to severe limitation of movement, flexion contractures, and severe mechanical deformities.

Systemic involvement: Clinical presentation

It is common to observe some signs and symptoms more indicative of a systemic disease, particularly those that are indicative of vasculitis. The most frequent sign is the formation of the rheumatoid nodules over pressure areas, such as the elbows. These nodules are an important clinical feature because, with rare exceptions, they are pathognomonic of RA in patients with chronic synovitis, and generally indicate a poor prognosis.

SYSTEMIC INVOLVEMENT: PATHOLOGICAL MANIFESTATIONS

In contrast with the necrotizing vasculitis associated with systemic lupus erythematosus (SLE), due almost exclusively to immune complex deposition, the vasculitis seen in RA is associated with granuloma formation. This indicates that cell-mediated immune processes are also likely to be involved. Regardless of the exact pathogenesis of the vasculitic process, rheumatoid patients with vasculitis usually have persistently elevated levels of circulating immune complexes, and generally, a worse prognosis.

Histopathological studies of rheumatoid nodules show fibrinoid necrosis at the center of the nodule surrounded by histiocytes arranged in a radial palisade. The central necrotic areas are believed to be the seat of immune complex formation or deposition. When the disease has been present for some time, small brown spots may be noticed around the nail bed or associated with nodules. These indicate small areas of endarteritis.

The overlap syndrome

The overlap syndrome describes a clinical condition in which patients show variable degrees of association of RA and SLE. The existence of this syndrome suggests that the demarcation between SLE and RA is not absolute, resulting in a clinical continuum between both disorders.

Clinically these patients present features of both diseases. Histopathological studies also show lesions characteristic of the two basic pathological components of RA and SLE (necrotizing vasculitis and granulomatous reactions). Serological studies in patients with the overlap syndrome demonstrate both antibodies characteristically found in SLE (e.g., anti-dsDNA) and antibodies typical of RA (rheumatoid factor, see discussion later in this chapter).

Other related diseases

Sjögren's syndrome can present as an isolated entity (primary) or in association with RA, SLE, and other collagen diseases (secondary). It is characterized by dryness of the oral and ocular membranes (Sicca syndrome), and the presence of rheumatoid factor and antibodies to Ro or La antigens.

Felty's syndrome is an association of RA with neutropenia caused by antibodies directed against neutrophils. The spleen is often enlarged, possibly reflecting its involvement in the elimination of antibody-coated neutrophils.

AUTOANTIBODIES IN RHEUMATOID ARTHRITIS

Rheumatoid factor and anti-immunoglobulin antibodies

The classical serological hallmark of RA is the detection of rheumatoid factor (RF) and other anti-immunoglobulin (anti-Ig) antibodies. By definition, classical RF is an IgM antibody to autologous IgG. The more encompassing designation of anti-Ig antibodies is applicable to anti-IgG antibodies of IgG or IgA isotypes.

Methods used for the detection of rheumatoid factor. RF and anti-Ig antibodies can be detected in the serum of affected patients by a variety of techniques:

- The **Rose-Waaler test** is a passive hemagglutination test that uses sheep or human erythrocytes coated with anti-erythrocyte antibodies as indicators. The agglutination of the IgG-coated red cells to titers greater than 16 or 20 is considered as indicative of the presence of RF. These tests detect mostly the classic IgM rheumatoid factor specific for IgG.
- The **latex agglutination test**, in which IgG-coated polystyrene particles are mixed with serum suspected of containing RF or anti-Ig antibodies (see Chapter 15). The agglutination of latex particles by serum dilutions greater than 1:20 is considered as a positive result. This test detects anti-Ig antibodies of all isotypes.

Diagnostic specificity of immunoglobulin antibodies. As with many other autoantibodies, the titers of RF are a continuous variable within the population studied. Thus, any level intending to separate the seropositive from the seronegative is arbitrarily chosen to include as many patients with clinically defined RA in the seropositive group, while excluding from it as many nonrheumatoid subjects as possible.

Even with these caveats, RF is neither specific nor diagnostic of RA. First, it is found in only 70%–85% of RA cases, while it can be detected in many other conditions, particularly in patients who have Sjogrën's syndrome. Also, RF screening tests can be positive in as many as 5% of apparently normal individuals, sharing the same V-region idiotypes (and by implication, the same V-region genes) as the antibodies detected in RA patients.

Physiological role of immunoglobulin antibodies. The finding of RF in normal individuals raises the concept that RF may have a normal, physiological role, such as to ensure the rapid removal of infectious antigen-antibody complexes from circulation. The synthesis of Ig antibodies in normal individuals follows some interesting rules:

- Ig antibodies are detected transiently during anamnestic responses to common vaccines, and in these cases, are usually reactive with the dominant Ig isotype of the antibodies produced in response to antigenic stimulation.
- Ig antibodies are also found in relatively high titers in diseases associated with persistent formation of antigen-antibody complexes such as subacute bacterial endocarditis, tuberculosis, leprosy, and many parasitic diseases.
- The titers of vaccination-associated RF follow very closely the variations in titer of the specific antibodies induced by the vaccine; similarly, the levels of RF detected in patients with infections associated with persistently elevated levels of circulating immune complexes decline once the infection has been successfully treated. In contrast, in patients with RA where the yet unknown triggers persist, the Ig antibodies remain high indefinitely.
- Infection-associated RF binds to IgG molecules whose configuration has been altered as a consequence of binding to exogenous antigens. The resulting RF-IgG-Ag complexes are large and quickly cleared from circulation. The

adsorption of IgG to latex particles seems to induce a similar conformational alteration of the IgG molecule as antigen binding, and as a result, IgG-coated latex particles can also be used to detect this type of RF.

The transient nature of Ig antibodies in normal individuals suggests that the regulatory component of the immune system works to terminate their existence, whereas in patients with RA, either the regulatory feedback is weak, or the B-cell clones that produce the Ig antibodies do not respond to regulatory cues. Indeed, central and peripheral B-cell tolerance checkpoints are defective in patients with RA.

Phenotype of B-cell precursors of RF-producing plasmablasts. In both mice and humans, the B lymphocytes capable of differentiating into RF-producing plasmablasts express CD5 in addition to the classical B-cell markers, such as membrane IgM and IgD, CR2, CD19, and CD20. CD5 is expressed by less than 2% of the B lymphocytes of a normal individual and was first detected in patients suffering from very active RA. It is considered a marker characteristic of autoimmune situations.

Pathogenic role of rheumatoid factor and Ig antibodies. RF titers are highly variable in patients with RA and do not correlate with the activity of the disease. Yet, high titers of RF tend to be associated with a more rapid progression of the articular component and with systemic manifestations, such as subcutaneous nodules, vasculitis, intractable skin ulcers, neuropathy, and Felty's syndrome. Thus, the detection of RF in high titers in a patient with symptomatic RA is associated with a poor prognosis.

The pathogenic properties of RF are likely to be derived from the biological characteristics of the antibodies involved. Classical IgM RF activates complement via the classical pathway, and the ability of RF to fix complement is of pathogenic significance, because it may be responsible, at least in part, for the development of rheumatoid synovitis.

The source of the anti-Ig antibodies that are likely to play an important role in causing the arthritic lesions is predominantly the synovium of the affected joints. The joints are the principal sites of RF production in RA patients, and it should also be noted that in some individuals, the locally produced anti-Ig antibodies are of the IgG isotype.

When this is the case, the joint disease is usually more severe, because anti-IgG antibodies of the IgG isotype have a higher affinity for IgG than their IgM counterparts; consequently, they form stable immune complexes that activate complement very efficiently.

Seronegative RA. Some patients with RA may have negative results on the screening tests for RA. True seronegative RA cases exist, particularly among agammaglobulinemic patients. In spite of their inability to synthesize antibodies, these patients develop a disease clinically indistinguishable from RF-positive RA. This is a highly significant observation since it argues strongly against the role of the RF or other serologic abnormalities as a major pathogenic insult in RA and suggests that the inflammatory response in the rheumatoid joint could be largely cell mediated. In some instances, negative serologies in patients with RA are falsely negative, but some patients with seronegative RA may have antibodies against citrullinated proteins.

Anticollagen antibodies

Antibodies reacting with different types of collagen have been detected with considerable frequency in connective tissue diseases such as **scleroderma**. In RA, considerable interest has been stimulated by the finding that antibodies elicited by injection of type II collagen with complete Freund's adjuvant into rats are associated with the development of a rheumatoid-type disease. However, the frequency of these antibodies in RA patients has been recently estimated to be in the 15%–20% range, which is not compatible with a primary pathogenic role. It is probable that the anticollagen antibodies in RA arise as a response to the degradation of articular collagen that could yield immunogenic peptides.

Anticitrullinated protein antibodies

The recently described autoantibodies to citrullinated proteins such as filaggrin and its circular form (cyclic citrullinated peptide) are highly sensitive and specific for RA. Citrullinated proteins, mostly fibrins, are localized in the synovial tissue of patients with RA, and the corresponding antibodies are locally produced in the joints. Cyclic citrullinated peptide (CCP) antibodies have been proposed as a serologic marker for early diagnosis of RA. Also, CCP antibody levels seem to have prognostic prediction of joint destruction.

Antinuclear antibodies

Antibodies against native, double-stranded DNA are conspicuously lacking in patients with classical RA, but antibodies against single-stranded DNA can be detected in about one-third of the patients. The epitopes recognized by anti-ssDNA antibodies correspond to DNA-associated proteins. The detection of anti-ssDNA antibodies does not have diagnostic or prognostic significance because these antibodies are neither disease specific nor involved in immune complex formation.

The reasons for the common occurrence of anti-ssDNA in RA and in many other connective tissue diseases are unknown. However, these antibodies may represent an indicator of immune abnormalities due to the persistence of abnormal B-lymphocyte clones that have escaped the repression exerted by normal tolerogenic mechanisms and are able to produce autoantibodies of various types. Some of these antibodies are simply cross-reactive. Other patients may have antibodies against heat shock proteins, peptidyl arginine deaminase 4, glucose-6-phosphate and high-mobility group box 1.

GENETIC FACTORS IN RHEUMATOID ARTHRITIS

HLA associations

The incidence of familial RA is low, and only 15% of identical twins are concordant for the disease. However, 70%–90% of Caucasians with RA express the human leukocyte antigen (HLA) DR4 antigen that is found in about 15%–25% of the normal population. Individuals expressing this HLA-DR4 are 6–12 times more at risk of having RA, but HLA-DR1 was also found to increase susceptibility to RA, and wide fluctuations in the frequency of these markers are seen between different patient populations.

HLA-DR4 subtypes. DNA sequencing of the β chain of the DR4 and DR1 molecules defined 5 HLA-DR4 subtypes: Dw4, Dw10, Dw13, Dw14, and Dw15. While Dw4, Dw10, Dw13, and Dw15 differ from each other in amino acid sequence at positions 67, 70, and 74 of the third hypervariable region of the β1 domain of the β chain, Dw4 and Dw14 have identical amino acid sequences at these positions and are associated with RA. The same amino acids are present in the Dw1 subtype of HLA-DR1. The prevalence of Dw4, Dw14, or Dw1 in the general population is 42%. Of these individuals, 2.2% develop RA. In contrast, the frequency of RA in individuals negative for these markers is only 0.17%, a 12.9-fold difference. Since most humans are heterozygous, a given individual may inherit more than one susceptibility allele. Individuals having both Dw4 and Dw14 have a much higher risk (seven to one) of developing severe RA. In contrast, individuals with the Dw10 and Dw13 markers, whose sequence differs in the critical residues (Table 19.2), seem protected against RA.

The interpretation of these findings hinges on the fact that amino acids 67–74 are located on the third hypervariable region of the DR4 and DR1 β chains. This region is part of a helical region of the peptide-binding pouch of the DRβ chain that interacts both with the side chains of antigenic peptides and with the T-cell receptor (TCR). Its

Table 19.2 HLA-DR subtypes and rheumatoid arthritis

Subtype	Critical residues on the third diversity region of β1				Predisposition to rheumatoid arthritis
	67	70	71	74	
DRB1*0101 (Dw1)	L	Q	R	A[a]	+
DRB1*0401 (Dw4)	L	Q	K	A	+
DRB1*0404 (Dw14)	L	Q	R	A	+
DRB1*0403 (Dw13)	L	Q	R	E	−
DRB1*0402 (Dw10)	I	D	E	A	−

[a] A, Ala; D, Asp; E, Glu; I, IsoLeu; K, Lys; L, Leu; Q, Gln; R, Arg.

configuration, rather than the configuration of any other of the hypervariable regions of the DR4 and DR1 β chains, seems to determine susceptibility or resistance to RA, depending on the charge of amino acids located on critical positions. In the case of Dw1 and Dw14, the sequence of the 70–74 motif is identical (QRRAA), while the homologous sequence in Dw4 (QKRAA) shows one single substitution (a basic arginine by an equally basic lysine). In contrast, the sequence of the same stretch of amino acids in protective alleles shows a higher degree of divergence. In Dw10 aspartic acid and glutamic acid replace the first two amino acids (glutamine and arginine or lysine), resulting in a total change in the charge and affinity of the peptide-binding pouch. In the case of Dw13, glutamic acid replaces alanine at position 74, again resulting in a marked charge difference relative to Dw1, 4, and 14.

It has been postulated that the structure of those DR4 and DR1 molecules that are associated with increased risk for the development of RA is such that they bind very strongly an "arthritogenic epitope" derived from an as-yet unidentified agent. Bacterial antigens, including heat-shock proteins, microbial or viral (e.g., Epstein–Barr virus [EBV]) proteins, as well as autologous proteins such as type II collagen or cartilage glycoprotein gp39 have been proposed as candidate sources for these peptides. The consequence of the binding of immunogenic peptides would be a strong and prolonged immune response that would be the basis of the inflammatory response in the joints. Obviously, the predominant localization of the inflammatory reaction to the periarticular tissues implies that the level of expression of the peptides in question must be higher in those tissues. The reverse would be the case for those DR4 molecules associated with protection against the development of RA.

Supporting this interpretation are several observations concerning the severity of the disease in patients bearing those HLA antigens and subtypes. For example, DR4 positivity reaches 96% in patients suffering from Felty's syndrome, the most severe form of the disease. More recent studies showed that RA patients who are DR4-Dw14 positive have a faster progression to the stages of pannus formation and bone erosion.

Genome-wide association studies (GWASs) have revealed linkage, besides the HLA genes, with many genes including *PTPN22, PADI4, CTLA4,*

STAT4, TRAF1, TNFAIP3, CD40, and others. It should be noted that several of the loci identified through GWASs have also been linked to other autoimmune diseases.

IMMUNOLOGICAL FACTORS IN PATHOGENESIS OF RHEUMATOID ARTHRITIS

Cell-mediated immunity abnormalities in rheumatoid arthritis

It is accepted that cell-mediated immune mechanisms play the main pathogenic role in RA. This conclusion is based on studies performed in the synovial fluid and on the hypertrophic synovium of the rheumatoid joints, both easily accessible to study by needle biopsy or aspiration. All of the essential cellular elements of the immune response are present in the joint, and the main challenge is to reconstitute the sequence of events that leads to the progressive destruction of joint tissues. A simplified summary of the interactions between immune cells that are believed to play a pathogenic role is illustrated in Figure 19.1.

The critical role of T lymphocytes. Immunohistologic studies of the inflammatory infiltrates of the synovial membrane show marked lymphocytic predominance (lymphocytes may represent up to 60% of the total tissue net weight). Among the lymphocytes infiltrating the synovium, CD4+ helper T lymphocytes outnumber CD8+ lymphocytes in a ratio of 5:1. The critical pathogenic role for Th lymphocytes is suggested by two important observations:

- RA is associated with specific DR alleles, and it is well accepted that major histocompatibility complex II (MHC-II) molecules present immunogenic peptides to Th lymphocytes.
- Increased concentrations of many lymphocyte-released cytokines are measurable in the synovial fluid, probably reflecting the activated state of infiltrating lymphocytes.

Most of the infiltrating CD4+ lymphocytes have the phenotype of a terminally differentiated memory helper T cell (CD4+, CD45RO+), which represent 20%–30% of the mononuclear cells in the synovium. They also express class-II MHC, consistent with chronic T-cell activation, but only 10%

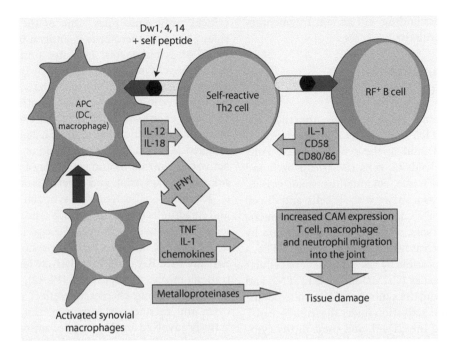

Figure 19.1 Pathogenesis of rheumatoid arthritis. In this diagram it is postulated that Th2 lymphocytes play the central role in the sequence of events that leads to the activation of synovial macrophages, which is the main effector system mobilized by this Th subpopulation. Not shown in the diagram is the role of rheumatoid factor as the mediator for complement and neutrophil-mediated articular and extra-articular inflammation.

express CD25, suggesting that they do not proliferate actively in the synovial tissues.

Synovial T cells express markers of activation (CD44, HLA-DR), but they cannot be stimulated further *in vitro*. The levels of the CD3ζ protein, important in CD3/TCR signaling, are decreased in T cells in the synovial fluid in RA patients. While IL17-producing T cells (Th17) are present in the synovial fluid, it is unclear whether the remaining T lymphocytes are Th1 or Th2. T cells in RA patients and particularly those found in the synovial fluid produce less interleukin-2 (IL-2) and IFNγ, whereas they produce more IL-1 tumor necrosis factor α (TNFα) and IL-10, all of which contribute to the inflammatory process.

Tregs (expressing FoxP3) have been considered to display limited function and to allow the inflammatory process to proceed uninhibited.

A variety of chemokines (RANTES, MIP1-α, MIP1-β, and IL-8), most of them produced by lymphocytes, can also be detected in the synovial fluid. These chemokines are probably responsible for the attraction of additional T lymphocytes, monocytes, and neutrophils to the rheumatoid joint.

T cells in the RA synovium also express CD40L, and are therefore able to deliver costimulating signals to B cells and dendritic cells (see discussion later in chapter).

A significant question that remains unanswered is, "What is the nature of the stimulus responsible for the activation of the T lymphocytes found in the synovial infiltrates?" Studies of the TCR Vβ genes expressed by the infiltrating T lymphocytes have shown that the repertoire is limited, i.e., only some T-cell clones appear to be activated, and the same clones are found in several joints of the same patient. An even more restricted profile was observed when the analysis was confined to the antigen-binding area of the Vβ chain (the CDR3 region). These findings suggest that antigenic stimulation through the TCR plays a critical role.

The long-term goal of these approaches, to identify the actual targets of the immune attack, remains elusive at this time. A major obstacle is our limited knowledge about the immunogenic peptides recognized by different TCR Vβ region families. Until some breakthrough happens in that area, our understanding will remain fragmentary and highly speculative.

Antigen presentation and dendritic cells

The autoimmune response that underlies the pathogenesis of RA is mostly localized to the synovial tissue and fluid in the synovial space. Fully differentiated dendritic cells (DCs) can be found in the synovial tissue, surrounding small vessels, and in close association with T cells and B-cell follicles. These DCs appear to be derived from circulating precursors, attracted to the synovium by chemokines such as MIP-1α, MCP, and RANTES, a process made possible by the expression of cellular adhesion molecules (CAMs) induced by TNF and IL-1. On reaching the synovium, DCs undergo differentiation and activation under the influence of T cells expressing the CD40L and some of the cytokines present in high concentrations in the synovial fluid, such as GM-CSF, TNF, and IL-1. Their differentiation in the synovium seems associated with an increased ability to present self-antigen, and, therefore, to stimulate autoimmune responses. Activated and differentiated DCs are also known to secrete IL-18, which, as discussed later, has pro-inflammatory activity, synergizes with IL-12 in the expansion of Th1 cells, and induces the synthesis and release of interferon-γ by activated Th1 cells.

B cells as local amplifiers of the autoimmune response

B cells expressing RF on their membrane can be found in the synovium of chronically inflamed joints. These RF+ B cells can bind immune complexes by the Fc portion of the antibodies, a process that results in B-cell activation and peptide presentation to T cells. In this role as antigen-presenting cells (APCs), RF+ B cells can activate multiple T-cell clones recognizing a wide variety of endogenous and exogenous peptides internalized as IC. Thus, RF+ B cells amplify intra-synovium immune responses and contribute to the exacerbation of the local inflammatory process.

Multiple roles of synovium macrophages

The synovial infiltrates are rich in activated monocytes, macrophages, and macrophage-derived synoviocytes that are believed to play several critical pathogenic roles. One of the significant roles played by these cells is antigen presentation to CD4+ lymphocytes. It is not unusual to see macrophage-lymphocyte clusters in the inflamed synovial tissue, and in those clusters, CD4+ lymphocytes are in very close contact with large macrophages expressing high levels of class-II MHC antigens. In addition, IL-12 and IL-18 mRNA and secreted IL-12 and IL-18 are found at biologically active concentrations and could play an important role in Th2 expansion and differentiation.

The other critical role of synovial monocytes and macrophages is to induce and perpetuate local inflammatory changes. Several lines of evidence support this role. First, the synovial fluid of patients with RA contains relatively large concentrations of phospholipase A2 (PLA2), an enzyme that has a strong chemotactic effect on lymphocytes and monocytes. Moreover, this enzyme is actively involved in the metabolism of cell membrane phospholipids, particularly in the early stages of the cyclooxygenase pathway, which leads to the synthesis of eicosanoids such as PGE2, one of a series of pro-inflammatory mediators generated from the breakdown of arachidonic acid. Thus, it is possible that these high levels of PLA2 reflect a hyperactive state of infiltrating macrophages engaged in the synthesis of PGE2 and other eicosanoids. Other factors locally released by activated macrophages include transforming growth factor-β (TGF-β), GM-CSF, and IL-18.

TGF-β further contributes to the predominance of Th2 activity over Th2 activity at the inflammatory sites.

GM-CSF induces the proliferation of several cell types in the monocyte-macrophage family, including DCs. It has been suggested that this overproduction of GM-CSF by all CD4 cells (macrophages and T lymphocytes) is responsible for the relatively large number of DCs found in the inflammatory lesion. This is a significant finding, because activated DCs release a variety of pro-inflammatory lymphokines, such as IL-1. Another prominent role of GM-CSF is to be a very strong inducer of the expression of MHC-II molecules (stronger than interferon-γ). Increased MHC-II expression is believed to be an important factor leading to the development of autoimmune responses and could help perpetuate a vicious circle of anti-self immune response by facilitating the persistent activation of Th2 cells and, consequently, the stimulation of synovial cells, monocytes, and DCs.

Interleukin-18, in addition to promoting differentiation of Th2 cells in synergism with IL-12, promotes the synthesis of interferon-γ, thus contributing indirectly to macrophage activation. In addition, mononuclear cells activated by IL-18 release GM-CSF, TNF, and prostaglandin E2, and show increased expression of inducible nitric oxide synthase. Therefore, IL-18 can be classified as a pro-inflammatory cytokine.

Matrix metalloproteinases are also secreted by activated macrophages, including collagenase, elastase, stromelysin, matrylisin, and gelatinase B, particularly when stimulated with IL-1 and TNF-α. Studies of biopsies of the rheumatoid synovium previously discussed found these two cytokines at levels high enough to deliver such stimulatory signals to monocytes and fibroblasts. The subsequent release of metalloproteinases is believed to have a primary role in causing tissue damage in the inflamed joints.

SUMMARY OVERVIEW OF PATHOGENESIS OF RHEUMATOID ARTHRITIS

Predisposing factors

Two important types of factors seem to have a strong impact in the development of RA.

Genetic factors. The link to HLA-DR4, and particularly with subtypes Dw4 and Dw14, as well as with the structurally related Dw1 subtype of HLA-DR1, was previously discussed in this chapter. It is currently accepted that such DR subtypes may be structurally fitted to present a peptide to autoreactive or cross-reactive helper T lymphocytes, thus precipitating the onset of the disease.

Hormonal factors. The role of hormonal factors is suggested by two observations:

- RA is three times more frequent in females than in males, predominantly affecting women from 30 to 60 years of age.
- Pregnancy produces a remission during the third trimester, sometimes followed by exacerbation after childbirth.

These observations suggest that hormonal factors may have a significant effect on the development of RA. However, to this day, the responsible factors have not been defined. A possible mechanism by which pregnancy would cause an improvement in the clinical picture has recently been suggested by the observation that estrogens potentiate B lymphocyte responses *in vitro*. This increased B-cell activity is likely to reflect a shift of predominant Th activity from Th1 to Th2, which is considerably less pro-inflammatory.

Precipitating factors

Three main mechanisms responsible for the escape from tolerance that must be associated with the onset of RA have been proposed:

- Decreased activity of downregulating T cells
- Nonspecific B-cell stimulation by microbial products (e.g., bacterial lipopolysaccharide) or infectious agents (e.g., viruses)
- Stimulation of self-reactive T lymphocytes as a consequence of the presentation of a cross-reactive peptide (possibly of infectious origin) by an activated APC (e.g., DC or RF+ B cell)

The genetic linkages discussed earlier in this chapter support the last theory. Also, the key role of T lymphocytes is supported by histological data (discussed earlier) and by the observations that HIV infection and immunosuppression for bone marrow transplantation, two conditions that depress T-helper lymphocyte function very profoundly, are associated with remissions of RA.

Environmental factors are presumed to contribute to disease development through epigenetic mechanisms or the formation of insulting autoantigens. For example, smoking has been shown to promote the formation of citrullinated proteins.

What are initiating factors of RA?

Although our understanding of the basic immune abnormalities and self-perpetuating circuits involved in RA has become more complete, there is considerable uncertainty about the factor(s) that may be responsible for the initiation of the disease. There is also very little knowledge about the factors that localize the disease to the joints in the initial stages. For example, there is experimental evidence supporting a critical role of DC, probably by promoting autoreactive T-cell activation, but there is no logical way to explain how the DC would be initially activated and localized to the synovial tissue. There are observations in animal models suggesting that arthritis can develop in the absence of autoreactivity to joint antigens, a model that could explain the association with infections such as those caused by *Proteus mirabilis* and EBV. What this model fails to provide is an explanation for the localization of the ensuing autoimmune reaction to the joints. In addition, the MHC molecules linked to RA appear to be able to recognize peptides derived from joint tissue proteins. If this is proven to be unquestionably the case, what remains to be explained is what triggers the initial activation of APCs in the joints to an extent that the recognition of self-peptides takes place in an environment conducive to the development of an immune response rather than maintaining the normal state of anergy.

THERAPY

Although we still do not have a complete understanding of the disease, we have made significant progress toward helping patients with RA to retain joint function and live normal lives. In addition, many of the complications of the disease (that is involvement of extra-articular tissues) have practically vanished. The current dogma is to treat the disease early (as early as possible), treat aggressively, and treat to target, that is, adjust the dose of the use drug so that the patient does not have any symptoms. Interestingly, the criteria for the diagnosis of the disease have become looser, allowing early diagnosis at the risk of false diagnosis.

Nonsteroidal anti-inflammatory drugs

The nonsteroidal anti-inflammatory drugs (NSAIDs) group includes, among others, aspirin, ibuprofen, naproxen, indomethacin, and the recently introduced COX-2 inhibitors. These compounds have as a common mechanism of action the inhibition of the cyclooxygenase pathway of arachidonic acid metabolism, which results in a reduction of the local release of prostaglandins. Their administration is beneficial in many patients with RA. Patients are advised of possible side effects, including upper gastrointestinal bleeding and hypertension.

Glucocorticoids

In more severe cases, in which the NSAIDs are not effective, glucocorticoids are indicated. However, the use of glucocorticoids in RA raises considerable problems, because in most instances, their administration masks the inflammatory component only as long as it is given. Thus, glucocorticoid therapy needs to be maintained for long periods of time at doses exceeding 20 mg/day, exposing the patient to very serious side effects, including muscle and bone loss that may become more devastating than the original arthritis.

Disease-modifying drugs

A variety of potent drugs have been used in attempts to reduce the intensity of the autoimmune reaction and/or the consequent inflammatory reaction and attenuate the clinical manifestations of the disease. This group includes a series of drugs that seems mainly to have anti-inflammatory effects, such as hydroxychloroquine, sulfasalazine, and a group of cytotoxic/immunosuppressive drugs that include methotrexate, azathioprine, chlorambucil, cyclophosphamide, leflunomide, and cyclosporine A. All of these agents have side effects, some more severe than others. Among those, methotrexate, administered in low weekly doses, is not associated with long-term side effects while controlling the inflammatory component of the disease and delaying the appearance of the chronic phase. The use of methotrexate in conjunction with hydroxychloroquine and sulfasalazine (triple therapy) has been found equally effective as the expensive biologics with minimal side effects.

Biological response modifiers

Considerable interest has been devoted in recent years to the use of biological response modifier (BRM) agents (discussed in detail in Chapter 24). Two basic types of BRMs have been used: those that try to suppress activated T-cell populations and those that have the neutralization of pro-inflammatory cytokines as their major mechanism of action. To date, there has been very limited success with BRMs targeting activated T cells, while the opposite has been true with BRMs that downregulate the effects of proinflammatory cytokines. Among the latter, recombinant humanized TNF-blocking antibodies and a recombinant form of a soluble TNF receptor have been most successful in clinical trials and have received U.S. Food and Drug Administration (FDA) approval. During the past 10 years or so, many additional biologics have been approved by the FDA, including B-cell depletors (rituximab), IL-1 inhibitors, and costimulatory molecule inhibitors (CTLA4-Ig). All biologics are used in conjunction with methotrexate or alone. Interestingly, at least a third of patients do not respond to each of the biologics. Still, biologic developers have not availed information to determine who among the patients will and will not respond. This fact underlines the heterogeneity of the pathogenic processes that lead to the expression of RA.

Reinduction of tolerance

Attempts to reinduce tolerance to cartilage antigens postulated to be involved in the autoimmune response by feeding animal cartilage extracts to RA patients have yielded promising results. However, the clinical benefits reported so far have been observed in short-term studies, and research is necessary to determine if the benefits persist in the long run. Also, additional studies are needed to better define the mechanism(s) involved in oral tolerization.

BIBLIOGRAPHY

Catrina AI, Svensson CI, Malmström V, Schett G, Klareskog L. Mechanisms leading from systemic autoimmunity to joint-specific disease in rheumatoid arthritis. *Nat Rev Rheumatol.* 2017;13:79–86.

Deighton C, Criswell LA. Recent advances in the genetics of rheumatoid arthritis. *Curr Rheumatol Rep.* 2006;8:394–400.

McInnes IB, O'Dell JR. State-of-the-art: Rheumatoid arthritis. *Ann Rheum Dis.* 2010;69:1898–1906.

McInnes IB, Schett G. The pathogenesis of rheumatoid arthritis. *N Engl J Med.* 2011;365(23):2205–2219.

McInnes IB, Schett G. Pathogenetic insights from the treatment of rheumatoid arthritis. *Lancet.* 2017;389(10086):2328–2337.

Samuels J, Ng YS, Coupillaud C, Paget D, Meffre E. Impaired early B cell tolerance in patients with rheumatoid arthritis. *J Exp Med.* 2005;201:1659–1667.

Schett G, Elewaut D, McInnes IB, Dayer JM, Neurath MF. How cytokine networks fuel inflammation: Toward a cytokine-based disease taxonomy. *Nat Med.* 2013;19:822–824.

Shaw AT, Gravallese EM. Mediators of inflammation and bone remodeling in rheumatic disease. *Semin Cell Dev Biol.* 2016;49:2–10.

Singh JA, Saag KG, Bridges SL Jr et al. 2015 American College of Rheumatology guideline for the treatment of rheumatoid arthritis. *Arthritis Rheumatol.* 2016;68:1–26.

Terao C, Raychaudhuri S, Gregersen PK. Recent advances in defining the genetic basis of rheumatoid arthritis. *Annu Rev Genomics Hum Genet.* 2016;17:273–301.

20

Overview of hypersensitivity

GABRIEL VIRELLA

INTRODUCTION

The immune response of vertebrates has evolved as a mechanism to eradicate infectious agents that succeed in penetrating natural anti-infectious barriers. However, in some instances, the immune response can be the cause of disease, both as an undesirable effect of an immune response directed against an exogenous antigen, or as a consequence of an autoimmune reaction. These undesirable immune responses define what is known as hypersensitivity, i.e., an abnormal state of immune reactivity that has deleterious effects for the host. A patient with hypersensitivity to a given compound suffers pathologic reactions as a consequence of exposure to the antigen to which he or she is hypersensitive. The term *allergy* is often used to designate a pathological condition resulting from hypersensitivity, particularly when the symptoms occur shortly after exposure.

Hypersensitivity reactions can be classified as immediate or delayed, depending on the time elapsed between the exposure to the antigen and the appearance of clinical symptoms. They can also be classified as humoral or cell-mediated, depending on the arm of the immune system predominantly involved. A classification combining these two elements was proposed in the 1960s by Gell and Coombs, and although many hypersensitivity disorders may not fit well into their classification, it remains popular because of its simplicity and obvious relevance to the most common hypersensitivity disorders.

The **Gell and Coombs classification of hypersensitivity reactions** considers four types of hypersensitivity reactions. Type I, II, and III reactions are basically mediated by antibodies with or without participation of the complement system; type IV reactions are initiated by a cell-mediated reaction (see Table 20.1). While in many pathological conditions mechanisms classified in more than one of these types of hypersensitivity reactions may be operative, the subdivision of hypersensitivity states into four broad types aids considerably in the understanding of their pathogenesis.

TYPE I HYPERSENSITIVITY REACTIONS (IgE-MEDIATED HYPERSENSITIVITY, IMMEDIATE HYPERSENSITIVITY)

Historical overview

Much of our early knowledge about immediate hypersensitivity reactions was derived from

Table 20.1 General characteristics of the four types of hypersensitivity reactions as defined by Gell and Coombs

Type	Clinical manifestations	Lag between exposure and symptoms	Mechanism
I (immediate)	Anaphylaxis, asthma, urticaria, hay fever	Minutes	Homocytotropic Ab (IgE)
II (cytotoxic)	Hemolytic anemia, cytopenias, Goodpasture's syndrome	Variable	Complement-fixing/ opsonizing Ab (IgG, IgM)
III	Serum sickness, Arthus reaction, vasculitis	6 hours[a]	Immune complexes containing complement-fixing Ab (mostly IgG)
IV (delayed)	Cutaneous hypersensitivity, graft rejection	12–48 hours	Sensitized lymphocytes

[a] For the Arthus reaction.

studies in guinea pigs. Guinea pigs immunized with egg albumin frequently suffer from an acute allergic reaction upon challenge with this same antigen. This reaction is very rapid (observed within a few minutes after the challenge) and is known as an anaphylactic reaction. It often results in the death of the animal in anaphylactic shock. If serum from a guinea pig sensitized 7–10 days earlier with a single injection of egg albumin and adjuvant is transferred to a nonimmunized animal that is challenged 48 hours later with egg albumin, this animal develops an anaphylactic reaction and may also die in anaphylactic shock. Because hypersensitivity was transferred with serum, this observation suggested that antibodies play a critical pathogenic role in this type of hypersensitivity.

PASSIVE CUTANEOUS ANAPHYLAXIS

The passive transfer of hypersensitivity can be less dramatic if the reaction is limited to the skin. Passive cutaneous hypersensitivity was induced in nonsensitized animals by intradermal injection of serum from a sensitized donor. That serum contained homocytotropic antibodies that became bound to the mast cells in and around the area where serum was injected. After 24–72 hours, the antigen in question was injected intravenously, mixed with Evans blue dye. When the antigen reached the area of the skin where antibodies were injected and became bound to mast cells, a localized type I reaction took place, characterized by a small area of vascular hyperpermeability that resulted in edema and redness. When Evans blue was injected with the antigen, the area of vascular

hyperpermeability had a blue discoloration due to the transudation of the dye.

The **Prausnitz–Küstner reaction** is a reaction with a similar principle that was practiced in humans and yielded similar results that contributed to our understanding of the immediate hypersensitivity reaction.

Clinical manifestations of immediate hypersensitivity

A wide variety of hypersensitivity states can be classified as immediate hypersensitivity reactions. Some have a predominantly cutaneous expression (hives or urticaria), some affect the airways (hay fever, asthma), and others are of a systemic nature. The latter are often designated as anaphylactic reactions, of which anaphylactic shock is the most severe form.

The expression of anaphylaxis is species specific. The guinea pig usually has bronchoconstriction and bronchial edema as the predominant expression, leading to death in acute asphyxiation. In the rabbit, on the contrary, the most affected organ is the heart, and the animals die of right heart failure. In man, allergic bronchial asthma in its most severe forms closely resembles the reaction in the guinea pig.

Most frequently, human type I hypersensitivity has a localized expression, such as the bronchoconstriction and bronchial edema that characterize bronchial asthma, the mucosal edema in hay fever, and the skin rash and subcutaneous edema that define urticaria (hives). The factor(s) involved in determining the target organs that will be affected in different types of immediate hypersensitivity reactions are not well defined, but the route of exposure to the challenging antigen seems an important factor. For example, allergic (extrinsic) asthma and hay fever are usually associated with inhaled antigens, while urticaria is seen as a frequent manifestation of food allergy. However, the manifestations of food allergy are very diverse, and, in addition to hives, can include a variety of symptoms affecting different organs and systems (Table 20.2).

Systemic anaphylaxis is usually associated with antigens that are directly introduced into the systemic circulation, as in the case of hypersensitivity to insect venom or to systemically administered drugs, such as penicillin and, more recently, monoclonal antibodies. However, orally ingested seafood and peanuts can also elicit anaphylactic reactions. Systemic anaphylactic reactions in humans can present in diverse forms, affecting different organs and systems (Table 20.3). Cardiovascular involvement is associated with the highest mortality rates.

Atopy. Some individuals have an obvious tendency to develop hypersensitivity reactions. The term *atopy* is used to designate this tendency of some individuals to become sensitized to a variety of allergens (antigens involved in allergic reactions), including pollens, spores, animal dander, house dust, and foods. These individuals, when skin tested, are positive to several allergens, and successful therapy must take this multiple reactivity into account. A genetic background for atopy is suggested by the fact that this condition shows familial prevalence.

Table 20.2 Common manifestations of food allergy

Nausea

Diarrhea

Abdominal cramps

Pruritic rashes

Angioedema

Asthma/rhinitis

Vomiting

Hives

Laryngeal edema

Anaphylaxis

Table 20.3 Common clinical manifestations of anaphylaxis

- Cardiovascular
  - Tachycardia then hypotension
  - Shock: $\leq 50\%$ intravascular volume loss
  - Myocardial ischemia
- Lower respiratory
  - Bronchoconstriction
  - Wheezing
  - Cough
  - Shortness of breath
- Upper respiratory
  - Laryngeal/pharyngeal edema
  - Rhinorrhea

Source: Adapted from Fisher, M.M., *Anaesth. Intens. Care*, 14, 17–21, 1986.

Pathogenesis

Immediate hypersensitivity reactions are a consequence of the predominant synthesis of specific IgE antibodies by the allergic individual; these IgE antibodies bind with high affinity to the membranes of basophils and mast cells. When exposed to the sensitizing antigen, the reaction with cell-bound IgE triggers the release of histamine through degranulation, and the synthesis of leukotrienes C4, D4, and E4. (This mixture constitutes what was formerly known as slow-reacting substance of anaphylaxis [SRS-A].) These substances are potent constrictors of smooth muscle and vasodilators and are responsible for the clinical symptoms associated with immediate hypersensitivity (see Chapter 21). In recent years, it has been shown, mainly through animal studies, that interleukin (IL)-13, released by Th2 cells, can induce clinical manifestations of asthma independently of IgE and eosinophils. Thus, cell-mediated, IgE-independent mechanisms may also play a pathogenic role in type I hypersensitivity reactions, as also discussed in Chapter 21.

CYTOTOXIC REACTIONS (TYPE II HYPERSENSITIVITY)

This second type of hypersensitivity involves, in its most common forms, complement-fixing antibodies (IgM or IgG) directed against cellular or tissue antigens. The clinical expression of type II hypersensitivity reaction depends largely on the distribution of the antigens recognized by the responsible antibodies.

Autoimmune hemolytic anemia and other autoimmune cytopenias

Autoimmune hemolytic anemia, autoimmune thrombocytopenia, and autoimmune neutropenia (discussed in greater detail in Chapter 22) are clear examples of type II (cytotoxic) hypersensitivity reactions in which the antigens are unique to cellular elements of the blood. Autoimmune hemolytic anemia is the best understood of these conditions.

Patients with autoimmune hemolytic anemia synthesize antibodies directed to their own red cells. Those antibodies may cause hemolysis by two main mechanisms:

- If the antibodies are of the IgM isotype, complement is activated up to C9, and the red cells can be directly hemolyzed (intravascular hemolysis).
- If, for a variety of reasons, the antibodies (usually IgG) fail to activate the full complement cascade, the red cells will be opsonized with antibody (and possibly C3b) and are taken up and destroyed by phagocytic cells expressing $Fc\gamma R$ and C3b receptors (extravascular hemolysis).

Intravascular hemolysis is associated with release of free hemoglobin into the circulation (hemoglobinemia), which may be excreted in the urine (hemoglobinuria). Massive hemoglobinuria can induce acute tubular damage and kidney failure, usually reversible. In contrast, extravascular hemolysis is usually associated with increased levels of bilirubin, derived from cellular catabolism of hemoglobin. All hemolytic reactions usually lead to the mobilization of erythrocyte precursors from the bone marrow to compensate for the acute loss. This is reflected by reticulocytosis and, in severe cases, by erythroblastosis.

Goodpasture's syndrome. The classical example of a type II hypersensitivity reaction in which the antibodies are directed against tissue antigens is Goodpasture's syndrome. The pathogenesis of Goodpasture's syndrome involves the spontaneous emergence of basement membrane autoantibodies that bind to antigens of the glomerular and alveolar basement membranes. Those antibodies

are predominantly of the IgG isotype. Using fluorescein-conjugated antisera, the deposition of IgG and complement in patients with Goodpasture's syndrome usually follows a linear, very regular pattern, corresponding to the outline of the glomerular or alveolar basement membranes.

Two types of observations support the pathogenic role of basement membrane antibodies:

- Elution studies yield immunoglobulin-rich preparations that, when injected into primates, can induce a disease similar to human Goodpasture's syndrome.
- Goodpasture's syndrome recurs in patients who receive a kidney transplant, and the transplanted kidney shows identical patterns of IgG and complement deposition along the glomerular basement membrane.

Once antigen-antibody complexes are formed in the kidney glomeruli or in the lungs, complement will be activated and, as a result, C5a and C3a will be generated. These complement components are chemotactic for polymorphonuclear (PMN) leukocytes; C5a also increases vascular permeability directly or indirectly (by inducing the degranulation of basophils and mast cells). Furthermore, C5a can upregulate the expression of cell adhesion molecules of the CD11b/CD18 family in PMN leukocytes and monocytes, promoting their interaction with ICAM-1 expressed by endothelial cells, thus facilitating the migration of inflammatory cells into the extravascular space. In the extravascular space, PMN leukocytes will recognize the Fc regions of basement membrane–bound antibodies, as well as C3b bound to the corresponding immune complexes (ICs), and will release their enzymatic contents that include a variety of metalloproteinases including collagenases and plasminogen activator. Plasminogen activator converts plasminogen into plasmin, which in turn can split complement components and generate bioactive fragments, enhancing the inflammatory reaction. Collagenases and other metalloproteinases cause tissue damage (i.e., destruction of the basement membrane) that may eventually compromise the function of the affected organ.

The pathological sequence of events after the reaction of basement membrane antibodies with their corresponding antigens is indistinguishable from the reactions triggered by the deposition of soluble ICs or by the reaction of circulating antibodies with antigens passively fixed to a tissue, considered as type III hypersensitivity reactions.

Nephrotoxic (Masugi) nephritis. This experimental model of immunologically mediated nephritis, named after the scientist who developed it, is induced by injection of heterologous basement membrane antibodies into healthy animals. Those antibodies combine with basement membrane antigens, particularly at the glomerular level, and trigger the development of glomerulonephritis.

This experimental model has been extremely useful in demonstrating the pathogenic importance of complement activation and neutrophil accumulation. For example, if instead of complete antibodies, one injects Fab or F(ab')$_2$ fragments generated from basement membrane antibodies that do not activate complement, the accumulation of neutrophils in the glomeruli fails to take place and tissue damage will be minimal to nonexistent. Similar protection against the development of glomerulonephritis is observed when animals are rendered C3 deficient by injection of cobra venom factor prior to the administration of anti–basement membrane antibodies, or when those antibodies are administered to animals rendered neutropenic by administration of cytotoxic drugs or neutrophil antibodies.

IMMUNE COMPLEX–INDUCED HYPERSENSITIVITY REACTIONS (TYPE III HYPERSENSITIVITY)

In the course of acute or chronic infections, or as a consequence of the production of autoantibodies, antigen-antibody complexes (also known as immune complexes [ICs]) are likely to be formed in circulation or in tissues on which the pertinent self-antigens or microbial antigens are expressed or have been adsorbed. Both scenarios can lead to inflammatory changes that are characteristic of the IC diseases.

Circulating ICs are usually adsorbed to red cells and cleared by the phagocytic system. In most cases, this will be an inconsequential sequence of events, but in cases where there is massive formation of circulating ICs (e.g., serum sickness), the clearance capacity of the phagocytic system is exceeded, and inflammatory reactions can be

triggered by the deposition of those ICs in tissues. A simplified sequence of events leading to IC-induced inflammation is shown in Figure 20.1.

The *in situ* formation of ICs is a more likely scenario as far as triggering tissue inflammation in conditions other than serum sickness. The adsorption of circulating antigens of microbial origin or those released by dying cells to a variety of tissues seems to be a relatively common event. If the same antigens trigger a humoral immune response, IC formation may take place in the tissues where the antigens are adsorbed, in which case, clearance by the phagocytic system may become impossible. In fact, tissue-bound ICs are very strong activators of the complement system and of phagocytic cells, triggering a sequence of events leading to tissue inflammation virtually identical to that observed in cases of *in situ* immune reactions involving the reaction of tissue antigens with the corresponding antibodies.

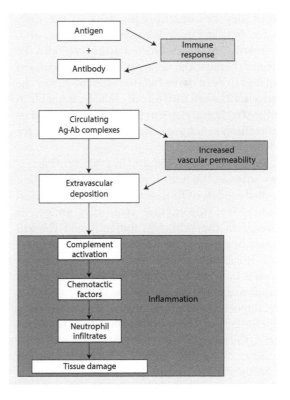

Figure 20.1 The sequence of events triggered by the deposition of soluble immune complexes that eventually results in inflammation and tissue damage.

Special manifestations of type III hypersensitivity

The Arthus reaction. Arthus, who observed that the intradermal injection of antigen into a previously sensitized animal results in a local inflammatory reaction, first described this reaction at the turn of the century. A human equivalent of this reaction can be observed in some reactions to immunization boosters in individuals who have already reached high levels of immunity.

The Arthus reaction is triggered by the combination of complement-fixing IgG antibodies (characteristically predominating in hyperimmune states in most species) and antigens immobilized in the extravascular space. The lag time between antigen challenge and the reaction is usually 6 hours, which is considerably longer than the time lag of an immediate hypersensitivity reaction, but considerably shorter than that of a delayed hypersensitivity reaction.

Arthus reactions are typically elicited in the skin. They are usually edematous in the early stages, but later may become hemorrhagic, and, eventually, necrotic. Deep tissues can also be affected, because the same pathogenic mechanisms can lead to deep tissue inflammation whenever the antigen, although intrinsically soluble, is unable to diffuse freely and remains retained in or around its penetration point (e.g., the perialveolar spaces for inhaled antigens).

Because it is easily induced in a variety of laboratory animals, the Arthus reaction is one of the best studied models of IC disease. Immunohistological studies have shown that soon after antigen is injected in the skin, IgG antibody and C3 will appear in perivascular deposits at the site of injection. This is followed by a massive influx of granulocytes, believed to result from activation of the complement system by the *in situ*-formed ICs. The importance of granulocytes was confirmed in experiments in which investigators tried to induce the Arthus in laboratory animals rendered neutropenic by administration of nitrogen mustard or antineutrophil serum. Under these experimental conditions, the inflammatory reaction is prevented, and the reaction does not develop.

In spite of their pathogenic role, granulocytes will actively engulf and catabolize the tissue-deposited ICs, eliminating the trigger for the inflammatory reaction. As the ICs are eliminated, the cellular infiltrate changes from a predominance of neutrophils and other granulocytes to a predominance of mononuclear cells, which is usually associated with the healing stage. The degree of healing depends on whether the exposure to the triggering antigen is a discrete event or repeated over time. Single or widely spaced exposure is usually followed by complete healing, while frequently repeated exposures tend to lead to irreversible damage.

Serum sickness. In the preantibiotic era, the treatment of rabies, bacterial pneumonia, diphtheria, and other infections involved the administration of heterologous antisera (usually obtained from horses) as a way to transfer immunity to the offending agents. In many instances, serotherapy appeared to be successful, and the patient improved, but a week to 10 days after the injection of heterologous antiserum, the patient developed what was termed as *serum sickness*—a combination of cutaneous rash (often purpuric), fever, arthralgias, mild acute glomerulonephritis, and carditis. Currently, serum sickness as a complication of passive immunotherapy with heterologous antisera is seen after injection of heterologous antisera to snake venom, after the administration of mouse monoclonal antibodies in cancer immunotherapy, and after the administration of heterologous (monoclonal or polyclonal) antilymphocyte sera in transplanted patients. But it can also be a side effect of some forms of drug therapy, particularly with penicillin and related drugs.

Serum sickness is extremely easy to reproduce in experimental animals through the injection of heterologous proteins. Basically, two types of experimental serum sickness can be induced:

- Acute, after a single immunization with a large dose of protein
- Chronic, after repeated daily injections of small doses of protein

While acute serum sickness is reversible, the chronic form, which closely resembles what is observed in human glomerulonephritis, is usually associated with irreversible tissue damage.

In all types of serum sickness, the initial event is the triggering of a humoral immune response, which explains the lag period of 7–10 days between the injection of heterologous protein (or drug) and the beginning of clinical symptoms. The lag period is shorter and the reaction more severe if there has been presensitization to the antigen in question.

As soon as antibodies are produced in sufficient amounts, they combine with the antigens (which at that time are still present in relatively large concentrations in the serum of the injected individual or experimental animal). Initially, the antigen-antibody reaction will take place in conditions of great antigen excess. The resulting complexes are too small to activate complement or be taken up by phagocytic cells and will remain in circulation without major consequences. As the immune response progresses and increasing amounts of antibody are produced, the antigen-antibody ratio will be such that intermediate-size ICs will be formed. The intermediate-size ICs are potentially pathogenic; they are large enough to activate complement and small enough to cross the endothelial barrier (particularly if vascular permeability is increased as a consequence of complement activation and release of C3a and C5a). Once they reach the extravascular space, inflammatory cells are recruited and activated and initiate the chain of events leading to tissue inflammation. As in the case of the Arthus reaction, the inflammatory changes associated with serum sickness do not take place or are very mild if complement or neutrophils are depleted.

The deposition of immune complexes can take place in different organs, such as the myocardium (causing myocardial inflammation), skin (causing erythematous rashes), joints (causing arthritis), and kidney (causing glomerulonephritis). Soluble immune complexes can also be absorbed by formed elements of the blood, particularly erythrocytes, neutrophils, and platelets. Although red blood cell (RBC) absorption is usually a protective mechanism, if the amounts and characteristics of RBC-absorbed ICs are such that the regulatory function of CR1 is overridden, hemolysis may take place. Thrombocytopenia and neutropenia can also result from the activation of the complement system by cell-associated ICs. Purpuric rashes due to thrombocytopenia are frequently seen in serum sickness.

DELAYED (TYPE IV) HYPERSENSITIVITY REACTIONS

In contrast to the other types of hypersensitivity reactions previously discussed, type IV or delayed hypersensitivity is a manifestation of cell-mediated immunity. In other words, this type of hypersensitivity reaction is due to the activation of specifically sensitized T lymphocytes rather than to an antigen-antibody reaction.

Tuberculin test as a paradigm of a type IV reaction

Intradermal injection of tuberculin or protein purified derivative (PPD) into an individual who has been previously sensitized (by exposure to *Mycobacterium tuberculosis* or bacillus Calmette-Guérin vaccination) is followed, 24 hours after the injection, by a skin reaction at the site of injection characterized by redness and induration. Histologically, the reaction is characterized by perivenular mononuclear cell infiltration, often described as "perivascular cuffing." Macrophages can be seen infiltrating the dermis. If the reaction is intense, a central necrotic area may develop. The cellular nature of the perivascular infiltrate, which contrasts with the predominantly edematous reaction in a cutaneous type I hypersensitivity reaction, is responsible for the induration.

Experimental studies

Experiments carried out with guinea pigs investigating the elements involved in transfer of delayed hypersensitivity were critical in defining the involvement of lymphocytes in delayed hypersensitivity. When guinea pigs are immunized with egg albumin and adjuvant, not only do they become allergic, as discussed earlier, they also develop cell-mediated hypersensitivity to the antigen. This duality can be demonstrated by passively transferring serum and lymphocytes from sensitized animals to unsensitized recipients of the same strain and challenging the passively immunized animals with egg albumin. The animals that received serum will develop an anaphylactic response immediately after challenge, while those that received lymphocytes will only show signals of a considerably less severe reaction after at least 24 hours have elapsed from the time of challenge.

Most of our knowledge about the pathogenesis of delayed hypersensitivity reactions derives from experimental studies involving contact hypersensitivity. Experimental sensitization through the skin is relatively easy to induce by percutaneous application of low-molecular-weight substances such as picric acid or dinitrochlorobenzene (DNCB). The initial application leads to sensitization. A second application will elicit a delayed hypersensitivity reaction in the area where the antigen is applied. In some cases, perhaps as a consequence of retention of the sensitizing substance in the dermis, a delayed reaction can be seen about 1 week after the contact. These instances may represent responses after primary sensitization.

Induction of contact hypersensitivity

The compounds used to induce contact hypersensitivity are not immunogenic by themselves. It is believed that these compounds couple spontaneously to an endogenous carrier protein, and as a result of this coupling, the small molecule will act as a hapten, while the endogenous protein will play the role of a carrier. A common denominator of the sensitizing compounds is the expression of reactive groups, such as Cl, F, Br, and SO_3H, which enable them to bind covalently to the carrier protein.

Spontaneous sensitization to drugs, chemicals, or metals, is believed to involve diffusion of the haptenic substance into the dermis, mostly through the sweat glands (hydrophobic substances appear to penetrate the skin more easily than hydrophilic substances), and once in the dermis, the haptenic groups will react spontaneously with "carrier" proteins to which they become covalently bound. By a pathway that has not been defined, antigen-presenting cells in the dermis (Langerhans cells, dendritic cells) take up the hapten-carrier conjugates and transport them to a draining lymph node, where a sensitizing peptide is presented in association with major histocompatibility complex (MHC)-II molecules to the CD4+ T lymphocytes in the environment. The predominant involvement of T lymphocytes in the antihapten responses of cutaneous expression is paradoxical if we consider that in most experimentally induced hapten-carrier responses, the hapten is recognized by B lymphocytes. Since the carrier protein is autologous and the T-cell receptors are not known to react with haptenic compounds, it seems likely that the reaction is triggered by a sensitizing peptide derived from an autologous protein carrier. The carrier protein is most likely modified as a consequence of the covalent binding of the sensitizing compound, which somehow must modify the configuration of an autologous peptide, rendering it immunogenic.

Effector mechanisms

The initial sensitization results in the acquisition of immunological memory. Later, when the sensitized individual is challenged with the same chemical, sensitized T cells will be stimulated into functionally active cells, releasing a variety of cytokines, which include IL-8, RANTES, and macrophage chemotactic proteins that attract and activate monocytes/macrophages, lymphocytes, basophils, eosinophils, and neutrophils. Other cytokines released by activated macrophages, particularly tumor necrosis factor (TNF) and IL-1, upregulate the expression of cell-adhesion molecules (CAMs) in endothelial cells, facilitating the adhesion of leukocytes to the endothelium, a key step in the extravascular migration of inflammatory cells. As a result of the release of chemokines and the upregulation of CAMs, a cellular infiltrate predominantly constituted by mononuclear cells, but also including granulocytes, forms in the area where the sensitizing compound has been reintroduced 24–48 hours after exposure. The tissue damage that takes place in this type of reaction is likely to be due to the effects of active oxygen radicals and enzymes (particularly metalloproteinases, collagenase, and cathepsins) released by infiltrating monocytes and tissue macrophages activated by the chemokines and other cytokines.

In severe cases, a contact hypersensitivity reaction may take an exudative, edematous, highly inflammatory character. The release of proteases from monocytes and macrophages may trigger the complement-dependent inflammatory pathways by directly splitting C3 and C5; C5a will add its chemotactic effects to those of chemokines released by activated mononuclear cells, and will also cause increased vascular permeability, a constant feature of complement-dependent inflammatory processes. It is not surprising, therefore, that a reaction which at the onset is cell mediated and associated to a mononuclear cell infiltrate, may, in time, evolve into a more classical inflammatory process with predominance of neutrophils and a more edematous character, less characteristic of a cell-mediated reaction.

Contact hypersensitivity in humans

Contact hypersensitivity reactions are observed with some frequency in humans due to spontaneous sensitization to a variety of substances (Figure 20.2):

- **Plant cathecols** (e.g., urushiol) are apparently responsible for the hypersensitivity reactions to poison ivy and poison oak.
- A variety of **chemicals** can be implicated in hypersensitivity reactions to cosmetics and leather.
- Topically used **drugs**, particularly sulfonamides, often cause contact hypersensitivity.
- **Metals** such as nickel can be involved in reactions triggered by the use of bracelets, earrings, or thimbles.

The diagnosis of contact hypersensitivity is usually based on a careful history of exposure to potential sensitizing agents and on the observation of the distribution of lesions that can be very informative about the source of sensitization. Patch tests using small pieces of filter paper impregnated with suspected sensitizing agents and taped to the back of the patient can be used to identify the sensitizing substance.

Jones-Mote reaction

Following challenge with an intradermal injection of a small dose of a protein to which an individual has been previously sensitized, a delayed reaction (with a lag of 24 hours), somewhat different than a classical delayed hypersensitivity reaction, may be seen. The skin appears more erythematous and less indurated, and the infiltrating cells are mostly lymphocytes and basophils, the latter sometimes predominating. The reaction has also been described, for this reason, as cutaneous basophilic hypersensitivity. Experimentally, it has been demonstrated that this reaction is triggered as a consequence of the antigenic stimulation of sensitized T lymphocytes.

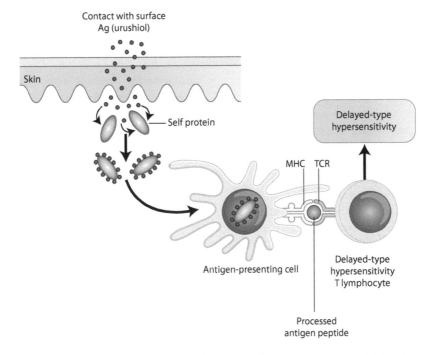

Figure 20.2 Poison ivy hypersensitivity is a manifestation of contact hypersensitivity that follows sensitization by topical drugs, cosmetics, or other types of contact chemicals. The causative agents, usually simple, low-molecular-weight compounds such as urushiol, found in poison ivy, poison oak, and other plants, are believed to behave as haptens. The development of sensitization depends on the penetrability of the agent and its ability to form covalent bonds with protein. Part of the sensitizing antigen molecule is thus represented by protein, usually the fibrous protein of the skin. The actual immunogen in contact hypersensitivity remains unidentified.

Homograft rejection

A most striking clinical manifestation of a delayed hypersensitivity reaction is the rejection of a graft. In classical chronic rejection, the graft recipient's immune system is first sensitized to peptides derived from alloantigens of the donor. After clonal expansion, activated T lymphocytes will reach the target organ, recognize the alloantigen-derived peptides against which they became sensitized, and initiate a sequence of events that leads to inflammation and eventual necrosis of the organ. This topic is discussed in detail in Chapter 25.

Systemic consequences of cell-mediated hypersensitivity reactions

Although type IV hypersensitivity reactions with cutaneous expression usually have no systemic repercussions, cell-mediated hypersensitivity reactions localized to internal organs, such as the formation of granulomatous lesions caused by chronic infections with mycobacteria, may be associated with systemic reactions. Cytokines released by activated lymphocytes and inflammatory cells play a major pathogenic role in such reactions. Proinflammatory cytokines, particularly IL-1, IL-6, and TNF, induce the release of prostaglandins in the hypothalamic temperature-regulating center and cause fever, thus acting as a pyrogenic factor. These cytokines can also cross-induce the others. For example, TNF can induce the release of IL-1 by endothelial cells and monocytes, and IL-1, in turn, can also induce the release of TNF. In addition, these cytokines activate the synthesis of acute-phase proteins (e.g., C-reactive protein) by the liver.

Prolonged release of TNF, in contrast, may have deleterious effects since this factor contributes to the development of cachexia. Cachexia develops because TNF inhibits lipoprotein lipase, and as a consequence, there is an accumulation of triglyceride-rich particles in the serum and a lack of the breakdown of triglycerides into glycerol and free fatty acids. This results in decreased incorporation of triglycerides into the adipose tissue and, consequently, a negative metabolic balance. The cells continue to break down stored triglycerides by other pathways to generate energy, and the used triglycerides are not replaced. Cachexia is often a preterminal development in patients with severe chronic infections or advanced malignancies.

BIBLIOGRAPHY

Cavani A. Breaking tolerance to nickel. *Toxicology*. 2005;209:119–121.

Dinarello CA. Review: Infection, fever, and exogenous and endogenous pyrogens: Some concepts have changed. *Innate Immunity*. 2004;10:201–222.

Graft DF. Insect sting allergy. *Med Clin North Am*. 2006;90:211–232.

Kavanaugh A. Adhesion molecules as therapeutic targets in the treatment of allergic and immunologically mediated diseases. *Clin Immunol Immunopathol*. 1996;80(3 part 2):S15–S22.

Larché M, Akdis CA, Valenta R. Immunological mechanisms of allergen-specific immunotherapy. *Nat Rev Immunol*. 2006;6:761–771.

Muller WA. Mechanisms of leukocyte transendothelial migration. *Annu Rev Pathol*. 2011;6:323–344.

Nagata M. Inflammatory cells and oxygen radicals. *Curr Drug Targets Inflamm Allergy*. 2005;4: 503–504.

Nangaku M, Couser WG. Mechanisms of immune-deposit formation and the mediation of immune renal injury. *Clin Exp Nephrol*. 2005;9:183–191.

Nankivell BJ, Chapman JR. Chronic allograft nephropathy: Current concepts and future directions. *Transplantation*. 2006;81:643–654.

Rael EL, Lockey RF. Interleukin-13 signaling and its role in asthma. *World Allergy Organ J*. 2011; 4:54–64.

Roychowdhury S, Svensson CK. Mechanisms of drug-induced delayed-type hypersensitivity reactions in the skin. *AAPS J*. December, 2005;7:E834–E846.

Schwiebert LM, Beck LA, Stellato C et al. Glucocorticosteroid inhibition of cytokine production: Relevance to antiallergic actions. *J Allergy Clin Immunol*. 1996;97:143–152.

Stone SF, Phillips EJ, Wiese MD, Heddle RJ, Brown SG. Immediate-type hypersensitivity drug reactions. *Br J Clin Pharmacol*. 2014;78:1–13.

Turnbull JL, Adams HN, Gorard DA. Review article: The diagnosis and management of food allergy and food intolerances. *Aliment Pharmacol Ther*. 2015;41:3–25.

Uzzaman A, Cho SH. Classification of hypersensitivity reactions. *Allergy Asthma Proc*. 2012;33(Suppl 1):96–99.

Vliagoftis H, Befus AD. Mast cells at mucosal frontiers. *Curr Mol Med*. 2005;5:573–589.

21

IgE-mediated (immediate) hypersensitivity

ALBERT F. FINN, JR. AND GABRIEL VIRELLA

INTRODUCTION

IgE-mediated hypersensitivity reactions are also known as immediate hypersensitivity reactions because of the short lag time (seconds to minutes) between antigen exposure and the onset of clinical symptoms. The initial symptoms of immediate hypersensitivity result from the release of pre-formed mediators stored in cytoplasmic granules of basophils and mast cells. The mediator release is triggered by the cross-linking of membrane-bound IgE with the corresponding antigen (also known as allergen, by being involved in allergic reactions).

MAJOR CLINICAL EXPRESSIONS

IgE-mediated allergic reactions can have a variety of clinical expressions, including anaphylaxis, asthma, urticaria (hives), and rhinitis (hay fever). Table 21.1 summarizes the morbidity and mortality data for the two most severe types of allergic reactions, anaphylaxis and asthma.

Anaphylaxis

Anaphylaxis is an acute systemic life-threatening IgE-mediated reaction usually affecting multiple organ systems. The time lag between exposure to the allergen and the onset of symptoms depends on the level of hypersensitivity and the nature of the antigen, intensity of exposure, and site of exposure to the antigen. In a typical case, symptoms begin within minutes after antigenic challenge. Generally, a latency longer than several hours after antigen exposure makes the diagnosis of anaphylaxis unlikely.

Multiple organ systems can be affected in anaphylactic reactions, including the skin (pruritus, flushing, urticaria, angioedema), respiratory tract (bronchospasm and laryngeal edema), and cardiovascular system (hypotension, cardiac arrhythmias, myocardial infarction).

As a rule, most of the acute manifestations subside within a few hours. However, similar symptoms of variable intensity may occur 6–12 hours later. This late-phase reaction results from cytokine release from activated basophils and mast cells, secondary immune cell activation, and further synthesis and release of mediators of inflammation.

When death occurs, it is usually due to laryngeal edema, intractable bronchospasm, hypotensive shock, or cardiac arrhythmias developing within the first few hours.

Table 21.1 Morbidity/mortality from systemic anaphylaxis and asthma in the United States

	Morbidity	Mortality
Systemic anaphylaxis		
All causes	50:100,000 persons/year	0.3–1.0 deaths million persons/year
Caused by insect bites	10:100,000 persons/year	10–80 per year
Asthma	More than 24 million persons	All ages:
	8.2% of all ages	1.7/100,000 per year
	9.6% of children	>65 years of age:
	7.7% of adults	10.5/100,000 per year

Atopy

Atopy is defined as a genetically determined state of IgE-related disease. Its most common clinical manifestations include rhinitis, asthma, and food allergy. Atopic dermatitis, although associated in about 75% of the cases with high IgE levels, is believed to be a consequence of Th2 and Tc2 cell activation resulting in the release of proinflammatory cytokines (IL-4, IL-5, IL-13, and IL-31).

Allergic asthma, by its potential severity and frequency, is one of the more important manifestations of atopy. However, not all cases of asthma are of proven allergic etiology. The differential characteristics of allergic (extrinsic) and nonallergic (intrinsic) asthma are summarized in Table 21.2. The major difference between both is the strong association of allergic asthma with demonstrable clinical allergy to relevant respirable allergens. These airborne allergens are inspired and reach the lower airways, where they cause chronic allergic inflammation.

Food allergies are common, can be caused by a variety of foodstuffs (Table 21.3), and have multiple clinical presentations (Table 21.4). Peanuts, tree nuts, and shellfish are often involved in the most severe reactions to food antigens, including anaphylactic reactions. Cow's milk, wheat, and egg are some of the more common food allergens. IgE-mediated allergic reactions to the galactose-α-1,3-galactose moiety that exists on proteins of nonprimate mammalian meat (beef, pork, lamb, etc.) following Lone Star tick (*Ambylomma americanum*) bite has become increasingly identified in the United States. It has been suggested that the tick may have previously bitten a nonprimate

Table 21.2 Characteristics of allergic (extrinsic) and nonallergic (intrinsic) asthma

	Allergic	Nonallergic
Symptoms	Shortness of breath and chest tightness with prolonged expiratory phase; may be associated with wheezing and cough	
Chest x-rays	Hyperlucency with increased AP distance (reflecting impaired expiratory capacity with air trapping), bronchial thickening	
Blood	Eosinophilia	Normal eosinophil count
Sputum	Eosinophilia	No eosinophils
Total IgE	Raised	Normal
Antigen-specific IgE	Raised	None
Pathology	Obstruction of airways due to smooth muscle hypertrophy with constriction and mucosal edema Hypertrophy of mucous glands Eosinophil infiltration	
Frequency		
	Children 80%[a]	20%
	Adults 60%[a]	40%

[a] Percentage of total number of bronchial asthma cases seen in each age range.

Table 21.3 **Common allergenic foods**

- Wheat
- Cow's milk
- Hen's eggs
- Legumes (peanuts and soybeans)
- Tree nuts (almonds, hazelnuts, walnuts, Brazil nuts, etc.)
- Mollusks (snails, mussels, oysters, scallops, clams, squid)
- Crustacea (shrimp, crawfish, lobster, etc.)
- Fish (cod, salmon, haddock, etc.)
- Nonprimate mammalian meat (beef, pork, lamb, etc.)

Table 21.4 **Clinical manifestations of food allergy**

- Flushing
- Pruritus (itching)
- Urticaria (hives) and angioedema (swelling)
- Stridor (laryngeal edema)
- Bronchospasm (wheezing)
- Abdominal cramps, nausea, vomiting, diarrhea
- Anaphylactic shock

mammal and could introduce a heterologous molecule in the human organism to facilitate the allergic reaction.

PATHOGENESIS

The pathogenesis of immediate hypersensitivity reactions involves a well-defined sequence of events:

- Induction of the adaptive immune response and synthesis of specific IgE antibodies.
- Binding of IgE antibodies to high-affinity $Fc_\varepsilon I$ receptors on basophils and mast cells. IgE remains affixed to the cell membrane and acts as an antigen receptor.
- Cross-linking of receptor-bound IgE by multivalent antigens. This initiates the release of preformed vasoactive compounds and the synthesis, and later release, of cytokines (e.g., IL-4, IL-5, IL-13) and other mediators of inflammation.
- The preformed substances released by basophils and mast cells have significant effects on target tissues, such as smooth muscle, vascular endothelium, and mucous glands. They also act as chemoattractants and may elicit central

nervous system–mediated reflexes (e.g., sneezing). Furthermore, activated basophils and mast cells can synthesize and release IL-4 and IL-13, and express the CD40 ligand. IL-4 synthesis and the expression of CD40L are both essential factors to stimulate IgE synthesis. The synthesis and release of IL-13 can facilitate processes that cause many of the symptoms associated with protracted allergic diseases, particularly chronic allergic asthma.

IgE antibodies

Prausnitz and Kustner published the first demonstration that serum contains a factor capable of mediating specific allergic reactions in 1921. The injection of serum from a fish-allergic person (Kustner) into Prausnitz's skin, and subsequent exposure of Prausnitz to fish antigen injected in the same site resulted in an allergic wheal and flare response.

In 1967, Ishizaka and collaborators isolated a new class of immunoglobulin, designated as IgE, from the serum of ragweed-allergic individuals. Several patients with IgE-producing plasmocytomas were subsequently discovered and provided a source of large amounts of monoclonal IgE that facilitated further studies of IgE structure and the production of anti-IgE antibodies.

IgE ANTIBODY RESPONSE

IgE is predominantly synthesized in perimucosal lymphoid tissues of the respiratory and gastrointestinal tract. In developing countries, the main antigenic stimuli for IgE synthesis are parasites (particularly nematodes). Levels of circulating IgE considered as normal in a developing country with endemic parasitism are two to three orders of magnitude higher than in the Western world. The vast majority of allergens, which are either ingested or inhaled, stimulate the same perimucosal cells. In the perimucosal tissues, only B lymphocytes with membrane IgE will differentiate into IgE-producing plasma cells. Those IgE-carrying B cells are only a small fraction of the total B-cell population in the submucosa but are overrepresented in the perimucosal lymphoid tissues compared to other lymphoid territories.

During the primary immune response to an allergen or a parasite, most of the IgE synthesized appears to be of low affinity. The changes occurring after a second exposure select out the synthesis of IgE of progressively higher affinity, probably as a consequence of somatic hypermutations and clonal selection. The expansion of affinity-optimized clones may be the reason why allergic reactions very seldom develop after the first exposure to an allergen. When an immediate hypersensitivity reaction appears to develop after what seems to be a first exposure to any given allergen, one must consider the possibility of cross-reaction between a substance to which the individual was previously sensitized and the substance that elicits the allergic reaction. Such cross-reactions are usually due to molecular mimicry and can be quite unpredictable.

Repeated exposures to parasites or allergens will stimulate the differentiation of memory cells, and the proportion of circulating high-affinity antigen-specific IgE will also increase with repeated exposures (Figure 21.1). In patients with severe seasonal allergies due to pollen, antigen-specific IgE may constitute up to 50% of the total IgE.

GENETIC CONTROL OF IgE SYNTHESIS

The study of total IgE levels in normal nonallergic individuals shows a distribution in three groups: high, intermediate, and low producers (Figure 21.2). Family studies further suggested that the ability to produce high levels of IgE is genetically controlled by gene loci independent of the HLA

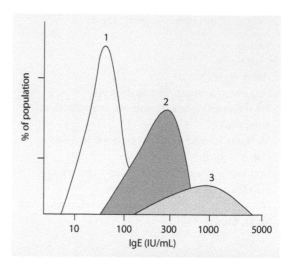

Figure 21.2 Distribution of IgE levels in a population of nonallergic individuals. Three subpopulations appear to exist: one constituted by low-responder individuals (1), one by high-responder individuals (3), and a third population of individuals with intermediate levels of IgE (2).

system. A candidate gene has been localized to chromosome 5(5q31-q33)—in close vicinity to the genes for IL-4, IL-5, and IL-13. The gene in question not only seems to influence the synthesis of IgE, but also determines bronchial hyperresponsiveness to histamine and other stimuli.

The tendency to develop allergic disorders in response to specific allergens is HLA linked. For instance, the ability to produce antigen-specific IgE after exposure to the Ra5 antigen of ragweed is observed more often in HLA B7, DR2 individuals than in the general population. Studies suggest that various major histocompatibility complex (MHC) class-II antigens are associated with high responses to many different allergens. The biological basis for the association between MHC-II molecules and the IgE-mediated allergic immune reaction is believed to be one of the many expressions of the control exerted by MHC-II–antigen presenting cells on the immune response. This theory is based on the assumption that the MHC-II repertoire determines what antigen-derived peptides are most efficiently presented to helper T cells. The genes controlling high IgE levels and high IgE antibody synthesis after exposure to allergens appear to have synergistic effects. For example, an HLA B7, DR2 individual who is also genetically predisposed to produce high levels of IgE may have

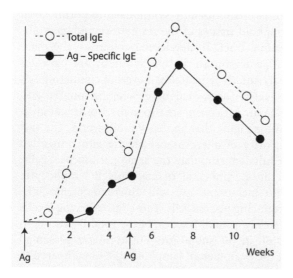

Figure 21.1 Longitudinal evolution of total IgE and antigen-specific IgE levels during an immune response to an allergen.

a more severe allergic disorder than an individual without this genetic combination.

T-B–cell cooperation in IgE antibody responses

The role of activated Th2 cells in type I IgE-mediated hypersensitivity reaction is critically important. Production of high levels of IgE has been shown to be dependent on the activation of IL-4–producing Th2 cells as well as on the delivery of coactivating signals involving CD28/CD80 and CD40/CD40L. IL-4 has been demonstrated to promote IgE synthesis by activated B lymphocytes. IL-5, which is produced at the same time by the same activated CD4 lymphocytes, is believed to play a role in the late phase of allergic reactions, which is discussed later in this chapter.

Both in humans and animal models, the production of allergen-specific IgE persists long after the second exposure. This may result from the capture of IgE-containing immune complexes by dendritic cells, which express the FcεRII (CD23). Membrane-bound immune complexes are known to persist for longer periods of time, constantly stimulating B cells and promoting the persistence of secondary immune responses and the differentiation of antibodies with increased affinity. At the same time, the internalization and processing of immune complexes containing the same antigen(s) and IgG antibody is likely to be the source of allergen-derived peptides that will continue to activate the Th2 subpopulation.

Interaction of IgE with cell surface receptors

Two types of Fc receptors reacting with IgE molecules have been characterized. A unique high-affinity receptor designated as Fc_ε-RI is expressed on the surface of basophils and mast cells. Most IgE antibodies interact with this receptor and become cell associated soon after secretion from plasma cells. This sequestration is partially responsible for the short, circulating half-life of IgE as a free molecule.

The structure of the Fc_ε-RI is unique among the characterized immune cell receptors. It is composed of three subunits: a heterodimer formed by the interaction of two chains (α and β), and a homodimer of a third type of chain (γ chain). The whole molecule is therefore designated as $\alpha\beta\gamma_2$ (Figure 21.3). The external domain of the α chain binds the Fc portion of IgE. The β and γ chains function as signal transduction units. Both of them contain immunoreceptor tyrosine-based activation motifs (ITAMs) (see Chapter 11). Cross-linking of the Fc_ε-RI results in activation of the protein kinase Lyn, which phosphorylates ITAM tyrosine residues, triggering a sequence of events that results in the activation of other protein kinases, such as Syk, as well as of the integral membrane linker molecule LAT. The phosphorylation of Syk and LAT is followed by activation of signaling cascades that eventually lead to the release of preformed granules and to the expression of a variety of genes coding for cytokines, enzymes, etc.

The interaction between the Fc_ε-RI and IgE is characterized by a very high affinity (association constants range from 10^8 to 10^{10} M^{-1}). Because of this high affinity, IgE binds rapidly and very strongly to cells expressing Fc_ε-RI and is released from these cells very slowly. Passively transferred IgE remains cell bound for several weeks in the skin of normal humans. IgE serves as an antigen receptor for mast cells and basophils. Receptor-bound IgE discriminates among antigens, binding exclusively those allergens to which the patient has become sensitized, but because the mast cells and basophils do not produce IgE molecules, there is no clonal restriction at the mast cell/basophil level.

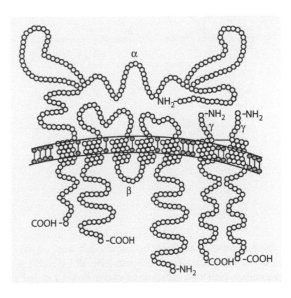

Figure 21.3 Primary structure of the Fcε-RI. (Modified from Metzger, H., *Clin. Exp. Allergy*, 21, 1, 1991.)

Therefore, if the patient produces IgE antibodies to more than one allergen, each basophil or mast cell may bind IgE antibodies of different specificities.

The interaction between one molecule of IgE and a single Fc_ε-RI does not result in cell activation, as there is no cross-linking of two IgE receptors simultaneously. The cross-linking of two IgE molecules affixed to two independent Fc receptors is essential for the induction of the release of intracellular mediators by basophils and mast cells (Figure 21.4). The physiological cross-linking agent is the allergen, which needs to be multivalent. Mast cells and basophils with IgE-anti-hapten antibodies on their membranes cannot be stimulated by soluble, univalent haptens, because those are unable to cross-link membrane IgE molecules. Cross-linking of receptor-bound IgE can also be induced with anti-IgE antibodies or with their divalent F(ab')2 fragments. Unoccupied receptors

may be cross-linked with aggregated Fc fragments of IgE. All of the types of cross-linking listed previously are equally efficient in activating IgE-carrying mast cells and basophils. Activation results in the release of granule contents into the extracellular compartment and activation of the synthesis of additional mediators.

Other receptors can be involved in basophil/mast cell activation, leading to the liberation of mediators. Basophils and mast cells also respond to C3a, C5a, basic lysosomal proteins, kinins, opioids, ionophores, and autoantibodies of the IgG isotype directed against the α subunit of the Fc_ε-RI. (These autoantibodies are detected in a large faction of the patients with chronic idiopathic urticaria.) It is apparent that there are multiple pathways for mast cell activation and that the participation of cell-bound IgE is not always needed.

A second receptor for IgE, Fc_ε-RII (CD23), is expressed on the membrane of lymphocytes, platelets, eosinophils, and dendritic cells and binds IgE with lower affinity than Fc_ε-RI. The role of Fc_ε-RII on dendritic cells has been previously discussed, and it is supposed to be involved in targeting eosinophils to parasites in one of the different variations of antibody-dependent cellular cytotoxicity; its role on platelets and lymphocytes is unclear.

Early and late phases in type I hypersensitivity

Early phase. After cross-linking of Fc receptor–associated IgE, mast cells and basophils undergo a series of biochemical and structural changes. The first change to be detected is the polymerization of microtubules, which is energy dependent (inhibited by 2-deoxyglucose), enhanced by the addition of 3–5 guanosine monophosphate (GMP), and inhibited by the addition of 3–5 adenosine monophosphate (AMP) and colchicine. The polymerization of microtubules allows the transport of the cytoplasmic granules to the cell membrane to which they fuse. This is followed by the release of the contents of the granules that contain a variety of preformed mediators (Table 21.5). *In vitro*, the sequence of events leading to the release of histamine, platelet-activating factor (PAF), and eosinophil chemotactic factor of anaphylaxis (ECFA) into the surrounding medium takes 30–60 seconds.

Histamine is the mediator responsible for many of the symptoms observed during the early phase

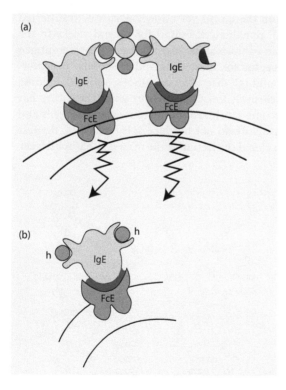

Figure 21.4 The conditions required for stimulation of mediator release by mast cells and basophils. (a) Reaction of membrane-bound IgE with a polyvalent antigen, leading to cross-linking of IgE molecules. This type of reaction leads to mediator release. (b) Reaction of membrane-bound IgE with a monovalent hapten. This reaction does not lead to mediator release.

Table 21.5 Mediators of immediate hypersensitivity produced by mast cells and basophils

Mediators	Structure	Actions
Stored		
Histamine	5-β-imidazolylethylamine (M.W. 111)	Smooth muscle contraction; increased vascular permeability; many others
Eosinophil chemotactic factors of anaphylaxis (ECF-A)	Acidic tetrapeptides (M.W. 360–390); Others (M.W. 500–3000)	Chemotactic for eosinophils
Proteolytic enzymes	Tryptase, chymase and other enzymes in human mast cells	Actions *in vivo* unknown, possibly include C' activation
Heparin	Acidic proteoglycan (M.W. ≈ 750,000)	Anticoagulant; C' inhibitor
Neutrophil chemotactic factor	Poorly characterized activity with M.W. >750,000	Chemotactic for neutrophils
Other granule proteins	Numerous poorly characterized peptides	*In vivo* significance not yet known
Newly synthesized (upon stimulation of mast cells or basophils)		
Slow-reacting substance of anaphylaxis (SRS-A)	Leukotrienes C4, D4, E4 (derived from arachidonic acid, M.W. 439–625)[a]	Smooth muscle contraction; increased vascular permeability; glandular hypersecretion
Prostaglandin D2	Cyclooxygenase product of arachidonic acid[b]	Smooth muscle contraction
Platelet-activating factor (PAF)	Phospholipid (M.W. 300–500)[c]	Platelet aggregation and release reaction; increased vascular permeability; eosinophil chemotaxis
Leukotriene B4	Eicosotetraenoate product of arachidonic acid (M.W. 336)	Chemotactic for eosinophils and neutrophils; neutrophil aggregation

[a] Also released by activated eosinophils.
[b] Produced exclusively by mast cells.
[c] Also stored as a preformed mediator.

of allergic reactions. Since the constricting effect of histamine on the smooth muscle lasts only 1 or 2 hours, this phase stops shortly after most of the granules have been emptied.

Platelet-activating factor (PAF), a phospholipid whose effects include platelet aggregation, chemotaxis of eosinophils, release of vasoactive amines, and increased vascular permeability (both due to a direct effect and to the release of vasoactive amines), is a second mediator involved in the early phase of the reaction. PAF is released by basophils, mast cells, neutrophils, and other cells. It may exist in preformed stores, but *de novo* synthesis is very rapid, so release takes place in a matter of seconds to a few minutes after cell stimulation.

Late phase. The cells remain viable after degranulation and proceed to synthesize other substances that will be released at a later time, causing the late phase of a type I hypersensitivity reaction. The mediators responsible for the late phase of the response are not detected until several hours after release of histamine and other preformed mediators. The long latency period between cell stimulation and detection of these mediators suggest that they are synthesized by mast cells after stimulation and/or by cells attracted by the previously mentioned chemotactic factors.

The main mediators involved in the late phase are the leukotrienes C4, D4, and E4 [LTC4, LTD4, LTE4]. This mixture of leukotrienes previously known as slow-reacting substance of anaphylaxis (SRS-A) reaches effective concentrations only 5 to 6 hours after challenge and have effects on target cells lasting for several hours. LTC4 and LTD4 are several-fold more potent than histamine in causing smooth muscle contraction, bronchovascular leak, and mucous hypersecretion in human bronchi.

Role of eosinophils in the late phase. Eosinophils are attracted to the site where an immediate hypersensitivity reaction is taking place by chemotactic factors released by basophils, mast cells, and Th2 lymphocytes, including the following:

- ECF-A and PAF, preformed chemotactic factors released during basophil or mast cell degranulation.
- Leukotriene B4, synthesized and released by stimulated basophils/mast cells.
- Interleukin-5, released by activated Th2 lymphocytes, mast cells, and eosinophils.

In many cases, the appearance of eosinophils signals the onset of internal negative feedback and control mechanisms that terminate the immediate hypersensitivity reaction. This effect is associated with the production and release of enzymes, particularly histaminase (which degrades histamine) and phospholipase D (which degrades PAF). Active oxygen radicals released by stimulated granulocytes, including eosinophils and perhaps neutrophils (which are also attracted by ECF-A and LTB4), cause the breakdown of leukotrienes. Histamine itself can contribute to the downregulation of the allergic reaction by binding to a type II histamine receptor expressed on basophils; the occupancy of this receptor leads to an intracellular increase in the level of cAMP, which inhibits further release of histamine (negative feedback).

In contrast, persistent eosinophil infiltrates are associated with intense inflammation that causes prolongation of symptoms. For example, asthmatic patients may develop a prolonged crisis during which the symptoms remain severe, and breathing becomes progressively more difficult, leading to a situation of increasing respiratory distress that can be refractory to the usual treatment.

In these patients, it is common to find very heavy peribronchial cellular infiltrates of the epithelium and lamina propria, with a prominent eosinophilic component, but containing also T lymphocytes, neutrophils, and plasma cells. The infiltrating lymphocytes are mostly activated CD4, $CD25^+$ T lymphocytes, whose cytokine mRNA pattern is typical of the Th2 subpopulation.

Three major cytokines released primarily by Th2 cells are believed to play significant roles in immediate hypersensitivity reactions, particularly in bronchial asthma:

- IL-4 is a critical factor in promoting Th2 cell differentiation, B-cell activation, and switch to IgE synthesis.
- IL-13, a cytokine related to IL-4, has been shown in experimental animal models to induce the pathophysiological features of asthma in an IgE and basophil-independent manner. It has also been shown that basophils also release this cytokine. These observations raise the interesting possibility that asthma symptoms may be triggered independently of the IgE-mediated pathway, and that activated Th2 cells may play a significant role in its pathogenesis (Figure 21.5).
- IL-5 released from the infiltrating activated Th2 lymphocytes seems to attract, retain, and activate eosinophils.
- IL-17, released by Th17 lymphocytes, is also involved in the pathogenesis of chronic inflammation in a variety of allergic disorders, including bronchial asthma.
- IL-25, of the IL-17 superfamily, IL-33, and thymic stromal lymphopoietin (TSLP) are several other cytokines elaborated by epithelial cells that contribute to allergic inflammation.

Activated eosinophils release leukotrienes and several toxic proteins: eosinophilic cationic protein (ECP), eosinophil-derived neurotoxin (EDN), eosinophil peroxidase (EPO), and major basic protein (MBP). ECP and MBP can cause ciliary dysfunction, bronchial epithelium injury, nonspecific bronchial hyperresponsiveness, and cellular denudation. This is believed to be a critical step in the pathogenesis of chronic airways inflammation that after decades may lead to chronic obstructive pulmonary disease with irreversible remodeling of the airways.

The severity of the clinical symptoms in an immediate hypersensitivity reaction is directly related to the amount of mediators released and produced, which in turn is determined by the number of "sensitized" cells stimulated by the antigen. The expression of early and late phases can be discriminated clinically. In the case of a positive immediate reaction elicited by a skin test, the

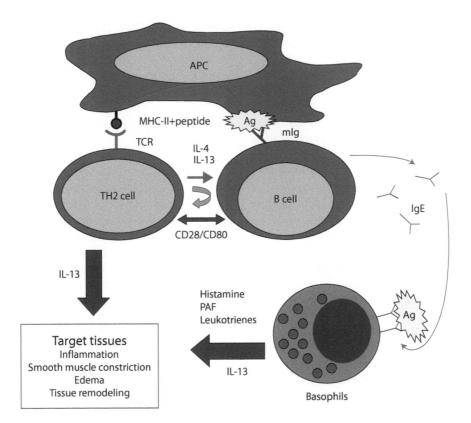

Figure 21.5 Representation of the pathways involved in immediate hypersensitivity. The classical pathway involves recognition of the allergens by B cells, synthesis of IgE antibodies favored by the predominant release of IL-4 and IL-13 released by activated Th2 cells. The IgE antibodies bind to high-affinity receptors on basophils and mast cells, and when cross-linked by the sensitizing antigen as a consequence of an ulterior exposure, degranulate and release histamine and other mediators, including IL-13. The IL-13 released by activated Th2 cells can also stimulate inflammatory cells in target tissues, inducing the same general symptoms of hypersensitivity without participation of histamine.

early phase resolves in 30–60 minutes, and the late phase generally peaks at 6–8 hours and resolves at 24 hours. In the case of an IgE-mediated asthma crisis, the early phase is characterized by shortness of breath, wheeze, and nonproductive cough and lasts 4–5 hours. If the exposure to the responsible airborne allergen is very intense, life-threatening bronchospasm may develop. With less intense or chronic exposure, the initial symptoms of wheezing and cough will linger for a few hours. Thereafter, the cough may produce sputum, and the dyspnea can become progressively less responsive to bronchodilators, signaling the onset of the late phase during which the airway obstruction may become more severe. In very severe cases, death may occur at this late stage because of intractable airway obstruction resulting from marked peribronchial inflammation associated with diffuse cellular infiltration of the airway mucosa and increased mucous secretion.

DIAGNOSTIC TESTS FOR IMMEDIATE HYPERSENSITIVITY

IgE levels and immediate hypersensitivity

The total IgE concentration, even in allergic individuals, is extremely low and generally not detectable by most routine assays used for the assay of IgG, IgA, and IgM. The concentration of specific IgE antibody to any given allergen is a very small fraction of the total IgE. The assay of such low concentrations became possible with the development of highly sensitive immunoassays. IgE levels are usually determined by solid-phase immunoassays.

A typical setup consists of absorbing a monoclonal anti-IgE antibody to solid phase (usually the wells of microtiter plates), wash, add calibration standards and samples with unknown concentrations of IgE, incubate, wash the unbound proteins, and then add a second IgE antibody labeled with an enzyme or with a fluorescent compound. When using enzyme-labeled antibodies, after adequate incubation, wash, and add a substrate that develops color when exposed to the enzyme-labeled antibody (Figure 21.6). After another period of incubation, stop the reaction and then measure color intensity in all samples, standards and controls. If a fluorescent-labeled antibody is used, measure the intensity of fluorescence instead. To determine the concentration of IgE in the patient's samples, the readings obtained from the standards with known IgE concentrations are used to establish a calibration curve. The results of IgE assays are expressed in nanograms/mL (1 ng $= 10^{-6}$ mg), or in International Units (1 IU $=2.5$ ng/mL); 180 IU/mL is considered as the upper limit for normal adults. Allergic individuals often have

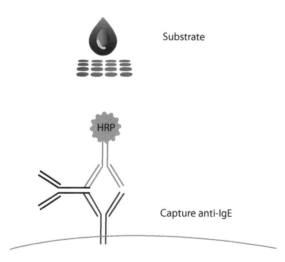

Figure 21.6 General principles of a capture enzymoimmunoassay for IgE quantitation. An immobilized anti-IgE antibody will bind IgE in the samples tested. After washing unbound proteins, an identical amount of enzyme-labeled antibody (in this diagram the enzyme is horseradish peroxidase, HRP) is added to every sample and allowed to bind to the captured IgE molecules. After the unbound labeled antibody is washed out, a substrate that is activated by HRP and generates color is added. The intensity of the color is directly proportional to the amount of captured IgE.

elevated levels of IgE. However, some asymptomatic individuals may also have elevated IgE levels. Therefore, a diagnosis of immediate hypersensitivity cannot be based solely on the determination of abnormally elevated IgE levels.

Assays for specific IgE antibodies

The **radioallergosorbent test (RAST)**, diagrammatically summarized in Figure 21.7, was the first solid-phase radioimmunoassay that determined antigen-specific IgE, which from the diagnostic point of view is considerably more relevant than the measurement of total serum IgE levels. In brief, a given allergen (ragweed antigen, penicillin, β-lactoglobulin, etc.) is covalently bound to polydextran beads. A patient's serum is added to beads coated with a single antigen; the antigen-specific IgE, if present, will bind to the immobilized antigen. After washing off unbound immunoglobulins, radiolabeled anti-IgE is added. The amount of bead-bound radioactivity counted after washing off unbound labeled antibody is directly related to the concentration of antigen-specific IgE present in the serum. This test has also been replaced by nonisotopic antigen-specific IgE assays that follow the same principle but use enzyme-labeled anti-IgE antibodies.

Skin tests. Although the antigen-specific IgE assays are helpful screening tests, they are expensive and may lack clinical specificity and sensitivity. Further, the range of antigens for which there are available tests is limited. The alternative method for diagnosis of specific allergies is provocation skin tests, which allow testing to a wide array of antigens. Although positive skin tests depend on the existence of allergen-specific IgE antibodies, they do not allow a direct quantitative assay of such antibodies; rather, they provide clinical information about their ability to mediate the hypersensitivity reaction in an individual patient.

The skin tests for immediate hypersensitivity are performed by introducing small amounts of purified allergens percutaneously or intradermally in known patterns. The patients are then observed for about 30 minutes to 1 hour. Classical IgE-mediated hypersensitivity reactions present as a wheal and flare at the site of the allergen exposure, which develops in a matter of minutes. In highly sensitized individuals, there is always a risk of anaphylaxis, even after minimal challenge.

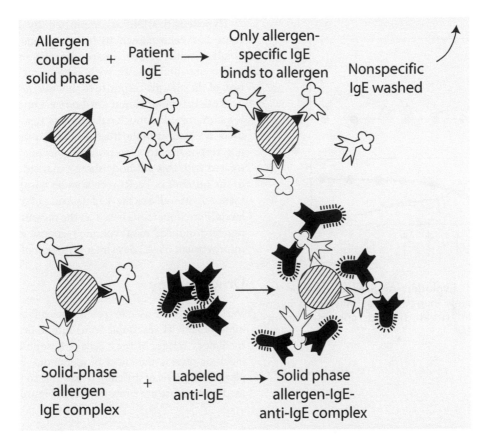

Figure 21.7 General principles of the radioallergosorbent test (RAST) for quantitation of specific IgE antibodies.

Because of this risk, trained professionals should always perform these tests in a properly equipped clinical facility.

PREVENTION AND THERAPY

Prevention

Environmental control, trying to prevent exposure to the allergen, is possible for individuals sensitized to a limited number of allergens; however, it cannot be easily achieved by individuals sensitized with multiple or ubiquitous allergens.

Hyposensitization (systemic allergen immunotherapy) is the standard of care in individuals with clinical insect venom IgE-mediated hypersensitivity and has beneficial results in patients suffering from seasonal pollen allergy (i.e., tree, grass, and weed pollen) and perennial allergies (i.e., dust mites, cat dander). Hyposensitization is achieved by subcutaneous injection of very small

quantities of the sensitizing antigen, starting at the nanogram level, and increasing the dosage on a weekly basis. This induces the production of IgG blocking antibodies, and an increase in the number of regulatory cells able to turn off the production of IgE antibodies, as reflected by a decline of serum IgE levels. Because both effects tend to be simultaneous, they appear to correlate with a decrease of the allergic symptoms (Figure 21.8). Conceptually, blocking antibodies of the IgG class in the systemic vascular and interstitial compartments should have a protective effect by combining with the antigen before it reaches the cell-bound IgE. In fact, a significant clinical improvement correlates better with an increase in blocking IgG than with a decrease in antigen-specific IgE. Recent observations suggest the shifting of regulatory lymphocytes (T4-helper) from a Th2 profile to a Th1 profile following hyposensitization with expected shifting of respective cytokine profiles from IL-4, IL-13 to IFN-γ.

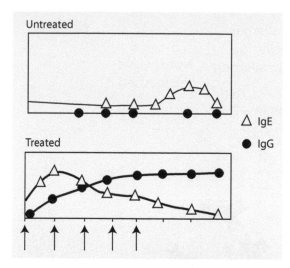

Figure 21.8 Evolution of allergen-specific IgE and IgG levels in patients submitted to hyposensitization (treated) and control patients (untreated).

Hyposensitization accomplished by the oral route has been shown to be efficacious as well. Small amounts of allergen are administered via the oral route sublingually, with subsequent attenuation of the allergic response to that allergen.

Anti-IgE monoclonal antibodies. Omalizumab is a humanized monoclonal antibody that has been used successfully in the treatment of chronic asthma not responsive to conventional therapy. Patients treated with this antibody show a marked decrease in the number of FcεRI receptors on basophils and mast cells as well as a marked decrease of serum IgE levels. Functional tests based on the measurement of ragweed-induced nasal volume response also show improvement 35–42 days after initiation of therapy.

Drug therapy

Various drugs are used to treat or prevent immediate hypersensitivity reactions. Some inhibit or decrease mediators' release by mast cells or basophils; others block or reverse the effect of mediators. The complex interactions of different drugs able to influence mediator release are summarized in Figure 21.9.

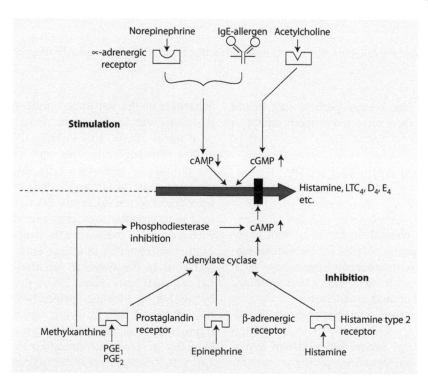

Figure 21.9 Major pathways leading to stimulation and inhibition of mediator-release by basophils and mast cells. (Modified from David, J., Rocklin, R.E. In: Rubinstein, E., Federman, D.D., eds., *Scientific American Medicine*, Section 6, Chapter IX, Scientific American, Inc., New York, 1983.)

TREATMENT OF IGE-MEDIATED ALLERGIC DISEASE

Limited allergic processes (seasonal rhinitis [hay fever] and perennial rhinitis) respond to antihistaminic compounds (oral and topical), which compete with histamine in binding to their type I receptors at the target cell level. Oral leukotriene antagonists block the effects of leukotrienes (see the next section). Topical corticosteroids can be directly employed to address the inflammation seen in nasal passages.

Systemic reactions (anaphylaxis) to foods, drugs, or insect stings often require very aggressive and urgent measures, particularly the administration of epinephrine (see the next section). Further, progression to anaphylactic shock can require more extensive resuscitative efforts if cardiovascular collapse ensues.

TREATMENT OF ALLERGIC ASTHMA

Bronchial asthma presents very complex therapeutic problems. Current therapy is based on the understanding that an initial acute bronchoconstrictive attack is followed by progressive inflammation in the airways and increased bronchial responsiveness. Each phase requires a different treatment. Relief of bronchoconstriction is the therapeutic goal of β-adrenergic agonists, methylxanthines, and anticholinergic compounds.

β-adrenergic receptor agonists (epinephrine, isoproterenol, and albuterol) increase cAMP levels by stimulating membrane adenylcyclase directly, inhibiting further degranulation of mast cells and basophils. As stated earlier, epinephrine is the drug of choice for treatment of severe allergic reactions such as anaphylaxis. Patients at risk of developing anaphylactic reactions are advised to carry a portable pressurized injecting device able to deliver a therapeutic dose of epinephrine by intramuscular injection. Epinephrine causes vasoconstriction with an increased heart rate, as well as bronchodilation. This results in an improvement in cardiovascular and respiratory function. However, the use of β-adrenergic receptor agonists in allergic asthma is limited by the fact that these compounds do not affect eosinophils, so that when patients have significant peribronchial eosinophilic inflammation, administration of β-agonists will have diminishing benefits. The patient will have a tendency to increase their use to try to achieve symptomatic relief. But since eosinophils and other immune cells are unaffected, the inflammation progresses and can reach a stage at which the patient is at risk of death or near death. A patient's increasing need for β-agonists should be considered an ominous sign of worsening lower airway inflammation.

Methylxanthines (e.g., theophylline) block phosphodiesterases, leading to a persistently high intracellular level of cAMP, which in turn inhibits histamine release. However, recent studies have led to question this interpretation because the levels of serum methylxanthine reached during the treatments are much lower than those needed to inhibit phosphodiesterases. Additionally, the required monitoring of blood levels due to their side effects and toxicity has diminished their regular use.

Anticholinergic drugs. Most cholinergic agents, raising intracellular levels of cyclic GMP, have an enhancing effect on mediator release: their use must be avoided in asthmatic patients since they aggravate the symptoms. On the opposite side, anticholinergic drugs that block vagal cholinergic tone may be useful but are not as efficient as β-agonists for acute bronchodilation.

In persistent asthma, treatment needs to focus on the chronic inflammatory reaction no longer responding to the agents useful for treatment in the early phase. Therefore, the treatment's goals are quite different and will include inhaled corticosteroids and cromolyn, as well as oral leukotriene-modifying drugs.

Glucocorticoids are anti-inflammatory drugs. They have no direct action on IgE synthesis or mast cell degranulation in the lung but strongly inhibit eosinophil degranulation and the elaboration of proinflammatory cytokines. Thus, the administration of corticosteroids inhibits the progression of the late phase and can indirectly reduce bronchial hyperresponsiveness. These effects can be achieved safely through administration by inhalation, delivering small intrabronchial concentrations that result in local anti-inflammatory effects with low daily doses. This lessens the risk of systemic side effects previously incurred with chronic systemic (oral or parenteral) administration. Glucocorticoids administered by inhalation are now recommended for the treatment of chronic persistent asthma. Systemic administration of glucocorticoids is reserved for the treatment of severe acute episodes, trying to prevent the development of the severe late-phase reactions, or for the treatment of severe recalcitrant inflammatory asthma.

Disodium cromoglycate (cromolyn) and nedocromil sodium, not shown in Figure 21.9, are examples of prophylactic drugs. Their mechanism of action is still unclear; however, it is believed that these drugs attenuate mast cell degranulation. Objectively, they decrease bronchoconstriction and have benefit, though limited, in helping to reduce the needs for glucocorticoids.

Leukotriene-modifying drugs are being employed in the treatment of asthma. These agents include lipoxygenase enzyme inhibitors, which downregulate the production of leukotrienes (zileuton), and leukotriene receptor antagonists that block the effects of leukotrienes (montelukast, zafirlukast). Presently they are used in mild forms of asthma, exercise-induced bronchospasm, or as adjuncts to inhaled glucocorticoids.

Monoclonal antibodies directed against molecular targets of the IgE-mediated inflammatory process have shown benefit in the treatment of allergic diseases. Omalizumab (anti-IgE mab) has the potential to interfere with the IgE-mediated mechanisms contributing to the pathogenesis of allergic asthma. It is administered systemically and patients require monitoring for adverse reactions. Possible reactions that may occur include local reactions at the site of injection and systemic reactions such as life-threatening anaphylaxis.

Anti-IL5 and anti-IL5 receptor antibodies are systemic agents aimed at the eosinophilic contribution to the allergic inflammatory process. These monoclonal antibodies are directed at the IL5 molecule directly (mepolizumab, reslizumab) or to its receptor (benralizumab). In both cases, disruption of the IL5-mediated eosinophil recruitment and activation is thought to attenuate the cellular inflammatory component seen in a subpopulation of asthmatics.

In patients with atopic dermatitis, anti-IL-31 monoclonal antibodies (nemolizumab, tralokinumab) and dupilumab, a monoclonal antibody that blocks the IL-4Rα receptor subunit shared by the receptor of both IL-4 and IL-13, are currently being evaluated with preliminary encouraging results.

BIBLIOGRAPHY

Abramovits W. Atopic dermatitis. *J Am Acad Dermatol.* 2005;53(Suppl. 1):S86–S93.

Chiricozzi A, Peroni P, Girolomoni G. Testing biologics and intracellular signaling inhibitors on pediatric atopic dermatitis: A stairway to modern therapeutic approaches. *Expert Opin Investig Drugs.* 2018;27:699–707.

Chiu AM, Kelly KI. Anaphylaxis: Drug allergy, insect stings, and latex. *Immunol Allergy Clin North Am.* 2005;25:389–405.

Commins SP, Satinover SM, Hosen J et al. Delayed anaphylaxis, angioedema, or urticaria after consumption of red meat in patients with IgE antibodies specific for galactose-α-1,3-galactose. *J Allergy Clin Immunol.* 2009;123:426–433.

D'Amato G. Role of anti-IgE monoclonal antibody (omalizumab) in the treatment of bronchial asthma and allergic respiratory diseases. *Eur J Pharmacol.* 2006;533:302–307.

Gupta RK, Gupta K, Dwivedi P. Pathophysiology of IL-33 and IL-17 in allergic disorders. *Cytokine Growth Factor Rev.* 2017;38:22–36.

Haitchi HM, Holgate ST. New strategies in the treatment and prevention of allergic diseases. *Expert Opin Investig Drugs.* 2004;13:107–124.

Hofmann MA, Kiecker F, Zuberbier T. A systematic review of the role of interleukin-17 and the interleukin-20 family in inflammatory allergic skin diseases. *Curr Opin Allergy Clin Immunol.* 2016;16:451–457.

Kubo M. Mast cells and basophils in allergic inflammation. *Curr Opin Immunol.* 2018;54:74–79.

Legendre DP, Muzny CA, Marshall GD, Swiatlo E. Antibiotic hypersensitivity reactions and approaches to desensitization. *Clinical Infectious Diseases.* 2014;58:1140–1148.

Li XM. Beyond allergen avoidance: Update on developing therapies for peanut allergy. *Curr Opin Allergy Clin Immunol.* 2005;5:287–292.

Lieberman P, Nicklas RA, Randolph C, Oppenheimer J. Anaphylaxis—A practice parameter update 2015. *Ann Allergy Asthma Immunol.* 2015;115:341–384.

Moorman JE, Rudd RA, Johnson CA et al. National surveillance for asthma—United States, 1980–2004. *MMWR Surveill Summ.* 2007;56:1–54.

Napolitano M, Marasca C, Fabbrocini G, Patruno C. Adult atopic dermatitis: New and emerging therapies. *Expert Rev Clin Pharmacol.* 2018;11:867–878.

National Asthma Education and Prevention Program. Expert panel report 3: Guidelines for the diagnosis and management of asthma-summary report 2007. *J Allergy Clin Immunol.* 2007;120(5 Suppl):S94–S138.

Poole JA, Matangkasombut P, Rosenwasser LJ. Targeting the IgE molecule in allergic and asthmatic diseases: Review of the IgE molecule and clinical efficacy. *J Allergy Clin Immunol.* 2005; 115:S376–S385.

Romano A, Torres MJ, Castells M, Sanz ML, Blanca M. Diagnosis and management of drug hypersensitivity reactions. *J Allergy Clin Immunol.* 2011;127:S67–S73.

Salvi SS, Krishna MT, Sampson AP, Holgate ST. The anti-inflammatory effects of leukotriene-modifying drugs and their use in asthma. *Chest.* 2001;119:1533–1546.

Sampson HA, Aceves S, Bock SA et al. Food allergy: A practice parameter update-2014. *J Allergy Clin Immunol.* 2014;134:1016–1025.

Strupka E, de Shazo R. Asthma in seniors, Part I: Evidence for underdiagnosis, undertreatment and increasing morbidity and mortality. *Am J Med.* 2007;122:6–11.

Tejedor Alonso MA, Moro-Moro M, Mugica-Garcia MV. Epidemiology of anaphylaxis. *Clin Exp Allergy.* 2015;45:1027–1039.

Wheatley LM, Togias A. Clinical practice—Allergic rhinitis. *N Engl J Med.* 2015;372:456–463.

Wills-Karp M, Luyimbazi J, Xu X et al. Interleukin-13: Central mediator of allergic asthma. *Science.* 1998;282:2258–2261.

Yssel H, Groux H. Characterization of T cell subpopulations involved in the pathogenesis of asthma and allergic diseases. *Int Arch Allergy Immunol.* 2000;121:10–18.

Zahran HS, Bailey C, Garbe P. Vital signs: Asthma prevalence, disease characteristics, and self-management education: United States, 2001–2009. *MMWR Morb Mortal Wkly Rep.* 2011;60: 547–552.

22

Immunohematology

GABRIEL VIRELLA AND ARMAND GLASSMAN

INTRODUCTION: BLOOD GROUPS

ABO system

The first human red cell antigen system to be characterized was the ABO blood group system. Specificity is determined by the terminal sugar in an oligosaccharide backbone structure. The terminal sugars of the oligosaccharides defining groups A and B are immunogenic. In group O, the precursor H oligosaccharide is not immunogenic. The red cells express A, B, both A and B, or neither, and antibodies are found in serum to antigens not expressed, as shown in Table 22.1.

The ABO group of a given individual is determined by testing both cells and serum. The subject's red cells are mixed with serum containing a known antibody, and the subject's serum is tested against cells possessing a known antigen. For example, the cells of a group A individual are agglutinated by anti-A serum but not by anti-B serum, and this serum agglutinates type B cells but not type A cells. The typing of cells as group O is done by exclusion. (A cell not reacting with anti-A or anti-B is considered to be of blood group O.)

The anti-A and anti-B isoagglutinins are synthesized as a consequence of cross-immunization with enterobacteriaceae that have outer-membrane oligosaccharides strikingly similar to those that define the A and B antigens. For example, a newborn with group A blood will not have anti-B in his or her serum, since it has had no opportunity to undergo cross-immunization. When the newborn's intestine is eventually colonized by the normal microbial flora, the infant will start to develop anti-B but will not produce anti-A because of his or her tolerance to his or her own blood group antigens (see Table 22.1).

The inheritance of the ABO groups follows simple Mendelian rules; with three common allelic genes: A, B, and O (A can be subdivided into A_1 and A_2), of which any individual will carry two, one inherited from the mother, and one from the father. The ABO system is the most important blood system for consideration in transfusion medicine as incompatible transfusions can result in immediate and fatal transfusion reactions.

Rh system

In the late 1930s, it was discovered that the sera of most women who gave birth to infants with hemolytic disease of the newborn contained an antibody that reacted with the red cells of their infants and with the red cells of 85% of Caucasians. A year later it was discovered that a reagent produced by

Table 22.1 The ABO system

Red cell antigen	Serum isoagglutinins	Blood group
A	Anti-B	A
B	Anti-A	B
A and B	None	AB
None	Anti-A and -B	O

injecting blood from the monkey *Macacus rhesus* into rabbits and guinea pigs agglutinated Rhesus red cells and appeared to have the same specificity as the neonatal antibody. Individuals whose cells reacted with the reagent were termed Rh-positive (for the Rhesus monkey); those whose cells were not agglutinated were termed Rh-negative. The Rh system is the second most important blood system in transfusion medicine.

Antigens of the Rh system. The Rh system is now known to have many antigens in addition to the one originally described, and several nomenclature systems were developed. For practical purposes, the **Fisher-Race** nomenclature is now used almost exclusively. Fisher and Race originally postulated that the Rh gene complex is formed by combinations of three pairs of allelic genes: *Cc, Dd, Ee.* This was later modified to a model that proposed a single genetic locus with three sub-loci. The possible combinations are as follows: *Dce, DCe, DcE, DCE, dce, dCe, dcE,* and *dCE.* Thus, a *DCe/DcE*

individual can only pass *DCe* or *DcE* to his offspring and no other combination. The original antigen discovered is called **D** and people who possess it are called **Rh-positive**. The allele "**d**" has never been discovered, so the symbol "d" is used to denote the absence of **D**. All individuals lacking the D antigen are termed **Rh-negative**. The most frequent genotype of D-negative individuals is *dce/dce*.

Recent studies analyzing DNA from donors of different Rh phenotypes have found that there are neither three loci nor one locus governing Rh but that there are two structural loci governing Rh in Rh(D)-positive individuals and only one present in Rh-negative persons. Therefore, one gene appears to encode the D protein, and the other governs the presence of the C, c, E, and e antigens.

Other blood groups

Several other blood group systems with clinical relevance have been characterized. Most transfusion reactions other than those caused by clerical error are due to alloimmunization to antigens of the Kell, Duffy, and Kidd systems, of which the Kell system is the most polymorphic. Occasionally, antibodies to these antigens may cause hemolytic disease of the newborn. Most cases of autoimmune hemolytic anemia involve autoantibodies directed to public antigens (antigens common to most, if not all, humans), such as the I antigen or core Rh antigens.

Table 22.2 Characteristics of some common blood group antigens and antibodies

Blood group	Antigen structure	Usual antibodies	Clinical significance	
			HTR	HDN
ABO	Carbohydrate	Anti-A, -B	Yes	Yes (Mild)
Rh	Protein	Anti-D, E, c	Yes	Yes
Kell	Protein	Anti-K	Yes	Yes
Kidd	Protein	Anti-Jk^a,-Jk^b	Yes	Few
Duffy	Glycoprotein	Anti-Fy^a,-Fy^b	Yes	Yes
MNS	Glycoprotein	Anti-M	Few	Few
P	Carbohydrate	Anti-P$_1$	Rare	No
Lewis	Carbohydrate	Anti-Le^a,-Le^b	Few	No
I	Carbohydrate	Autoanti-I	No^a	No*

Abbreviations: HTR, hemolytic transfusion reaction; HDN, hemolytic disease of the newborn.

* The clinical significance of anti-I antibodies relates to a special form of autoimmune hemolytic anemia, known as cold agglutinin disease.

There are over 200 blood group antigens in addition to those of the ABO and Rh systems. Some of the most important blood groups are seen in Table 22.2. Blood group antigenic determinants are either carbohydrate or protein in nature. Upon exposure to foreign carbohydrate antigens, IgM antibodies are predominantly produced, while IgG antibodies predominate after immunization to protein-borne blood group antigens. Some blood groups have known associated biological functions such as the Duffy glycoprotein that is the receptor for *Plasmodium vivax*, which causes malaria. The Duffy glycoprotein also has recently been shown to be a chemokine receptor able to bind both C-X-C and C-C chemokines, and for this reason has been renamed as Duffy antigen receptor for chemokines. Its function on the mature red cell membrane is not known. Another known function of some blood groups is transport. The Kidd protein is the urea transporter. Many carbohydrate antigens bind bacteria such as the P antigen that binds *Escherichia coli* and the Lewis system Le^b antigen on gastric epithelial cells, which binds *Helicobacter pylori,* the organism implicated in gastritis, gastric ulcers, and gastric carcinoma.

SEROLOGICAL PRINCIPLES OF BLOOD TRANSFUSION

Laboratory determination of blood types

REAGENTS

Most reagents used for blood group typing consist of monoclonal antibodies, usually of mouse origin, used individually or blended, directed against the different blood group antigens. A major advantage of the use of monoclonal antibodies is their specificity, minimizing the possibility of false-positive reactions due to additional contaminating antibodies found in human serum reagents. An important disadvantage derives from the fact that monoclonal antibodies react with a single epitope, and the blood group antigens have multiple epitopes. Thus, individuals missing the epitope recognized by the antibody may be typed as negative. Using a blend of monoclonal antibodies, each one of them recognizing a different epitope of a given antigen, significantly reduces this problem.

TESTS

Direct hemagglutination is the simplest, preferred test. It is easy to perform with typing reagents containing IgM antibodies that directly agglutinate cells expressing the corresponding antigen. Reagents containing IgG antibodies can also be used in a direct hemagglutination test. Protein is added in relatively high concentration to the reagent with the purpose of dissipating the repulsive forces that keep the red cells apart. As a consequence, IgG antibodies can directly agglutinate the red cells.

In general, reagents containing IgG antibodies are used in an indirect antiglobulin test (see discussion later in chapter), as a way to induce the agglutination of red cells coated with the corresponding antibodies.

**Direct and indirect antiglobulin (Coombs')
tests**. In 1945, **Coombs, Mourant,** and **Race** described the use of anti-human globulin serum to detect red cell bound nonagglutinating antibodies. There are two basic types of antiglobulin or Coombs' tests.

The **direct antiglobulin test** is performed to detect *in vivo* sensitization of red cells or, in other words, sensitization that has occurred in the patient (Figure 22.1). The test is performed by adding anti-human IgG and/or anti-human complement (to react with complement components bound to the red cells as a consequence of the antigen-antibody reaction) to the patient's washed red cells. If IgG antibody (and/or complement) is/are bound to the red cells, agglutination (positive result) is observed after addition of the antiglobulin reagent and centrifugation. The direct

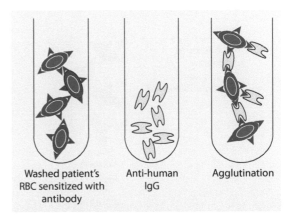

Washed patient's RBC sensitized with antibody   Anti-human IgG   Agglutination

Figure 22.1 Direct Coombs' test using anti-IgG antibodies.

antiglobulin test is an aid in diagnosis and investigation of hemolytic disease of the newborn, autoimmune hemolytic anemia, drug-induced hemolytic anemia, and hemolytic transfusion reactions.

The indirect antiglobulin test detects *in vitro* sensitization, i.e., sensitization that has been allowed to occur in the test tube under optimal conditions (Figure 22.2). Therefore, the test is used to investigate the presence of nonagglutinating red cell antibodies in a patient's serum. The test is performed in two steps (hence the designation of *indirect*). In the first step, a serum suspected of containing red cell antibodies is incubated with normal red blood cells. In the second step, after washing unbound antibodies, anti-human IgG (and/or anticomplement) antibodies are added to the red cells as in the direct test. The indirect antiglobulin test is useful in detecting and characterizing red cell antibodies using test cells of known antigenic composition (antibody screening), cross-matching, and phenotyping blood cells for antigens not demonstrable by other techniques. Antigen phenotyping has been simplified by the advent of monoclonal reagents that makes it possible to type many red cell antigens by direct agglutination.

Compatibility testing. Before a blood transfusion, a series of procedures need to be done to establish the proper selection of blood for the patient. Basically, those procedures try to establish the compatibility between donor and recipient ABO and Rh systems, and to rule out the existence of antibodies in the recipient's serum that could react with transfused red cells. To establish the ABO and Rh compatibility between donor and recipient, both the recipient and the blood to be transfused are typed. To rule out the existence of

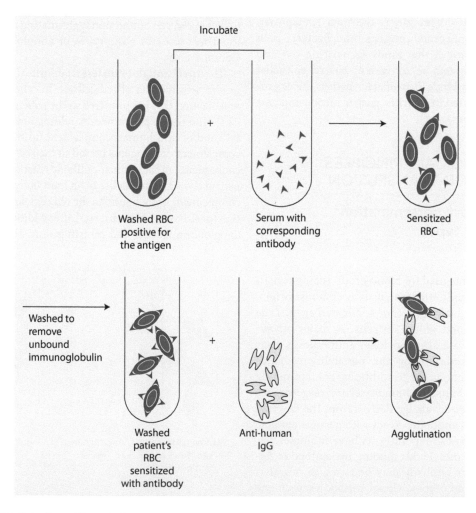

Figure 22.2 Indirect Coombs' test.

antibodies (other than anti-A or anti-B), a general antibody screening test is performed with group O red cells of known composition. The O$^+$ cells are first incubated with the patient's serum to check for agglutination; if this test is negative, an indirect antiglobulin (Coombs') test is performed.

CROSS-MATCH

The most direct way to detect antibodies in the recipient's serum that could cause hemolysis of the transfused red cells is to test the patient's serum with the donor's cells (major cross-match). The complete cross-match also involves the same tests as the antibody screening test previously described.

An abbreviated version of the cross-match is often performed in patients with a negative antibody screening test. This consists of immediately centrifuging a mixture of patient's serum and donor cells to detect agglutination; this primarily checks for ABO incompatibility.

Alternatives to tube testing. Newer methods that represent alternatives to the traditional tube test are being increasingly utilized in larger blood banks. These methods require little training, offer greater standardization, and use a micro sample. The reactions are stable and may be rechecked by another technologist.

The gel test uses six microtubes in a card, replacing six test tubes. In each microtube, a column of dextran acrylamide gel particles functions as a filter that traps agglutinates upon centrifugation. This technique may be used for antiglobulin tests where gels containing antiglobulin serum are used to trap sensitized but unagglutinated red cells. The red cells in a negative test will all centrifuge to the bottom of the microtube. The gel test is adaptable to typing, antibody screening, antibody identification, and cross-matching.

Solid-phase red cell adherence assays use immobilized antibody for the direct test. The red cells to be typed are added to antibody-coated wells in a polystyrene tray. The red cells will adhere in a monolayer across the well in a positive test and will settle to the bottom in a negative test. The indirect test uses red cells or red cell membranes of known phenotype, immobilized as a monolayer in the bottom of test wells. In order to demonstrate that a patient's serum has an antibody directed against a red cell sample, indicator red cells coated with anti-IgG are added after incubating patient's serum with the immobilized cells or cell membranes,

and washing to remove unbound antibodies. The indicator cells will efface across the well when an antibody has bound to the immobilized red cells. Automated solid-phase techniques are being used by some blood centers.

Implications of positive antibody screening for transfusion. Donor blood found to contain clinically significant red cell antibodies is generally not transfused. If a patient (recipient) has a positive antibody screening test due to a clinically significant antibody, the antibody is identified using a panel of cells of known antigenic composition, and antigen-negative blood is selected for transfusion.

BLOOD TRANSFUSION REACTIONS

Transfusion reactions may occur due to a wide variety of causes (Table 22.3). Among them, the most severe are those associated with hemolysis, which may be life threatening. A list of the causes of fatal transfusion reactions reported to the U.S. Food and Drug Administration (FDA) from 2012 to 2016 is reproduced in Table 22.4. The most common fatal reactions are nonimmunological in nature and include transfusion-related acute lung injury and transfusion-associated circulatory overload.

Intravascular hemolytic reactions ("immediate" transfusion reactions)

The binding of preformed IgM antibodies to the red cells triggers intravascular hemolytic transfusion reactions because IgM antibodies are very effective in causing the activation of the complement system. Massive complement activation by red cell antibodies causes intravascular red cell lysis, with release of hemoglobin into the circulation. Most intravascular reactions are due to ABO incompatibility. The direct antiglobulin test may be negative if all donor cells are quickly lysed.

Table 22.3 Immunological classification of transfusion reactions

A. Nonimmune
B. Immune
   1. Red cell incompatibility
   2. Incompatibilities associated with platelets and leukocytes
   3. Incompatibilities due to anti-allotype antibodies (anti-Gm or Am antibodies)

Table 22.4 Transfusion-associated fatalities by complication, FY2012–FY2016

Complication	FY12 number	FY12 %	FY13 number	FY13 %	FY14 number	FY14 %	FY15 number	FY15 %	FY16 number	FY16 %	Total number	Total %
Anaphylaxis	2	5	–	0	2	7	2	5	5	12	11	6
Contamination	3	8	5	13	1	3	5	14	5	12	19	10
HTR (ABO)	3	8	1	3	4	13	2	5	4	9	14	8
HTR (non-ABO)	5	13	5	13	4	13	4	11	1	2	19	10
Hypotensive reaction	–	0	–	0	1	3	1	3	1	2	3	2
TACO	8	21	13	34	5	17	11	30	19	44	56	30
TRALI	17	45	14	37	13	43	12	32	8	19	64	34

Source: Reproduced from *Fatalities Reported to FDA Following Blood Collection and Transfusion Annual Summary for FY2016.* U.S. Food and Drug Administration, Silver Spring, MD.
Abbreviations: HTR, hemolytic transfusion reaction; TACO, transfusion-associated circulatory overload; TRALI, transfusion-related acute lung injury.

Due to the massive release of soluble complement fragments (e.g., C3a and C5a) with anaphylatoxin properties, the patient may suffer generalized vasodilatation, hypotension, and shock. Because of the interrelationships between the complement and clotting systems, disseminated intravascular coagulation may occur during a severe transfusion reaction. As a consequence of the release of free heme, a pro-oxidant and pro-inflammatory catabolite released from degraded hemoglobin, the patient may develop acute tubular necrosis, leading to acute renal failure.

Extravascular hemolytic reactions ("delayed" transfusion reactions)

Extravascular hemolytic reactions are caused by the opsonization of red cells with IgG antibodies. IgG red cell antibodies can activate complement but do not cause spontaneous red cell lysis. Red cells opsonized with IgG (often with associated C3b) are efficiently taken up and destroyed by phagocytic cells, particularly splenic and hepatic macrophages.

These reactions are usually less severe than intravascular transfusion reactions. In addition, transfusion reactions may be delayed when an anamnestic response in a patient with undetectable antibody is the precipitating factor. Typically, a positive direct antiglobulin (Coombs') test will be noted after transfusion in association with a rapidly diminishing red cell concentration.

Clinical presentation of transfusion reactions

The most common initial symptom in a hemolytic transfusion reaction is fever, frequently associated with chills. Red or wine-colored urine (due to hemoglobinuria) may be noted. With progression of the reaction, the patient may experience chest pains, dyspnea, hypotension, and shock. Renal damage is indicated by back pain, oliguria, and in most severe cases, anuria.

During surgery, the only symptom may be bleeding and/or hypotension. Generalized bleeding is the most serious manifestation of disseminated intravascular coagulation. Treatment includes immediate cessation of the transfusion, support of vital signs, and active prevention of possible renal failure.

Laboratory investigation

Immediately after a hemolytic transfusion reaction is suspected, the following procedures must be done:

- A clerical check to detect any errors that may have resulted in the administration of a unit of blood to the wrong patient.
- Confirmation of intravascular hemolysis by visual or photometric comparison of pre- and postreaction plasma specimens for free hemoglobin (the prereaction specimen should be light yellow, and the postreaction sample should have a pink/red discoloration).
- Direct antiglobulin (Coombs') test on pre- and postreaction blood samples.

If any of these procedures gives a positive result supporting a diagnosis of intravascular hemolysis, additional serological investigations are indicated, including the following:

- Repeat ABO and Rh typing on patient and donor samples.
- Repeat antibody screening and cross matching.
- If an anti–red cell antibody is detected, determine its specificity using a red cell panel in which group O red cells of varied antigenic composition are incubated with the patient's serum to determine which red blood cell (RBC) antigen(s) are recognized by the patient's antibody(ies).

Additionally, one or several of the following confirmatory tests may be performed.

- Measurement of unconjugated bilirubin on blood drawn 5–7 hours after transfusion (the concentration should rise as the released hemoglobin is processed).
- Determination of free hemoglobin and/or hemosiderin in the urine (neither is normally detected in the urine).
- Measurement of serum haptoglobin (if hemolysis is not apparent upon visual inspection of the serum).
- Culture of the unit(s) for bacterial contamination and serological studies to rule out other microbial contaminants (viruses, parasites).

Nonhemolytic immune transfusion reactions

Antileukocyte antibodies. When a patient has antibodies directed to leukocyte antigens, a transfusion of any blood product containing cells expressing those antigens can elicit a febrile transfusion reaction. Leukocyte-depleted blood products should be used for transfusions in patients with recurrent febrile reactions.

Special problems are presented by patients requiring platelet concentrates that have developed anti-HLA antibodies or antibodies directed to platelet-specific antigens (HPA antigens). In such cases, it will be necessary to give HLA- or HPA-matched platelets, since platelets will be rapidly destroyed if given to a sensitized individual with circulating antibodies to the antigens expressed by the donor's platelets.

Transfusion of blood products containing antibodies to leukocyte antigens expressed by the patient receiving the transfusion can induce intravascular leukocyte aggregation. These aggregates are usually trapped in the pulmonary microcirculation, causing acute respiratory distress, and, in some cases, noncardiogenic pulmonary edema. This condition is recognized clinically as transfusion-associated related lung injury. A similar situation may emerge when granulocyte concentrates are given to a patient with antileukocyte antibodies reactive with the transfused granulocytes.

Anti-IgA antibodies. The transfusion of any IgA-containing blood product into a patient with preformed anti-IgA antibodies can cause an anaphylactic transfusion reaction. These are rare events; transfusion reactions are not usually observed when the antibody titers (determined by passive hemagglutination) are low. Anti-IgA antibodies are mostly detected in immunodeficient individuals, particularly those with IgA deficiency.

It is very important to test for anti-IgA antibodies in any patient with known IgA deficiency that is going to require a transfusion, even if the patient has never been previously transfused. If an anti-IgA antibody is detected, it is important to administer packed red cells with all traces of plasma removed by extensive washing. If plasma products are needed, they should be obtained from IgA-deficient donors.

HEMOLYTIC ANEMIAS

Several pathogenic scenarios can result in hemolysis, as summarized in Table 22.5.

Hemolytic disease of the newborn (erythroblastosis fetalis)

PATHOGENESIS

Immunological destruction of fetal and/or newborn erythrocytes is likely to occur when IgG antibodies are present in the maternal circulation

---

Table 22.5 Immune hemolytic anemias

Alloantibody-induced immune hemolytic anemia
    Hemolytic transfusion reactions
    Hemolytic disease of the newborn
Autoimmune hemolytic anemias (AIHA)
    Warm antibody AIHA
        Idiopathic (unassociated with another disease)
        Secondary (associated with chronic lymphocytic leukemia,
            lymphomas, systemic lupus erythematosus, etc.)
    Cold antibody AIHA
        Idiopathic cold hemagglutinin disease
        Secondary cold hemagglutinin syndrome
        Associated with *Mycoplasma pneumoniae* infection
        Associated with chronic lymphocytic leukemia, lymphomas, etc.
Immune drug-induced hemolytic anemia

Source: Modified from Petz, LD et al. In: Vyas, G.N., Stites, D.P., Brechter, G., eds., *Laboratory Diagnosis of Immunologic Disorders*, 1974; Grune & Stratton, New York.

directed against the corresponding antigen(s) present on the fetal red blood cells (only IgG antibodies can cross the placenta and reach the fetal circulation).

The two types of incompatibility most usually involved in hemolytic disease of the newborn are anti-D and anti-A or -B antibodies. Anti-A or anti-B antibodies are usually IgM, but in some circumstances, IgG antibodies may develop (usually in group O mothers). This can be secondary to immune stimulation (some vaccines contain blood group substances or cross-reactive polysaccharides) or may occur without apparent cause for unknown reasons.

Mechanism of Sensitization

Although the exchange of red cells between mother and fetus is prevented by the placental barrier during pregnancy, about two thirds of all women, after delivery (or miscarriage) have fetal red cells in their circulation. If the mother is Rh-negative and the infant Rh-positive, the mother may produce antibodies to the D antigen. The immune response is usually initiated at term, when large amounts of fetal red cells reach maternal circulation. In subsequent pregnancies, even the small number of red cells crossing the placenta during pregnancy are sufficient to elicit a strong secondary response, with switch to the production of IgG antibodies. As IgG antibodies are produced in larger amounts, they will cross the placenta, bind to the Rh-positive cells, and cause their destruction in the spleen through Fc-mediated phagocytosis. Usually the first child is not affected, since the red cells that cross the placenta after the 28th week of gestation do so in small numbers and are unlikely to elicit a primary immune response.

IgG anti-D antibodies do not appear to activate the complement system, perhaps because the D antigenic sites on the red cell surface are too separated to allow the formation of IgG doublets with sufficient density of IgG molecules to induce complement activation. Complement, however, is not required for phagocytosis that can be mediated by the Fc receptors in monocytes and macrophages.

Epidemiology

Prior to the introduction of immunoprophylaxis the frequency of clinically evident hemolytic disease of the newborn was estimated to be about 0.5% of total births, mostly due to anti-D, with a mortality rate close to 6% among affected newborns. Recent figures are considerably lower: 0.15%–0.3% incidence of clinically evident disease, and the perinatal mortality rate appears to be declining to about 4% of affected newborns. Due to the introduction of immunoprophylaxis, the proportion of cases due to anti-D antibodies decreased, while the proportion of cases due to other Rh antibodies, and to antibodies to antigens of other systems, increased proportionately.

Clinical presentation

The usual clinical features of this disease are anemia and jaundice present at birth, or more frequently, in the first 24 hours of life. In severe cases, the infant may die *in utero*. Unless treated appropriately, other severely affected children who survive until the third day develop signs of central nervous system damage, attributed to the high concentrations of unconjugated bilirubin (kernicterus). The peripheral blood shows reticulocytes and circulating erythroblasts (hence the term "erythroblastosis fetalis").

Immunological diagnosis

A strongly positive direct Coombs' (antiglobulin) test on cord RBC is invariably found in cases of Rh incompatibility, although 40% of the cases with a positive reaction do not require treatment. In ABO incompatibility, the direct antiglobulin test is usually weakly positive and may be confirmed by eluting antibodies from the infant's red cells and testing the eluate with A and B cells.

Prevention

Rh hemolytic disease of the newborn is rarely seen when mother and infant are incompatible in the ABO systems. In such cases, the ABO isoagglutinins in the maternal circulation appear to eliminate any fetal red cells before maternal sensitization occurs. This observation led to a very effective form of prevention of Rh hemolytic disease of the newborn, achieved by the administration of anti-D IgG antibodies (Rh immune globulin) to Rh-negative mothers.

The therapeutic anti-D preparation is manufactured from the plasma of previously immunized mothers with persistently high titers, or from male donors immunized against Rh-positive RBC. Its mechanism of action is not entirely clear, but a recently proposed mechanism to explain the immunotherapeutic effect of intravenous gamma globulin in idiopathic thrombocytopenia has some interesting parallels. According to this postulate, illustrated in Figure 22.3, it is possible that Rh immune globulin may downregulate anti-D-producing B cells as a consequence of co-ligation of surface immunoglobulin and FcIIγR (by the Fc region of red-cell bound anti-D).

The schedule of administration involves two separate doses. Antepartum administration of a full dose of Rh immune globulin at the 28th week of pregnancy is recommended, in addition to postpartum administration. The rationale for this approach is to avoid sensitization due to prenatal spontaneous or post-traumatic bleeding. Prenatal anti-D prophylaxis is also indicated at the time that a Rh-negative pregnant woman is submitted to amniocentesis and must be continued at 12-week intervals until delivery to maintain sufficient protection. The postpartum dose is administered in the first 72 hours after delivery of each Rh incompatible infant (before sensitization has had time to occur). The risk of immunization with a postpartum dose alone is 1%–2%. Antepartum administration decreases the risk to 0.1%.

The recommended full dose is 300 μg IM that can be increased if there is laboratory evidence of severe feto-maternal hemorrhage (by tests able to determine the number of fetal red cells in maternal peripheral blood, from which one can calculate the volume of feto-maternal hemorrhage). Smaller doses (50 μg) should be given after therapeutic or spontaneous abortion in the first trimester.

Treatment

To prevent serious hemolytic disease of the newborn in their infants, pregnant women who have a clinically significant antibody in the maternal circulation directed against a fetal antigen are carefully monitored. Amniocentesis is usually performed if the antibody has an antiglobulin titer greater than 16 or if the woman has a history of a previously affected child. The amniotic fluid is examined for bile pigments at appropriate intervals, and the severity of the disease is assessed according to those levels. An alternate approach is to monitor the fetus by percutaneous umbilical blood sampling (PUBS) which allows for direct hematologic and biochemical measurements by removing blood from the umbilical vessel using ultrasound guidance.

If fetal maturity has been established, labor may be induced, and if necessary, the baby can be exchange-transfused after delivery. If fetal lung maturity is inadequate (judged by the lecithin/sphyngomyelin ratio in amniotic fluid), intrauterine transfusion may be performed by transfusing O, Rh-negative red cells to the fetus.

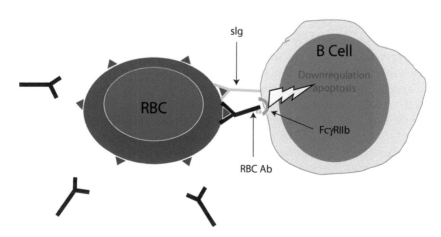

Figure 22.3 One of the postulated mechanisms of Rhogam in the prevention of hemolytic disease of the newborn. The co-ligation of the O+ antigen by the B-cell receptor (sIg) and of the Fc of the Rhogam antibody to the FcγRIIb on the B cell would result in downregulation or apoptosis.

AUTOIMMUNE HEMATOLOGICAL DISORDERS (AIHDs)

AIHDs are the result of inherent immunological mechanisms encumbering or eliminating one or more of the elements of the hematopoietic process. Immune destruction of or reduction of functioning red blood cells results in autoimmune hemolytic anemia (AIHA). Immune impairment and reduction in the number of platelets results in immune thrombocytopenia (ITP). Autoimmune neutropenia (ANP) may involve any of the myeloproliferative or lymphoproliferative cell lines including stem cells. Multiple cell lines may be involved as in Evans Syndrome.

Autoimmune hemolytic anemia (warm antibody type)

This is the most common form of autoimmune hemolytic anemia. It can be idiopathic (often following overt or subclinical viral infection) or secondary, as shown in Table 22.5.

Pathogenesis. Warm autoimmune hemolytic anemia is due to the spontaneous emergence of IgG antibodies that may have a simple Rh specificity such as anti-e, or uncharacterized specificities common to almost all normal red cells ("public" antigens, thought to be the core of the Rh substance). In many patients, one can find antibodies of multiple specificities. The end result is that the serum from patients with autoimmune hemolytic anemia of the warm type is likely to react with most, if not all, of the red cells tested. These antibodies usually cause shortening of red cell life due to the uptake and destruction by phagocytic cells in the spleen and liver.

Diagnosis. Diagnosis relies on the demonstration of antibodies coating the red cells or circulating in the serum at 37°C. RBC-fixed antibodies are detected by the direct antiglobulin Coombs' test and the search for antibodies in serum is carried out by the indirect antiglobulin test, using patient's serum or antibody eluted from affected red blood cells tested against a panel of erythrocytes which have known antigens on their surface (Table 22.6).

TREATMENT

Corticosteroids have been classically considered as the first line treatment, but recent data suggests that the combination of corticosteroids with Rituximab (CD20 monoclonal antibody) induces a higher percentage of clinical responses with longer duration of remission. In patients not responding to pharmacotherapy splenectomy may be considered.

Autoimmune hemolytic anemia associated with cold agglutinins

Cold agglutinins are classically IgM antibodies (very rarely IgA or IgG) and react with red cells at temperatures below normal body temperature.

In chronic, idiopathic, cold agglutinin disease, the antibodies are in the vast majority of cases of

Table 22.6 Typical results of serological investigations in patients with autoimmune hemolytic anemia

	Cells			Serum	
	Direct Coombs' test				
	Antibody to	Positivity rate	Antibody isotope	Serologic characteristics	Ab specificity
Warm AIHA	IgG	30%	IgG	Positive indirect Coombs' test (40%)	Rh system antigens ("public")
	IgG + C'	50%		Agglutination of enzyme treated RBC (80%)	
Cold agglutinin disease	C' C'	20%	IgM	Monoclonal IgMκ agglutinates RBC to titers >1024 at 4°C	I antigen

Source: Modified from Petz LD et al. In: Vyas, G.N., Stites, D.P., Brechter, G., eds., *Laboratory Diagnosis of Immunologic Disorders*, 1974; Grune & Stratton, New York.

the IgMk isotype and react with antigens of the I/i public antigen system, most commonly the I antigen. The fetus expresses the "i" antigen, common to primates and other mammalians, which is the precursor of the "I" specificity. The newborn expresses "i" predominantly over "I"; in the adult, the situation is reversed.

Because the affinity of IgM antibodies is low, the reactivity with red cells is enhanced by cold temperatures (for this reason, these autoantibodies are known as cold agglutinins). Clinical disease is seen during the winter months, when the temperatures of cold exposed areas drop below 37°C. The sera of patients with suspected cold agglutinin disease is tested at 4°C on a direct hemagglutination test using O positive red cells as antigens.

Monoclonal cold agglutinins can be also detected in cases of IgM-producing B cell malignancy (Waldenström's macroglobulinemia), when the IgM paraprotein behaves as a cold agglutinin. The titers of cold agglutinins in such cases are very high, and usually the patient will have symptoms attributable to the cold agglutinin. In patients with symptomatic idiopathic cold agglutinin disease the cold agglutinin titers may be equally high, but there is no evidence of B-cell dyscrasia other than the presence of the monoclonal anti-I cold agglutinin and an increase in the numbers of lymphoplasmacytic cells in the bone marrow, which could be considered as indicative of a monoclonal gammopathy of unknown significance. Less clear in significance, but clinically important is the fact that the majority of patients presenting with cold agglutinins may also have lymphoproliferative disorders or other types of malignancy, that should be ruled out in each individual case.

In contrast, the cold agglutinins associated with some infectious diseases (e.g., mycoplasma pneumonia and infectious mononucleosis), are also predominantly IgM, but contain both κ and λ light chains, suggesting their polyclonal origin.

Hemolysis in patients with post-infectious cold agglutinin disease is usually mild. In those cases the cold agglutinins are present in relatively low titers and have low thermal amplitude, i.e., they do not react at temperatures close to normal body temperature and hemolysis is due to opsonization of red cells through C3b receptors. When cold agglutinins are present in high titers and react at temperatures close to normal body temperature (i.e., 35°C) ischemia of cold-exposed areas and

intravascular hemolysis can take place. Cold-induced ischemia is caused by massive intracapillary agglutination areas where the temperature drops below the critical level for agglutination.

Clinical presentation. Hemolysis is usually mild, and in most cases the clinical picture is dominated by symptoms of cold sensitivity (Raynaud's phenomenon, vascular purpura, and tissue necrosis in exposed extremities). When the cold agglutinin titers are very high, intravascular hemolysis can be of sufficient magnitude to cause acute tubular necrosis secondary to the toxicity of hemoglobin and its degradation products.

Laboratory diagnosis. Testing for cold agglutinins is usually done by incubating a series of dilutions of the patient's serum (obtained by clotting and centrifuging the blood at 37°C immediately after drawing) with normal group O RBC at 4°C. Titers up to the hundreds of thousands can be observed in patients with cold agglutinin disease. Intermediate titers (below 1000) are when the cold agglutinins are associated with an infectious disease.

Drug-induced hemolytic anemia

Three different types of immune mechanisms may play a role in drug-induced hemolytic anemias. It is important to differentiate between drug-induced hemolytic anemia and warm autoimmune hemolytic anemia since cessation of the drug alone will usually halt the drug-induced hemolytic process.

Immune Complex Mechanism (Drug Dependent Antibody Mechanism). Traditionally this mechanism has been thought to be due to the formation of soluble immune complexes between the drug and the corresponding antibodies that is followed by non-specific adsorption to red cells and complement activation. Alternatively the neoantigen concept proposes that the drug binds transiently with the red cell forming a "non-self" epitope that stimulates antibody formation. The distinction between this mechanism and the drug adsorption mechanism, where a stable bond is formed between the drug and the cell membrane, may be more apparent than real. When IgM antibodies are predominantly involved, intravascular hemolysis is frequent and the direct Coombs' test is usually positive. IgG antibodies can also form immune complexes with different types of antigens and be adsorbed onto red cells and platelets.

In vitro, such adsorption is not followed by hemolysis or by phagocytosis of red cells, but *in vivo* it has been reported to be associated with intravascular hemolysis.

The absorption of IgG-containing immune complexes to platelets is also the cause of drug-induced thrombocytopenia. Quinine, quinidine, digitoxin, gold, meprobamate, chlorothiazide, rifampin, and the sulfonamides have been reported to cause this type of drug-induced thrombocytopenia.

Drug adsorption mechanism. This mechanism proposes that the adsorbed drug functions as hapten and the RBC as carrier, and an immune response against the drug ensues. The antibodies, usually IgG, are present in high titers, and may activate complement after binding to the drug adsorbed to the red cells, inducing hemolysis (Figure 22.4) or phagocytosis. Penicillin (when administered in high doses by the IV route) and cephalosporins can induce this type of hemolytic anemia. Some cephalosporins (such as cephalothin) also have been shown to modify the red cell membrane that becomes able to adsorb proteins non-specifically, a fact that can lead to a positive direct Coombs' test but not to hemolytic anemia.

Autoimmunity-induction mechanism. The drug used as an example of this form of drug induced hemolytic anemia is α-**methyldopa** (Aldomet). Ten to 15% of the patients receiving the drug will have a positive Coombs' test, and 0.8% of the patients develop clinically evident hemolytic anemia. It is particularly interesting from the pathogenic point of view in that it is indistinguishable from a true warm autoimmune hemolytic anemia. Alpha methyldopa

is unquestionably the trigger for this type of anemia, but the antibodies are of the IgG1 isotype and react with Rh antigens. It is believed that the drug changes the membrane of red cell precursors, causing the formation of antibodies reactive with a modified Rh precursor. Once formed, the anti-red cell antibodies will react in the absence of the drug, as true autoantibodies. Alpha methyldopa is seldom used clinically because of this complication.

Other drugs such as L-dopa, procainamide and some nonsteroidal anti-inflammatory drugs can also act by this mechanism. Both α-methyldopa and L-dopa also stimulate the production of antinuclear antibodies.

Treatment

Blood transfusions may be necessary in emergency situations but are made difficult when there are autoantibodies to red cell antigens widely represented in the population. The serum from a patient with cold or warm-type AIHA typically agglutinates all the red cells in an antibody identification panel. It is most important to determine if there are clinically significant underlying alloantibodies that may be masked by autoantibody. The patient's red cells may be pretreated in a manner to enhance removal of autoantibody from the serum. After one or more autoadsorptions the adsorbed serum may be used for alloantibody detection and crossmatching.

Glucocorticoids and rituximab, by themselves or in combination, are the first line of treatment in patients with chronic symptomatic warm AIHA. Other immunosuppressive drugs such as azathioprine, cyclosporine, and mycophenolate can be tried in patients not responding to glucocorticoids. Splenectomy can be useful in individuals who do not respond to glucocorticoids, when there is a marked predominance of red cell sequestration in the spleen. In such cases splenectomy leads to a longer half-life of the patient's red cells.

Glucocorticoids and splenectomy are generally ineffective in treating cold agglutinin disease. Patients should be kept warm, especially their extremities. If pharmacological intervention is deemed necessary, a combination of rituximab and fludarabine has been shown to be effective in 76% of the patients in which it was used.

In cases of drug-induced hemolytic anemia the offending drug should be withdrawn, and hemolysis should resolve.

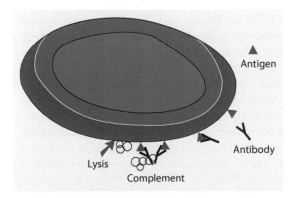

Figure 22.4 Pathogenesis of drug-induced hemolytic anemia as a consequence of adsorption of a drug to the red cell membrane.

AUTOIMMUNE THROMBOCYTOPENIAS

Thrombocytopenia is defined as a decrease in the platelet count below the ambulatory "normal" level, which varies from approximately 150,000–450,000 platelets per μL of blood. Thrombocytopenia is usually considered clinically significant at levels <50,000/μL, although petechiae and spontaneous bleeding may not occur until much lower levels (<20,000/μL). Causes of thrombocytopenia include reduced or absent bone marrow production, splenomegaly, bacterial or viral infections, malignancies and aberrant immune responses. Autoimmune thrombocytopenias to be discussed are immune thrombocytopenic purpura (ITP), thrombotic thrombocytopenia (TTP) and heparin induced thrombocytopenia (HIT). The basic pathogenesis of these entities is generation of autoimmune antibodies to one or more of the approximate 24 specific human platelet antigens (HPA), identified as glycoproteins of Group I, II or III, or proteins associated with thromboses.

Immune thrombocytopenic purpura (ITP)

Immune thrombocytopenic purpura, also known as Idiopathic Thrombocytopenia, may have an acute or a chronic clinical course. Acute ITP often follows a viral infection in children or adolescents and is due to the formation of immune complexes containing viral antigens that become adsorbed to the platelets or to the production of anti-viral antibodies that cross-react with platelets. Platelet destruction can be due to irreversible aggregation caused by immune complexes, when anti-platelet antibodies are involved, or to complement-induced lysis or phagocytosis.

Chronic ITP occurs in adults, is caused by autoantibodies that react with platelets and lead to their destruction by phagocytosis, lasts longer than six months, can go through periods of remissions and exacerbations and does not often have an obvious infection as a precursor.

As many as 60% of patients with ITP have demonstrable antibodies to platelet membrane antigens of the glycoprotein IIb-IIIa or Ib-IX groups. The antibodies are of the IgG isotype and render the coated platelets vulnerable to opsonization and phagocytosis by reticuloendothelial cells

of the spleen and liver. Diagnosis of ITP is usually made by clinical history and physical examination findings, low platelet count, and exclusion of active infections, malignancies and other blood and/or bone marrow abnormalities. Laboratory testing for antiplatelet antibodies can be performed and it has approximately 80% specificity but is considered unnecessary for the majority of patients in the most recent guidelines.

CLINICAL PRESENTATION

Clinically, ITP is characterized by easy and exaggerated bleeding mucosal and subcutaneous bleeding secondary to thrombocytopenia.

The acute forms of ITP are seen mainly in children, often in the phase of recovery after a viral exanthem or an upper respiratory infection, and usually run a course of 2–6 months with complete resolution.

In contrast, chronic ITP is an adult disease, often associated with other autoimmune diseases. The bone marrow is usually normal, but in some cases an increase in megakaryocytes may be seen, representing an attempt to compensate for the excessive destruction in the peripheral blood. The spleen may be enlarged due to platelet sequestration by phagocytic cells.

TREATMENT OF CHRONIC ITP

Administration of corticosteroids, by themselves, or associated with rituximab or with a combination of rituximab and cyclosporine are considered as the first line of treatment. Thrombopoietin receptor agonists (thrombopoietin, romiplostim and eltrombopag) appear to also be effective but their evaluation is still in progress. Intravenous gamma globulin (IVIg) and anti-D immunoglobulin were considered as the therapy of choice in the past. Their primary mechanism of action is believed to be the blocking of Fc receptors in phagocytic cells, which would inhibit the ingestion and destruction of antibody-coated platelets. This mechanism is most likely to explain the rapid increase in platelet counts seen after therapy with IVIg is initiated. However, the effects are relatively short-lived, and the use of these agents is now relegated either to cases in which there is an urgent need to raise the platelet numbers or cases not responding to the first-line agents mentioned above.

Splenectomy is usually reserved for patients that do not respond to pharmacological agents and in whom the spleen is the major site for platelet sequestration and destruction.

Thrombotic Thrombocytopenia (TTP) is a rare coagulation disease that exists in acquired (most commonly) and inherited forms. The acquired form is caused by antibodies that inhibit ADAMTS13, a metalloproteinase with thrombospodin type I motif enzyme that cleaves large multimers of von Willebrand factor (vWF). In the absence of ADAMTS13 activity, thrombosis due to the residual large multimers of vWF result in the formation of small platelet clots which adhere to endothelial surfaces blocking vessels. The circulating red blood cells passing through the clots are subjected to sheer stress Platelets are consumed in the thrombi resulting in the combination of thrombocytopenia and thrombosis and the sheer stress of the red cell results in the formation of schistocytes, anemia, and renal failure.

The trigger for the formation of ADAMTS13 antibody generation is usually unknown although there have been associations with some medications, pregnancy, lupus erythematosus and other autoimmune diseases, some neoplasias and human immunodeficiency disease. The very rare form of inherited TTP is associated with autosomal recessive inheritance of the absence of ADAMTS13. The diagnosis is most usually based on clinical and laboratory parameters but can be confirmed by determining ADAMTS13 levels (less than 5% of normal values are diagnostic).

Treatment consists of plasmapheresis or administration of fresh frozen plasma to replenish ADAMTS13, and corticosteroids or rituximab to reduce the synthesis of ADAMTS13 antibodies. Transfusion of packed red blood cells is contraindicated until the thrombotic process is under control as the presence of additional red cells may exacerbate the coagulopathy.

Heparin Induced Thrombocytopenia (HIT) is the clinical presentation of paradoxical thrombocytopenia secondary to the use of heparin for anticoagulation. The cause of this disease is the development of antibodies to heparin administered as an anti-thrombotic agent. The antibodies react with complexes of heparin and platelet factor 4, activate the plalets to release intracellular particles leading to thrombosis, which result in thrombocytopenia thus leading to a combination of thrombosis and thrombocytopenia. Treatment includes stopping heparin and the use of alternate anticoagulants to control the thrombotic processes.

AUTOIMMUNE NEUTROPENIA

Human granulocytes are known to have five sets of human neutrophil antigens. Antibodies to one or more of these antigens can result in immune neutropenia. Alloimmune neutropenia can be seen in neutrophil incompatible fetal-maternal conditions and post blood or bone marrow transfusions. Primary autoimmune neutropenia is caused by autoantibodies to neutrophil antigens and is usually seen in children. Secondary autoimmune neutropenia may be associated with a variety of autoimmune diseases, including patients with rheumatoid arthritis, usually in association with splenomegaly (Felty's Syndrome), and also with some lymphoproliferative disorders. Treatment includes administration of granulocyte stimulating factor and immunosuppression when indicated.

AUTOIMMUNE COAGULOPATHIES

Autoimmune coagulopathies occur as primary or secondary clinical conditions. Most often are secondary to a variety of autoimmune diseases, lymphoproliferative disorders and may also be drug-induced. The coagulopathy is caused by antibodies that bind to the functional epitopes of specific coagulation factors, neutralizing their activity or enhancing their clearance. Either mechanism results in a hemorrhagic state. The autoantibodies are against factors V, VIII, XI, XII, and other coagulation proteins. The most commonly involved target of these antibodies is factor VIII. Of interest, autoantibodies to coagulation factors are often polyclonal. They are mostly of the IgG1 and/or IgG4 types, but IgA and IgM immunoglobulins have also been reported. The antibodies bind to functional epitopes of the factors resulting in enhanced clearance or blocking of activity. Testing for factor activity reveals prolongation of clotting. Clinically the patient may manifest mild bleeding to severe hemorrhage.

Acquired hemophilia A

While congenital F VIII deficiency (hemophilia A) is an X-linked recessive hemorrhagic disease primarily of women because of its sex chromosome linkage, acquired hemophilia A, due to the production of autoantibodies to F VIII occurs more frequently in men, but may also affect women. The incidence of acquired F VIII problems increases with age. The median age for acquired hemophilia A (AHA) is in the seventh decade. An increase among women during pregnancy or after partum is also noted.

Approximately one-half of the cases of AHA are idiopathic, while the other half are associated with autoimmune disorders, lymphomas and other malignancies, pregnancy, and drug induced. Diagnosis includes identification of the antibody and assessment of its titer. The laboratory hallmark for the diagnosis of AHA is a prolonged activated partial thromboplastin time (APTT), not corrected after mixing with normal plasma. Lack of correction of bleeding indicates an autoantibody inhibitor. Similar tests with specifically prepared plasma can be used to identify specific inhibitors. After the identification of the inhibitors is made qualitatively a quantitative titer can be sought by available tests. The attempts at quantitation are directed at guiding the proper dose of replacement factor to overcome the inhibitor. Recombinant Factor VIII preparations are FDA-approved for that purpose. Drug-induced and pregnancy-related forms of this disease may resolve by withdrawing the causative drug or spontaneously. In cases in which autoantibodies are the cause of the disease, immunosuppression is indicated. A combination of corticosteroids and cyclophosphamide has been considered as the optimal treatment, but there is a recent trend to replace cyclophosphamide with rituximab.

Antiphospholipid antibody syndrome

The antiphospholipid antibody syndrome is a constellation of clinical findings that are the result of antibodies produced against the phospholipids that are an integral part of the plasma membrane of all cells, including blood cells and blood vessel endothelial cells. These antibodies injure endothelial cells initiating the coagulation cascade that results in consumption of platelets, coagulation factors and hemolysis. Clinical manifestations can include stroke, myocardial infarction, kidney damage, deep vein thrombosis and problems in pregnancy. The antibody can cause a false positive VDRL test due to the cross-reaction with cardiolipin. More recent testing methods look for the presence of antibodies specific beta-2 glycoprotein and lupus anticoagulant. Not all patients with positive antibody testing will have clinical evidence of antiphospholipid antibody syndrome. Treatment is based on the administration of anticoagulants. Treatment with immunosuppressive drugs has not been proven to be effective.

BIBLIOGRAPHY

Arndt PA, Garratty G. The changing spectrum of drug-induced hemolytic anemia. *Semin Hematol.* 2005;42:137–144.

Brinc D, Lazarus AH. Mechanisms of anti-D action in the prevention of hemolytic disease of the fetus and newborn. *Hematology Am Soc Hematol Educ Program.* 2009;185–191.

Chaudhuri A, Zbrzezna V, Polyakova J, Pogo AO et al. Expression of the Duffy antigen in K562 cells. Evidence that it is the human erythrocyte chemokine receptor. *J Biol Chem.* 1994; 269:7835–7838.

Ching E. Solid phase red cell adherence assay: A tubeless method for pretransfusion testing and other applications in transfusion science. *Transfus Apher Sci.* 2012;46:287–291

Fatalities Reported to FDA Following Blood Collection and Transfusion Annual Summary for FY2016. U.S. Food and Drug Administration, Silver Spring, MD

Franchini M, Vaglio S, Marano G, Mengoli C et al. Acquired hemophilia A: a review of recent data and new therapeutic options. *Hematology.* 2017;22:514–520.

Harmening DE. *Modern Blood Banking and Transfusion Practices*, 4th ed. 1999; F. A. Davis Co., Philadelphia.

Hendrickson JE, Delaney M. Hemolytic disease of the fetus and newborn: Modern practice and future investigations. *Transfus Med Rev.* 2016;30:159–164.

Hill QA, Stamps R, Massey E, Grainger JD et al. The diagnosis and management of primary autoimmune haemolytic anemia. *Brit J Haematol.* 2017;176:208–220.

Lambert MP, Gernsheimer TB. Clinical updates in adult immune thrombocytopenia. *Blood.* 2017;129:2829–2835.

Lovecchio F. Heparin-induced thrombocytopenia. *Clin Toxicol.* 2014;52:579–583.

Mollison PL, Engelfriet CP, Contreras M. *Blood Transfusion in Clinical Medicine*, 10th ed. 1997; Blackwell Science Ltd, Oxford.

Patel S. Diagnosis and treatment of immune-mediated and non–immune-mediated hemolytic disease of the newborn. In *Hematology, Immunology and Infectious Disease: Neonatology Questions and Controversies* (Ohls RK, Maheshwari A Eds.), 2nd ed. 2012; Elsevier, pp. 75–88.

Petz LD, Garraty G.In: Vyas GN, Stites DP, Brechter G. (Eds.), *Laboratory Diagnosis of Immunologic Disorders*, 1994; Grune & Stratton, New York.

Petz LD, Swisher S, Kleinman S, Spence RK et al. (Eds.), *Clinical Practice of Transfusion Medicine*, 3rd ed. 1996; Churchill Livingstone, New York.

Rossi EC, Simon TL, Moss GE, Gould SA (Eds.), *Principles of Transfusion Medicine*, 2nd ed. 1996; Williams & Wilkins, Baltimore.

Silberstein LE (Ed.), *Molecular and Functional Aspects of Blood Group Antigens*. 1995; Amer. Ass. Blood Banks, Bethesda, MD.

Swiecicki PL, Hegerova LT, Gertz MA. Cold agglutinin disease. *Blood.* 2013;122:1114–1121.

23

Pathogenic role of antigen-antibody complexes

GABRIEL VIRELLA AND GEORGE C. TSOKOS

INTRODUCTION

The formation of circulating antigen-antibody complexes (immune complexes, ICs) is one of the natural events that characterize the immunologic response against soluble antigens. Normally, ICs formed by soluble proteins and their respective antibodies are promptly eliminated from circulation by phagocytic cells without any detectable adverse effects on the host. However, there are well-characterized clinical and experimental situations in which it has been proven that ICs play a pathogenic role.

In the late 1800s and early 1900s, passive immunization with equine antisera was a common therapy for severe bacterial infections. It was often noted that 1–2 weeks after administration of the horse antisera, when the symptoms of acute infection had often disappeared, patients complained of arthralgia and exanthematous rash, and had proteinuria and an abnormal urinary sediment, suggestive of glomerulonephritis. von Pirquet coined the term *serum sickness* to designate this condition.

Several decades later, Cochrane and Kopfler published the seminal study of the pathogenic role of ICs in rabbits in which serum sickness was induced by injection of a single dose of an heterologous protein. As summarized in Figure 23.1, after the lag time necessary for antibody production, soluble ICs were detected in serum, serum complement levels decreased, and the rabbits developed glomerulonephritis, myocarditis, and arthritis. The onset of disease coincided with the disappearance of circulating antigen, while free circulating antibody appeared in circulation soon after the beginning of symptoms.

Both the experimental one-shot serum sickness and human serum sickness are usually transient and will leave no permanent sequelae. However, if the organism is chronically exposed to antigen (as in autoimmune diseases or chronic infections), irreversible lesions will develop.

The formation of an IC does not have direct pathological consequences. The pathogenic consequences of IC formation depend on the ability of those ICs to leave the intravascular compartment, become tissue-fixed, and activate effector systems, such as the complement system or inflammatory cells able to release enzymes and cytokines. Also, ICs may form directly in tissues where the antigens are formed or trapped. In either case, the pro-inflammatory properties of ICs are related to their physicochemical characteristics.

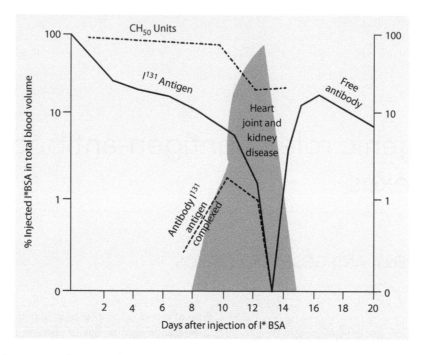

Figure 23.1 Sequence of events that takes place during the induction of acute serum sickness in rabbits. Six days after injection of radiolabeled BSA, anti-BSA antibodies start being produced and form complexes with the antigen, which appears to be eliminated from the circulation. The decline of free antigen coincided with the detection of immune complexes containing radiolabeled BSA. The maximal concentration of immune complexes precedes shortly a decrease in complement levels and the appearance of histological abnormalities on the heart, joints, and kidney. After the antigen is totally eliminated, the antibody becomes detectable, and the pathological lesions heal without permanent sequelae. (Reproduced with permission from Cochrane, C.G., Koffler, D., *Adv Immunol.*, 16, 185, 1973.)

Physicochemical characteristics of pathogenic immune complexes

Size, affinity of the Ag.Ab reaction, and class and subclass of antibodies involved in IC formation are among the most important determinants of the pathogenic significance of ICs.

In the case of circulating ICs, very large Ag.Ab aggregates containing IgG1 or IgG3 antibodies will activate complement very effectively but are usually nonpathogenic. This is due to a combination of facts: very avid ingestion and degradation by phagocytic cells and difficulty in diffusing across the endothelial barrier. Very small complexes formed in antigen excess, even when involving IgG1 and IgG3 antibodies, are able to diffuse easily into the extravascular compartment but are usually nonpathogenic because of their inability to activate complement. Actually, the most potentially pathogenic circulating ICs are those of intermediate size, particularly when complement-fixing

antibodies (IgG1, IgG3) of moderate to high affinity are involved in their formation. Under the appropriate circumstances, these ICs may be deposited in the subendothelial space and trigger inflammatory reactions. ICs formed *in situ* between tissue-fixed antigens and freely diffusible antibodies of the IgG1 and IgG3 class are most likely pro-inflammatory. Due to their large size, IgM antibodies are predominantly intravascular and are rarely involved in the formation of ICs in tissues.

Immune complex formation and cell interactions

Circulating ICs may be deposited in various tissues where they cause inflammation and tissue damage. The mechanisms allowing or preventing extravascular deposition of ICs are rather complex and involve interactions with a variety of cells and tissues.

Circulating ICs can bind to platelets and red cells. Human platelets express Fc receptors, specific for all IgG subclasses, and CR4, which binds the C3dg fragment of C3. Red blood cells (RBCs) express CR1, through which C3b-containing IC can be bound. In addition, IC can bind to RBC through nonspecific interactions of low affinity, which do not require the presence of complement. IC binding to RBC is believed to be an important mechanism for clearance of soluble IC from the systemic circulation. Experimental work in primates and metabolic studies of labeled ICs in humans show that RBC-bound ICs are maintained in the intravascular compartment until they reach the liver, where they are presented to phagocytic cells. The phagocytic cells have Fc receptors able to bind the IC with greater affinity than the red cells; as a consequence, the ICs are removed from the RBC membrane, while the red cells remain undamaged (Figure 23.2).

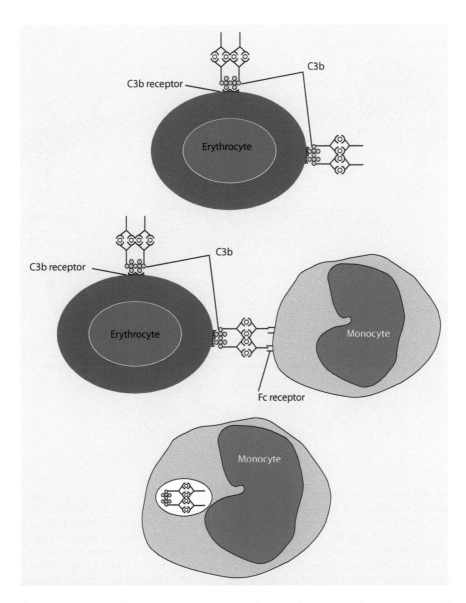

Figure 23.2 Protective role of erythrocytes against the development of immune complex disease. Erythrocytes can adsorb circulating IC through C3b receptors or through nonspecific interactions. RBC-adsorbed ICs persist in circulation until the ICs are stripped from the RBC surface by phagocytic cells expressing Fc receptors, which bind the IC with greater avidity. Once taken up by phagocytic cells, the ICs are degraded, and this uptake is responsible for their disappearance from circulation.

INTERACTIONS WITH ANTIGEN-PRESENTING CELLS AND INFLAMMATORY CELLS

While the interaction of ICs with phagocytic cells can be a protective mechanism, it can also be a pathogenic factor. In systemic lupus erythematosus (SLE), it has been demonstrated that DNA-containing ICs bind to CD32 (FcγRIIa) expressed on the surface of plasmacytoid dendritic cells, become internalized, and activate the DNA-binding toll-like receptor-9 (TLR9) located in the endosomal compartments. Thus, the interaction with a surface receptor (FcγRIIa) and an intracellular receptor (TLR9) cause the activation of dendritic cells that, in turn, will present antigen to lymphocytes and propagate an unwanted response.

C3bi opsonized ICs bind to complement receptor-3 (CR3), and FcγR receptors present on polymorphonuclear leukocytes (Figure 23.3).

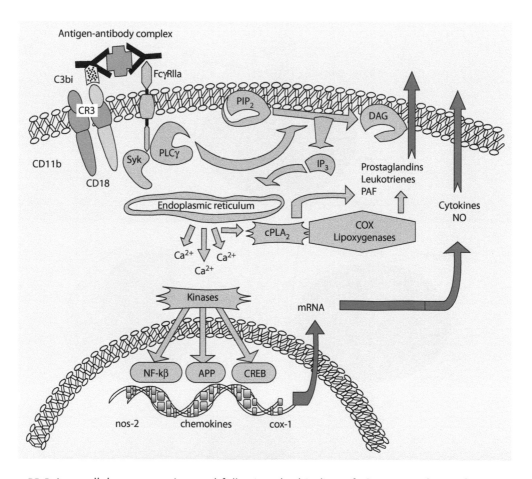

Figure 23.3 Intracellular events triggered following the binding of IC to Fc and complement receptor binding cells. ICs containing IgG antibodies and associated C3bi bind to Fcγ receptors and CR3 expressed by circulating monocytes, macrophages, PMNs, and tissue-residing cells. FcγRIIa binding triggers the activation of src kinase Syk and PLCγ (phospholipase γ). CR3 binding activates various kinases including Syk. PLCγ leads to increased release of free calcium (Ca²⁺) in the cytoplasm, which is involved in the activation of various processes. Syk activates a series of kinases including mitogen-activated kinases. Subsequently, cytoplasmic phospholipase A2 (cPLA2) followed by activation of lipooxygenase and cyclooxygenases that lead to the production of leukotrienes and prostaglandins, respectively. In the nucleus, various (nuclear factor κB, NFκB; activating protein, 1-AP1; cAMP; response element binding protein, CREB) transcription factors become activated which increase the transcription rate of genes such as NOS (nitric oxide synthase) 2 and COX (cyclooxygenases) chemokines. Understanding of the involved pathways has prompted investigators to consider additional interventions (such as blocking the activity of Syk or blocking the effect of chemokines) to treat IC-associated diseases.

Binding to these receptors results in the activation of a variety of phospholipases (such as phospholipase A2, PLA2) and kinases (e.g., Fyn, Lyn, and Syk). As a consequence of PLA2 activation, platelet-activating factor (PAF) is synthesized, and arachidonic acid is released and converted into proinflammatory prostaglandins and leukotrienes. The activation of membrane-associated kinases eventually leads to the expression of genes encoding proinflammatory cytokines and nitric oxide synthase.

TISSUE DEPOSITION OF CIRCULATING IMMUNE COMPLEXES

Some of the most frequent localization of deposited IC is around the small vessels of the skin, particularly in the lower limbs, the kidney glomeruli, the choroid plexus, and the joints. Our understanding of the mechanisms responsible for extravascular deposition of ICs is incomplete. A major obstacle to such deposition is the endothelial barrier, which is poorly permeable even to intermediate-size ICs. The first step in tissue deposition of ICs is likely to be the interaction with vascular receptors. C1q receptors, expressed by endothelial cells, and Fc receptors, expressed on the renal interstitium and by damaged endothelium, could play a role in IC immobilization. The frequent involvement of the kidney in IC-associated disease may be a consequence of the existence of C3b receptors in the renal glomerular epithelial cells, Fc receptors in the renal interstitium, and a collagen-rich structure (the basement membrane) that can also be involved in nonspecific interactions with antigens or antibodies. Regional factors may influence the selectivity of IC deposition. For example, the preferential involvement of the lower limbs in IC-related skin vasculitis may result from the simple fact that the circulation is slowest and the hydrostatic pressure highest in the lower limbs.

Any pathogenic sequence involving the deposition of circulating IC has to account with increased vascular permeability in the microcirculation, allowing the diffusion of small to medium-sized soluble ICs to the subendothelial spaces (Figure 23.4). After ICs are immobilized, they are in an ideal situation to activate monocytes or granulocytes, causing the release of vasoactive amines and cytokines. The retention of soluble ICs diffusing through the endothelium should be determined by interaction with extravascular structures. For example, in the kidney, C3b receptors of the renal epithelial cells and Fc receptors in the renal interstitium could play the role.

FORMATION OF IMMUNE COMPLEXES IN SITU

Direct injection of antigen into a previously immunized laboratory animal or human can result in local IC formation with extravascular antibody. Examples include the Arthus reaction (antigen injected into the dermis) and hypersensitivity pneumonitis (inhaled antigen forms IC with extravascular antibody).

Other types of ICs formed *in situ* include those formed when antibodies react with antigens present on the cell surface membrane of circulating or tissue cells. ICs formed on cell membranes can lead to the destruction of the cell, either by promoting phagocytosis or by causing complement-mediated lysis. This mechanism is responsible for the development of various immune cytopenias.

Autoantibodies may also bind to basement membrane antigens, as in Goodpasture's syndrome, or may react with an antigen that has become adsorbed to a basement membrane due to charge interactions, such as seems to be the case of the glomerular deposition of DNA-anti-DNA IC in patients with SLE.

Another example is the formation of ICs involving modified low-density lipoprotein (LDL) and corresponding antibodies in vessel walls. LDL is modified in a variety of ways in vessel walls, and although present in circulation (where it becomes involved in the formation of circulating IC), it is also present in the subendothelial space, available to form ICs with transudated IgG antibodies. In general, *in situ* formation of ICs appears as the most likely mechanism leading to deposition of ICs in tissues.

INFLAMMATORY CIRCUITS TRIGGERED BY IMMUNE COMPLEXES

The development of inflammatory changes after extravascular formation or deposition of ICs is not observed when serum sickness is induced in experimental animals depleted of neutrophils or complement. Activated phagocytic cells and the soluble compounds released as a consequence of their activation also play important roles (Table 23.1), particularly in chronic conditions (see discussion later in the chapter). Complement components play a significant role as the source of opsonins and

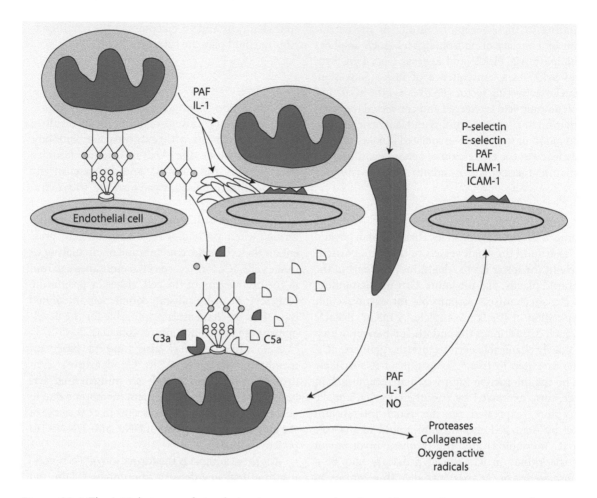

Figure 23.4 The initial stages of circulating immune complex deposition require a sequence of events, which enables circulating ICs and inflammatory cells to cross the endothelial barrier. In this representation of such a hypothetical sequence the first event is the binding of circulating ICs containing IgG antibodies and associated C1q to C1q receptors on the endothelial cell. The immobilized ICs are then able to interact with circulating cells expressing Fcγ receptors, such as PMN leukocytes. Such interaction results in PMN activation and release of mediators, such as platelet-activating factor (PAF) and IL-1. These two mediators have a variety of effects: PAF induces vasodilatation and activates platelets, which form aggregates and release vasoactive amines. The resulting increased vascular permeability allows circulating IC to cross the endothelial barrier. IL-1 activates endothelial cells and induces the expression of selectin molecules that interact with glycoproteins and sialoglycoproteins on the leukocyte membrane. This interaction slows down PMNs along the endothelial surface, a phenomenon known as "rolling." As endothelial cells continue to receive activating signals, they start expressing membrane-associated PAF, which interacts with PAF receptors on neutrophils, ICAM-1, which interacts with leukocyte integrins of the CD11/CD18 family, and VCAM-1, which interacts with VLA (very late antigen)-1, upregulated on PMN leukocytes as a consequence of the occupancy of Fc receptors. This promotes firm adhesion of leukocytes to endothelial cells. At the same time, the ICs, which diffuse to the subendothelial space, activate complement and generate chemotactic factors, such as C5a and C3a. Adherent PMN leukocytes are attracted to the area and insinuate themselves between endothelial cells, reaching the area of IC deposition. Interaction with those extravascular ICs with associated C3b delivers additional activation signals to already primed granulocytes, resulting in the release of metalloproteinases (including proteases and collagenases), oxygen active radicals, and nitric oxide. These compounds can cause tissue damage and can further increase vascular permeability, and in doing so contribute to the perpetuation of an inflammatory reaction.

Table 23.1 Elements involved in immune complex–mediated immunopathology

A. Cells
- *Polymorphonuclear leukocytes.* PMN-depleted animals do not develop arthritis or Arthus reaction.
- *Monocytes/macrophages.* Monocyte depletion in experimental glomerulonephritis decreases proteinuria.

B. Soluble factors (circulating and released locally)
- *Complement fragments.* Complement-depleted animals develop less severe forms of serum sickness.
- *Lymphokines/cytokines.* Corticosteroids reduce interleukin release and have beneficial effects in the treatment of immune complex disease.
- *Lysosomal enzymes (e.g., matrix metalloproteinases).* The main mediators of PMN-induced tissue damage.
- *Prostaglandins.* Important mediators of the inflammatory reaction; their synthesis is inhibited by aspirin and most nonsteroidal anti-inflammatory agents.
- *Nitric oxide and products of the respiratory burst.* These compounds can affect vascular permeability and induce cell and tissue damage because of their oxidative properties.

chemotactic factors, while activated granulocytes can release a wide variety of proteolytic enzymes that mediate tissue damage.

Activation of the complement cascade results in the generation of chemotactic and pro-inflammatory fragments, such as C3a and C5a. These complement components have strong pro-inflammatory effects, mediated by a variety of mechanisms:

- C5a increases vascular permeability directly as well as indirectly (by causing the release of histamine and vasoactive amines from basophils and mast cells).
- C5a enhances the expression of the CD11/CD18 complex on neutrophil membranes, increasing their adhesiveness to endothelial cells.
- C5a and C3a are chemotactic for neutrophils, attracting them to the area of IC deposition and stimulating their respiratory burst and release of granule constituents.

The combination of chemotaxis, increased adherence, and increased vascular permeability plays a crucial role in promoting extravascular emigration of leukocytes. It needs to be stressed that the inflammatory process triggered by ICs is usually associated with extravascular granulocyte infiltrates. The migration of neutrophils and other granulocytes is regulated by a series of interactions with endothelial cells, known as the adhesion cascade.

The initial event in the cascade involves the upregulation of selectins (P-selectin and E-selectin) on endothelial cells, which can be caused by a variety of stimuli (e.g., histamine, thrombin, bradykinin, leukotriene C4, free oxygen radicals, or cytokines). The consequence of this upregulation is the slowing down (rolling) and loose attachment of leukocytes (which express a third selectin, L-selectin, which binds to membrane oligosaccharides on endothelial cells). These initial interactions are unstable and transient.

The endothelial cells, in response to persistent activating signals, express PAF and intercellular adhesion molecule (ICAM)-1 on the membrane. Neutrophils express constitutively a PAF receptor that allows rolling cells to interact with membrane-bound PAF. The interaction of neutrophils with PAF, as well as signals received in the form of chemotactic cytokines such as interleukin (IL)-8 (which can also be released by endothelial cells), activate neutrophils and induce the expression of integrins—CD11a/CD18, LFA-1 and related molecules, and the very late antigen-4 (VLA-4).

The interaction between integrins expressed by neutrophils and molecules of the immunoglobulin superfamily expressed by endothelial cells (ICAM-1 and related antigens bind LFA-1 and related molecules; VCAM-1 binds VLA-4) causes firm adhesion of inflammatory cells to the endothelial surface, which is an essential step leading to their extravascular migration. VLA-4 is also expressed on the membrane of lymphocytes and monocytes, and its interaction with endothelial VCAM-1 allows the recruitment of these cells to the site of inflammation.

The interactions between integrins and their ligands are important for the development of vasculitic lesions in patients with SLE and other systemic autoimmune disorders and of purulent exudates in infection sites. As discussed in Chapter 29, patients with genetic defect in the expression of CD18 and related CAMs fail to form abscesses because their neutrophils do not express these molecules and fail to migrate.

The actual transmigration of leukocytes into the subendothelial space seems to involve yet another set of CAMs, particularly one member of the immunoglobulin superfamily known as PECAM (platelet endothelial cell adhesion molecule) that is expressed both at sites of intercellular junction and on the membranes of leukocytes. PECAM-1 interacts with itself, and its expression is upregulated on both endothelial cells and leukocytes by a variety of activating signals. The egression of leukocytes from the vessel wall is directed by chemoattractant molecules released into the extravascular space and involves diapedesis through endothelial cell junctions.

As leukocytes begin to reach the site of IC deposition, they continue to receive activating signals. Their activation brings about the release of additional chemotactic factors and continuing upregulation of CAMs on endothelial cells, intensifies the efflux of phagocytic cells to the subendothelial space, and creates the conditions needed for self-perpetuation of the inflammatory process. All polymorphonuclear leukocytes express Fcγ receptors and C3bi (CR3) receptors that mediate their binding and ingestion of IC. This process is associated with activation of a variety of functions and with the release of a variety of cytokines, enzymes, and other mediators. As previously mentioned, one important mediator released by activated neutrophils is PAF, which will promote the self-perpetuation of the inflammatory process by increasing vascular permeability (directly or as a consequence of the activation of platelets, which release vasoactive amines), inducing the upregulation of the CD11/CD18 complex on neutrophils, and inducing monocytes to release IL-1 and tumor necrosis factor (TNF), which activate endothelial cells and promote the upregulation of adhesion molecules (E and P selectins) and the synthesis of PAF and IL-8.

Furthermore, as granulocytes try to engulf large IC aggregates or immobilized IC, they become activated and release their enzymatic contents, including metalloproteinases with protease and collagenase activities and oxygen active radicals. These compounds can damage cells, digest basement membranes and collagen-rich structures, and contribute to the perpetuation of the inflammatory reaction by causing direct breakdown of C5 and C3 and generating additional C5a and C3a. The formation of C3b promotes the formation of C3 convertase and further activation complement, thus continuing to amplify the pro-inflammatory reaction. As the inflammatory reaction continues to intensify, clinical manifestations emerge. The clinical manifestations of IC disease depend on the intensity of the inflammatory reaction and on the tissue(s) predominantly affected by IC deposition.

While the involvement of neutrophils and complement in acute inflammatory processes induced by ICs has been well-documented, chronic inflammatory processes, such as the smoldering vascular inflammation characteristic of atherosclerosis, are usually associated with infiltrates of activated macrophages, probably reflecting more complex pathogenic pathways with participation of activated Th1 cells, and predominantly extravascular formation of IC involving modified lipoproteins and the corresponding IgG antibodies.

Influence of antigen in pathological effects of immune complexes

The consensus about the pathogenic consequences of ICs has centered on their pro-inflammatory effects consequent to the activation of the complement system and phagocytic cells. However, it has been recently demonstrated that the nature of the antigen involved in IC formation has a modulatory effect on the macrophage response. ICs containing low-density lipoprotein (LDL) with different degrees of modification and ICs containing keyhole limpet hemocyanin were compared for their ability to release pro-inflammatory cytokines, release matrix metalloproteinases, and induce apoptosis. In general, all types of tested ICs induced similar levels of released IL-6 and MCP-1, but ICs containing highly oxidized LDL induced significantly higher degrees of apoptosis as well as of release of

TNF and matrix metalloporoteinase-1. These findings correlated with clinical observations showing that patients with circulating IC containing high levels of highly modified LDL were at a significantly higher risk for acute cardiovascular events, such as myocardial infarction.

HOST FACTORS THAT INFLUENCE DEVELOPMENT OF IMMUNE COMPLEX DISEASE

The development of IC disease in experimental animals is clearly dependent on host factors. If several rabbits of the same strain, age, weight, and sex are immunized with identical amounts of a given heterologous protein by the same route, only a fraction of the immunized animals will form antibodies, and of those, only some will develop IC disease. The magnitude of the response primarily depends on genetic factors. The extent of tissue involvement is likely to depend on the general characteristics of the antibodies produced (such as affinity, complement-binding ability, capacity to interact with cell receptors) as well as on the functional state of the reticuloendothelial system of the animal.

The affinity and number of available Fcγ receptors on professional phagocytic cells (PMN leukocytes, monocytes, and macrophages) are important in the expression of IC disease. If ICs are predominantly taken up by those cells in tissues where they abound, such as the liver and spleen, the likelihood of developing tissue inflammation is limited. Thus, it follows that blocking the Fc-mediated clearance of IC would result in longer IC circulation time and increased pathogenicity, and this concept is supported by observations in patients with SLE and rheumatoid arthritis. Those patients have decreased ability to clear antibody-sensitized red cells, indicating a general inability to clear circulating ICs that would facilitate tissue deposition and the development of inflammatory lesions.

The importance of the interaction of IC with tissue Fcγ receptors has been highlighted by experiments carried out in animal models of atherosclerosis. One of the models utilized apolipoprotein E–deficient mice, predisposed to develop atherosclerosis, with an additional genetic deletion of the γ chain of the Fcγ receptors, which results in inhibition of signaling after occupancy of the receptors. The mice deficient in the γ chain of the Fc receptors showed a significant attenuation

of vascular inflammation and development of atherosclerosis compared with the animals with functional Fcγ receptors. A second model, using diabetic LDL receptor–negative mice, showed that administration of F(ab')$_2$ fragments of anti-oxidized LDL, which form ICs unable to interact with Fcγ receptors, showed similar attenuation of vascular inflammation and of the development of atherosclerosis.

The ability to interact with complement receptors may also be an important determinant of pathogenicity. C1q, C3b, C3bi, C3c, and C3d readily associate with IC. This allows IC to bind to cells expressing the corresponding complement receptors. As mentioned previously, the binding of IC to CR1 expressed on the surface membrane of red cells facilitates their clearance for the circulation. In patients with SLE and other IC diseases, the number of CR1 on the surface of red cells is decreased, and this contributes to decreased IC clearance. This decreased CR1 expression has been claimed to be genetically determined in SLE. However, it is possible that the decrease may not be numerical, but functional. In other words, in patients with high concentrations of circulating IC, CR1 may be saturated, and this may result in the blocking of receptors by the IC, impairing IC clearance.

DETECTION OF SOLUBLE IMMUNE COMPLEXES

Many techniques have been proposed for the detection of soluble ICs. In general, these techniques are based on either the physical properties (e.g., precipitation with polyethylene glycol [PEG] or precipitation at cold temperatures) or the biologic characteristics of the IC. The latter techniques make use of various properties of ICs such as their ability to bind C1q or their binding to cells that express CR1 and CR2 (Raji cell assay).

Detection of cryoglobulins

Circulating ICs are often formed in antigen excess, with low-affinity antibodies, and remain soluble at room temperature. However, if the serum containing these IC is cooled to 4°C for about 24 hours, the stability of the antigen-antibody reaction increases, and eventually there is sufficient cross-linking to

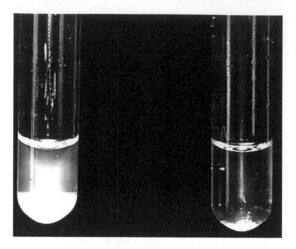

Figure 23.5 Cryoglobulin screening. Two test tubes were filled with sera from a patient (left) and a healthy volunteer (right). After 48 hours at 4°C, a precipitate is obvious in the patient's serum but is not present in the control.

result in the formation of large aggregates that precipitate spontaneously (Figure 23.5). Because antibodies are the main constituents of these cold precipitates, and because antibodies are globulins, the precipitated proteins are designated as cryoglobulins. Serum separated from blood drawn, clotted, and centrifuged at 37°C is used for the detection of cryoglobulins. The proper characterization of a cryoprecipitate requires redissolution of the precipitated proteins at 37°C, followed by identification of their constituents by appropriate immunochemical assays. Based on immunochemical characterization, cryoglobulins can be classified in two major types:

Monoclonal cryoglobulins: Containing immunoglobulin of one single isotype and one single light-chain class, are usually detected in patients with plasma cell malignancies and in some cases of idiopathic cryoglobulinemia. Monoclonal cryoglobulins are essentially monoclonal proteins with abnormal thermal behavior, and their existence has no correlation with IC formation or any special diagnostic significance besides the possibility of creating conditions favorable for the development of the hyperviscosity syndrome (see Chapter 27).
Mixed cryoglobulins: Contain two or three immunoglobulin isotypes, one of which (usually IgM)

can be a monoclonal component (with one single light-chain type and one single heavy-chain class), while the remaining immunoglobulins are polyclonal. Complement components (C3, C1q) can also be found in the cryoprecipitates containing mixed cryoglobulins. Mixed cryoglobulins represent cold-precipitable ICs. One of the immunoglobulins present in the precipitate is an antibody that reacts with the other immunoglobulin(s) that constitute the cryoglobulin. The most frequent type of mixed cryoglobulin is IgM-IgG, in which IgM is a rheumatoid factor. It is believed that, at least in some cases, the IgM antibody is directed to determinants expressed by IgG antibodies bound to their corresponding antigens (Figure 23.6). Evidence supporting the involvement of infectious agents in the formation of mixed cryoglobulins has been obtained by identifying antigens and/or antibodies in the cryoprecipitates, particularly antigens derived from hepatitis B and C viruses.

Assays based on interactions with complement

One of the techniques used for general screening of IC is based on the binding of C1q. It is usually performed on a solid base platform, in which purified C1q is immobilized in the wells of a microtiter plate and when an IC-containing sample is added to the C1q-coated well, the IC contained in the added sample will be bound to the immobilized C1q. To determine whether ICs are bound to C1q, radiolabeled or enzyme-labeled anti-human IgG antibodies are added to the wells; their retention on the plate is directly proportional to the IC captured by the immobilized C1q. Alternative immunoassays using monoclonal anti-C1q antibodies were also developed.

Precipitation of soluble immune complexes with polyethylene glycol

Low concentrations (3%–4%) of polyethylene glycol (PEG) cause preferential precipitation of IC relative to monomeric immunoglobulins. As a screening technique, PEG precipitation is nonspecific. But if the antigen involved in IC formation is

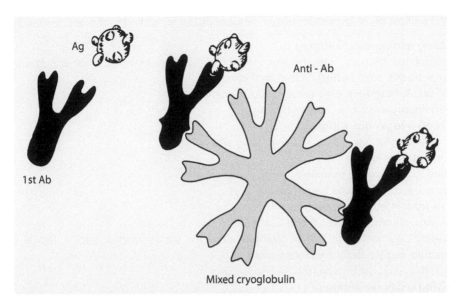

Figure 23.6 **Pathogenesis of mixed cryoglobulins.** Initially, an antimicrobial antibody (e.g.,) of the IgG class is produced. This antibody, as a consequence of binding to the antigen, exposes a new antigenic determinant, which is recognized by an IgM antiglobulin. The combination of this IgM with the first IgG antibody and the microbial antigen constitutes the mixed cryoglobulin. Viral antigens and corresponding antibodies (e.g., HBsAg and Anti-HBsAg) have been characterized in cryoprecipitates from patients with mixed cryoglobulins, both with and without a history of previous viral hepatitis B infection. It is believed that this mechanism, antiviral IgG combined with an IgM anti-antibody, accounts for over 50% of the cases of essential or idiopathic cryoglobulinemia (cryoglobulinemia appearing in patients without evidence of any other disease).

not precipitable in its soluble form, its finding on a PEG precipitate can be considered as evidence of the presence of circulating IC involving that particular antigenic protein. Also, PEG precipitation is often used as the initial step of IC isolation protocols.

All of the assays previously described have a significant drawback: their lack of specificity. For that reason, they have been considered of limited value in clinical practice.

Assays based on characterization of the antigen(s) involved in immune complex formation

The characterization of antigens and antibodies in PEG-precipitated IC has been proven to be more clinically valuable than the nonspecific assays, particularly as biomarkers for the progression of cardiovascular disease. However, those assays involve many steps, and there has not been any successful attempt to develop simplified assays that could be used in diagnostic laboratories, so they have been performed exclusively as part of research studies.

ROLE OF IMMUNE COMPLEXES IN HUMAN DISEASE

Classification of immune complex diseases

ICs have been implicated in human disease either through demonstration in serum or through identification in tissues where lesions are found. Most often the antibody moiety of the IC is detected, and knowledge about the antigens involved is still very fragmentary. However, one of the most common classifications of IC disease, proposed by a committee sponsored by the World Health Organization, is based on the nature of the antigens involved (Table 23.2).

Table 23.2 A classification of immune complex diseases (ICDs) according to the antigen involved

1. **ICD involving endogenous antigens**
   - *Immunoglobulin antigens*, e.g., rheumatoid arthritis, hypergammaglobulinemic purpura
   - *Nuclear antigens*, e.g., systemic lupus erythematosus
   - *Specific cellular antigens*, e.g., tumors, autoimmune diseases
   - *Modified lipoproteins*, e.g., atherosclerosis
2. **ICD involving exogenous antigens**
   - *Medicinal antigens*, e.g., serum sickness, drug allergy
   - *Environmental antigens*
     - Inhaled, e.g., extrinsic alveolitis
     - Ingested, e.g., dermatitis herpetiformis
   - *Antigens from infectious organisms*
     - Viral, e.g., chronic hepatitis B and C, HIV/AIDS
     - Bacterial, e.g., poststreptococcal glomerulonephritis, subacute endocarditis, leprosy, syphilis
     - Protozoan, e.g., malaria, trypanosomiasis
     - Helminthic, e.g., schistosomiasis, onchocerciasis
3. **ICD involving unknown antigens**
   This category includes most forms of chronic immune complex glomerulonephritis, vasculitis with or without eosinophilia, and many cases of mixed cryoglobulinemia

Clinical expression of immune complex disease

The clinical expression of IC disease depends on the target organs where the deposition of IC predominates:

- The kidney is very frequently affected (SLE, mixed cryoglobulinemia, chronic infections, poststreptococcal glomerulonephritis, purpura hypergammaglobulinemia, serum sickness, etc.), usually with glomerulonephritis as the prevailing feature.
- The joints are predominantly affected in rheumatoid arthritis.
- The skin is affected in cases of serum sickness, mixed cryoglobulinemia, purpura, and vasculitis.
- The large vessels are affected by the subendothelial formation of antigen-antibody complexes containing oxidized LDL and the corresponding antibodies, leading to the development or progression of atherosclerosis.
- The lungs are affected in extrinsic alveolitis.

The reasons why the target organs can vary from disease to disease are not clear. In some cases, such as in extrinsic alveolitis, the route of exposure to the antigen is a major determinant for the involvement of the lungs. The kidneys, due to their physiological role and to the existence of complement and Fc receptors in different anatomical structures, appear to be an ideal organ for IC trapping. In rheumatoid arthritis, ICs appear to be present not only in the circulation but also (and probably formed) in and around the joints, and although they do not appear to be the initiating factor for the disease, their potential for perpetuating the inflammatory lesions is unquestionable. The skin manifestations are obviously easy to detect, but the same patients may have involvement of other organs and tissues, e.g., vasculitis associated with chronic hepatitis B virus infection.

THERAPEUTIC APPROACHES TO IMMUNE COMPLEX DISEASE

The most common types of therapy in IC disease are based on four main approaches:

- Eradication of the source of persistent antigen production (e.g., infections).
- Turning off the inflammatory reaction (using corticosteroids and nonsteroidal agents).
- Suppression of antibody production using immunosuppressive drugs such as cyclophosphamide, azathioprine, cyclosporine, or CD20 antibodies (e.g., rituximab). This is the mainstay of IC disease treatment, particularly when autoimmune reactions are present.

- Removal of soluble IC from the circulation by plasmapheresis, a procedure that consists of the removal of blood (up to 5 L each time), separation and reinfusion of red cells, and replacement of the patient's plasma by normal plasma or plasma-replacing solutions. Plasmapheresis appears most beneficial when associated with the administration of immunosuppressive drugs; by itself, it can even induce severe clinical deterioration perhaps related to changes in the immunoregulatory circuits.

In the last few years, there has been considerable interest in applying emerging basic concepts on the pathogenesis of inflammation to the treatment of a variety of conditions in which IC formation or deposition may play an important role. Four major approaches have been tried:

- Blocking critical cytokines, such as TNF. This has been done either with monoclonal antibodies reacting with pro-inflammatory cytokines, with cytokine receptor antagonists, or with recombinant cytokine receptors. A TNF-receptor-Fc fusion protein that blocks the effects of TNF is widely used in the treatment of rheumatoid arthritis.
- Interruption of the interaction between leukocyte integrins and endothelial cell adhesion molecules. Humanized anti-ICAM-1 (and other cell-cell interaction-facilitating molecules) as well as soluble forms of these molecules have been successfully tested in animal models.
- Inhibition of the complement activation cascade using soluble forms of regulatory proteins (C1q inhibitor, MCP, DAF, CR1) and antifactor antibodies (anti-C5 antibody) with the goal of inhibiting the production of C3a and C5a (see Chapter 9).
- Administration of F(ab)′2 fragments of oxidized LDL IgG antibody has been shown to attenuate vascular inflammation and plaque formation in diabetic LDL receptor–deficient mice, suggesting possible medical application.

BIBLIOGRAPHY

Bamoulid J, Staeck O, Crépin T et al. Antithymocyte globulins in kidney transplantation: Focus on current indications and long-term immunological side effects. *Nephrol Dial Transplant*. 2017;32:1601–1608.

Chen M, Daha MR, Kallenberg CG. The complement system in systemic autoimmune disease. *J Autoimmun*. 2010;34:J276–J286.

de Silva HA, Ryan NM, de Silva HJ. Adverse reactions to snake antivenom, and their prevention and treatment. *Br J Clin Pharmacol*. 2016;81:446–452.

Ferri C, Zignego AL, Pileri SA. Cryoglobulins. *J Clin Pathol*. 2002;55:4–13.

Hebert LA. The clearance of immune complexes from the circulation of man and other primates. *Am J Kidney*. 1991;17:352–361.

Hernández-Vargas P, Ortiz-Muñoz G, López-Franco O et al. Fcγ receptor deficiency confers protection against atherosclerosis in apolipoprotein E knockout mice. *Circ Res*. 2006 24;99:1188–1196.

Jancar S, Crespo MS. Immune complex-mediated tissue injury: A multistep paradigm. *Trends Immunol*. 2005;26:48–55.

Lopes-Virella MF, Virella G. Modified LDL immune complexes and cardiovascular disease. *Curr Med Chem*. 2019;26:1680–1692.

Means TK, Latz E, Hayashi F, Murali MR, Golenbock DT, Luster AD. Human lupus autoantibody-DNA complexes activate DCs through cooperation of CD32 and TLR9. *J Clin Invest*. 2005;115: 407–417.

Nourshargh S, Alon R. Leukocyte migration into inflamed tissues. *Immunity*. 2014;41:694–707.

Nydegger UE. Immune complex pathophysiology. *Ann NY Acad Sci*. 2007;1109:66–83.

Ragab G, Hussein MA. Vasculitic syndromes in hepatitis C virus: A review. *J Adv Res*. 2017;8: 99–111.

Tecklenborg J, Clayton D, Siebert S, Coley SM. The role of the immune system in kidney disease. *Clin Exp Immunol*. 2018;192:142–150.

Tsokos GC. Lymphocytes, cytokines, inflammation, and immune trafficking. *Curr Opin Rheumatol*. 1995;7:376–383.

Van Hoeyveld E, Bossuyt X. Evaluation of seven commercial ELISA kits compared with the C1q solid-phase binding RIA for detection of circulating immune complexes. *Clin Chem*. 2000; 46:283–285.

Virella G, Wilson K, Elkes J et al. Immune complexes containing malondialdehyde (MDA)

LDL induce apoptosis in human macrophages. *Clinl Immunol.* 2018;187:1–9.

Warren JS, Ward PA. Immune complex diseases. In: *Encyclopedia of Life Sciences.* Published online: April 2017. doi: 10.1002/9780470015902. a0002164.pub3

Yanchun L, Zhongyang L, Yan H et al. F(ab′)2 fragments of anti-oxidized LDL IgG attenuate vascular inflammation and atherogenesis in diabetic LDL receptor-deficient mice. *Clin Immunol.* 2016;173:50–56.

24

Immune system modulators

RICHARD M. SILVER AND STEPHEN ELMORE

INTRODUCTION

Immune system modulators are agents that alter the activity of an individual's immune response, either up or down, until the desired immunity level is reached. Typical targets for such modulators include the major components of the immune response (T and B lymphocytes) as well as cellular products (including cytokines and chemokines). The goal is to selectively "fine-tune" the function of the various parts of the immune system to promote better health in the patient. Immunomodulation can be broken down into two general scenarios:

1. *Immunosuppression*: Therapies that act to dampen the immune response. This is useful in conditions where T and B cells have become activated against one's own body, such as in autoimmune diseases, or when trying to prevent organ rejection following transplantation. Such immunosuppression can be generalized or more selective in nature.
2. *Immunopotentiation*: Boosting the immune system function of the patient, either by stimulating the original immune system to respond better (such as with immunizations) or by introducing protective immune system components into the body to stimulate a more robust response (i.e., immunoglobulins).

IMMUNOSUPPRESSION

Suppression of the immune system remains the most effective therapeutic approach to controlling autoimmune diseases, as well as preventing organ rejection following transplant. Initially, such therapies were focused on general immunosuppression, allowing for a broad, nonspecific downregulation of the immune system, usually targeting humoral or cell-mediated responses. Recently, however, newer agents have been developed that are more selective in terms of their immune activity. These targeted immunosuppressive therapies limit the impact on the immune system, resulting in a greater response to the therapy while decreasing overall side effects. Newer agents are being introduced to the market at a rapid pace, treating previously recalcitrant diseases and providing a pathway for the development of similarly specified therapies in other fields, including oncology.

IMMUNOSUPPRESSIVE DRUGS: PHARMACOLOGICAL AND IMMUNOLOGICAL ASPECTS

Glucocorticoids

Glucocorticoids, or corticosteroids, remain one of the oldest and most widely used of the immunosuppressive agents. This class of drugs acts on the immune systems in a number of ways.

Induction of apoptosis. At high doses, glucocorticoids can produce lymphopenia via activation of an endonuclease that leads to apoptosis. The steroid binds to a glucocorticoid-cytoplasmic receptor, after which the resulting complex translocates to the nucleus. There, it binds to glucocorticoid-responsive elements of regulatory DNA sequences, where one of two possible actions may occur: proteins that normally inhibit endonuclease are downregulated, allowing greater endonuclease activity, or specific caspases are upregulated and act directly to degrade the endonuclease inhibiting protein.

Downregulation of cytokine synthesis. Glucocorticoids downregulate cytokine production by preventing the expression of genes encoding cytokine production. Again, the exact process is not known, but two mechanisms are hypothesized. In the first, the glucocorticoid-cytoplasmic receptor complex prevents a protein, AP-1, from interacting with promoters that allow for the transcription of cytokine genes. A second hypothesis suggests that the steroid-receptor complex itself binds to promoters to upregulate production of the NFκB inhibitory protein IKB. With increased inhibition of NFκB, cytokine production is diminished.

Anti-inflammatory effects. Glucocorticoids provide a variety of anti-inflammatory effects. As noted previously, glucocorticoids can decrease production of cytokines involved in the inflammatory cascade. As the synthesis of cytokines declines, a similar reduction in the expression of cell-adhesion molecules (CAMs) on the walls of blood vessels occurs. This, in turn, means that fewer neutrophils and T lymphocytes engage in inflammatory responses, instead remaining sequestered in the bone marrow and lymph nodes. The glucocorticoid-receptor complex, in addition to the previously noted effects, can also decrease production of phospholipase A2. The downregulation of this protein results in diminished synthesis of leukotrienes, prostaglandins, and platelet-activating factor, known mediators of inflammation. Finally, glucocorticoids can decrease the production of nitric oxide (NO) leading to less vasodilation.

Nonsteroidal anti-inflammatory drugs

Nonsteroidal anti-inflammatory drugs (NSAIDs) work by inhibiting prostaglandin and thromboxane synthesis via inhibition of cyclooxygenase (COX), which acts on arachidonic acid to form these products; as a result, they do not result in direct immunosuppression. There are two functional isoforms of COX in humans; COX-1 is constitutively expressed in the vast majority of cells, while COX-2 occurs predominantly in inflamed tissue only. The ability to inhibit COX-2 forms the basis of the anti-inflammatory effect of NSAIDs. Initially, the only such agents available were nonselective NSAIDs, which target COX-1 and COX-2 equally. Examples include aspirin, ibuprofen, indomethacin, and naproxen. While these agents work to lower inflammation by inhibiting COX-2, they can also predispose patients to adverse side effects, including gastrointestinal side effects and gastric ulcer formation, through their inhibition of COX-1. It was thought that the development of selective COX-2 inhibitors would provide the same level of anti-inflammatory effect while avoiding many of the harmful side effects. Three COX-2 inhibitors were eventually approved for use in the United States, including celecoxib, rofecoxib, and valdecoxib. Studies with celecoxib demonstrated that it provided similar analgesic relief in patients with rheumatoid arthritis as the nonselective NSAID naproxen, while having a lower incidence of gastric ulcers. However, the selective COX-2 agents were subsequently found to increase the risk of cardiovascular events in a dose-dependent fashion, and both rofecoxib and valdecoxib were removed from the market due to these risks, leaving celecoxib (celebrex) as the only agent in this class available for use in the United States. The addition of low-dose aspirin to celecoxib therapy has been shown to lessen the cardiovascular risk associated with COX-2 inhibition, and with a lower risk for gastrointestinal toxicity when compared to traditional nonselective COX inhibitors, e.g., ibuprofen and naproxen.

Cell cycle–specific alkylating agents

Cell cycle–specific agents work by interfering with the cell-division cycle, resulting in cell death. A number of medications fall into this category, including methotrexate, azathioprine, mycophenolate mofetil (MMF), and leflunomide.

METHOTREXATE

A folic acid analogue, methotrexate binds to and interferes with dihydrofolate reductase, resulting in decreased thymidine production and preventing DNA replication. As T lymphocytes interact with antigen-presenting cells (APCs), they enter the S-phase of the cell cycle in an attempt to proliferate. Through its actions, methotrexate prevents this. Unfortunately, its interference with S-phase activity is not limited to T lymphocytes, and instead acts on all rapidly dividing cells. As a result, methotrexate can cause bone marrow suppression resulting in cytopenias, as well as diarrhea, nausea and vomiting, stomatitis, and hair loss when cells in the bone marrow, gastrointestinal (GI) tract, and skin are impacted. The use of folic acid supplementation (typically 1 mg per day) may help to limit such toxicity. Several other major side effects are associated with use of methotrexate. Hepatotoxicity, including elevated serum transaminases and development of hepatic fibrosis and cirrhosis, has been noted in psoriatic arthritis patients treated with methotrexate. Although also seen in rheumatoid arthritis patients, hepatotoxicity appears less common, though this may be in part due to adjustments in the dose of methotrexate administered. Rarely, methotrexate can contribute to pulmonary toxicity in the form of interstitial pneumonitis. Methotrexate is also classified as a teratogen, capable of causing central nervous system (CNS) abnormalities in the developing fetus as well as leading to spontaneous abortion. Other side effects include skin rashes, headaches, and increased infection rates.

Methotrexate is used in the treatment of multiple diseases, including serving as the primary disease-modifying antirheumatic drug in the treatment of rheumatoid arthritis and psoriatic arthritis, as well as in treating certain types of malignancy (breast cancer, acute lymphoblastic leukemia). Other conditions in which methotrexate is used include juvenile idiopathic arthritis, polymyalgia rheumatica, antineutrophil cytoplasmic antibody (ANCA) associated vasculitis, and myositis. While using the medication, lab monitoring of blood counts and liver and renal function are carried out every 8–12 weeks once the patient is on a stable dose. Individuals are asked to limit alcohol intake while on the medication (given the risk of hepatotoxicity) and are generally advised to hold the medication during periods of serious infection.

AZATHIOPRINE

A prodrug of 6-mercaptopurine, azathioprine, following administration, is taken up by hepatocytes and red blood cells, where glutathione acts to metabolize it. The now formed 6-mercaptopurine is then further broken down into thiopurine ribonucleosides and nucleotides that act to inhibit the purine synthesis pathways. This, in turn, prevents T- and B-lymphocyte proliferation. The most common side effects of azathioprine include GI disturbances, such as diarrhea and nausea, bone marrow suppression, as well as an increased risk of developing non-Hodgkin's lymphoma with prolonged use. Previously, azathioprine was used alongside cyclosporine and prednisone to prevent rejection in solid organ transplant recipients, although the use of MMF (vide infra) has overtaken this role. Azathioprine is still commonly used in the treatment of systemic lupus erythematosus and is one of the few lupus medications that are safe to continue during pregnancy. Other diseases in which azathioprine has been used successfully include polymyositis and dermatomyositis, ANCA-associated vasculitis, and Crohn's disease.

MYCOPHENOLATE MOFETIL

MMF also works to decrease T- and B-lymphocyte proliferation by inhibiting inosine monophosphate dehydrogenase, an enzyme essential for the synthesis of guanine via the de novo pathway. While other cells are able to compensate for guanine production via a salvage pathway, T and B lymphocytes are entirely dependent on the de novo pathway and are thus unable to replicate. Side effects of MMF are similar to those seen with azathioprine, including GI intolerance, cytopenias, and hepatotoxicity. Like other immunosuppressive agents, use of this agent does increase the risk of infection. Mycophenolate serves as treatment for a number of conditions. It has become one of the primary prophylactic agents to prevent rejection following solid organ transplant. In terms of autoimmune diseases, it plays a role in the treatment of lupus nephritis as well as preventing progression of lung fibrosis in scleroderma-associated interstitial lung disease (SSc-ILD). Frequent lab work to monitor cell counts and liver and renal function is required, as is the need to avoid pregnancy, as mycophenolate is a teratogenic agent.

LEFLUNOMIDE

This agent works to impair the *de novo* pathway of pyrimidine synthesis, specifically targeting and inhibiting dihydro-orotate dehydrogenase. Side effects of leflunomide are similar in nature to those appreciated with methotrexate but can be more prolonged due to the longer half-life of the medication. Other side effects include headache, dizziness, skin rash, and hypertension. In addition, leflunomide is also teratogenic. Leflunomide has found a role in the treatment of rheumatoid arthritis, with trials demonstrating that it has a similar efficacy as methotrexate and sulfasalazine. Other diseases where leflunomide has been used include psoriatic arthritis, juvenile idiopathic arthritis, and several forms of vasculitis.

CYCLOPHOSPHAMIDE

Cyclophosphamide is an alkylating agent that inhibits both the cellular and humoral immune responses. After administration, cyclophosphamide is broken down into active metabolites that prevent DNA replication, causing the death of both dividing and nondividing T and B lymphocytes. Initially, cyclophosphamide was administered as a daily oral agent. However, intravenous (IV) cyclophosphamide pulses are now favored, as the IV form has a lower risk of toxicity, including fewer incidents of hemorrhagic cystitis and bladder cancer. The IV dosing for cyclophosphamide is typically carried out on an intermittent basis (usually every few weeks to monthly, depending on the cycle utilized). Side effects associated with cyclophosphamide include hematologic abnormalities (particularly leukopenia), nausea and vomiting, and diminished fertility in both male and female patients, in addition to the previously mentioned bladder toxicity. The use of Mesna, a sulfhydryl compound, administered before and after IV cyclophosphamide infusions, may lower the risk of bladder toxicity by binding to and neutralizing the toxic effects of acrolein and other urotoxic by-products of cyclophosphamide. Cyclophosphamide has found a role in the treatment of several autoimmune diseases resistant to steroid and other immunosuppressive treatment, including lupus nephritis, SSc-ILD, and ANCA-associated vasculitides.

Inhibitors of signal transduction: Cyclosporine, tacrolimus, and sirolimus

Immunophilins belong to a class of drugs synthesized from fungal metabolites that have some immunosuppressive properties. There are two classes: macrocyclic peptides, including the agent cyclosporine, and macrocyclic lactones, such as tacrolimus and sirolimus. Immunophilins work by inhibiting the signal transduction that lymphocytes rely on for activation and proliferation. As they act on signal transduction, these agents have no impact on lymphocyte precursors and thus avoid the side effects of leukopenia and lymphopenia seen with cytotoxic medications.

CYCLOSPORINE A

Derived from the fungus *Tolypocladium inflatum*, cyclosporine A is a cyclic undecapeptide that works to selectively inhibit T lymphocytes by suppression of humoral T-cell dependent and cell-mediated responses. It binds to the cytosol-based protein cyclophilin to form a complex that goes on to bind to and inactivate calcineurin. Normally, calcineurin activates nuclear factor of activated T cells (NF-AT). NF-AT, in turn, upregulates expression of interleukin-2 (IL-2), a pro-inflammatory cytokine. The inactivation of calcineurin thus downregulates production of IL-2, as well as a number of other cytokines produced via the Ca^{2+} associated T-cell activation pathway, including IL-3, IL-4, interferon-γ (IFN-γ), and tumor necrosis factor (TNF). The predominant targets of cyclosporine are CD4$^+$ helper T cells, but cyclosporine also impedes the differentiation of Foxp3T regulatory cells and also both directly and indirectly inhibits the activation of cytotoxic T-cell precursors.

Cyclosporine's role in medicine has expanded over the years. It has a prominent place in transplant medicine as a means to prolong the life of organ transplants and grafts. Studies have demonstrated that the use of cyclosporine decreases the incidence and severity of graft-versus-host disease in bone marrow transplant recipients. Cyclosporine works well with other immunosuppressive medications, enabling clinicians to use smaller doses of these medications to achieve their goal of immunosuppression. In terms of autoimmune diseases, cyclosporine is occasionally used in the treatment of lupus nephritis as well as psoriasis, rheumatoid arthritis, ulcerative colitis, and as part of the acute treatment of the macrophage activation syndrome. Cyclosporine does have its fair share of side effects, including hypertension, hypercholesterolemia, hepatotoxicity, hirsutism, and gingival hyperplasia. Although used in renal transplant recipients, cyclosporine can cause nephrotoxicity, especially if the daily dose exceeds 5 mg/kg. Use of cyclosporine can also increase rates of cytomegalovirus infection in transplant recipients. It has been associated with an increased incidence of lymphoproliferative syndromes as well.

TACROLIMUS

Tacrolimus is another fungal metabolite that targets FK506 binding protein (FKBP) in cells. The formed complex acts similarly to the cyclophilin-cyclosporine complex to inactivate calcineurin and prevent NF-AT activation. This results in similar effects as demonstrated with cyclosporine. Although initially used in liver transplant recipients, tacrolimus, like cyclosporine, is used in other organ transplants as well. Tacrolimus has many of the same side effects as cyclosporine, albeit less severe, along with additional concerns for GI intolerance and neurotoxicity.

SIROLIMUS

Although similar in nature to tacrolimus, sirolimus (rapamycin) instead binds to both FKBP as well as to the mammalian target of rapamycin (mTOR, previously FKBP-sirolimus associated protein or FRAP). The ensuing complex then works to inactivate specific kinases that are normally activated by the binding of IL-2 and IL-4 to their respective receptors. As a result, IL-2 and IL-4 responsive cells are unable to progress through replication. Like cyclosporine and tacrolimus, sirolimus is used for prophylaxis against organ transplant rejection.

Kinase inhibitors: Tofacitinib

Tyrosine kinases have recently been identified to be significant mediators of intracellular signaling and regulatory pathways. When certain ligands bind to an associated cell-surface receptor, these kinases are triggered to phosphorylate particular amino acids, thus activating proteins. These can then translocate to the nucleus to allow for transcription of particular genes. Although a number

of tyrosine kinases exist, the JAK kinase family has emerged as a particularly effective target for treating rheumatoid arthritis and perhaps other autoimmune diseases as well. Tofacitinib is an orally administered small molecule JAK kinase inhibitor that works on JAK1 and JAK3. Blockade of these signals leads to a reduction in a number of cytokines and interferons involved in the inflammatory processes important to the pathogenesis of rheumatoid arthritis. Side effects of tofacitinib include increased infection risk, especially with herpes zoster, as well as cytopenias, elevated serum transaminases, and hyperlipidemia. Tofacitinib is approved for the treatment of rheumatoid arthritis, psoriatic arthritis, and ulcerative colitis, and is administered as a once-daily extended-release pill or a twice-daily regular dose. Baricitinib is another small molecule JAK1 and JAK2 inhibitor that was recently approved for the treatment of patients with moderate-to-severe rheumatoid arthritis. Studies of tofacitinib, baricitinib, and other JAK inhibitors for the treatment of other autoimmune diseases, e.g., systemic lupus erythematosus, are currently underway.

Immunosuppressive polyclonal antibody preparations

Polyclonal antibody preparations are used in the treatment of acute solid organ transplant rejection episodes that fail treatment with corticosteroid. Two main agents fall into this category: antithymocyte globulin (equine antiserum) and thymoglobulin (rabbit antiserum). Each agent is formed by injecting their respective animal host with human T lymphocytes, then harvesting and sterilizing the serum. This, in turn, is administered to the patient. Although the serum contains antibodies directed against the T lymphocytes facilitating the rejection episode, it also contains antibodies against other cellular components in the blood, resulting in a variety of cytopenias. It also can trigger a serum-sickness response because of the heterologous nature of horse and rabbit antibodies.

Immunosuppressive monoclonal antibodies and other biological response modifiers

Monoclonal antibodies represent one of most groundbreaking developments in immunology of the past century. By taking advantage of the ability of B lymphocytes to produce antibodies directed against specific antigens, newer agents are being developed that can have a more selective impact on the immune response. To produce monoclonal antibodies, an animal host (typically murine) is immunized with a specific antigen against which antibodies are to be formed. The mature B cells that develop are then harvested and combined with a line of immortal myeloma cells, forming hybridomas that continually replicate. These hybridomas are then screened to select the lines producing the desired antibody. In order to prevent an immune response or even a hypersensitivity reaction from occurring due to the use of a fully murine monoclonal antibody, efforts have been made to produce genetically modified antibodies that are either chimeric (antibodies that combine the antigen-binding region derived from the murine cells with a human Ig constant region) or fully humanized. These efforts help to decrease the development of antibodies directed against the monoclonal antibody. A number of agents have been developed to assist in the treatment of organ rejection, malignancy, and a variety of different autoimmune conditions.

Monoclonal antibodies that block costimulatory signals: Abatacept

Abatacept is a fusion protein consisting of the Fc portion of human IgG bound to a CTLA-4 domain that targets T cell activation. Normally, T cells bind with APCs via a cell-to-cell interaction that includes a number of costimulatory signals encountering one another. Abatacept acts on one such costimulatory process, preventing CD-28 from binding to B7-1 and B7-2 molecules on the APC. As a result, the T cell, despite being bound to the APC, cannot sustain activation, and the immune response is downregulated. Patients receive the medication either as a monthly infusion or as a weekly self-administered injection. Side effects include infusion site reactions, increased risk of infection, as well as possible increased risk of malignancy similar to that seen with other biologic agents. Abatacept has been used primarily in the treatment of rheumatoid arthritis in patients who have failed a tumor necrosis factor inhibitor agent, but it can be used as monotherapy and is also approved for the treatment of patients with psoriatic arthritis or juvenile idiopathic arthritis.

Monoclonal antibodies directed against CD20

Rituximab is a chimeric monoclonal antibody directed against CD20, which is expressed on pre–B lymphocytes, mature B lymphocytes, and some populations of dendritic cells and malignant plasma cells, but not on stem cells or mature plasma cells. By binding to CD20, rituximab induces B-cell death by a variety of mechanisms: apoptosis induction, complement-mediated cytotoxicity, and antibody-dependent cellular cytotoxicity. As a consequence, the numbers of CD20$^+$ B cells are reduced, subsequently diminishing the production of autoantibodies. The impact of rituximab lasts for several months before wearing off and allowing a new population of B cells to arise. Rituximab has been used in a variety of conditions, including treatment of B-cell lymphomas, follicular cell lymphoma, refractory rheumatoid arthritis, various forms of vasculitis, idiopathic thrombocytopenic purpura, and systemic lupus erythematosus. In several autoimmune diseases, it has been demonstrated that the combination of corticosteroids with rituximab leads to better clinical results than those obtained with each of the drugs by themselves.

Cytokine modifiers

As mentioned earlier, the development of monoclonal antibodies has allowed for the development of immunosuppressive drugs that have more selective targets. In particular, a number of cytokines have emerged as primary targets given the large role some play in mediating the immune response. By binding to cytokines themselves or their receptors, these cytokine modifiers can prevent pro-inflammatory effects from occurring, thus limiting the role of inflammation in a number of disease states.

TUMOR NECROSIS FACTOR INHIBITORS

TNF has been implicated as one of the primary cytokines responsible for inflammation in several diseases, including rheumatoid arthritis, psoriatic arthritis, and ankylosing spondylitis. Several different medications have been developed to inhibit TNF in a number of ways. Etanercept exists as an artificial, plasma-based version of the TNF receptor that binds to TNF before it is able to interact with cell-bound receptors and initiate the inflammatory cascade. It is typically administered as a weekly subcutaneous injection. Infliximab is a monoclonal anti-TNF antibody that is a murine/human hybrid. It functions by binding and neutralizing TNF in the plasma and is given as an IV infusion every 6–8 weeks. Due to its chimeric nature, however, use of this medication can lead to development of antichimeric antibodies that can lower the functional level of the drug, making it less effective. Adalimumab differs in that it is a fully humanized monoclonal antibody to TNF. This theoretically lowers the immunogenicity of the molecule. Adalimumab is given as a subcutaneous injection every 7–14 days. Similar to adalimumab, golimumab also is a monoclonal antibody, and its longer half-life allows the medication to be given on a monthly basis subcutaneously or every 2 months intravenously. Finally, certolizumab is another TNF inhibitor, in this case a pegylated F(ab′)$_2$ fragment of anti-TNF antibody. Its half-life is shorter (11 days) and thus it needs to be administered initially every 2 weeks and every 4 weeks for maintenance of its effects.

The TNF inhibitors all share certain side effects, including infusion/injection site reactions and increased risk of infection. Several studies have suggested that these agents may increase the risk of certain types of cancer, including lymphoma and nonmelanoma skin cancers. TNF inhibitors may worsen heart failure. Rarely, these medications can lead to a demyelinating process, and thus they are contraindicated in patients with multiple sclerosis. Finally, TNF inhibitors are one class of agents known to potentially cause drug-induced lupus. All TNF inhibitors have been approved for the treatment of rheumatoid arthritis, psoriatic arthritis, and ankylosing spondylitis. Infliximab, adalimumab, and certolizumab also are approved in the treatment of Crohn's disease, while infliximab and adalimumab are used for ulcerative colitis.

INTERLEUKIN-1 INHIBITORS: ANAKINRA, RILONACEPT, CANAKINUMAB

The cytokine interleukin-1β (IL-1β) provokes a number of immune and inflammatory responses, including its role in Th17 cell differentiation, promoting cartilage destruction, inducing fever, and stimulating production of other cytokines. IL-1β is initially produced in an inactivated form (pro-IL-1β) before becoming activated by the inflammasome, a multiprotein complex that forms in cells to cleave cytokines into their biologically active forms. Several agents have been developed to target IL-1β in order to impede its actions. Anakinra is a soluble IL-1 receptor antagonist, while canakinumab is a "human" monoclonal antibody produced in transgenic mice directed against IL-1. Both agents are able to prevent the interaction of IL-1 with its receptor, thus inhibiting the inflammatory response. Rilonacept, also known as IL-1 Trap, is a dimeric fusion protein consisting of the ligand-binding domains of the human IL-1 receptor (IL-1R1) and IL-1 receptor accessory protein (IL-1RAcP) linked to the Fc portion of IgG1 that binds and neutralizes IL-1. Side effects include infusion reactions, increased risk of infection, and a small increase in the risk of lymphoma. Anakinra and canakinumab are used in the treatment of Still's disease (both systemic-onset juvenile idiopathic arthritis [JIA] as well as the adult-onset form of Still's disease), cryopyrin-associated and other forms of periodic syndromes such as familial Mediterranean fever, hyperimmunoglobulin-D syndrome, and TNF receptor–associated periodic syndrome. Anakinra is also approved for use in rheumatoid arthritis and is being explored as a treatment for acute polyarticular gout.

INTERLEUKIN-6 ANTAGONISTS: TOCILIZUMAB, KEVZARA

Similar to IL-1β, IL-6 plays a role in several inflammatory conditions. Excessive IL-6 results in enhanced T-cell differentiation, increased IL-17 production, as well as fever, fatigue, and other constitutional symptoms. Tocilizumab and Kevzara are humanized monoclonal antibodies against IL-6 that bind to both the soluble and membrane-bound IL-6 receptor. Tocilizumab is typically administered either as a weekly subcutaneous injection or as a monthly IV infusion. Kevzara is administered as a weekly subcutaneous injection. As typical of other biologic medications, IL-6 blockade can be associated with increased rates of infections. Other side effects include an increased risk of diverticular perforation in those with underlying diverticulosis, infusion reactions, and hyperlipidemia, the significance of which is still being evaluated. Tocilizumab has been approved for use in patients with rheumatoid arthritis, systemic-onset JIA, adult-onset Still's disease, and more recently, giant cell arteritis. Kevzara has been approved for use in adult patients with moderately to severely active rheumatoid arthritis who have had an inadequate response or intolerance to one or more disease-modifying antirheumatic drugs (DMARDs).

Work continues on the identification and characterization of other cytokines that may play important roles in autoimmune diseases, leading to the development of effective and safe agents that downregulate such effects. Two of the newer cytokine inhibitors target IL-17 and IL-23. IL-17 has been implicated as contributing to bone and cartilage destruction in inflammatory arthritis via activation of osteoclasts, as well as working with several of the previously mentioned cytokines to increase the inflammatory response. Secukinumab is a monoclonal antibody against IL-17A that has been approved for the treatment of ankylosing spondylitis and psoriatic arthritis. It is administered as a monthly injection. It has many of the same contraindications and risks as other biologic medications. IL-23 is produced by a number of immune cells and appears to play a role in the production of many pro-inflammatory cytokines. Ustekinumab is a monoclonal antibody that blocks this cytokine and thus its multiple downstream actions. Ustekinumab is approved for use in the treatment of psoriatic arthritis and Crohn's disease and is administered as a subcutaneous injection every 12 weeks.

ADVERSE EFFECTS OF PROLONGED IMMUNOSUPPRESSION

The alteration of the body's natural immune and inflammatory processes is not without consequence. The impact of inhibiting such responses creates a number of widespread effects that go beyond simply increasing the risk for infections. Although side effects for each individual agent were previously noted, several generalized effects are listed as follows.

1. *Infection:* As one would expect, the act of suppressing the immune system can predispose an individual to increased susceptibility to infection, and this risk of infection remains one of the most common side effects of these medications. Patients on the previously discussed medications can develop both common as well as opportunistic infections. In particular, viral pathogens appear to be a particular concern, given the depression of cellular immunity. Rates of varicella zoster infection are higher in immunosuppressed individuals, although the overall course is often the same. However, disseminated spread of these diseases can occur with potentially fatal consequences, and both strong vigilance as well as aggressive treatment are needed should such infections develop, with recommendations to hold immunosuppressive medications until the infection resolves. In addition, live vaccines are contraindicated for individuals receiving immunosuppressive medications due to concern for possible dissemination. Inactivated vaccines, however, can be safely administered.

2. *Bone marrow suppression:* The most common toxicity associated with immunosuppressive agents remains bone marrow suppression, as many of these agents act on the marrow to reduce hematopoiesis and other cellular processes. The degree and severity of suppression are often related to the dose utilized and can be mitigated by frequent lab monitoring and reductions in the dose as needed. In particular, neutropenia is often associated with severe infections that can be fatal. Symptoms usually occur once white blood cell counts dip below 3000 cells/mm^3. Holding of the immunosuppressive agent is recommended until recovery of counts occurs. Other agents, such as granulocyte-colony stimulating factor, can be used to speed recovery of severely depressed neutrophil counts.

3. *Neoplasms:* Our understanding of the immune system's role in preventing development of malignancy continues to grow, and a great deal of speculation has occurred as to the risk of cancer in patients who are chronically immunosuppressed. Many of the agents used for the treatment of autoimmune conditions can be used as chemotherapeutic agents for certain malignancies. However, these same agents can also serve as potential carcinogens for other types of malignancies. Further complicating the picture is the fact that certain autoimmune conditions carry increased malignancy risks by themselves, such as an increased risk of lymphoma and leukemia in patients with rheumatoid arthritis compared to the general

population. For patients receiving immunosuppression following solid-organ transplantation, common malignancies include non-Hodgkin's lymphoma, several different forms of skin cancer including basal and squamous cell carcinoma, Kaposi sarcoma, and hepatobiliary carcinoma. While continued studies are needed to evaluate the overall increased risk of malignancy, ultimately concerns regarding potential malignancy development must be weighed against the many potential benefits these medications can have on the lives of those living with autoimmune conditions.

IMMUNOPOTENTIATION

Immunopotentiation refers to the process of attempting to increase and maximize an individual's given immune response. A number of agents exist that attempt to do so, either through their own actions or by adjusting the immune system's own components. One such group of agents includes the biological response modifiers (BRMs), a series of soluble compounds (usually cytokines and interferons) that enhance communication among the various aspects of the immune system. In contrast to hormones, BRMs act in the immediate area at which they are secreted. Their nature, timing of their secretion, along with their concentrations, are critical for potentiating the immune response. The cellular sources of these BRMs consist of the majority of cell types that make up the immune system. Examples of BRMs produced by T lymphocytes include IL-2, IL-3, IL-4, IL-5, IL-10, GM-CSF, and IFN-γ. Macrophages also produce a number of BRMs, including IL-1, IL-6, IL-8, IL-12, IFN-α, and TNF.

Clinical applications

INTERLEUKIN-2

IL-2 was recognized as having potential antitumor effects following a mouse model study in which the use of IL-2 resulted in regression of a number of sarcomas and melanomas. In human trials, individuals suffering from disseminated melanoma and renal cell carcinoma also demonstrated a positive result when receiving high-dose IL-2. However, this accounted for only around 15% of individuals receiving the medication. Of those who did respond, though, almost half had a complete (i.e., full regression) response to the medication that lasted for several years. Unfortunately, IL-2 use is associated with a number of side effects that limit its utility; these include severe nausea/vomiting, renal failure, hypotension, and altered mental status. Use of IL-2 in the treatment of melanoma has largely been supplanted by the development of newer, more targeted therapies utilizing checkpoint inhibitors.

INTERFERON-α

Interferon (IFN)-α binds to specific cell surface receptors and, through its signaling cascade, activates transcription of a number of effector proteins that stimulate an antiviral and antitumor response. In addition, IFN-α may also modulate oncogenes directly and interfere with the synthesis of proteins needed by tumor cells for growth and survival. Finally, IFN-α has also been shown to stimulate expression of certain cell surface markers on tumor cells, helping to target them for destruction by other immune system components. Interferon therapy, particularly using pegylated IFN-α, has found a role in the treatment of chronic myeloid leukemia, melanoma, and chronic hepatitis B and C, although the introduction of new therapeutic agents for the treatment of hepatitis B and C has significantly reduced the use of IFN-α in those diseases.

HEMATOPOIETIC GROWTH FACTORS

Although primarily known for their ability to promote neutrophil recovery in neutropenia, G-CSF (filgrastim) or GM-CSF (sargramostim) also have been shown to reduce the frequency and severity of infection. This is due to both stimulation of neutrophil production as well as enhancement of the activity of neutrophils, e.g., phagocytosis, chemotaxis, and superoxide production. These agents are often used following chemotherapy to blunt the neutrophil nadir and shorten the duration of neutropenia. Typical protocols call for a 10–14 day course following chemotherapy. Other hematopoietic factors include erythropoietin and IL-11, a key regulator of multiple events in hematopoiesis, most notably the stimulation of megakaryocyte maturation.

INTRAVENOUS IMMUNOGLOBULINS

Gamma globulins represent one of the oldest forms of immunopotentiation, providing a means to easily transfer passive immunity. Intravenous immuno-globulin (IVIG) consists of concentrated polyclonal immunoglobulins, of which over 90% are IgG. IVIG is used in a number of medical conditions. For patients suffering from primary or secondary immune deficiencies, IVIG restores the circulating IgG concentrations. IVIG also helps to modulate the immune response for autoimmune disorders, e.g., immune thrombocytopenic purpura, severe polymyositis, dermatomyositis, and Kawasaki syndrome. In these conditions, autoantibodies bind to cells or tissues and activate complement and phago-cytic cells, causing cell death and/or tissue damage. IVIG can help modulate the immune response by saturating Fc receptors on phagocytes, prevent-ing them from engaging in phagocytosis, as well as providing anti-idiotype antibodies against the paratopes of autoantibodies, thus inhibiting the autoantibodies from binding to their targets.

CANCER IMMUNOTHERAPY

The immune system has been recognized for some time for its antitumor role. A number of cell pop-ulations that make up the immune system help to combat malignant cells, including CD8+ and CD4+ T lymphocytes, natural killer cells, and macrophages. The relationship of the immune system with malignant cells and how cancerous cells are able to avoid destruction occurs through a series of interactions. Initially, the cells making up the innate and adaptive immune systems tar-get and destroy cells expressing tumor-associated antigens. However, a balance can develop whereby the rate of malignant cell destruction is matched by further malignant cell replication. As the tumor cells continue to divide, they may eventually fur-ther mutate and gain the ability to avoid detection by the immune system. This is accomplished via a number of processes. Malignant cells may lose the tumor antigens or major histocompatibility com-plex (MHC) class I molecules recognized as tar-gets by the immune system, as well as encourage production of cytokines that inhibit the actions of cytotoxic T cells. In addition, cancerous cells can increase expression of immune checkpoint mol-ecules on their surface, encouraging self-tolerance of these tissues.

Inhibition of checkpoint molecules has become an emerging goal of anticancer therapy in recent years. In particular, inhibitors targeting

programmed cell death receptor 1 (PD-1) and cytotoxic T-lymphocyte–associated protein 4 (CTLA-4, CD152) have demonstrated efficacy in combating certain types of cancer. Nivolumab, a PD-1 inhibitor, has become an important agent in the treatment of non-small cell lung cancer, uro-thelial and renal cell carcinoma, and, in combina-tion with the CTLA-4 inhibitor ipilimumab, is the first-line treatment now for metastatic melanoma. Together, these medications have improved overall survival times and outcomes for previously rapidly fatal illnesses.

The success of checkpoint inhibitors is not with-out consequences, however. Checkpoint inhibitors have been implicated in a number of immune-related adverse drug events, which result when the now amplified immune system acts on otherwise normal tissue. Common associated side effects include skin rash and mucocutaneous changes, fatigue, diarrhea, hepatotoxicity, and inflamma-tory arthritis and myositis. As these symptoms are due to increased activity of the immune system, they are best combated with immunosuppression. In general, high-dose steroids (e.g., Prednisone 0.50–2 kg/mg/day) are the first-line treatment, depending on severity. Should symptoms fail to respond, infliximab has emerged as an effective treatment. Checkpoint inhibitors are typically held during symptoms, with a decision regarding resumption of these inhibitors based on the overall severity of their reaction.

BIBLIOGRAPHY

Balato A, Scala E, Balato N et al. Biologics that inhibit the Th17 pathway and related cytokines to treat inflammatory disorders. *Expert Opin Biol Ther.* 2017;17:1363–1374.

Burton CM, Andersen CB, Jensen AS et al. The incidence of acute cellular rejection after lung transplantation: A comparative study of anti-thymocyte globulin and daclizumab. *J. Heart Lung Transplant.* 2006;25:638–647.

Choy EHS, Panayi GS. Cytokine pathways and joint inflammation in rheumatoid arthritis. *N Eng J Med.* 2001;344:907–916.

Coenen JJ, Koenen HJ, van Rijssen E et al. Rapamycin, and not cyclosporin A, preserves the highly suppressive CD27+ subset of human CD4+CD25+ regulatory T cells. *Blood.* 2006; 107:1018–1023.

Davis BP, Ballas ZK. Biologic response modifiers: Indications, implications, and insights. *J Allergy Clin Immunol.* 2017;139:1445–1456.

Dhimolea E. Canakinumab. *MAbs.* 2010;2:3–13.

Edwards J, Szczepanski L, Szechinski J et al. Efficacy of B-cell targeted therapy with rituximab in patients with rheumatoid arthritis. *N Engl J Med.* 2004;350:2572–2580.

FitzGerald GA, Patrono C. The coxibs, selective inhibitors of cyclooxygenase-2. *N Eng J Med.* 2001;9:433–442.

Floros T, Tarhini AA. Anticancer cytokines: Biology and clinical effects of interferon-α2, interleukin (IL)-2, IL-15, IL-21, and IL-12. *Semin Oncol.* 2015;42:539–548.

Gonzales NR, De Pascalis R, Schlom J, Kashmiri SV. Minimizing the immunogenicity of antibodies for clinical application. *Tumour Biol.* 2005; 26:31–43.

Hardinger KL, Schnitzler MA, Koch MJ et al. Thymoglobulin induction is safe and effective in live-donor renal transplantation: A single center experience. *Transplantation.* 2006;81:1285–1289.

Ito Y, Kaneko N, Iwasaki T et al. IL-1 as a target in inflammation. *Endocr Metab Immune Disord Drug Targets.* 2015;15:206–211.

Kovarik J. From immunosuppression to immunomodulation: Current principles and future strategies. *Pathobiology.* 2013;80:275–281.

Luchetti MM, Benfaremo D, Gabrielli A. Biologics in inflammatory and immunomediated arthritis. *Curr Pharm Biotech.* 2017;18:989–1007.

O'Mahony D, Bishop MR. Monoclonal antibody therapy. *Front Biosci.* 2006;11:1620–1635.

Schwartz DM, Kanno Y, Villarino A, Ward M, Gadina M, O'Shea JJ. JAK inhibition as a therapeutic strategy for immune and inflammatory diseases. *Nat Rev Drug Disc.* 2017;16: 843–862.

Tocheva AS, Mor A. Checkpoint inhibitors: Applications for autoimmunity. *Curr Allergy Asthma Rep.* 2017;17:72.

Tocut M, Brenner R, Zandman-Goddard G. Autoimmune phenomena and disease in cancer patients treated with immune checkpoint inhibitors. *Autoimmun Rev.* 2018;17:610–616.

Watad A, Amital H, Shoenfeld Y. Intravenous immunoglobulin: A biological corticosteroid-sparing agent in some autoimmune conditions. *Lupus.* 2017;26:1015–1022.

Weiner GJ. Rituximab: Mechanism of action. *Semin Hematol.* 2010;47:115–123.

25

Transplantation immunology

SATISH N. NADIG AND JANE C. KILKENNY

INTRODUCTION

The replacement of defective organs with transplants was seemingly one of the impossible dreams of medicine for many centuries. Its realization required a multitude of important steps: surgical asepsis, development of surgical techniques for vascular anastomosis, understanding of the cellular basis of the rejection phenomena, and introduction of drugs and antisera effective in the control of rejection.

By the early 1970s, tissue and organ transplantation emerged as a major area of interest for surgeons and physicians. Solid-organ transplants since have become routine in most industrialized countries. Currently, kidney and bone marrow transplants are performed most frequently, followed by liver, heart, pancreas, lung, and small bowel transplants, in order of decreasing frequency. Transplantation of trachea, extremities, uterus, and facial tissue are also performed in investigational situations. Other tissues and organs will certainly follow.

The success of an organ transplant is a function of several variables. These include technical advancements, advances in preservation, increased understanding of the immune system, and pharmacologic advances to prevent and treat rejection. However, the magnitude of the immunological response against the graft is the major determinant of acceptance or nonacceptance (rejection) of a technically perfect graft. The likelihood of acceptance or rejection is closely related to the extent of genetic differences between the donor and recipient of the graft. Although transplantation of organs between animals of the same inbred strain or between homozygous (syngeneic) twins is successful and does not elicit an immune rejection response, transplants between distantly related individuals (allogeneic) or across species barriers (xenogeneic) are always rapidly rejected.

Thankfully, significant progress in the development of new immunosuppressive drugs and administration regimens has had a significant impact in transplantation outcome. The significant increases in graft survival rate are not a consequence of better donor-recipient matching but rather a reflection of better medical management.

DONOR-RECIPIENT MATCHING

Prevention of rejection is more desirable than trying to treat established rejection. This is achieved both by careful matching of donor and recipient and by manipulation of the recipient's immune response peri- and posttransplant. To successfully match donor and recipient, antigenic differences between the two must be avoided. Although many different antigenic systems show allotypic variation, in transplantation practice, only the ABO blood groups and the human leukocyte antigen (HLA) system are routinely typed.

ABO incompatibility is generally considered a contraindication to transplantation in the United States since it can lead to an accelerated rejection response, called hyperacute rejection (see later), which likely represents a recipient response to A and B antigens expressed on vascular endothelium of the transplanted organ. However, some groups have reported successful grafting of HLA-compatible but ABO-incompatible organs, after removing anti-A and/or anti-B isohemagglutinins from the recipient by plasmapheresis or by extracorporeal immunoadsorption in conjunction with antibody induction therapy with thymoglobulin. It currently accounts for one-fourth of living donor kidney transplants in Germany and almost one-third of kidney transplants in Japan. In extremely urgent cases of liver transplantation, ABO matching is sometimes ignored, and reasonable graft function and survival can be seen in this setting as well.

HLA matching is also done routinely, with the goal of matching donor and recipient antigenicity as closely as possible. However, the practical significance of HLA matching varies depending on the organ to be transplanted. In kidney transplantation, HLA matching is important since there is a positive correlation between the number of HLA antigens common to the donor and recipient and the survival of the transplanted kidney (Table 25.1).

It follows that when grafting kidneys from living relatives, HLA-identical sibling grafts have the best outcome, followed by haploidentical grafts, which, in turn, outperform haplotype-incompatible grafts. Likewise, cadaveric kidney transplants recipient-matched for HLA-A, -B, and -DR achieve survival rates similar to those obtained with transplants between two haplotype-matched living, related individuals. Major histocompatibility complex (MHC) class-II matching appears also to be somewhat important for survival of pancreatic grafts.

Another more important facet of the donor-recipient matching process involves screening the recipient's serum for cytotoxic antibodies directed against the donor's lymphocytes. The presence of these antibodies heralds a recipient who is already immune to potential donor tissue. This screen is achieved by means of a cross-match, in which the recipient's serum is tested against lymphocytes from the potential donor(s) as well as against a cell panel of known phenotypes (known as a Rope test or panel reactive antigens [PRAs]), followed by flow cytometry. This test is useful to prevent rapid rejection of the grafted tissue or organ.

In bone marrow transplantation, HLA typing is very important, but this type of transplant presents a unique problem not encountered with solid-organ transplants. With bone marrow transplants, it is necessary to avoid both the rejection of the grafted tissue by the host and the damage

Table 25.1 Five-year graft survival rates among various levels of human leukocyte antigen mismatched donors

		N	Average percentage (%) survival at 5 years	95% CI
Level of HLA mismatch	0	3,877	82.8	(81.7, 83.8)
	1	1,341	84.1	(82.3, 85.7)
	2	4,071	83.1	(82.1, 84.1)
	3	8,328	80.8	(80.0, 81.5)
	4	10,205	77.7	(77.1, 78.4)
	5	12,136	75.9	(75.2, 76.5)
	6	6,334	75.8	(74.9, 76.7)

Source: Based on data as of April 20, 2018. Department of Health and Human Services, Health Resources and Services Administration, Healthcare Systems Bureau, Division of Transplantation, Rockville, MD; United Network for Organ Sharing, Richmond, VA; University Renal Research and Education Association, Ann Arbor, MI.

Note: Kaplan-Meier graft survival rates for transplants performed 2008–2015.

Abbreviations: 95% CI, 95% confidence interval; HLA, human leukocyte antigen.

of host tissue by the transplanted lymphocytes, a phenomenon called graft-versus-host disease (GVHD) (discussed later). A living relative of the recipient is therefore usually the preferred marrow donor. An identical twin is the optimal choice for a donor, followed by an HLA-identical sibling (with six identical specificities for HLA-A, -B, and -DR) and a haplotype-identical relative (with three identical specificities for HLA-A, -B, and -DR) in order of preference. Mixed lymphocyte cultures can also be used preoperatively to screen for the GVHD reaction, which can emerge even in HLA-identical siblings due to incompatibilities in nontested, minor antigenic systems. With this technique, cultures are set up by mixing the recipient's lymphocytes with lymphocytes from potential donors. A well-matched donor-recipient pair should react minimally to one another and translate into a low probability for GVHD to occur.

In the case of liver transplantation, HLA matching is not as important for graft acceptance and survival. The acceptance of liver transplants among heterozygous pigs was reported in the 1960s by Roy Calne. Transplanted livers are not so readily accepted by humans, but the patients require lower degrees of immunosuppression than patients receiving other organs. The reasons for the easier acceptance of liver transplants are poorly understood. Two important factors may be the remarkable regenerative capacity of the liver or its relatively small antigen load. Unless the recipient has a high level of panel reactive antigens, HLA matching is also not generally performed in the case of heart, lung, and small bowel transplantation because of the scarcity of available donors for these organs.

GRAFT REJECTION

Graft rejection is the consequence of an immune response mounted by the recipient against the graft, due to incompatibility between tissue antigens of the donor and recipient. Cells that express class-II MHC antigens (such as passenger leukocytes, in the case of solid-organ transplants) play a major role in sensitizing the immune system of the recipient and heightening the potential for graft rejection. These cells also may shed antigen as blood flows through the implanted organ, activating alloreactive helper T lymphocytes from the recipient. This results in the production of interleukin (IL)-2, which leads to clonal expansion, and in turn, multiple immunological and inflammatory phenomena—some mediated by activated T lymphocytes and others mediated by antibodies—which can converge to cause graft rejection.

Rejection episodes are traditionally classified as hyperacute, accelerated, acute, and chronic, based primarily on the time elapsed between transplantation and the rejection episode, and on the type of protein and cellular response, as determined by tissue biopsy of the affected organ.

Hyperacute (early) rejection

Hyperacute rejection is a rare occurrence in modern transplantation. It occurs within the first minutes to hours posttransplantation and is mediated by preformed antibodies against ABO or MHC antigens present on the grafted organ. It is also possible that antibodies directed against other alloantigens, such as vascular endothelial antigens, may play a role in this type of rejection. Upon antibody binding to antigen on the transplanted organ, rejection can be caused either by activation of the complement system, which results in the chemotactic attraction of granulocytes and the triggering of inflammatory cascades, and/or by antibody-dependent cellular cytotoxicity (ADCC).

A major pathological feature of hyperacute rejection is the formation of massive intravascular platelet aggregates, which leads to microvascular thrombosis, and ultimately to tissue ischemia and necrosis. The formation of platelet thrombi probably results from several factors, including release of platelet-activating factor (PAF) from immunologically damaged endothelial cells and/or from activated neutrophils.

Hyperacute rejection episodes are irreversible and uniformly result in graft loss. With proper ABO blood group verification and cross-matching prior to transplantation, this type of rejection is almost always avoidable. However, it must be noted that the major limitation to xenogeneic transplantation (e.g., pig to human) is hyperacute rejection by antibodies to cellular, animal-specific antigens, that exist in humans, prior to any known exposure to xenogeneic tissues (natural antibodies).

Acute rejection

Acute rejection usually occurs within the first few days to months after transplantation and is generally due to inadequate immunosuppression due to noncompliance or early immunosuppression underdosing. Currently, less than 10% of transplanted kidneys experience clinically significant acute cellular rejection episodes leading to graft loss at 1 year. When taking place in the first few days after grafting, it may correspond to a secondary (second set) immune response, implying that the recipient has been previously carried a sensitization to the HLA antigens present in the donated organ as a consequence of a previous antigen exposure, such as transplant, pregnancy, or blood transfusions. This particular phenomenon is known as an accelerated acute rejection. When acute rejection occurs beyond the first week after grafting, it usually corresponds to a first set, or primary, response.

Acute rejection is predominantly mediated by T lymphocytes and by both CD8+ cytotoxic lymphocytes and T-helper-1 (Th1) CD4+ lymphocytes.

In organs that are undergoing acute rejection, the cellular infiltrates are mostly composed of monocytes and both CD4+ and CD8+ T lymphocytes. The infiltrates also contain small populations of B lymphocytes, natural killer (NK) cells, neutrophils, and eosinophils, all of which contribute to rejection through secretion of inflammatory cytokines. IL-2 and IL-4 signal expansion of specific CD8+ T cells and B cells, interferon (IFN)-γ upregulation of MHC-II antigens on the graft, and chemotactic agents, such as IL-8 and complement fragments (C3a and C5a), attract additional immune cells to the transplanted organ.

In most cases, acute rejection if detected early can be reversed by increasing the dose of immunosuppressive agents or by briefly administering additional immunosuppressants.

The initial diagnosis of acute rejection is usually based on clinical suspicion. Abnormal laboratory studies or functional deterioration of the grafted organ are the main bases for considering the diagnosis of acute rejection. Confirmation usually requires a biopsy of the grafted organ. There are established histological criteria (Banff criteria) for the classification of acute rejection in transplanted organs. A hallmark finding in graft undergoing acute rejection is a heavy mononuclear cell infiltration of the affected organ or tissue.

Given the risk of complications associated with biopsy, there are several noninvasive approaches for diagnosis of acute rejection in kidney transplant recipients. These include *in vivo* imaging (contrast-enhanced ultrasound [US], intravascular US, and magnetic resonance imaging), gene-expression profiling, and analysis of blood and urine samples (specifically for urine biomarkers such as CXCL0/CXCL10). While some of these methods show promise in clinical trials, none have replaced the gold standard of biopsy.

Chronic rejection

Chronic rejection, including chronic allograft nephropathy in the setting of kidney transplantation, is characterized by an insidiously progressive loss of function of the grafted organ. In all transplanted organs with chronic rejection, there is arterial intimal thickening, called transplant arteriosclerosis or transplant vasculopathy. Both immune (HLA mismatch, inadequate immunosuppression, acute rejection episodes) and non-immune-mediated (ischemia time, brain-dead donors, ischemia/reperfusion injury) stimuli may upregulate pathways that lead to progressive graft failure.

Transplant arteriosclerosis is the hallmark of chronic graft dysfunction affecting transplanted organs in the long term. Fibroproliferative lesions lead to neointimal thickening in transplanted allografts. This then causes luminal narrowing, which causes graft ischemia and ultimately graft failure. A variety of cells, such as granulocytes, monocytes, and platelets, have an increased tendency to adhere to injured vascular endothelium. The expression of PAF on the membrane of endothelial cells may be one of the major factors determining the adherence of neutrophils and platelets. In addition, experimental models have shown the presence of macrophage attractants, such as RANTES (regulated on activation, normal T cell expressed and secreted), which cause these cells to enter tissues and secrete offending proinflammatory cytokines. A variety of interleukins and soluble factors are also released by activated leukocytes at the level of the damaged vessel walls, including IL-1, IL-6, tumor necrosis factor (TNF), macrophage chemoattractant protein-1, and platelet-derived growth factor. In addition, growth factors, especially basic fibroblast growth factor and TGF-β, are also secreted at the level of the damaged endothelium. A layer of platelets and fibrin covers the damaged endothelium while proliferating fibroblasts and smooth muscle cells can be found in the subendothelial space. The end result is a proliferative lesion in the vessels as a consequence of the inflammatory nature of the process, which progresses toward fibrosis and occlusion. Also, the growth factors contribute to progressive vascular hypertrophy. In addition, continuous production of alloantibodies by activated B cells exacerbates the arteriopathy and perpetuates the graft dysfunction. At the same time, a number of adhesion molecules are upregulated with brain death, ischemia reperfusion injury, and acute rejection. The resulting cytokine release due to these early donor factors contributes to the upregulation of MHC-II molecules and adhesion molecules, such as intercellular adhesion molecules-1 and vascular cell adhesion molecule (VCAM)-1, which perpetuate the adhesion and damage pathways and continue the chronic rejection cycle.

In summary, although the exact etiology of chronic rejection is not completely understood, a variety of factors are believed to play significant roles. Further research is currently ongoing to define and potentially modulate these factors in order to lessen the detrimental effects of the chronic rejection process. However, it should be noted that with the current immunosuppressive therapies available, kidney graft loss is rarely the cause of death of a graft recipient.

Antibody-mediated rejection

Antibody-mediated rejection can occur in either the acute or chronic phase as it is due to production of donor-specific antibodies directed to the endothelial lining of organ allografts. The interaction between donor-specific antibodies and endothelial cells leads to complement activation triggering the attraction and activation of neutrophils and other leukocytes that result in allograft injury. Treatment of antibody-mediated rejection is based on removing these donor-specific antibodies with plasmapheresis, immunoadsorption, or use of B-cell toxic antibodies, such as rituximab (CD20 monoclonal antibody).

IMMUNOSUPPRESSION

The ideal transplantation should take place among genetically identical individuals. This is only possible in the rare event of transplantation between identical twins. Thus, the success of clinical transplantation depends heavily on the use of nonspecific immunosuppressive agents that, by

decreasing the magnitude of immunological rejection responses, prolong graft survival. Operational tolerance is defined as the immunologic acceptance of a transplanted organ while maintaining global functioning and efficacy of the immune system. Immunosuppressive regimens have been developed to impact pathways in T-cell activation by recipient antigen-presenting cells (APCs). These immunosuppressive drugs and pathways are shown in Figure 25.1. These therapies have been improved over time to be more specific and less toxic to the host immune system.

Chemical immunosuppression

GLUCOCORTICOIDS

Historically, the first available immunosuppressive drugs used to treat and prevent rejection were glucocorticoids. They have multiple effects on the immune system and are nonspecific with actions that include lymphocyte apoptosis, inhibition of antigen-driven T-lymphocyte proliferation, inhibition of IL-1 and IL-2 release, and inhibition of chemotaxis. Because of the side effects associated with the use of glucocorticoids in relatively large doses for long periods of time (as required in transplantation), they are usually administered together with other immunosuppressant drugs, allowing the reduction of steroid doses below levels causing major side effects. In addition, more recent combination protocols are more frequently being used so as to completely avoid corticosteroids due to their morbidity with chronic use.

ANTIMETABOLITES

Antimetabolites are mostly used in the prevention of rejection episodes. All of these agents inhibit DNA replication, lymphocyte proliferation, and the expansion of antigen-reactive clones of lymphocytes:

- **Azathioprine (Imuran)** undergoes metabolic conversion into 6-mercaptopurine, which inhibits purine nucleotide synthesis and prevents lymphocyte proliferation (both T and B). This therapy is toxic (associated with inflammatory bowel disease, autoimmune disease, bone marrow suppression, and pancreatitis) and currently very infrequently used.
- **Mycophenolate mofetil (CellCept)** is converted to mycophenolic acid, which is an

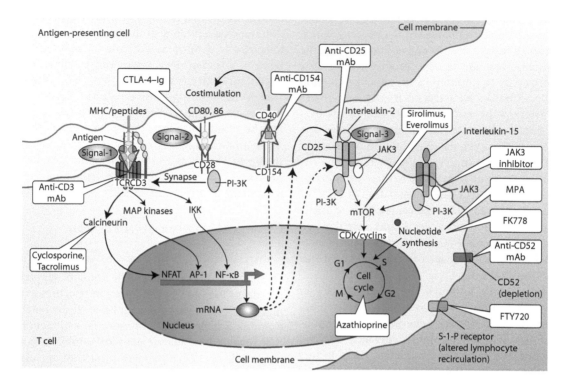

Figure 25.1 T-cell activation requires three signals to initiate an effector response: (1) antigen presentation of non-self MHC, (2) costimulation, and (3) regulation of cytokine signaling. These three signals are the targets of the immunosuppressive drugs used in induction, maintenance, as well as treatment of rejection episodes. (Reproduced with permission from Mulholland, M.W. et al., eds., *Greenfield's Surgery*, 6th ed., Wolters Kluwer, Philadelphia, PA, 2017: 519.)

inhibitor of inosine monophosphate dehydrogenase, a critical enzyme for the synthesis of guanosine. This process is required for *de novo* synthesis of purines, upon which lymphocytes are critically dependent for proliferation, whereas other cells can utilize salvage pathways. Therefore, mycophenolate inhibits lymphocyte proliferation and inhibits the production of antibodies. This agent has virtually replaced azathioprine as a maintenance immunosuppressant and is often used in suppression of autoimmune conditions. It has recently been associated with gastrointestinal toxicity. A newer antimetabolite, mycophenolic acid (MPA) has emerged as an option in solid-organ transplantation. MPA has less myelosuppressive activity compared to azathioprine, but side effects are common.

- **Cyclophosphamide (Cytoxan)** is an alkylating agent, which modifies DNA and prevents lymphocyte replication. This drug is rarely used in solid organ transplantation. It is used in refractory rejection when more mainstream therapies fail.

CALCINEURIN INHIBITORS

Calcineurin inhibitors disrupt regulatory T-cell signaling and lead to the inhibition of activity of transcriptional activators controlling the expression of IL-2 and other lymphokine genes in helper T cells. Thus, the onset of both cellular and humoral immune responses is inhibited and the activity of cytotoxic T cells markedly depressed.

Cyclosporine A (CsA) (Sandimmune, Neoral) was the first calcineurin inhibitor identified, and the discovery of CsA in 1983 marks the beginning of a new era in transplantation and has made possible the transplantation of other solid organs with increasing success. CsA is particularly helpful in the prevention of rejection, usually administered in association with glucocorticoids, because it allows their use in lower doses, or even their discontinuation.

CsA itself has marked toxicity. It is nephrotoxic (and that raises considerable problems in patients receiving kidney transplants, in which it will be necessary to differentiate between acute rejection and CsA toxicity) and commonly causes hypertension. Less frequently, it causes tremor, hirsutism, and gum hyperplasia. Monitoring of circulating cyclosporine levels is essential to minimize the toxic effects of this drug, as well as monitoring of renal function.

Tacrolimus (Prograf, FK506) has a mechanism of action similar to CsA, although it is 10 times more potent. It is able to reverse rejection episodes in patients unresponsive to some other immunosuppressive agents. Tacrolimus is used in a fashion similar to that as CsA, in combination with glucocorticoids and antimetabolites. It also has toxic effects including nephrotoxicity and neurotoxicity. In addition, a form of insulin-dependent posttransplant diabetes mellitus is reported in 20% of patients. This complication is largely reversible but necessitates careful monitoring of blood glucose levels, as well as renal function and potassium levels. It has become the mainstay of maintenance immunosuppression.

INHIBITORS OF THE MAMMALIAN TARGET OF RAPAMYCIN (mTOR)

Like calcineurin inhibitors, mTOR inhibitors lead to decreased IL-2 production. Rapamycin (Sirolimus, Rapamune) is a unique compound that is structurally similar to tacrolimus. However, its mechanism of action seems to be related to cell-cycle inhibition. Rapamycin works by binding to FK506 binding proteins, thereby inhibiting T-cell proliferation by blocking both calcium-dependent and -independent pathways. In addition, it downregulates the humoral immune response, thereby decreasing potentially cross-reactive antibody formation. Sirolimus is currently used largely in calcineurin inhibitor-free regimens. Sirolimus, in conjunction with mycophenolate and/or steroids subsequent to an immune induction-blocking antibody, has been shown very recently to be less nephrotoxic and reduce the incidence of chronic allograft nephropathy, by reducing the kidney insult induced by the calcineurin inhibitors. It should be noted that preliminary evidence has shown that sirolimus can potentiate the nephrotoxic effects of CsA and tacrolimus. However, sirolimus coupled with steroids and/or mycophenolate shows a paradoxical synergistic effect in preventing chronic allograft nephropathy. Sirolimus is also used in calcineurin inhibitor withdrawal regimens, where immunosuppression is initiated with a calcineurin inhibitor, such as CsA, to prevent early acute rejection. This agent is later withdrawn, and immunosuppression is maintained with sirolimus. It is also currently sometimes used instead of CellCept or Imuran. However, side effects caused by rapamycin include pancytopenia and hyperlipidemia, and these side effects are often magnified in regimens that include mycophenolate. Of particular interest here is that the hyperlipidemia exacerbates any underlying coronary artery disease, which is the leading cause of death among patients with functioning kidney allografts.

Certican (everolimus), when used in conjunction with CsA, has been shown to greatly decrease the incidence of cardiac vasculopathy posttransplant. It also has reduced nephrotoxicity.

Biological response modifiers

This group includes a variety of biological compounds that have been found to be useful in the prevention and treatment of graft rejection. It should be noted that induction therapy is now the standard of care for kidney transplantation, reducing acute rejection percentages to single digits or very low teens. It is also hoped that combinations of biological response modifiers and immunosuppressive agents may lead to tolerization protocols applicable to humans. Tolerance induction to kidney and pancreas grafts, for example, has been successfully accomplished in a variety of animal models, but so far human tolerization remains an elusive target.

ANTITHYMOCYTE AND ANTILYMPHOCYTE GLOBULINS

Antithymocyte and antilymphocyte globulins were among the earliest successful therapeutic agents used in the management of graft rejection. These reagents are γ-globulin fractions separated from the sera of animals (rabbits, goats, or horses) injected with human thymic lymphocytes or human peripheral blood lymphocytes. Therefore, they are polyclonal and are directed against numerous cell surface epitopes on platelets, T and B cells, NK cells, macrophages, as well as adhesion molecules. They are very effective in the prevention and reversal of rejection episodes, and their mechanism of action is related to the destruction or inhibition of recipient lymphocytes. Their main drawbacks have been related to difficulty in obtaining standardized preparations, reactivity with other cell types, and frequent sensitization of the patients, which often leads to serum sickness when the globulins are administered repeatedly. However, the serum sickness has been greatly reduced by abandoning the horse preparation in favor of the rabbit preparation. Currently, the rabbit preparation is the most widely used and exhibits less batch variation than preparations from previous species. Thymoglobulin is used in situations where reversal of aggressive rejection is necessary, as well as cases where the patient is resistant to immunosuppression with steroids. Finally, this preparation is also used for pregraft induction, a process that involves suppression of immune cell proliferation prior to host exposure to graft antigens.

ANTI-T-CELL MONOCLONAL ANTIBODIES

Anti-T-cell monoclonal antibodies obtained from mice and directed against human T cells, particularly those reacting with the CD3 marker (muromonab CD3, OKT3), have been extensively used in the management of transplanted patients. Their mechanisms of action are multiple. CD3 monoclonal antibodies cause depletion of CD3$^+$ T lymphocytes , and it is likely that the depletion is due to complement-mediated lysis, opsonization, and ADCC. CD3 monoclonal antibodies also cause downmodulation of CD3 on the cell surface of otherwise viable T cells and may induce T-cell anergy.

These antibodies are predominantly used for the treatment of acute rejection. In addition, some groups use the monoclonal antibody as treatment immediately before transplantation to prevent rejection. As with antilymphocyte and antithymocyte globulins, the possibility of using monoclonal antibodies to treat repeated episodes of rejection is limited by the sensitization of the patients receiving the antibody. It must be noted that in spite of concomitant immunosuppression, up to 30% of patients become sensitized to various antibody preparations. However, changing to a different monoclonal antibody can meet with success in hypersensitive patients. In addition, the modern humanized versions of these antibodies are less immunogenic.

Besides serum sickness, monoclonal and polyclonal antibodies can cause what is known as the cytokine syndrome, which presents with fever, chills, headaches, vomiting, diarrhea, muscle cramps, and vascular leakage and transudation.

Experimental data suggest that the syndrome is caused by massive cytokine release from T cells activated as a consequence of the binding of these antibodies to the lymphocyte membrane. The main cytokines responsible for this clinical syndrome are TNF, IL-10, IL-6, and IFN-γ. This syndrome can cause pyrexia, hypotension, and rigors similar to systemic sepsis. This condition can lead to life-threatening pulmonary edema if the patient is fluid overloaded or death. The symptoms can be ameliorated by infusion of antihistamines, glucocorticoids, and anti-inflammatory agents prior to the use of CD3 monoclonal antibodies, and continuous infusion throughout the treatment if necessary.

Both monoclonal and polyclonal antilymphocyte antibody preparations are strongly immunosuppressive, so the risk of developing life-threatening infections or posttransplant lymphoproliferative disorder (PTLD) is markedly higher in patients treated with them (see subsequently). This condition is secondary to transformation by Epstein–Barr virus (EBV) and can be life-threatening. As a result, treatment with these agents usually does not exceed 14 days, and repeated courses of antibody treatment are usually contraindicated.

OTHER MONOCLONAL ANTIBODIES

- **Anti-IL-2R monoclonal antibodies (Daclizumab/Simulect, Basiliximab/Zenapax)** are also approved for use in transplantation for the prevention of rejection. Currently, these agents are used in all solid-organ transplants. They are used as induction agents, and they are shown to markedly reduce rejection in the vast majority of cases, especially in the instance of kidney transplantation.
- **Anti-CD52 monoclonal antibodies (Alemtuzumab/Campath)**. Antibodies directed against the CD52 cell surface protein (found on lymphocytes, NK cells, monocytes, macrophages, and cells of the male reproductive system) are often also used as inductions agents. The specific binding to the surface of the lymphocytes causes their specific lysis, thereby depressing the immune response to antigens encountered in the transplant process. In addition to allowing opportunistic infection and often causing rigors, fever, and nausea, other side effects include lymphopenia, thrombocytopenia, anemia, and bone marrow hypoplasia.

COSTIMULATION BLOCKADE

Naïve CD4+ and CD8+ T cells must become activated to acquire effector functions, which results in graft damage. Activation of a naïve T cell is a tightly regulated process that requires three distinct signals. If one signal is activated without the others, the resultant signal is anergic. Given this, costimulation pathways have been targeted by various types of biologics.

- The engagement of APC-derived CD80/86 (B7 molecules) with CD28 on T cells is integral to positive costimulation. CD 80 and CD 86 interact preferentially with CTLA4 when compared to CD28. **LEA29Y (belatacept)** is an immunoglobulin fusion protein that has a twofold greater ligation capacity for both CD80 and CD86.
- **Basiliximab** is a chimeric mouse/human IgG1 monoclonal antibody to the α chain of CD25 (IL2 receptor). It has been used to reduce acute rejection rates without nephrotoxic side effects.

HUMANIZED AND CHIMERIC MONOCLONAL ANTIBODIES

The problem of sensitization can be minimized by the use of genetically engineered monoclonal antibodies of reduced immunogenicity. These antibodies are obtained by combining the antigen-binding regions of a murine monoclonal antibody with the constant regions of human IgG (see Chapter 24). These humanized or chimeric monoclonals can be administered for more prolonged periods of time without the occurrence of sensitization. However, they are considerably more expensive.

Immunosuppression side effects

Effective long-term immunosuppression is inevitably associated with a state of immunoincompetence. Two major types of complications may result from this: infections and neoplasia. The timeline for these complications is shown in Table 25.2.

OPPORTUNISTIC INFECTIONS

The immunosuppressed patient is susceptible to a wide variety of infections, particularly caused

Table 25.2 The timeline of common infections after transplantation

<1 Month	1–6 Months	>6 Months

• Infection with antimicrobial-resistant species
  • MRSA
  • *Candida* (non-*albicans*)
  • VRE
• Donor-derived infection (uncommon)
  • HSV
  • HIV
  • Rhabdovirus
  • LCMV
  • *Trypanosoma cruzi*
• Recipient-derived infection
  • *Aspergillus*
  • *Pseudomonas*
	• With PCP and antiviral prophylaxis
	  • HCV infection
	  • Adenovirus
	  • Polyomavirus BK infection
	  • *Clostridium difficile*
	  • *Cryptococcus neoformans*
	  • *Mycobacterium tuberculosis*
	• Without prophylaxis
	  • Herpesviruses (HSV, VZV, CMV, EBV)
	  • HBV
	  • Pneumocystis
	  • *Listeria*
	  • *Nocardia*
	  • *Toxoplasma*
	  • *Strongyloides*
	  • *Leishmania*
	  • *Trypanosoma cruzi*
		• Infection with *Nocardia, Rhodococcus* species
		• Infection with *Aspergillus*, atypical molds, *Mucor* species
		• Community-acquired pneumonia
		• UTI
		• Late viral infections
		  • CMV (colitis and retinitis)
		  • Hepatitis (HBV, HCV)
		  • HSV encephalitis
		  • JC polyomavirus infection (PML)
		  • Community-acquired (SARS, West Nile virus infection)

Source: Modified from Fishman, J.A., *N England J Med.*, 357, 2601–2614, 2007.
Abbreviations: CMV, cytomegalovirus; EBV, Epstein–Barr virus; HBV, hepatitis B virus; HCV, hepatitis C virus; HIV, human immunodeficiency virus; HSV, herpes simplex virus; LCMV, lymphocytic choriomeningitis virus; MRSA, methicillin-resistant *Staphylococcus aureus*; PCP, *Pneumocystis carini* (jiroveci) pneumonia; PML, progressive multifocal leukoencephalopathy; SARS, severe acute respiratory syndrome; UTI, urinary tract infection; VRE, vancomycin-resistant enterococci; VZV, varicella zoster virus.

by infectious agents that are not often seen as pathogens in immunocompetent individuals, such as cytomegalovirus, herpes viruses of the herpes group (EBV, herpes simplex virus, varicella-zoster virus), *Pneumocystis jiroveci, Toxoplasma gondii*, and fungi (e.g., *Candida* spp. and *Aspergillus* spp.). The risk of opportunistic infection is highest in the first three months after transplant when the immunosuppression is most severe. Cytomegalovirus (CMV) infections are particularly ominous because this virus can further interfere with the host's immune competence and may also trigger rejection in a nonspecific way.

The incidence of infections in transplant patients can be reduced by prophylactic therapy with intravenous γ-globulin, which is part of most post bone marrow transplant protocols, since those patients are probably the most profoundly immunosuppressed. Bone marrow and solid-organ transplant patients also usually receive prophylactic antibiotics such as trimethoprim-sulfamethoxazole (for *Pneumocystis* and bacterial pneumonia, urinary tract infections, and cholangitis prophylaxis), ganciclovir or acyclovir (for herpes and CMV prophylaxis), and clotrimazole or fluconazole (for candidiasis).

MALIGNANCIES

Either as a consequence of the oncogenic properties of some immunosuppressive agents or as a consequence of disturbed immunosurveillance, the incidence of three main types of malignancy is significantly increased in transplant patients. In patients with survival times following transplantation of 10 years or longer, the frequency of skin cancer (squamous or basal cell carcinoma) may be up to 40%, although the lesions are no more invasive than in normal individuals. Rates of cervical cancer are also increased in immunosuppressed patients. Along with the increased rates of other anogenital cancers, the reasoning behind the increase involves the decreased immune surveillance against transforming oncogenic viruses. An additional 5% of patients may develop other types of malignancies, including EBV-associated posttransplant lymphoproliferative disorder, as discussed earlier. Thanks to careful monitoring of EBV infection status, this number has decreased from approximately 20%.

PTLD is a feared complication of transplant because it carries high morbidity and mortality. The cumulative 3-year incidence is 0.5% in adults and 1.5% in pediatric kidney transplants. More than 90% are non-Hodgkin's lymphomas, and most are of recipient B-cell origin. Risk factors include EBV+ donor and EBV– recipient, CMV+ donor and CMV– recipient, pediatric recipients (as they are more likely to be EBV-naïve), and intensity of immunosuppression.

Decreased immune surveillance against transforming oncogenic viruses has been suggested as the reason for the increased incidence of neoplasia in immunosuppressed patients. Thus, the predominance of skin and cervical cancer and PTLD among transplant patients may relate to the inability of the immune system to respond to papillomaviruses and EBV, which are etiologic agents for these malignances, respectively. Some of these PTLDs are reversible with interruption or reduction of immunosuppressive therapy or treatments that include agents such as Rituximab, a monoclonal antibody directed against the CD20 epitope on B cells. Others, however, are true malignant lymphomas that may spread to areas usually spared in non-transplanted patients, such as the brain. Common cancers such as colon, lung, and breast do not show increased frequently in transplant patients. This suggests that immune surveillance does not influence some of the most common cancers.

OTHER SIDE EFFECTS

The most widely used immunosuppressives have specific side effects that may have a significant negative impact on the quality of life of transplanted patients. Glucocorticoids can cause, among other side effects, obesity, insulin-resistant diabetes, cataracts, avascular necrosis of the femoral head, and thinning of the skin. Antimetabolites are associated with decreased blood counts and bone marrow depression. Cyclosporine and tacrolimus cause hypertension, nephrotoxicity, and neurotoxicity.

The use of combinations of different immunosuppressive drugs usually reduced the incidence and degree of side effects, because each drug that is part of the combination can be used at relatively well-tolerated doses. However, the ultimate goal of transplantation researchers is to develop protocols that would not require maintenance immunosuppression.

GRAFT-VERSUS-HOST DISEASE

Whenever a patient with a profound immunodeficiency (primary, secondary, or iatrogenic) receives a graft of an organ rich in immunocompetent cells, there is a risk that GVHD may develop. GVHD is a significant problem in infants and children with primary immunodeficiencies, in which a bone marrow transplant is performed with the goal of reconstituting the immune system, as well as in adults receiving a bone marrow transplant as part of a therapeutic protocol for aplastic anemia or for a hematopoietic malignancy. Small bowel, heart, lung, and even liver transplantation rank second in risk of causing GVHD, since these organs have a substantial amount of lymphoid tissue. In contrast, transplantation of organs such as the heart and kidneys, poor in endogenous lymphoid tissue, very rarely results in graft-versus-host (GVH) reaction. The probability of developing GVHD is greatest in the 2- to 3-month period immediately following transplantation, when immunosuppression is high.

Pathogenesis

Two elements are essential for the development of a GVHD: the immune system of the recipient needs to be severely compromised, and the transplanted organ or tissue needs to contain viable immunocompetent cells. The deficiency of the immune system may be congenital or acquired. For example, patients receiving bone marrow transplants receive cytotoxic and immunosuppressive therapy, and their immune system is completely or partially destroyed to avoid rejection of the transplanted bone marrow.

When a graft containing cells from an immunocompetent donor is placed into an immunoincompetent host, the transplanted cells can recognize as non-self the host antigens. In response to these antigenic differences, the donor T lymphocytes become activated, proliferate, and differentiate into helper and effector cells that attack the host cells and tissues, producing the signs and symptoms of GVHD. The crucial role played by the donor T cells in GVHD is demonstrated by the fact that their elimination from a bone marrow graft avoids the reactions (see subsequently). However, as the GVHD evolves and reaches its highest intensity, the majority of the cells infiltrating the different tissues affected by the GVH reaction are of host origin and include T and B lymphocytes as well as monocytes and macrophages. The proliferation of host cells is a result of the release of high concentrations of nonspecific mitogenic and differentiation factors by activated donor T lymphocytes.

It is important to note that several groups have reported findings suggesting that a low-grade GVHD may actually accelerate bone marrow engraftment and has a beneficial impact in patients receiving bone marrow grafts as part of their treatment for leukemia (graft versus leukemia effect).

Pathology

The initial proliferation of donor T cells takes place in lymphoid tissues, particularly in the liver and spleen (leading to hepatomegaly and splenomegaly). Later, at the peak of the proliferative reaction, the skin, liver, and intestinal walls are heavily infiltrated leading to severe skin rashes or exfoliative dermatitis, hepatic insufficiency, and severe diarrhea or even intestinal perforation. The splenic involvement results in a loss of function, not unlike that seen in splenectomized patients. The patients often develop *Streptococcus pneumoniae* bacteremia, and antibiotic prophylaxis may be necessary.

Treatment

All immunosuppressive drugs used in the prevention and treatment of rejection have been used for treatment of GVHD. In addition, thalidomide, the sedative drug that achieved notoriety due to its teratogenic effects, has been used successfully for the control of chronic GVHD unresponsive to traditional immunosuppressants.

Prevention

Once a GVH reaction is initiated, its control may be extremely difficult. Thus, great emphasis is placed on preventing GVH reactions. Besides the administration of immunosuppressive drugs, other approaches have been tried with variable success.

Autologous stem cell transplantation using purified CD34+ cells and allogeneic umbilical cord stem cell transplantation (stem cells obtained from cord blood after delivery) are also associated with a lower risk of GVH reactions. Umbilical cord stem cell transplantation is also associated with reduced graft-versus-leukemia effect but at a cost of higher frequency of relapses.

ROAD TO TOLERANCE: STEM CELLS AND CHIMERISM

Although blood transfusions were generally avoided in potential transplant recipients due to the fear of sensitization to HLA, blood groups, and other antigens, in the early 1980s it was reported that kidney graft survival was longer in patients who had received blood prior to transplantation. This led to attempts to precondition transplant recipients with multiple pretransplant transfusions. Some investigators suggested that the tolerizing effect of blood transfusions was due to the transfer of donor-derived hematopoietic stem cell precursors. This could lead to the establishment of a low level of donor-derived cells within the recipient bone marrow and peripheral blood and result in a state of microchimerism. The microchimeric state could then induce tolerance to the donor tissues and, consequently, result in improved graft survival. While pretransplant transfusions have been very much abandoned—with improvements in matching and immunosuppression protocols the transfusion effect became less and less evident—there is considerable interest in developing protocols to induce a more complete tolerance state that could allow suspension or significant dose reduction of immunosuppressive drugs. It has long been known that chimerism induces tolerance to organ and tissue transplants. Hematopoietic cell chimerism is defined by the presence of donor hematopoietic cells in the circulation of the recipient. Complete chimerism is when all the hematopoietic cells in the recipient are of donor origin. Mixed chimerism is a variable number of donor cells in the recipient. And microchimerism is when the donor cells in the recipient are below the level of detection from flow cytometry and can only be identified by polymerase chain reaction. Mixed chimerism is the goal of the current tolerance induction trials. The Stanford protocol has been used to induce tolerance in HLA-matched kidneys, allowing cessation of immunosuppressive therapy in a majority of their study participants (80% of participants). Work continues on these approaches

to determine if early observations are reproducible in larger groups of patients.

BIBLIOGRAPHY

Adu D, Cockwell P, Ives NJ, Shaw J, Wheatley K. Interleukin-2 receptor monoclonal antibodies in renal transplantation: Meta-analysis of randomised trials. *BMJ*. 2003;326:789–794.

Bakr MA. Induction therapy. *Exp Clin Transplant*. 2005;3:320–328.

Beniaminovitz A, Itescu S, Lietz K et al. Prevention of rejection in cardiac transplantation by blockade of the interleukin-2 receptor with a monoclonal antibody. *N Engl J Med*. 2000;342:613–619.

Cailhier JF, Laplante P, Hebert MJ. Endothelial apoptosis and chronic transplant vasculopathy: Recent results, novel mechanisms. *Am J Transplant*. 2006;6:247–253.

Caillard S, Agodoa LY, Bohen EM et al. Myeloma, Hodgkin disease, and lymphoid leukemia after renal transplantation: Characteristics, risk factors and prognosis. *Transplantation*. 2006;81: 888–895.

Calne RY. "It can't be done." *Nature Med*. 2012; 18:1493–1495.

Campbell P. Clinical relevance of human leukocyte antigen antibodies in liver, heart, lung, and intestine transplant. *Curr Opin Organ Transplant*. 2013;18:463–469.

deWeerd AE, Betjes MGH. ABO-Incompatible kidney transplant outcomes: A meta-analysis. *Clin J Am Soc Nephrol*. 2018;1:1234–1243.

Djamali A, Kaufman DB, Ellis TM et al. Diagnosis and management of antibody-mediated rejection: Current status and novel approaches. *Am J Transplant*. 2014;14:255–271.

Elster EA, Hale DA, Mannon RB et al. The road to tolerance: Renal transplant tolerance induction in non-human primate studies and clinical trials. *Transplant Immunol*. 2004;13:87–99.

Erpicum P, Hanssen O, Weekers L et al. Non-invasive approaches in the diagnosis of acute rejection in kidney transplant recipients, part II: Omics analyses of urine and blood samples. *Clin Kidney J*. 2017;10:106–115.

Hanssen O, Erpicum P, Lovinfosse P et al. Non-invasive approaches in the diagnosis of acute rejection in kidney transplant recipients. Part I. In vivo imaging methods. *Clin Kidney J*. 2017 Feb;10:97–105.

Heeger PS, Dinavahi R. Transplant immunology for the non-immunologist. *Mt Sinai J Med.* 2012;79:376–387.

Larsen CP, Pearson TC, Adams AB et al. Rational development of LEA29Y (belatacept), a high affinity variant of CTLA4-IG with potent immunosuppressive properties. *Am J Transplant.* 2005;5:443–453.

Lee TC, Savoldo B, Rooney CM et al. Quantitative EBV viral loads and immunosuppression alterations can decrease PTLD incidence in pediatric liver transplant recipients. *Am J Transplant.* 2005;5:2222–2228.

Nadig SN, Wieckiewicz J, Wu DC et al. In vivo prevention of transplant arteriosclerosis by ex vivo-expanded human regulatory T cells. *Nat Med.* 2010;16:809–813.

Nankivell BJ, Chapman JR. Chronic allograft nephropathy: Current concepts and future directions. *Transplantation.* 2006;81:643–654.

Peggs KS, Mackinnon S. Immune reconstitution following hematopoietic stem cells transplantation. *Brit J Haematol.* 2004;124:407–420.

Saliba F, Dharancy S, Lorho R et al. Conversion to everolimus in maintenance liver transplant patients: A multicenter, retrospective analysis. *Liver Transpl.* 2011;17:905–913.

Scandling JD, Busque S, Lowsky R et al. Macrochimerism and clinical transplant tolerance. *Hum Immunol.* 2018;79:266–271.

Shimabukuro-Vornhagen A, Gödel P, Subklewe M et al. Cytokine release syndrome. *J Immunother Cancer.* 2018;6:56. doi: 10.1186/s40425-018-0343-9

Snanoudj R, de Preneuf H, Creput C et al. Costimulation blockade and its possible future use in clinical transplantation. *Transplant Int.* 2006;19:639–704.

Yakupoglu YK, Kahan BD. Sirolimus: A current perspective. *Exp Clin Transplant.* 2003;1:8–18.

26

Tumor immunology

JUAN CARLOS VARELA

INTRODUCTION

The immune system can survey, recognize, and destroy tumor cells. Complex cross talk between the immune system, tumor cells, and their microenvironment determines the fate of neoplastic processes. Similar to responses to infections, the immune system mounts a well-orchestrated, multistep, acute inflammatory response that targets and destroys tumor cells. However, tumors have developed mechanisms to evade the immune system at every step of the antitumoral immune response. Furthermore, while acute inflammatory responses can lead to tumor eradication, it is now well defined that chronic inflammation can play a significant role in the pathogenesis of several types of cancer.

Over the past few decades, one of the most important endeavors of tumor immunologists has been to better elucidate the mechanisms that lead to tumor evasion of immune recognition and destruction. The knowledge obtained from these studies has been translated into immune-based treatments for many different types of cancer. The field of cancer immunotherapy has evolved quickly and has revolutionized the treatment of cancer in recent years. Control and even cure of several types of cancers that were not possible before are now within reach using novel immunotherapeutic approaches.

In this chapter, we review the mechanisms involved in the immune response to tumors, the immune evasion strategies used by tumors, and the current state of cancer immunotherapy in the treatment of cancer patients.

Natural immune response to cancer

The immune response to tumors consists of a number of well-orchestrated steps that ultimately lead to tumor recognition, targeting, and killing. This process was termed the *cancer immunity cycle* by Chen and Mellman in 2013. While many different cell types are involved in this process, T cells and dendritic cells (DCs) play central roles in the anticancer response. The cancer immunity cycle consists of seven steps that lead to a self-renewing process (Figure 26.1).

TUMOR CELL ANTIGEN RELEASE

Initiation of the process requires the release of tumor antigens into the tumor microenvironment. In general, there are two types of tumor antigens: (1) tumor-associated antigens (TAAs) and (2) tumor-specific antigens (TSAs). TAAs are derived from proteins that are expressed not only by tumors but also by other normal tissues. The difference is that in tumors these proteins are either overexpressed or have undergone some kind of posttranslational modification. For example, a common TAA is derived from the protein mucin-1 (MUC1). MUC1 is a heavily glycosylated transmembrane protein that is expressed on the apical

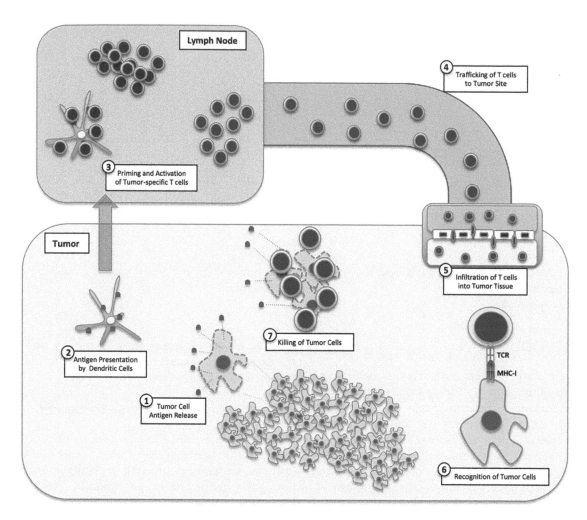

Figure 26.1 *Mechanism of an antitumor immune response.* The immune system elicits a coordinated response against tumors. This process has been termed the cancer immunity cycle (MHC-I, major histocompatibility complex I; TCR, T-cell receptor). (Adapted from Chen, D., Mellman, I., *Immunity*, 39, 1–13, 2013.)

surface of glandular epithelial cells. In tumor cells, MUC1 is overexpressed, underglycosylated, and its expression is no longer limited to the apical surface of cells. These changes in the expression pattern lead to generation of tumor-associated MUC1 antigens that are immunogenic. The immune system can mount a response against these antigens, but there is risk of cross-reactivity with normal tissues. TSAs (also known as neoantigens) are derived from "neoproteins" that are only expressed by the tumor itself. These proteins are different from normal proteins as a result of tumor-specific mutations. Neoantigens derived from these proteins are tumor specific, and immune responses to these types of antigens target only the tumor while sparing normal tissues. Clinical responses mediated by T lymphocytes targeting neoantigens have been identified in different types of cancers.

ANTIGEN PRESENTATION BY DENDRITIC CELLS

After TAAs or TSAs are released into the tumor microenvironment, they are taken up by DCs. Tumor antigens are processed and presented by DCs on class-I and class-II major histocompatibility complex (MHC) molecules. As these antigens are being processed, DCs traffic to lymph nodes where they will be presented to T cells.

PRIMING AND ACTIVATION OF TUMOR-SPECIFIC T LYMPHOCYTES

The interaction between DCs and T cells at this point in the process is critical for the development of anticancer responses. In addition to the recognition of tumor antigens presented on MHCs on the surface of DCs by the T-cell receptor (TCR) on the surface of T cells, costimulatory signals must be delivered to the T cell. The nature of the costimulatory signals determines whether an effective antitumor T-cell response will be elicited or whether regulatory T cells will be generated resulting in the development of tolerance (see section, Immune Evasion in Cancer). In general, the optimal anticancer T-cell response should include a combination of effector CD8$^+$ T cells and helper CD4$^+$ T cells.

TRAFFICKING TO TUMOR SITE

Activated, antitumor T cells must then traffic to the site of the tumor or its metastases (in the case of solid tumors) or to the bone marrow or affected lymph node(s) in the case of hematological malignancies. This trafficking is mainly mediated by chemokines including CCL2, CCL5, CXCL9, and CXCL10. The trafficking process can be influenced by the type and location of the tumor, and it is another possible target to promote immune evasion.

INFILTRATION INTO TUMOR TISSUE

The precise mechanisms for T-cell infiltration into tumor tissue are not fully elucidated. In general, T cells must adhere to the endothelium of tumor vasculature via adhesion molecules and extravasate across the endothelium into the tumor stroma. T cells that successfully traffic into tumors are called tumor-infiltrating lymphocytes (TILs). There is a significant correlation between the amount of TILs seen in a tumor biopsy and the response to immune therapies in several different types of cancer. The tumor vasculature and tumor stroma make up the tumor microenvironment and represent a major hurdle to the successful outcome of anticancer immune responses due to their ability to produce immune-suppressive substances such as inhibitory cytokines and growth factors.

RECOGNITION OF TUMOR CELLS

Following successful infiltration into the tumor, tumor-specific CD8$^+$ T cells bind and recognize cancer cells via TCR-MHC complex interactions. The antitumor T-cell responses are specific for the antigen/MHC complex that was originally presented by the DCs in the lymph nodes, and any changes in this complex will prevent the binding and recognition of tumor cells.

KILLING OF TUMOR CELLS

Once T cells recognize and bind to tumor cells, tumor cell killing occurs via the classical mechanisms of T cell–mediated killing, mainly induction of apoptotic pathways via Fas-ligand and activation of the perforin/granzyme pathway. The killing of tumor cells leads to the release of tumor antigens, and the cancer immunity cycle restarts in a self-renewing fashion.

Immune evasion in cancer

CANCER IMMUNOEDITING

It is now well understood that the immune system is not only able to survey and control neoplastic processes, but that by applying this immune pressure it also transforms the tumor and its microenvironment. Cancer immunoediting is the general process by which tumor cells "edit" themselves and/or their microenvironment in response to an antitumor immune response leading to cancer progression. Immune selection leads to the generation of tumor escape variants, and there are multiple mechanisms that lead to the immune evasion by tumors as outlined in Figure 26.2.

DYSREGULATION OF DENDRITIC CELL FUNCTION

DCs play a central role in the antitumor response; therefore, tumors have developed a number of inhibitory mechanisms aimed at DCs. Studies of tumor-derived DCs have shown they are not fully mature and express high levels of coinhibitory molecules. These changes lead to an inability of DCs to effectively prime and activate tumor-reactive T cells. Evidence suggests that these changes in DCs are triggered by soluble mediators produced by the tumor and the tumor microenvironment. Vascular endothelial growth factor (VEGF), transforming growth factor β (TGFβ), IL-10, IL-6, and macrophage colony-stimulating factor (M-CSF) have all been shown to affect the maturation and function of DCs. Furthermore, tumor-derived DCs have high expression of inhibitory molecules that can

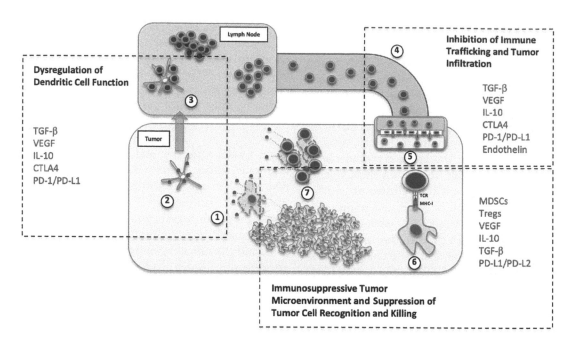

Figure 26.2 *Immune evasion mechanisms in cancer.* Tumors have evolved a number of mechanisms to evade the natural immune response to cancer. This schematic represents the broader immune evasion mechanisms that affect each step of the cancer immunity cycle. In addition, relevant cytokines, growth factors, proteins, and cell types involved are listed. (MHC-I, major histocompatibility complex I; TCR, T-cell receptor.)

inhibit T-cell priming and activation of T cells via two pathways. First, tumor-derived T cells express high levels of programmed death ligand 1 (PD-L1). PD-L1 is an inhibitory ligand that binds to the programmed death-1 (PD-1) receptor on T cells and blocks T-cell function. Second, tumor-derived DCs engage the cytotoxic T lymphocyte–associated molecule 4 (CTLA-4) pathway. CTLA-4 is expressed on activated T cells, and when it binds its ligands (CD80/CD86) on the surface of tumor-derived DCs leads to T-cell inactivation.

INHIBITION OF IMMUNE TRAFFICKING AND TUMOR INFILTRATION

Tumors also target the processes of immune trafficking and immune cell tumor infiltration as a means to evade the immune response. Chemokine function has been found to be abnormal in the setting of cancer. Evidence has shown that tumors produce mediators that inhibit chemokines, and it has been found that tumors can also produce chemokines with aberrant posttranslational modifications that can recruit inhibitory immune cells to the tumor site, such as myeloid-derived suppressor cells (MDSCs).

Infiltration of tumors by immune cells is mediated by adhesion molecules on endothelial cells in the tumor vasculature. Tumor growth dysregulates adhesion molecule function by production of VEGF. In a normal state, tumor necrosis factor (TNF) promotes the expression of adhesion molecules on endothelial cells. However, in the presence of VEGF, the effect of TNF is abrogated. Many types of tumor also produce high levels of endothelin (ET). ET has also been found to affect endothelial cells leading to dysregulation of adhesion molecules. Additionally, tumor vasculature can affect the infiltration of tumor-reactive cells by expressing molecules that can directly kill T cells (e.g., Fas ligand) or by expressing immune-inhibitory molecules such as PD-L1, IL-10, and TGFβ.

IMMUNOSUPPRESSIVE TUMOR MICROENVIRONMENT

Once tumor-reactive T cells are able to traffic and infiltrate into tumors, they encounter an extremely hostile tumor microenvironment. Physiological factors such as high levels of lactic acid, increased reactive oxygen species, and hypoxia affect immune cell functioning. Furthermore, there are increased populations of suppressive immune cells such as MDSCs and regulatory T cells (Tregs) that inhibit T-cell function. Tumor cells, cells in the tumor stroma, and suppressive immune cells in the tumor microenvironment produce a number of inhibitory molecules that suppress the immune system and allow tumor scape. Examples of these molecules include VEGF, IL-10, TGFβ, and prostaglandins.

SUPPRESSION OF TUMOR CELL RECOGNITION AND KILLING

There are several mechanisms utilized by tumor cells to prevent recognition and attack by tumor-reactive T cells. Tumor cells have been shown to downregulate the expression class-I MHC molecules and can also modulate expression of tumor antigens in response to immune pressure. Tumor cells can also express molecules that can directly kill T cells such as Fas ligand. In addition, a significant mechanism by which tumor cells protect themselves is by overexpression of PD-L1 and PD-L2 (overexpression of these molecules has significant therapeutic implications, see later section on checkpoint inhibitors). Secretion of immunosuppressive mediators such as IL-10 and TGFβ at the immune synapse also leads to decreased anti-tumor effects.

Cancer immunotherapy

Harnessing the power of the immune system to target and destroy cancer has been the central goal of tumor immunologists for decades. Our knowledge of the mechanisms used by tumors to evade the immune system has allowed us to target specific immune escape strategies and develop immune therapies that are changing the treatment landscape in oncology. Along with chemotherapy, surgery, and radiation, immunotherapy is now becoming the fourth pillar of treatment for many malignancies. The following is a discussion of the current cancer immunotherapies used in the clinical care of cancer patients.

ALLOGENEIC HEMATOPOIETIC STEM CELL TRANSPLANTATION

Allogeneic **hematopoietic stem cell transplantation** (HSCT) is the only curative option for many patients with hematological malignancies such as acute leukemias, lymphoma, and some cases of multiple myeloma. The goal of transplant is to generate a donor-derived allogeneic immune response against a patient's hematological cancer; this response is known as the graft-versus-tumor effect. Unlike other immune therapies, allogeneic HSCT does not target a specific immune evasion mechanism or a specific tumor target, but it aims to break tolerance against cancer at a much broader level. Allogeneic HSCT is an intensive process, and the treatment-related mortality can be as high as 30%. The success rate of allogeneic transplant varies depending on the disease, but in all cases, the possibility of success outweighs the chances of transplant-related mortality. One of the most serious complications from allogeneic HSCT is graft-versus-host disease (GVHD). GVHD occurs when the donor's immune system recognizes the patient's tissues as foreign and mounts an immune response against those tissues. Our ability to prevent and control GVHD has dramatically improved over the last two decades, but it remains a significant cause of morbidity and mortality in transplant patients.

CYTOKINES AND INTERFERON

Interferon and certain cytokines (e.g., IL-2, IL-15) are pro-inflammatory mediators that have been shown to play a role in anticancer immune responses. In the 1970s there was great excitement for the use of interferon-α in the treatment of several types of cancer. Unfortunately, treatment with interferon did not fulfill its promise due to its side-effect profile and lack of efficacy. Today, therapy with interferon-α is limited to the treatment of some patients with melanoma and renal cell carcinoma, although its use is becoming less common with the development of newer immunotherapies.

IL-2 is a strong agonist of T cells. It has been extensively used as a treatment for melanoma and renal cell carcinoma with mixed results. However, this treatment modality provides proof of principle that immune therapies can activate the immune system to target and destroy tumor cells. Today, IL-2 has also been replaced by newer immune therapies, but it is still used in specific cases of melanoma and renal cell carcinoma. Most recently, IL-15 has also been used in the treatment of cancer. IL-15 has shown activity in the treatment of lung cancer and some hematological malignancies.

MONOCLONAL ANTIBODIES

Monoclonal antibodies (MAbs) have become an integral part of cancer therapy. MAbs target surface proteins on tumor cells and can lead to tumor destruction by a number of ways: (1) direct cytotoxicity by activating the complement system leading to tumor cells lysis, (2) induction of antibody-dependent cellular cytotoxicity (ADCC), (3) binding to stimulatory receptors that can activate signaling pathways leading to growth arrest and death, or (4) binding to growth factors or their receptors and blocking the positive effect of those growth factors on tumor cells.

There are several examples of MAbs that have had a great impact on the treatment of cancer (Table 26.1). Rituximab, an anti-CD20 antibody, is widely used in most treatment regimens for lymphoma; trastuzumab, an anti-HER2 antibody, is used for the treatment of epidermal growth factor 2 positive breast cancer; and bevacizumab, an anti-VEGF antibody, leads to the inhibition of the beneficial effects of VEGF on tumors and is used in many different types of cancer.

Most recently, additional modifications have been made to MAbs to enhance their efficacy. A new generation of antibodies, termed *antibody-drug conjugates* (ADCs), consists of a MAb linked to a toxin or a radioisotope. Three examples of widely used ADCs are (1) brentuximab vedotin: an anti-CD30 antibody linked to monomethyl auristatin E (MMAE, a microtubule disrupting agent) used in the treatment of Hodgkin lymphoma; (2) gemtuzumab ozogamicin: an anti-CD33 antibody linked

to a calicheamicin (a cytotoxic agent) used in the treatment of acute myeloid leukemia (AML); and (3) inotuzumab ozogamicin: an anti-CD22 antibody linked to a calicheamicin used in the treatment of acute lymphoblastic leukemia (ALL).

MODULATORS OF IMMUNE CHECKPOINTS

Tumor cells "hijack" the PD-1/PD-L1 and the CTLA-4 regulatory pathways of T cells to evade the immune system. Our understanding of these mechanisms has led to one of the most significant advances in cancer immunotherapy: The development of checkpoint inhibitors (CPIs). CPIs are monoclonal antibodies that bind to PD-1, CTLA-4, PD-L1, or PD-L2 and lead to immune activation. Colloquially speaking, the use of CPIs "takes the breaks of the immune system" and circumvents one of the immune evasion mechanisms that results in tumor survival and growth. The first successful CPI was ipilimumab, a monoclonal antibody targeting CTLA-4. It was approved for use in melanoma. Pembrolizumab and nivolumab are CPIs that bind and block PD-1. They are approved for use in a number of different types of cancer. Table 26.2 summarizes the current CPIs that are being used to treat cancer patients. CPIs have revolutionized the treatment of cancer; however, not all patients respond to treatment. Currently, efforts are directed toward identifying biomarkers that can predict response. Of interest, it is now clear that response to CPIs is

Table 26.1 Monoclonal antibodies in clinical practice[a]

Antibody name	Target	Disease
Monoclonal antibodies		
Rituximab	CD20	B-cell lymphomas
Trastuzumab	HER2	Breast cancer, metastatic gastric cancer
Bevacizumab	VEGF	Cervical cancer, colorectal cancer I, non-small cell lung cancer, ovarian cancer, renal cell carcinoma, glioblastoma
Cetuximab	EGFR	Colorectal, head and neck cancer
Daratumumab	CD38	Multiple myeloma
Alemtuzumab	CD52	Chronic lymphocytic leukemia
Antibody-drug conjugates		
Brentuximab vedotin	CD30	Hodgkin lymphoma, CD30+ T-cell lymphomas
Gemtuzumab ozogamicin	CD33	Acute myeloid leukemia
Inotuzumab ozogamicin	CD22	Acute lymphoblastic leukemia
Trastuzumab emtansine	HER2	Metastatic breast cancer

Abbreviations: EGFR, epidermal growth factor receptor; HER2, human epidermal growth factor receptor 2.
[a] Selected list of monoclonal antibodies and antibody-drug conjugates that are widely used in the treatment of cancer.

Table 26.2 Checkpoint inhibitors in clinical practice

Antibody name	Target	Disease
Ipilimumab	CTLA-4	Melanoma, colorectal cancer, renal cell carcinoma
Nivolumab	PD-1	Melanoma, colorectal cancer, head and neck cancer, hepatocellular carcinoma, Hodgkin's lymphoma, non-small cell lung cancer, renal cell carcinoma, urothelial carcinoma, small cell lung cancer
Pembrolizumab	PD-1	Cervical cancer, gastric cancer, head and neck cancer, Hodgkin's lymphoma, melanoma, non-small cell lung cancer, primary mediastinal large B-cell lymphoma, urothelial carcinoma, Merkel cell carcinoma, microsatellite instability-high cancer
Atezolizumab	PD-L1	Non-small cell lung cancer, urothelial carcinoma
Avelumab	PD-L1	Merkel cell carcinoma, urothelial carcinoma
Durvalumab	PD-L1	Non-small cell lung cancer, urothelial carcinoma

Abbreviations: CTLA-4, cytotoxic T-lymphocyte associated protein 4; PD-1, programmed cell death protein 1; PD-L1, programmed death-ligand 1.

directly related to the presence of T cells within the tumor, suggesting that combining CPIs with other immune therapies promoting T-cell trafficking and tumor infiltration could be of benefit.

ADOPTIVE CELL THERAPY

Adoptive cell therapy (ACT) involves the isolation, *ex vivo* manipulation, and reinfusion of T cells into cancer patients in order to treat their disease (Figure 26.3). The initial purpose behind ACT was to isolate T cells and expand them *ex vivo* in order to circumvent the immunosuppressive mechanisms present in cancer patients. In theory, delivery of already activated and expanded T cells would lead to more efficient T cell–mediated tumor killing. The concept has been studied for several decades, but it was not until the last 5 years that this treatment modality became more widely used. In 2017, the first ACT regimen was approved for use in patients with ALL. There are two types of ACT protocols, those involving the use of genetically engineered T cells and those involving nonengineered T cells.

ACT of nongenetically engineered T cells

Initial protocols were developed using tumor-infiltrating lymphocytes (TILs). The rationale was that T cells found in the tumor were already tumor-reactive and were being suppressed by inhibitory tumor mechanisms. Isolation of TILs from tumor fragments, followed by *ex vivo* expansion and reinfusion into patients has led to response rates of 50% in melanoma patients. These studies provided

proof of principle for this therapy, but broad application of this approach has been limited due to the complex manufacturing process. Currently, ACT using TILs is a viable option, but much work is being done to simplify and streamline the ACT process. In addition, ACT protocols using endogenous peripheral T cells from cancer patients are also being developed.

ACT of genetically engineered T cells

Given the complex manufacturing process involved with ACT using TILs, alternative options were sought for optimization of ACT protocols. The use of genetically engineered T cells has significantly improved ACT protocols leading to broader clinical application. The most common genetically engineered T cells are chimeric antigen receptor T cells (CAR T cells). CAR T cells are generated by isolating T lymphocytes from the blood of cancer patients and transducing them *ex vivo* using a retroviral vector. The vector delivers a construct that consists of an antigen-binding domain (an antibody fragment), a T-cell signaling domain (CD3), and a T-cell costimulation domain (CD28, 41BB) (Figure 26.4). Because in the CAR construct the binding domain is directly linked to the T-cell activation domain and the costimulatory domain, CAR T cells do not require TCR-MHC interactions. They are activated simply by binding to their tumor targets. Once CAR T cells are transduced and expanded *ex vivo*, they are infused back into the patient. Inside the patient, CAR T cells bind to tumor cells via their binding domain, and they

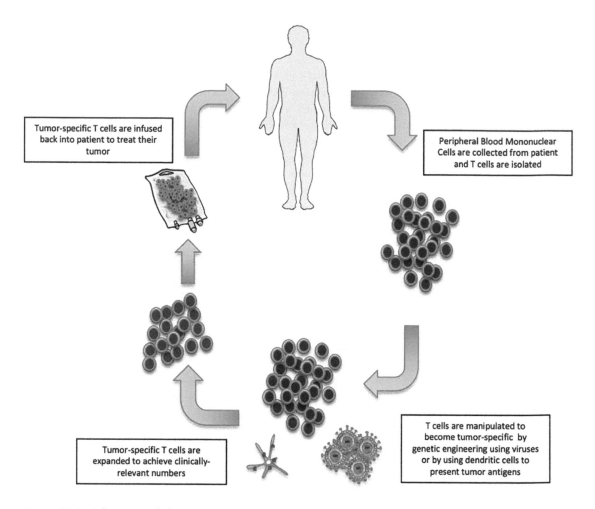

Figure 26.3 *Adoptive cell therapy (ACT).* The general process of ACT.

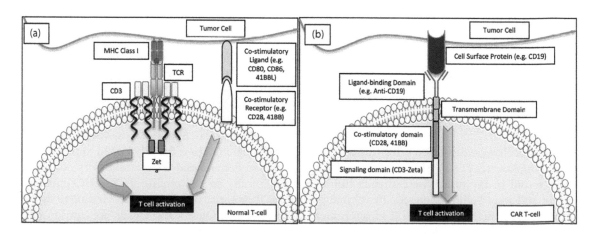

Figure 26.4 *Chimeric antigen receptor (CAR) T cells.* (a) The immune synapse during recognition of tumors by normal T cells. (b) The immune synapse during recognition of tumor cells by CAR T cells.

are immediately activated leading to tumor killing. Clinical response to CAR T-cell treatment has been very impressive with overall response rates in the 70%–80% range for ALL and diffuse large B-cell lymphoma patients. Currently, there are two approved CAR T-cell products: (1) tisagenlecleucel and (2) axicabtagene ciloleucel. Both are CAR T cells targeting CD19 and are approved for treatment of ALL and diffuse large B-cell lymphoma.

Bispecific T-cell engagers

With the growing interest and positive clinical results using T-cell therapies in the treatment of cancer, alternative methods have been developed to target tumors using T cells. Blinatumomab is a bispecific monoclonal antibody that is able to bind to T cells (via CD3) and tumor cells (via CD19); it belongs to a class of molecules called bispecific T-cell engagers (BiTEs) (Figure 26.5). Blinatumomab acts

as a link between non-tumor-reactive T cells and tumor cells. Once blinatumomab binds T cells via CD3, it activates them; binding to CD19 (a molecule overexpressed in ALL and many lymphomas), blinatumomab brings T cells in close proximity to tumor cells where a cytolytic synapse forms and tumor cells are killed via classical T-cell killing pathways. The advantage of such an approach is that tumor-reactive T cells are not required, and T-cell activation does not require TCR-MHC complex interaction. Blinatumomab is used for the treatment of ALL and is currently being studied for treatments of different types of lymphomas. In addition, additional bispecific T-cell engagers are being developed to target other types of cancer.

CLOSING REMARKS

Our understanding of the immune responses against cancer and the mechanisms that tumors utilize to evade those immune responses has allowed us to develop novel and effective cancer immunotherapies. Current immune therapies have achieved unprecedented results in the treatment of cancer patients. As we look ahead, there are many approaches either in clinical trials or preclinical investigations that will likely improve on the current approaches. Combination therapies (e.g., checkpoint inhibitors with cytokine complexes, CAR-T cells combined with checkpoint inhibitors, BiTEs with checkpoint inhibitors) are the next logical step in therapy development. New targets for CAR T cells and BiTEs are currently in clinical trials and showing very encouraging results. Novel strategies to enhance ACT protocols are being developed. One of the most promising and exciting approaches in the field of cancer immunotherapy is the development of neoantigen-specific therapies. By determining tumor-specific mutations and identifying immunogenic neoepitopes, therapies such as vaccines or T-cell therapies can be developed, opening the door for the development of personalized, tumor-specific immune therapies.

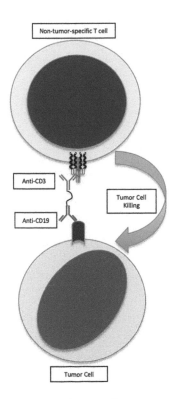

Figure 26.5 *Bispecific T-cell engagers (BiTEs).* Blinatumomab, a CD3/CD19 BiTE and its mechanism of action: Binding to the CD3 receptor complex activates the engaged T cell, and CD19+ tumor cells are brought into close proximity to the engaged T cell via binding to CD19 resulting in tumor cell killing.

BIBLIOGRAPHY

Appelbaum F. Haematopoietic cell transplantation as immunotherapy. *Nature*. 2001;411:385–389.

Chen D, Mellman I. Oncology meets immunology: The cancer immunity cycle. *Immunity*. 2013;39: 1–13.

Ferrara J, Levine J, Reddy P, Holler E. Graft-versus-host disease. *Lancet.* 2009;373:1550–1561.

Huehls A, Coupet T, Sentman C. Bispecific T cell engagers for cancer immunotherapy. *Immunol Cell Biol.* 2015;93:290–296.

June C, O'Connor R, Kawalekar O et al. CAR T cell immunotherapy for human cancer. *Science.* 2018;359:1361–1365.

June C, Riddell S, Schumacher T. Adoptive cellular therapy: A race to the finish line. *Sci Transl Med.* 2015 Mar 25;7(280):280ps7. doi: 10.1126/scitranslmed.aaa3643.

Kalos M, June C. Adoptive transfer for cancer immunotherapy in the era of synthetic biology. *Immunity.* 2013;39:49–60.

Mittal D, Gubin M, Schreiber R, Smyth M. New insights into cancer immunoediting and its three component phases—Elimination, equilibrium and escape. *Curr Opin Immunol.* 2014; 27:16–25.

Motz G, Coukos G. Deciphering and reversing tumor immune suppression. *Immunity.* 2013;39: 61–73.

Mukherjee A, Waters A, Babic I et al. Antibody drug conjugates: Progress, pitfalls and promises. *Hum Antibodies.* 2018;27:1–10.

Perica K, Varela JC, Oelke M, Schneck J. Adoptive T cell immunotherapy for cancer. Rambam Maimonides. *Med J.* 2015;6(1):e0004. doi: 10.5041/RMMJ.10179.

Ribas A, Wolchok J. Cancer immunotherapy using checkpoint blockade. *Science.* 2018;359:1350–1355.

Singh A, McGuirk J. Allogeneic stem cell transplantation: A historical and scientific overview. *Cancer Res.* 2016;76:6445–6451.

Singh S, Kumar N, Dwiwedi P et al. Monoclonal antibodies: A review. *Curr Clin Pharmacol.* 2018; 13:85–99.

Vinay D, Ryan E, Pawelec G et al. Immune evasion mechanisms in cancer: Mechanistic basis and therapeutic strategies. *Semin Cancer Biol.* 2015;35:185–198.

Wrangle J, Patterson A, Johnson C et al. IL-2 and beyond in cancer immunotherapy. *J Interferon Cytokine Res.* 2018;38:45–68.

27

Lymphocyte and plasma cell malignancies

JUAN CARLOS VARELA AND GABRIEL VIRELLA

INTRODUCTION

Lymphocytes are frequently affected by neoplastic mutations, perhaps as a consequence of their intense mitotic activity. Lymphocyte malignancies can be broadly classified into B-cell and T-cell malignancies. B-cell malignancies (or dyscrasias) are identified by the production of abnormally high amounts of homogeneous immunoglobulins (or fragments thereof) resulting from the monoclonal proliferation of immunoglobulin-secreting B cells or plasma cells, or by the proliferation of lymphocytes or lymphocyte precursors expressing specific B-cell markers. T-cell malignancies (or dyscrasias) are defined as proliferations of lymphocytes or their precursors expressing T-cell membrane markers.

B-CELL DYSCRASIAS

Malignant proliferations of B cells can involve undifferentiated lymphocytes (leukemias, lymphomas) or immunoglobulin-producing cells (plasma cell dyscrasias). Plasma cell dyscrasias usually are associated with the presence of high levels of immunoglobulins with single heavy- and light-chain isotypes. Because of the homogeneity of these proteins, it is assumed that a malignant clone of plasma cells generates them, and they are designated as monoclonal proteins. Monoclonal proteins or paraproteins, in practical terms, are defined by the fact that they are constituted by large amounts of identical molecules, carrying one single heavy-chain class and one single light-chain type (Figure 27.1), or, in some cases, by isolated heavy or light chains of a single type. It must be noted that monoclonal proteins may be detected in patients without overt signals of malignancy (some mutations may lead to clonal expansion without uncontrolled cell proliferation).

Plasma cell and plasma cell precursor dyscrasias

In general, the diagnosis of a plasma cell or a plasma cell precursor dyscrasia relies on the demonstration of a monoclonal protein. As stated previously, a monoclonal protein has to be defined by its homogeneity in heavy and/or light chains, and this information can be obtained by serum electrophoresis, immunochemical techniques, such as immunofixation (Figures 27.1 and 27.2), or by determination of an increase of one type of light chains (in serum or urine) exceeding by 100-fold

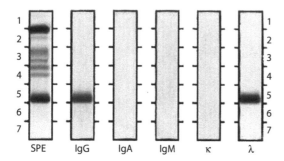

Figure 27.1 Immunoblot of the serum protein of a patient with multiple myeloma. The lane labeled SPE was fixed and stained after electrophoresis and shows an homogeneous fraction in the γ-globulin region, near the bottom part of the separation region. The remaining lanes were blotted with the following antisera: anti-IgG, anti-IgA, anti-IgM, anti-kappa chains (κ), and anti-lambda chains (λ). Notice that the antisera specific for IgG and for λ chains reacted with the homogeneous fraction, which therefore was identified as an IgGλ monoclonal protein. (Immunoblot courtesy of Dr. Sally Self, Department of Pathology and Laboratory Medicine, Medical University of South Carolina.)

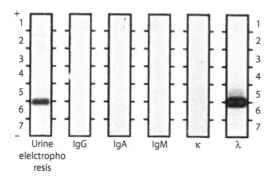

Figure 27.2 Immunoblot of the urine of patient with multiple myeloma. The far left lane was stained for total protein and shows a homogeneous band that reacted exclusively with anti-λ chain antiserum. (Immunoblot courtesy of Dr. Sally Self, Department of Pathology and Laboratory Medicine, Medical University of South Carolina.)

or more the levels of the other type (e.g., a κ:λ ratio equal to or greater than 100, or vice versa). Immunofixation is widely used to diagnose specific B-cell dyscrasias, including multiple myeloma, light-chain disease, Waldenström's macroglobulinemia, and the heavy-chain diseases, discussed later in this chapter.

- A monoclonal protein in serum and/or urine can be detected in 97% of the cases of multiple myeloma. The distribution of monoclonal proteins among the different immunoglobulin classes closely parallels the relative proportions of those immunoglobulins in normal serum: 60%–70% of the monoclonal proteins are typed as IgG, 20%–30% as IgA, 1%–2% as IgD, and, very rarely one monoclonal protein can be typed as IgE. A single light-chain type is found in these paraproteins, and the ratio between the normal and abnormal light-chain types (measured either in serum or urine) should be ≥100. For example, IgG paraproteins can be either κ or λ. The finding of a heterogeneous increase of IgG or any other immunoglobulin (i.e., an increase of both IgGκ and IgGλ molecules) is not compatible with a diagnosis of multiple myeloma, but rather indicative of reactive plasmacytosis.

In the urine, the most frequent finding is the elimination of free light chains, κ or λ (Bence-Jones proteins, see Figure 27.2). These light chains are usually found in addition to a monoclonal immunoglobulin detectable in serum, or, in some cases the serum has two abnormal bands, one is a complete monoclonal protein, and the other corresponds to free light chains of the same type carried by the complete protein (Figure 27.3). In about 20%–30% of patients with multiple myeloma, the only abnormal proteins to be found are the free monoclonal light chains in the urine. Some authors give the designation of light-chain disease to the form of multiple myeloma in which the only detectable paraprotein consists of free light chains.

In some instances, plasma cell dyscrasias do not result in the secretion of paraproteins. In rare cases of multiple myeloma, for example, the neoplastic mutation alters the synthetic process so profoundly that no paraproteins are produced.

Note that the finding of a monoclonal protein does not give a very precise diagnostic indication. For example, the isolated finding of homogeneous free light chains (Bence-Jones protein) in the urine may correspond to one of the following B-cell dyscrasias: (1) light-chain disease, (2) chronic lymphocytic leukemia, (3) lymphocytic lymphoma, smoldering multiple myeloma (SMM), or

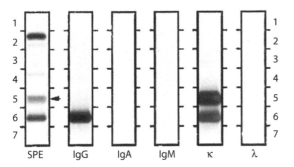

Figure 27.3 Immunoblot study of the serum proteins of a patient with multiple myeloma. The serum protein electrophoresis (SPE, left lane) reveals several proteins, including albumin (top) and two homogeneous fractions (bottom). The bottom fraction on SPE reacted both with an antiserum specific for IgG heavy chains and anti-κ chains and is thus identifiable as complete IgGκ. The second homogeneous protein seen in SPE (arrow) reacted only with anti-κ chains. Thus, this fraction is identifiable as free κ chains (Bence-Jones protein, κ type), and its presence in serum suggests that the patient has kidney deficiency. (Immunoblot courtesy of Dr. Sally Self, Department of Pathology and Laboratory Medicine, Medical University of South Carolina.)

(4) monoclonal gammopathy of undetermined significance (MGUS). The precise diagnosis depends on a combination of clinical and laboratory data, as discussed in detail later in this chapter.

Other B-cell dyscrasias

B-lymphocyte malignancies include leukemias and lymphomas. Chronic lymphocytic leukemias involve malignant B-cell proliferations in the vast majority of cases, but only one-third show paraproteins; the remainder have monoclonal cell surface immunoglobulins only.

B-cell acute lymphocytic leukemias show rearrangements of their immunoglobulin heavy-chain genes in chromosome 14, and the malignant cells may synthesize μ chains, but those remain intracytoplasmic, and there is no detectable monoclonal protein in serum or urine.

Hodgkin's lymphoma, Burkitt's lymphoma, and other non-Hodgkin lymphomas associated with immunosuppression (e.g., HIV infections, posttransplant immunosuppression) are not associated with the synthesis of monoclonal proteins.

Physiopathology of B-cell dyscrasias

DIRECT PATHOLOGICAL CONSEQUENCES OF MALIGNANT B-CELL PROLIFERATION

Symptoms related to malignant cell proliferation: Depending on the type of proliferating B cell, patients may present with a variety of symptoms directly resulting from the expansion of a malignant B-cell population, including the following:

- Enlargement of lymph nodes, spleen, and liver, as seen in lymphomas and some leukemias.
- Proliferation of malignant cells in the bone marrow (characteristic of B-cell leukemias, multiple myeloma, and some lymphomas) can cause profound anemia, thrombocytopenia, and leukopenia. Furthermore, leukemic invasion of peripheral blood is the hallmark of B-cell leukemias and plasma cell leukemias.
- Compressive and obstructive symptoms resulting from the proliferation of plasma cells in soft tissues. Oropharyngeal plasmacytomas often lead to obstructive symptoms. Heavy-chain-producing intestinal lymphomas, when grossly nodular, can lead to intestinal obstruction. In addition, bulky B-cell lymphomas (both Hodgkin's and non-Hodgkin's) can cause obstructive symptoms, for example, B-cell lymphomas affecting the mediastinum can cause Pancoast syndrome and thoracic outlet syndrome.
- Intestinal malabsorption, typical of α-chain disease, results from extensive infiltration of the intestinal submucosa by malignant B cells, causing total disruption of the normal submucosal architecture.
- Compression fractures of vertebral bodies or pathological fractures of other bones are often a presenting symptom associated with plasma cell dyscrasias.

General metabolic disturbances are responsible for some major pathological manifestations of B-cell dyscrasia, such as bone destruction, renal insufficiency, anemia, and secondary immunodeficiency.

Bone destruction results from a combination of osteoclast hyperactivity and depressed osteoblast function, proliferation, and activation. Several osteoclast activation factors released by plasma cells and stromal cells have been proposed as responsible for osteoclast activation, including the ligand for the receptor activator of NF-κB (RANKL), macrophage inflammatory protein 1α (MIP-1α), vascular endothelial growth factor (VEGF), hepatocyte growth factor (HGF), tumor necrosis factor (TNF), IL-6, IL-1β, and lymphotoxin-α. On the other hand, the production of osteoprotegerin, which inhibits the effects of RANKL, is depressed. In addition, conditions for osteoblast proliferation and differentiation are adverse, as a result of the release of soluble factors by malignant plasma cells (Dickkopf-1, Dkk-1) and T cells (IL-3, IL-7) that suppress osteoblast differentiation. The end result of this imbalance is localized or disseminated bone reabsorption.

Renal insufficiency can result from a diversity of factors, such as hypercalcemia (secondary to bone reabsorption), hyperuricemia, deposition of amyloid substance in the kidney, clogging of glomeruli or tubuli with paraprotein (favored by dehydration), and plasmacytic infiltration of the kidney.

Anemia (normochromic, normocytic) is frequent and is basically due to decreased production of red cells. A moderate shortening of red cell survival is also common.

Immunodeficiency is a paradoxical feature of many B-cell malignancies. It often develops in patients who have marked increases in their concentrations of circulating immunoglobulins. This is particularly obvious in patients with multiple myeloma, who have an increased tendency for pyogenic infections. In reality, if the levels of residual normal immunoglobulins are measured, they are found to be low. Also, these patients show decreased antibody production after active immunization. The depression of the humoral immune response in patients with multiple myeloma appears to be multifactorial:

- In IgG myeloma, the large amounts of IgG secreted by the malignant cells are likely to have a negative feedback effect, depressing normal IgG synthesis (see Chapter 6).
- A more general mechanism of suppression of the humoral response seems to be a consequence of impaired B-cell responses caused by a variety of factors, including deficient antigen presentation by dendritic cells and release of immunosuppressive cytokines such as TGF-β and IL-17. Furthermore, in more advanced stages of multiple myeloma, the number of normal plasma cells in the bone marrow shows a significant depression.
- Other abnormalities that may contribute to the predisposition to infections are defects in neutrophil responses and impairment of Fcγ receptor functions in phagocytes, which are more likely to exist in patients with renal failure. Anemia also seems to predispose to infections, for unknown reasons.

In chronic lymphocytic leukemia (CLL), in addition to a depression of humoral immunity (milder than that seen in multiple myeloma), there is a depression of T-cell counts and function. Viral and fungal infections as well as cases of disseminated infection after administration of live attenuated viral vaccines have been reported in patients with this type of leukemia. Recent studies have demonstrated that T cells from patients with CLL stimulated *in vitro* with anti-CD3 plus IL-2 express the costimulatory molecule CD28 at lower levels and for a shorter time than cells from normal controls, while they express higher levels for longer periods of time of the downregulatory molecule CTLA-4 (CD152). These findings could explain why CLL patients have impaired cell-mediated immune responses.

SERUM HYPERVISCOSITY

Some plasma cell dyscrasias may present with a constellation of symptoms known as the hyperviscosity syndrome. This is a direct result of increased serum viscosity, caused by high concentrations of monoclonal proteins. Serum viscosity is directly related to protein concentration. IgM and polymeric IgA, due to their molecular complexity and high intrinsic viscosity, lead to disproportionate increases of blood viscosity (Figure 27.4). Not surprisingly, the hyperviscosity syndrome is a frequent manifestation of Waldenström's macroglobulinemia, a B-cell dyscrasia defined by the synthesis of monoclonal IgM. However, the hyperviscosity syndrome is also observed in multiple myeloma patients, mainly in those with polymeric IgA paraproteins, and occasionally in IgG myeloma, when the concentrations of IgG are very high. The symptoms of serum hyperviscosity are related to high protein concentration, expanded plasma volume, and sluggishness of circulation. Table 27.1 lists the main signs and symptoms of the syndrome. Typical funduscopic changes are shown in Figure 27.5.

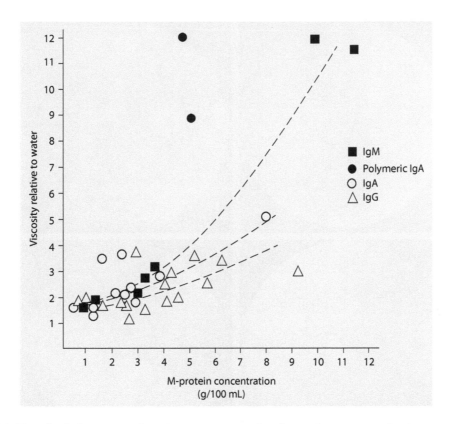

Figure 27.4 Plot of relative serum viscosity versus monoclonal protein concentration in sera containing IgG, IgA, and IgM monoclonal proteins. The highest viscosity values were determined in sera containing IgM or polymeric IgA monoclonal proteins.

Table 27.1 Clinical manifestations of the hyperviscosity syndrome

Ocular
  Variable degrees of vision impairment
  Funduscopic changes
  Dilation and tortuosity of retinal veins ("string-of-sausage" appearance)
  Retinal hemorrhage and "cotton-wool" exudates
  Papilledema
Hematologic
  Mucosal bleeding (oral cavity, nose, gastrointestinal tract, urinary tract)
  Prolonged bleeding after trauma or surgery
Neurological
  Headaches, somnolence, coma
  Dizziness, vertigo
  Seizures, EEG changes
  Hearing loss
Renal
  Renal insufficiency (acute or chronic) due to
    (a) clogging of the glomerular vessels with paraprotein and
    (b) diminished concentrating and diluting abilities
Cardiovascular
  Congestive heart failure secondary to expanded plasma volume

Source: Modified from Bloch, K.J., Maki, D.G., *Sem. Hematol.*, 10, 113, 1974.

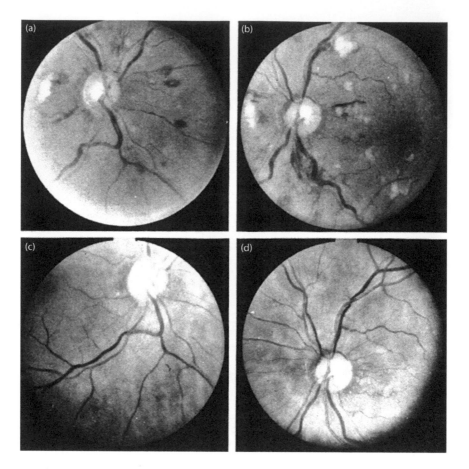

Figure 27.5 Funduscopic examination of a patient with hyperviscosity syndrome. (a, b) Pictures obtained from the right and left eyes, respectively, at the time of admission. Flame-shaped hemorrhages, "cotton-wool" exudates, and irregular dilation of retinal veins are evident. (c, d) Pictures obtained from the same eyes after 5 months of therapy, showing total normalization. (From Virella, G. et al., *Brit. J. Haematol.*, 30, 479, 1975. Reproduced with authorization of the publisher.)

PATHOLOGICAL CONSEQUENCES OF IMMUNOLOGICAL ACTIVITY OF PARAPROTEIN

Most paraproteins have unknown and inconsequential antibody activities, but in some exceptional cases, the reactivity of a monoclonal protein may be directly responsible for some of the manifestations of the disease:

- **Cold agglutinin disease** results from the synthesis of large concentrations of monoclonal IgM (IgM-κ in more than 90% of the cases) with cold agglutinating properties and has been described in detail in Chapter 22.
- **Hyperlipidemia** is a rare feature of some cases of multiple myeloma in which the monoclonal protein has autoreactivity with ApoB. More

frequently, those are IgA monoclonal proteins, but cases of IgG monoclonal proteins with the same reactivity have also been reported. In all cases, the patients have pronounced increases in serum lipid and lipoprotein levels. The exact physiopathologic mechanisms involved in these rare cases have not been established.

Clinical presentations, diagnosis, and management of plasma cell dyscrasias

Plasma cell dyscrasias include three main diseases: MGUS, smoldering myeloma, and multiple myeloma. Each of these diseases is associated with the presence of monoclonal paraproteins and plasma cells in the bone marrow, but only multiple myeloma is associated with end-organ damage as described later.

MONOCLONAL GAMMOPATHY OF UNDETERMINED SIGNIFICANCE

Clinical presentation and diagnosis. The designation of MGUS is used when a monoclonal protein is found in an asymptomatic individual or in a patient with a disease totally unrelated to B-lymphocyte or plasma cell proliferation (solid tumors, chronic hepatobiliary disease, different forms of non-B-cell leukemia, rheumatoid arthritis, neurological disorders, etc.).

Scandinavian authors conducting extensive population studies have given an average figure for the incidence of MGUS of about 1%, by far the most common form of B-cell dyscrasia. The incidence seems to increase in the elderly, up to about 20% in 90-year-old and older individuals.

Management. The majority of MGUS patients are asymptomatic as it relates to the paraprotein. They are monitored for progression into smoldering myeloma or multiple myeloma via serum/urine electrophoresis and blood chemistries. In general, there are three risk factors that increase the risk of progression in MGUS patients: (1) the presence of non-IgG paraprotein, (2) a monoclonal protein spike of $\geq$1.5 g/dL, and (3) an abnormal free light-chain ratio (κ:λ ratio of <0.26 or >1.65). These patients require closer monitoring and may need a deeper evaluation with a bone marrow biopsy to evaluate progression of disease.

SMOLDERING MYELOMA

Clinical presentation and diagnosis. Smoldering myeloma is defined by the presence of a monoclonal spike of >3 g/dL and/or the presence of 10%–60% plasma cells in the bone marrow in the absence of any signs of end-organ damage. It is an intermediate state between MGUS and multiple myeloma. A large percentage of patients are asymptomatic, and those with symptoms typically present with weakness and/or fatigue. Similar to patients with MGUS, there are three risk factors that increase the risk of progression to multiple myeloma: (1) serum monoclonal protein spike of $\geq$3 g/dL, (2) more than 10% clonal plasma cells in the bone marrow, and (3) an abnormal free light-chain ratio (κ:λ ratio of <0.125 or >8).

Management. Current guidelines do not recommend treatment for smoldering myeloma outside of a clinical trial. The goal of management is to monitor for progression into multiple myeloma and institute treatment promptly. The progression of smoldering myeloma into multiple myeloma is characterized by the appearance of end-organ damage (i.e., lytic bone lesions, severe anemia, hypercalcemia, renal failure).

MULTIPLE MYELOMA

Clinical presentation and diagnosis. The most frequent presenting clinical symptoms of multiple myeloma are (1) fatigue and weakness secondary to anemia; (2) bone pain and pathological fractures, in the long bones, skull, or spinal column, as a consequence of bone erosion; (3) acute renal failure; and (4) hypercalcemia. In addition, patients are at increased risk for infection (most frequently Gram-negative organisms and *Streptococcus pneumoniae*). Less frequently, patients may present with malaise, headaches, or other symptoms related to hyperviscosity. In many cases, anemia is the leading feature, and the diagnosis is established when the cause of anemia is investigated. Hemoglobin levels below 7.5 g/dL are usually associated with poor prognosis. Symptoms related to hyperviscosity (see Table 27.1) may also lead to hospitalization.

Recurrent infections and renal failure, which are often seen in advanced stages of the disease, are among the most common causes of death. Infection is associated with an increased risk of death, and the prognosis of a multiple myeloma patient with renal failure, particularly when his or her blood urea nitrogen exceeds 80 mg/dL, is also poor.

Diagnosis. The diagnosis of multiple myeloma relies on the finding of clonal bone marrow plasmacytosis ($\geq$10% clonal cells as defined by flow cytometry) or biopsy proven plasmacytoma lesions, plus one or more of the following myeloma defining events:

- **Evidence of end-organ damage as determined by**
  - Hypercalcemia (serum calcium >11 mg/dL)
  - Renal insufficiency (estimated creatinine clearance <40 mL/min)
  - Anemia (hemoglobin <10 g/dL)
  - Osteolytic bone lesions. These lesions can appear in the x-ray as multiple punched-out areas in a given bone or in multiple bones without peripheral osteosclerosis (Figure 27.6). Rarely, a single bone lesion may be detected in one patient; however, such a "solitary bone plasmacytoma" is in fact rarely

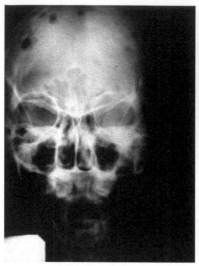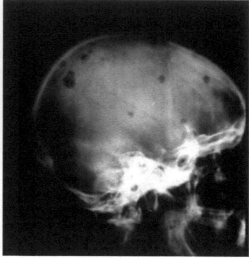

Figure 27.6 X-ray of the skull of a patient with multiple myeloma showing typical osteolytic lesions. (Courtesy of Dr. S. Richardson.)

solitary, and bone marrow aspiration will reveal diffuse plasmacytosis in most cases. Exceptionally, a patient with monoclonal gammopathy and diffuse plasmacytosis can present with no evident bone lesions, or with generalized osteoporosis. Imaging techniques with higher resolution than x-rays may reveal lesions not otherwise detected.

Or

- **Evidence of a biomarker associated with likely progression to end-organ damage as determined by:**
  - ≥60% clonal plasma cells in the bone marrow
  - Free light-chain ratio (involved/uninvolved) of >100
  - Radiographical evidence of more than one bone lesion

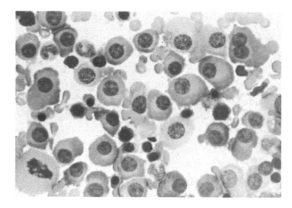

Figure 27.7 Plasma cell infiltration of the bone marrow in a patient with multiple myeloma. Note the binucleated plasma cell in the upper right corner of this picture.

Bone marrow plasmacytosis with clonal cells ≥60% is rare, but when present carries a very poor prognosis. Bone marrow aspirates show massive infiltration of plasma cells with a more or less mature appearance (Figure 27.7). The clonal nature of multiple myeloma plasma cells is indirectly proven by the detection of a monoclonal protein in the serum and/or urine, but there are phenotypic characteristics of clonal malignant plasma cells that can be detected by flow cytometry and allow a more precise estimate of the numbers of clonal cells. In general, malignant plasma cells do not express some of the markers expressed by normal plasma cells (CD19, CD45) or express them weakly (CD27, CD38, CD81) and express markers not detected or detected in very low levels in normal plasma cells (CD20, CD28, CD56, CD117, CD200). The level of expression of these markers has prognostic implications. For example, normal expression of CD27 in clonal plasma cells has a better prognosis, the opposite being true when CD27 is not expressed. The expression of CD81 in clonal plasma cells is also associated with poor prognosis. In contrast, the expression of CD117 is associated with better prognosis.

The revised international staging system (R-ISS) is broadly used to stage multiple myeloma. It takes several parameters into consideration: serum albumin, β-2 microglobulin, lactate dehydrogenase (LDH) levels, and cytogenetic abnormalities. The serum albumin concentration reflects the general metabolic state of the patient and the levels of circulating β-2 microglobulin are an apparent indicator of the B-cell proliferation rate. Cytogenetic aberrations are common in multiple myeloma. Some seem not to have an impact on prognosis, but others do.

Normal levels of LDH, serum albumin levels ≥3.5 g/dL, and β-2 microglobulin levels <3.5 mg/L (stage 1) are associated with the best prognosis (median survival of 62 months), while high levels of LDH, β-2 microglobulin levels ≥5.5 mg/L, and chromosome 17 deletions and/or translocations between chromosomes 4 and 14 (stage 3) are indicative of poor prognosis (median survival of 29 months). Other parameters indicative of poor prognosis (survival <12 months) are β-2 microglobulin levels >10 mg/L, serum creatinine >4 mg/L, serum albumin <2.5 g/L, ratio between free monoclonal light chains of one type and free light chains of the opposite type ≥100, and platelet count <130,000/µL.

Management. Multiple myeloma is not curable, but it can be controlled for many years, even decades, with the current treatment strategies. The initial recommended treatment of multiple myeloma consists of induction with a three-drug chemotherapy regimen followed by consolidation with autologous stem cell transplantation. The most common three-drug regimen used for induction of patients with standard or high-risk multiple myeloma consists of bortezomib (a proteasome inhibitor), lenalidomide (an immunomodulatory agent), and dexamethasone. The goal of induction therapy is to reduce the tumor burden and achieve a remission prior to stem cell transplantation. Once remission is achieved, the patients are given GCSF to mobilize stem cells from the bone marrow to the peripheral blood, and CD34+ stem cells are harvested. Patients are subsequently conditioned with high doses of melphalan (an alkylating agent) and the collected CD34 stem cells are infused back into the patient. Stem cell transplantation is considered successful when the level of monoclonal protein is reduced by >90%. To achieve this goal, a second stem cell transplantation may be required. Maintenance therapy after the transplant is recommended to prolong the relapse-free survival of patients. Most commonly, lenalidomide is given after autologous transplant for patients with standard risk, and a proteasome inhibitor such as bortezomib is given to patients with high-risk disease. Median relapse-free survival for multiple myeloma patients who undergo induction chemotherapy, followed by autologous stem cell transplant and posttransplant maintenance is 5–6 years for standard-risk patients and 2–3 years for high-risk patients. Management of relapsed or refractory disease consists of treatment with multidrug regimens. Different combinations of proteasome inhibitors (bortezomib, carfilzomib, ixazomib), immunomodulatory agents (lenalidomide, pomalidomide), and chemotherapy agents (cyclophosphamide) have been studied in clinical trials, but there is no clear standard of care. Immunotherapy with daratumumab, a monoclonal antibody against CD38, has also been incorporated into treatment regimens.

Hypercalcemia is usually treated with glucocorticoids, but biphosphonates such as pamidronate and zoledronic acid have been found to be highly effective, Biphosphonates are also used successfully to reduce bone destruction and avoid pathological fractures. Recent reports of severe oral adverse effects, especially painful necrosis of the jaw bones, associated with several products of this group in patients receiving chemotherapy, raise issues about the long-term use of biphosphonates in patients with multiple myeloma and other malignancies affecting the bones.

Plasmapheresis, which consists in replacing the patient's plasma with normal plasma or a plasma-replacing solution, is indicated in cases with hyperviscosity. The reduction on viscosity secondary to the reduction in the circulating levels of monoclonal protein caused by chemotherapy takes time, and the rapid correction of hyperviscosity may be essential for proper management. The rapidly beneficial effects of plasmapheresis are illustrated in Figure 27.5, which shows the normalization of retinal changes observed after plasmapheresis.

Other supportive measures include hemodialysis or peritoneal dialysis in cases with renal insufficiency, and antibiotic therapy and prophylactic administration of gammaglobulin in patients with recurrent infections.

PLASMA CELL LEUKEMIA

Plasma cell leukemia is the designation applied to cases in which large numbers of plasma cells can be detected in the peripheral blood (exceeding 5%–10% of the total white blood cell count). Besides the leukemic picture in the peripheral blood, the remaining clinical and laboratory features of plasma cell leukemia are usually indistinguishable from those of multiple myeloma. The prognosis is generally poor; this may reflect a higher degree of de-differentiation on the part of malignant plasma cells that abandon their normal territory.

WALDENSTRÖM'S MACROGLOBULINEMIA

Waldenström's macroglobulinemia (also known as lymphoplasmacytic lymphoma) is a B-cell proliferative disorder characterized by bone marrow infiltration and IgM monoclonal gammopathy. A Swedish physician, Jan Waldenström, after whom the disease was named, first described it.

Clinical presentation and diagnosis. Waldenström's macroglobulinemia is clinically characterized by a constellation of symptoms that include weakness and anemia, easy bruising, fever, headache, night sweats, weight loss, hyperviscosity-related symptoms (Table 27.1), hepatomegaly, splenomegaly, and lymphadenopathy. Neuropathy can also be present in these patients, apparently as a result of having an IgM monoclonal protein that binds to the myelin sheath and causes demyelination.

Symptoms suggestive of multiple myeloma, such as bone pain, bone lesions, or "spontaneous" fractures, are rare. The immunosuppression is also milder than in multiple myeloma. Hypercalcemia, leukopenia, thrombocytopenia, and azotemia are rarely seen. Renal insufficiency, when present, is usually a manifestation of serum hyperviscosity and can be reversed by plasmapheresis and/or peritoneal dialysis. In general, the disease has a much more benign evolution than multiple myeloma, with median survival rates ranging from 5 to 10 years.

The two main diagnostic features of Waldenström's macroglobulinemia are the presence of an IgM monoclonal protein and the pleomorphic infiltration of the bone marrow with predominance of small lymphocytes, plasmacytoid cells, and mature plasma cells. Mast cells can also be prominent. Most infiltrating lymphocytes and lymphoplasmacytic cells express B-cell markers (CD19, 20, 22).

Management. Waldenström's macroglobulinemia frequently follows a benign course. Patients without evidence of end-organ damage are considered as having smoldering disease (IgM MGUS) and should be closely followed up, but do not require treatment. Poor prognosis is associated with a variety of parameters, such as age ($\geq$65), anemia, high β-2 microglobulin levels and the MYD88 L265P mutation. In patients with high levels of circulating IgM, serum hyperviscosity can be the cause of a variety of complications, some of them life-threatening (Table 27.1). In such cases, emergency plasmapheresis should be performed to correct the hyperviscosity, followed by the administration of one of the drug regimens recommended for symptomatic patients or patients with poor prognosis indicators.

Combinations of rituximab, a CD20 monoclonal antibody, with cyclophosphamide and dexamethasone, or with newer drugs, such as bendamustine (an alkylating agent) or bortezomib are widely used with good results. However, bortezomib administration is associated with the development of neuropathy in about 50% of patients, and its replacement by carfilzomib (a non-neurotoxic proteasome inhibitor) has been recommended. For younger patients with Waldenström macroglobulinemia, autologous stem cell transplant and rarely allogeneic transplantation can be highly efficacious.

Heavy-chain diseases

Some B-cell dyscrasias are associated with the exclusive production of heavy chains (or fragments thereof) or with the synthesis of abnormal heavy chains that are not assembled as complete immunoglobulin molecules and are excreted as free heavy chains. Both types of abnormality can be on the basis of a heavy-chain disease. The heavy-chain diseases are classified according to the isotype of the abnormal heavy chain as γ, α, μ, and δ. (A single case of δ-chain disease has been reported, and ε-chain disease has yet to be described.)

α-CHAIN DISEASE

This is the most common and best-defined heavy-chain disease. It affects patients in all age groups, even children, and is more frequent in the Mediterranean countries, particularly affecting individuals of Jewish or Arab ancestry.

Clinically, it is indistinguishable from the Mediterranean-type abdominal lymphoma, characterized by diarrhea and malabsorption unresponsive to gluten withdrawal, with progressive wasting and death. Intestinal x-ray may show changes suggestive of diffuse infiltration of the small intestine, such as thickened mucosal folds. Intestinal biopsy reveals diffuse infiltration of the submucosa by reticulolymphocytic cells.

Diagnosis relies on the demonstration of free α chains, usually in serum. Routine electrophoresis usually fails to show a monoclonal component, but immunofixation shows an abnormal IgA band that does not react with antisera specific for light chains.

γ-CHAIN DISEASE

This was the first form of heavy-chain disease discovered. Clinically, it appears as a lymphoma with lymphadenopathy, splenomegaly, and hepatomegaly. Bone marrow and lymph node biopsies show lymphoplasmacytic proliferation. The diagnosis is based on the immunochemical demonstration of free γ chains in the serum and/or urine.

μ-CHAIN DISEASE

This variant of heavy-chain disease is found less frequently than either γ- or α-heavy-chain diseases, and clinically, it is indistinguishable from chronic lymphocytic leukemia or lymphocytic lymphoma, with marked Bence-Jones proteinuria and small amounts of free μ chains detectable in the serum and sometimes also in the urine.

LEUKEMIAS AND LYMPHOMAS

Nomenclature

The malignant proliferation of leukocytes can be classified by a variety of criteria. One first important distinction is made between leukemia and lymphoma. It should be noted that it is not rare for a patient to have features of both types of processes, but the clinical classifications of lymphocyte malignancies are useful and widely used.

Leukemia refers to any malignant proliferation of leukocytes in which the abnormal cell population can be easily detected in the peripheral blood and in the bone marrow. Leukemias may involve any type of hematopoietic cell, including granulocytes, red cells, and platelets. Leukemias are often classified as acute or chronic, based on their clinical evolution and morphologic characteristics that are closely related. Acute leukemias follow a very rapid progression toward death if left untreated. Many immature and atypical cells can be seen in

the peripheral blood of patients with acute leukemias. Chronic leukemias have a more protracted evolution; differentiated cells predominate in the peripheral blood of patients with chronic leukemia. Leukemic states may evolve from a chronic form to an acute disease, and the type of proliferating cell may also change during the course of the disease. For example, transition from a chronic granulocytic stage to an acute and very often fatal lymphoblastic leukemia is characteristic of myelocytic leukemia.

Lymphoma refers to localized lymphocyte malignancies, often forming solid tumors, predominantly affecting the lymph nodes and other lymphoid organs (e.g., spleen). Lymphomas are always lymphocytic malignancies.

Classification of lymphocytic leukemias and lymphomas

All malignant proliferations of cells identifiable as lymphocytes are classified as either T- or B-cell malignancies, based on a variety of characteristics:

- Identification of the malignant cells as immunoglobulin-producing cells allows their classification as B-cell malignancies.
- Cell membrane markers are widely used to classify malignant lymphocyte proliferations.
- Cytogenetic studies and molecular genetic procedures are the basis of further subclassifications with prognostic and therapeutic implications. The classifications have increased in complexity, and their full discussion can be found specialty publications and hematology textbooks. In this chapter, we limit our discussion to paradigmatic entities and center our discussion on aspects that tie together basic and clinical science.

Chronic lymphocytic leukemia

CLL is a B-cell malignancy and the most common form of leukemia in the Western hemisphere. The disease usually has a late onset (median age of diagnosis is 65 years) and relatively benign course (median survival of 10 years). In the vast majority of cases, the leukemic cells are small or medium-sized lymphocytes, expressing CD5 and CD23 and low levels of surface immunoglobulins (low levels of sIgM can be detected in >95% of the patients).

Central to its pathogenesis seems to be an overexpression of the *bcl-2* gene, which inhibits apoptosis.

CLINICAL PRESENTATION AND DIAGNOSIS

Clinical symptoms are often absent or very mild. Malaise, fatigue, or enlargement of the lymphoid tissues felt by the patient are the most frequent presenting complaints. Physical diagnosis shows enlargement of the lymph nodes, spleen, and liver. Viral infections, such as herpes and herpes zoster, and fungal infections are frequent in these patients, pointing to a T-cell deficiency that is confirmed by the finding of reduced numbers of T cells and reduced responses to T-cell mitogens. The prognosis is determined by the frequency of severe opportunistic infections. Recent data suggest that patients with mutated immunoglobulin, variable heavy-chain gene, or expressing a specific heavy-chain variable region gene (VH3-21) have significantly lower survival rates, probably reflecting that cells with higher degrees of biological abnormalities are less likely to respond to therapy.

Diagnosis is established by a variety of approaches, including morphological studies and identification of specific cell membrane markers (CD5, CD23). Bence-Jones proteins can be detected in the concentrated urine of approximately one-third of the patients. Rarely, IgM monoclonal proteins may be detected in serum. Most patients are hypogammaglobulinemic.

MANAGEMENT

A large proportion of patients with CLL is asymptomatic and does not require any treatment but rather close surveillance. Patients are monitored for the development of findings that indicate the need for treatment. These include the following: (1) symptoms such as fever, night sweats, chills, weakness, and weight loss; (2) rapid lymphocytosis (doubling within 6 months); (3) extranodal involvement; (4) evidence of bone marrow failure secondary to involvement by CLL; and (5) repeated infections. Treatment consists of combination chemotherapy; the most common regimens include bendamustine/rituximab (monoclonal antibody to CD20), fludarabine/cyclophosphamide/Rituximab, and single-agent treatment with ibrutinib (a Bruton's tyrosine kinase inhibitor). Cure is not achieved with the aforementioned regimens, but prolonged disease control is possible. To date, the only known curative treatment for CLL is allogeneic stem cell transplantation. However, this approach can be highly toxic and is reserved for younger, fitter patients.

Hairy cell leukemia

CLINICAL PRESENTATION AND DIAGNOSIS

Hairy cell leukemia is a rare lymphoid B-cell malignancy, predominantly affecting middle-age males (median age of diagnosis: 55 years). The clinical presentation is nonspecific and includes malaise, fatigue, and frequent infectious episodes. The physical examination usually shows splenomegaly and, sometimes, generalized lymphadenopathy. Laboratory data show pancytopenia, anemia being most frequent, followed by thrombocytopenia, and leukopenia. The diagnosis is based on the finding of atypical lymphocytes with numerous finger-like (or hairy) projections in the peripheral blood (the name of the disease derives from the morphological characteristics of the abnormal lymphocytes). The abnormal cells express light-chain membrane immunoglobulins, often of several isotypes (IgG3 often predominating), and also express classical B-cell markers (CD19, CD20, CD22).

MANAGEMENT

The mainstay of therapy for hairy cell leukemia is the use of the purine nucleoside analogue 2-chlorodeoxyadenosine (cladribine). The combination of cladribine and rituximab has also been shown to be effective. In addition, deoxycoformycin (Pentostatin), an inhibitor of adenosine deaminase, and interferon-α are therapeutically useful in hairy cell leukemia.

Acute lymphoblastic leukemia

CLINICAL PRESENTATION AND DIAGNOSIS

Acute lymphoblastic leukemia (ALL) is the result of a wide array of mutations that affect hematopoietic stem cells and result in the proliferation of lymphoblasts, which spill into the peripheral blood. At the same time, normal hematopoiesis is negatively affected, and the patients develop anemia, neutropenia, and thrombocytopenia. Bone marrow failure is the most frequent cause of morbidity and mortality.

ALL is most common in childhood, and the majority of cases occur between 2 and 10 years of

Table 27.2 Classification of acute lymphoblastic leukemia based on immunophenotyping

Group	Tdt	HLA-DR	CD19	CD20	sIg	Ig gene rearrangement	CD3	CD5	CD4/ CD8	TCR gene rearrangement
Early pre-B cell	+	+	+	−	−	+	−	−	−	−
Pre-B cell	+	+	+	+	−	+	−	−	−	−
Mature B cell	−	+	+	+	+	+	−	−	−	−
T cell	+	−	−	−	−	−	+	+	+	+

age. Childhood ALL generally responds well to chemotherapy (overall cure rates of 80%, expected to rise to 90% in the near future), but the same is not true for adults with ALL.

Death usually occurs as a consequence of the massive lymphocytic proliferation in the bone marrow, where the proliferating cells overwhelm and smother the normal hematopoietic cells.

ALL can be classified by immunophenotyping (Table 27.2). The large majority (about 95%) of acute ALL is B cell–derived because the proliferating cells express the CD19 B-cell marker and have rearranged immunoglobulin genes. The remaining 5% of these leukemias are of the T-cell type, express T-cell markers (CD3, CD4, CD8), and have rearranged TCR genes. In addition, leukemic cells of patients with ALL may express enzymes of the purine salvage pathway, particularly terminal deoxynucleotidyl transferase (Tdt), not expressed by mature B lymphocytes but reexpressed in about 80% of all cases of this type of leukemia, when the proliferating populations correspond to earlier stages of T-cell and B-cell differentiation. The measurement of the expression of Tdt is clinically useful because its levels fall during remission and increase again before a clinically apparent relapse.

T-cell acute lymphocytic leukemia has usually a worse prognosis than B-cell acute lymphocytic leukemia. In addition, the two main types of ALL (B cell and T cell) respond differently to cytotoxic drugs.

Chromosomal and genetic abnormalities are common in ALL, and some of them have defined prognostic implications. For example, hyperdiploidy, trisomy-4, -10, -17, and translocation t(12,21), the most common translocation in ALL, are associated with good prognosis, while hypodiploidy, trisomy-5, rarer translocations such as t(1;19) and t(9;22)—the Philadelphia chromosome more frequently associated with acute myeloid leukemia—are associated with poor prognosis. The coexpression of myeloid and lymphoid characteristics by the leukemic cells was also considered as a poor prognosis indicator, but therapeutic progress has blunted the differences. In the end, prognosis is established based on a sum of clinical, immunological, and genetic data.

MANAGEMENT

The treatment of ALL has significantly changed over the past 20 years. In general, children, adolescents, and young adults (<40 years old) with ALL can be treated, and in many instances cured, with just chemotherapy. Chemotherapy regimens for ALL are complex and have several "phases" of treatment expanding several months. Adults >40 years old are treated with induction chemotherapy followed by an allogeneic stem cell transplant for those patients who are eligible. This combination of chemotherapy and transplant is the only known curative treatment for ALL in adults. The treatment of relapsed/refractory ALL in children and adults has seen the most dramatic advances with the development of immune therapies targeting CD19, a molecule expressed by the majority of ALL cells. The two main immunotherapies used for the treatment of ALL are chimeric antigen receptor T cells (CAR T cells) and blinatumomab, a bispecific T-cell engager (BiTe). (See Chapter 26 for more information regarding these therapies.)

Adult T-cell leukemia/lymphoma

Etiology. Adult T-cell leukemia (ATLL) has the unique feature of being caused by an infectious agent, the human T-lymphotropic virus 1 (HTLV-I) human retrovirus. It has a very unique geographic distribution, closely associated to the prevalence of HTLV-I in the population, with particularly high incidence in Japan and the Caribbean basin (where the rates of infection reach endemic proportions); the virus has also been reported, although with lower frequency, in the southeastern United States as well as in Central and South America.

HTLV-1 is predominantly transmitted through infected cells, and there are three main routes of transmission: breastfeeding, sexual transmission, and parenteral transmission through blood or blood products containing live infected cells. The receptor for HTLV-1 is the glucose transporter type 1, whose expression on T cells is enhanced by TGF-β. After penetrating T cells, the virus integrates, and the infected cell number increases because the virus promotes proliferation and inhibits apoptosis. The HTLV-I–associated T-cell leukemia develops 10–20 years after infection with the virus, but it only develops in a small fraction of the HTLV-I-infected individuals (4%–5% of the seropositive individuals).

HTLV-1 is an exogenous retrovirus, fully able to replicate and to be transmitted horizontally. Its genome contains a transforming gene, *tax*, whose gene product (Tax protein) is a transcriptional activator of the viral LTR, thus promoting HTLV-I gene expression and genomic replication. In addition, Tax activates the nuclear binding protein NF-κB, leading to the permanent overexpression of IL-2 receptors (CD25), and it also induces the activation of the IL-2 promoter. IL-13, IL-15, and the IL15Rα are also upregulated. These changes, associated with direct activating effects of Tax on cyclin-dependent kinases that control cell cycle, could explain the T-cell proliferation associated with HTLV-1. In addition, Tax removes controls that normally would counteract this effect, by inactivating p53 and the Rb gene product. Thus, Tax has both proliferative and antiapoptotic effects. However, the long latency between HTLV-1 and the detection of adult T-cell leukemia suggests that other factors must be involved in the final transforming events, which seem to be due to DNA damage caused by Tax. Of note is the fact that fully transformed cells often do not express Tax, suggesting that once the cells have become immortalized and chromosomal aberrations have developed, Tax is no longer required.

CLINICAL PRESENTATION AND DIAGNOSIS

ATLL can present as an acute or chronic condition, with or without lymphomatous characteristics. The acute presentation is the most common. The chronic as well as the smoldering forms usually evolve to assume acute characteristics. Clinical findings include lymphadenopathy, hepatosplenomegaly, osteolytic lesions, and hypercalcemia, secondary to osteoclast activation caused by the excessive release of monocyte colony-stimulating factor (M-CSF) by leukemic cells, and skin lesions. The most common skin lesions are erythroderma and skin ulcerations, and they are associated with a dense lymphocytic infiltration of the dermis and epidermis. It is believed that increased venous permeability, probably caused by an increased local concentration of IL-2 and other interleukins, is responsible for the formation of cellular infiltrates, which, in turn, interfere with proper oxygenation of tissues, leading to localized ischemia and necrosis. Some patients present with Sézary syndrome, an exfoliative erythroderma with generalized lymphadenopathy and circulating atypical cells. The skin is the original site of malignant cell proliferation, and the phase of cutaneous lymphoma can last many years with little evidence of extracutaneous dissemination. The leukemic evolution is associated with the invasion of the periphery by malignant cells. Occasionally the skin lesions are similar to those that are classically described as mycoses fungoides, where the infiltrating cells in the skin are also CD4$^+$ but no leukemic stage seems to develop.

Patients with ATLL are often immunocompromised, as a consequence of several factors, including the shedding of IL-2 receptors from the membrane of the leukemic cells that adsorb IL-2 and block its activating effect on normal T cells. In addition, in ATL the proliferating CD4$^+$ cells function as suppressor-inducers and turn on cells with suppressor activity.

Diagnosis is based on morphological and phenotypical characteristics of the malignant lymphocytes and confirmation of HTLV-1 infection. The peripheral blood lymphocytes in the more aggressive forms of disease, including Sézary syndrome with leukemic evolution, are often large, with a characteristic polylobulated nucleus (Sézary cells, flower cells).

The phenotype of ATLL malignant cells is characterized by the expression of activated T-cell markers, including CD2, CD3, CD4, CD25, and MHC-II. Tdt is not expressed.

MANAGEMENT

Patients with smoldering or chronic ATLL should be treated with anti-viral therapy, combining zidovudine (AZT) and IFNα. Patients with active disease are treated with combinations of chemotherapeutic agents associated with GM-CSF.

T- and B-cell lymphomas

Most lymphomas are B-cell derived, and they can be grouped in two large groups: Hodgkin's lymphoma and non-Hodgkin's lymphoma. All groups can be subclassified by a variety of criteria. We refer the readers to hematology publications for the full details about classification and management of lymphomas.

HODGKIN'S LYMPHOMA

Hodgkin's lymphoma (HL) has been finally classified as a B-cell lymphoma in the vast majority of the cases, based on evidence of B-cell receptor rearrangement of the Reed–Sternberg cells characteristic of the disease, which are very dedifferentiated and do not express markers that allow their phenotypic definition as B cells. T-cell Hodgkin's lymphomas also exist but are a rarity, seen in only 1%–2% of the cases.

The Reed–Sternberg cells show constitutive expression of NF-κB and are resistant to apoptosis, as a consequence of the expression of the products of at least two antiapoptotic genes and of a mutated Fas protein (CD95). In addition, these cells produce IL-13 and express the corresponding receptor, creating conditions for an autocrine proliferation circuit. In about 40% of the cases of classical Hodgkin's lymphoma, there is evidence of infection with the Epstein–Barr virus (EBV), and two of the viral-encoded transforming proteins of the EBV (LMP1 and LMP2a) are expressed by infected Reed–Sternberg cells. Thus, at least in this 40% of cases, it is possible that EBV infection may play a role in the oncogenic transformation.

A significant feature of Hodgkin's lymphoma is the formation of large cellular infiltrates around the Reed–Sternberg cells, which follow different morphological patterns (basis of the classification of the disease into four subtypes). The infiltrating cells are nonclonal and seem to be attracted by chemokines released by the Reed–Sternberg cells. There is a close interaction between the Reed–Sternberg cells and the infiltrating nonclonal cells

that is essential for the continuing proliferation of the malignant cells.

NON-HODGKIN'S LYMPHOMA

Non-Hodgkin's lymphoma (NHL) is a designation that encompasses a very heterogeneous group of malignancies affecting the lymphoid tissues. Although they can be divided into B-cell and T-cell lymphomas, the vast majority (90%) are B-cell malignancies. They can be classified by a variety of criteria. The two most common histological entities are follicular lymphoma and diffuse large B-cell lymphoma. Burkitt's lymphoma is usually discussed separately because of the clear association of its African endemic form with EBV.

Follicular lymphomas are usually indolent, presenting with lymphadenopathy, and as the disease progresses, fever, night sweats, and weight loss may develop. The bone marrow is usually infiltrated, and normal hematopoiesis may be compromised. Hepatosplenomegaly is frequently detected. Large B-cell lymphomas are more aggressive, and although lymphadenopathy is present in most patients, extranodal proliferation (gastrointestinal tract, skin, sinuses, thyroid, central nervous system) is common. Systemic symptoms are also more frequent in patients with this type of lymphoma.

Chromosomal translocations are common in non-Hodgkin's lymphoma and are usually associated with the expression of antiapoptotic genes and/or genes that promote cell proliferation.

Management depends largely on staging, which is based on the histological features and extent of diffusion of the malignancy. Positron emission tomography is the preferred technique for staging. Treatment involves radiation therapy and/or chemotherapy in a variety of combinations according to the extent of lymphatic tissue involvement. Patients with follicular lymphomas usually experience long survival, but only a minority is truly cured. Diffuse large B-cell lymphomas are treated with combinations of chemotherapeutic agents and rituximab. The rate of cure is about 50%.

Burkitt's lymphoma, a distinct subtype of NHL, is endemic in certain areas of Africa and sporadic in the United States, has been characterized as a B-cell lymphoma expressing monotypic surface IgM. Endemic Burkitt's lymphoma is epidemiologically linked to infection of the B-lymphocytes with the EBV. The malignant B cells in Burkitt's lymphoma usually express a single EBV gene product, the nuclear antigen EBNA-1, which is essential for establishment of latency but has no known transforming properties. It is possible that the EBV infection has as its main role promoting a state of active B-cell proliferation that may favor the occurrence of the translocations involving the region of chromosome 8 coding for *c-myc*. Similar translocations are also found in sporadic Burkitt's lymphoma, not linked to EBV infection. A common consequence of the translocations is the overexpression the c-myc gene, often mutated, which is believed to be a major factor contributing to the uncontrolled B-cell proliferation characteristic of this disease.

Clinically, Burkitt's lymphoma is usually characterized by the development of a large tumor, either in the angle of the jaw and neck (epidemic form) or in the abdomen (endemic form). Burkitt's lymphoma responds well to chemotherapy, and most adults with the disease are cured.

B-cell lymphomas are frequently detected in immunodeficient or iatrogenically immunosuppressed patients. In posttransplant situations (posttransplant lymphoproliferative disorder [PTLD]), the overall incidence is 1%–2%, with highest rates after heart, heart-lung, intestinal transplantation, and allogeneic stem cell transplantation in T-cell depleted patients. In the majority, there is evidence of association with viral infection, particularly EBV. A variety of EBV-coded proteins may be expressed on the malignant cells, including six different nuclear antigens and three different membrane proteins. Of the proteins coded by nuclear antigens, EBNA-2 protein has immortalizing properties, transactivating the cyclin-2 gene and others, EBNA-LP impairs the function of the products of two tumor suppressor genes, p53, and the retinoblastoma gene product, and the latent membrane protein 1 (LMP-1) is considered as a transforming gene whose activity seems to be mediated by the activation of a Ca^{2+}/calmodulin-dependent protein kinase. In addition, host cell molecular alterations are present in PTLD, including translocation and overexpression of *c-MYC*, rearrangement of BCL-6, and p53 mutations.

Patients with AIDS are at increased risk for the development of common as well as some rare types of lymphomas. The risk seems not to be as high for Hodgkin's disease as it is for non-Hodgkin's lymphoma. Among the rare types of lymphomas that affect AIDS patients, it is worth mentioning the association with Kaposi's sarcoma and primary effusion lymphoma, both caused by the human herpes virus type 8 (HHV-8). The incidence of lymphoma is related to the degree of immunodepression of the patient, and since the introduction of highly active antiretroviral therapy (HAART), the frequency of HIV-infected patients with very low CD4 counts has decreased, and with this there has been an associated decrease in the frequency of lymphoid malignancies, with the exception of Hodgkin's lymphoma. Furthermore, patients who develop lymphoid malignancies but are treated with HAART can tolerate chemotherapy, and their survival is close to that of the general population.

BIBLIOGRAPHY

Attal M, Lauwers-Cances V, Hulin C et al. Lenalidomide, bortezomib, and dexamethasone with transplantation for myeloma. *N Engl J Med.* 2017;376:1311–1320.

Capello D, Rossi D, Gaidano G. Post-transplant lymphoproliferative disorders: Molecular basis of disease and pathogenesis. *Hematol Oncol.* 2005;23:61–67.

Carbone A, Gloghini A. AIDS-related lymphomas: From pathogenesis to pathology. *Brit J Haematol.* 2005;130:662–670.

Gentile M, Mauro FR, Guarini A, Foa R. New developments in the diagnosis, prognosis and treatment of chronic lymphocytic leukemia. *Curr Opin Oncol.* 2005;17:597–604.

Gertz MA. Waldenström macroglobulinemia: 2018 update on diagnosis, risk stratification, and management. *Am J Hematol.* 2018;93:511.

Grassmann R, Aboud M, Jeang K-T. Molecular mechanisms of cellular transformation by HTLV-1 tax. *Oncogene* 2005;24:5976–5985.

Guo Z, Li H, Geng Y et al. Using both lactic dehydrogenase levels and the ratio of involved to uninvolved free light chain levels as risk factors improves risk assessment in patients with newly diagnosed multiple myeloma. *Am J Med Sci.* 2018;355:350–358.

Kantarjian H, Stein A, Gökbuget N et al. Blinatumomab versus chemotherapy for advanced acute lymphoblastic leukemia. *N Engl J Med.* 2017;376:836–847.

Kyle RA, Remstein ED, Therneau TM et al. Clinical course and prognosis of smoldering (asymptomatic) multiple myeloma. *N Engl J Med.* 2007; 356:2582–2590.

Palumbo A, Avet-Loiseau H, Oliva S et al. Revised international staging system for multiple myeloma: A report from international myeloma working group. *J Clin Oncol.* 2015;33:2263–2269.

Park JH, Rivière I, Gonen M et al. Long-term follow-up of CD19 CAR therapy in acute lymphoblastic leukemia. *N Engl J Med.* 2018;378:449–459.

Rajkumar SV, Dimopoulos MA, Palumbo A et al. International Myeloma Working Group updated criteria for the diagnosis of multiple myeloma. *Lancet Oncol.* 2014;15:e538–e548. doi: 10.1016/S1470-2045(14)70442-5

Rajkumar SV, Kyle RA. Multiple myeloma: Diagnosis and treatment. *Mayo Clin Proc.* 2005; 80:1371–1382.

Rajkumar SV, Kyle RA, Buadi FK. Advances in the diagnosis, classification, risk stratification, and management of monoclonal gammopathy of undetermined significance: Implications for recategorizing disease entities in the presence of evolving scientific evidence. *Mayo Clin Proc.* 2010;85:945–948.

Randolph TR. Advances in acute lymphoblastic leukemia. *Clin Lab Sci.* 2004;17:235–245.

Ravandi F, O'Brien S. Chronic lymphoid leukemias other that chronic lymphocytic leukemia: Diagnosis and treatment. *Mayo Clin Proc.* 2005;80:1660–1674.

Romano A, Conticello C, Cavalli M et al. Immunological dysregulation in multiple myeloma microenvironment. *Biomed Res Int.* 2014;20:12993–13005.

Soh KT, Tario JD, Wallace PK. Diagnosis of plasma cell dyscrasias and monitoring of minimal residual disease by multiparametric flow cytometry. *Clin Lab Med.* 2017;37:821–853.

Terpos E, Dimopoulos MA. Myeloma bone disease: Pathophysiology and management. *Ann Oncology.* 2005;16:1223–1231.

Wahner-Roedler DL, Kyle RA. Heavy chain diseases. *Best Pract Res Clin Haematol.* 2005;18:729–746.

Yared JA, Kimball AS. Optimizing management of patients with adult T cell leukemia-lymphoma. *Cancers (Basel).* 2015;7:2318–2329.

28

Diagnosis of immune deficiency diseases

JOHN W. SLEASMAN AND GABRIEL VIRELLA

INTRODUCTION

Immunodeficiency diseases are a major cause of mortality and morbidity worldwide. Immune-deficient states can be subdivided into primary immune deficiency diseases due to a hereditary or intrinsic defect in the immune system or secondary immune deficiency as the result of infection, such as HIV, administration of cytotoxic drugs, as with cancer chemotherapy, or metabolic states, such as undernutrition, that compromise the immune system. Primary immune deficiencies (PID) provide valuable insight into the nature of the immune response and the physiology of the human immune system. Any assessment of the immune system relies on a careful and targeted assessment of immunity using laboratory-based assays that are both accurate and precise.

CLINICAL AND LABORATORY DIAGNOSIS OF IMMUNE DISORDERS

Most immune-deficient states are classified on the basis of the major component of immunity impacted. In general, the immunity is subdivided in the innate and adaptive immune responses with considerable overlap in between the two. Innate immune consists primarily of nonspecific defense mechanisms mediated by a variety of antimicrobial substances, pattern recognition receptors, phagocytic cells, and the complement system (see Chapter 14), while adaptive immunity is antigen specificity and memory. Adaptive immunity consists of humoral and cellular immune responses, which can be measured by enumeration of lymphocyte subpopulations, antibody responses, or tests of cellular function. Defects in each of these components are associated with characteristic clinical presentations that provide clues into the nature of the disorder. A careful and systematic assessment of the clinical presentation, family history, and laboratory evaluation will lead to the precise nature of the immunodeficiency allowing for prompt and effective initiation of therapeutic interventions.

General considerations

The clinical diagnosis of a probable immunodeficiency disease is based on a variety of clinical criteria (summarized in Table 28.1), such as history of recurrent infections, the pattern of infections, age of onset of symptoms, length of treatment needed to clear infections, autoimmunity, malignancy, and types of infecting organism(s), particularly when involving opportunistic or unusual organisms. The

Table 28.1 Clinical features suggestive of primary immunodeficiency

1. Defects predominantly related to antibody mediate immunity
   - Recurrent bacterial sinopulmonary infections, particularly involving encapsulated organisms (e.g., *Haemophilus influenzae, Streptococcus pneumoniae*)
   - Chronic enteroviral gastroenteritis or chronic giardiasis
   - Recurrent serious bacterial infections (pneumonia, meningitis, sepsis, osteomyelitis, septic arthritis)
2. Clinical features suggestive of a defect in cell-mediated immunity
   - Recurrent severe or persistent viral infection
   - Failure to thrive in an infant or adult
   - Chronic or severe mycotic infections (e.g., fungal pneumonia, mucocutaneous candidiasis)
   - Severe infections with opportunistic organisms (e.g., *Pneumocystis jirovecii* pneumonia, cryptosporidiosis, toxoplasmosis, atypical mycobacteria)
   - Viral-induced malignancy (Kaposi sarcoma, Epstein–Barr virus driven lymphoma)
   - Autoimmune cytopenia, symptoms of graft-versus-host disease
3. Clinical features suggestive of a defect in phagocytic function
   - Poor wound healing or delayed separation of the umbilical cord
   - Soft tissue abscesses and lymphadenitis
   - Chronic gingivitis, chronic periodontal disease, or mucosal ulcerations
   - Infections with catalase positive microorganisms (e.g., *Staphyococcus aureus, Serratia marcescens, Aspergillus* spp., *Candida* spp.)
4. Clinical features suggestive of a defect innate immunity of the complement system
   - Angioedema of face, hands, gastrointestinal tract
   - Autoimmune disease (e.g., glomerulonephritis, hemolytic uremic syndrome, rheumatoid arthritis)
   - Recurrent infections in the absence of fever
   - Disseminated *Neisseria* infections

clinical history should include a complete family history to determine if there are patterns of inheritance such as autosomal-dominant, recessive, or X-linked patterns of inheritance. Questions should include history of infant deaths due to infections, familial patterns of autoimmune disease, recurrent pneumonia, or spontaneous angioedema among family members. The physical exam should explore findings associated with immune disorders such as failure to thrive and growth retardation, eczema, easy bruising or bleeding, abnormal hair and dentition, skeletal abnormalities, congenital heart disease, hypocalcemia, or albinism. When undertaking the evaluation of a possible immune deficiency, both primary and secondary causes should be considered. Secondary causes would include HIV infection, undernutrition, environmental toxins, or immune suppressive drugs. Nonimmune causes of recurrent infections include cystic fibrosis, occult malignancy, sickle cell anemia, and ciliary dyskinesia. Laboratory results should be interpreted in the context of the patient's age. Finally, if no obvious diagnosis can be made after the initial evaluation, a follow-up plan for evaluation and further referral should be implemented. Over half of patients evaluated for recurrent infections will have normal immune systems based on standard immune testing. Most of these cases will be due to exposures to infections in day care settings or in the work environment. Recurrent sinopulmonary infections are also a manifestation of allergic diseases such as asthma and allergic rhinitis. Only about 10% of patients evaluated for recurrent infections ultimately have a known primary immune deficiency disease.

Clinical signs suggesting specific disorders in immunity

Disorders of particular arms of immunity have common clinical signs indicating the nature of the immune disorder (Figure 28.1). The clinical history is the starting point for the laboratory evaluation to identify the precise immune defect.

ANTIBODY DEFICIENCY

Defective antibody production is the most common cause of PID accounting for over half of

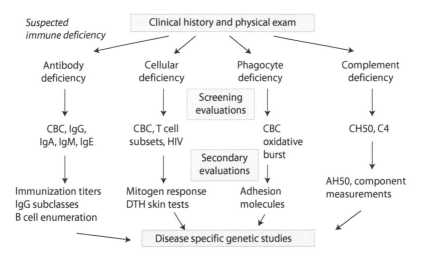

Figure 28.1 Diagnostic steps in evaluating for primary immune deficiency first involve a careful clinical history and physical exam to determine the principal component of the immune system impacted by the disorder. Screening evaluations for antibody, cellular, phagocytic, and complement disorders represent the first steps, and secondary evaluations are performed based on the screening results. Definitive diagnosis is made on the basis of disease-specific genetic screening. (AH50, alternative hemolytic complement 50; CBC, complete blood count; CH50, total hemolytic complement 50.)

all cases (see Chapter 29). Clinical manifestations of a congenital antibody deficiency are primarily recurrent of severe bacterial sinopulmonary infections beginning after the first year of life as passively acquired maternal antibody wanes. Infections with *Haemophilus influenzae*, *Streptococcus pneumoniae*, and other encapsulated bacterial organisms are most common. The lack of secretory IgA results can increase susceptibility to chronic enterovirus and parasitic infections such as chronic *Giardia* enteritis. Severe antibody deficiency carries a risk of serious systemic bacterial infections such as pneumonia, bacterial meningitis, *Pseudomonas* sepsis, osteomyelitis, and septic inflammatory arthritis.

CELLULAR IMMUNE DEFICIENCY

Clinical symptoms resulting from primary defects in cellular immunity or combined defects in cellular and antibody immunity can begin during the first year of life or in the case of HIV infection, following viral infection (Chapter 30). Symptoms consist of failure to thrive in a child, wasting syndrome in an adult, chronic mucocutaneous candidiasis, chronic viral infections such as cytomegalovirus or herpes simplex virus, *Pneumocystis jirovecii* pneumonia, and

unexplained autoimmune disease such as hemolytic anemia or thrombocytopenia. Children and adults with defective cellular immunity are at increased risk for malignancy, particularly B-cell lymphomas or lymphoproliferative diseases driven by Epstein–Barr virus.

PHAGOCYTIC CELL DEFICIENCY

Defective phagocytic cell function commonly is associated with recurrent or chronic infections of the soft tissues such as cellulitis, lymphadenitis, and osteomyelitis. Abscesses and granulomas of the liver, lung, and spleen are also common. Oral and periodontal disease is common including chronic necrotizing gingivitis, oral ulcers, and dental abscesses. Poor wound healing, which may manifest as delayed separation of the umbilical cord (more than 6 weeks after birth), is characteristic of primary phagocytic cell defects. Specific defects in neutrophil oxidative burst result in systemic infections with catalase-positive organisms such as *Staphylococcus aureus*, *Serratia* spp., *Aspergillus* spp., *Escherichia coli*, and *Pseudomonas aeruginosa*. Infections are often deep-seated in tissues and can occult clouding the initial clinical presentation that may solely consist of fever of unknown origin.

INNATE IMMUNITY AND COMPLEMENT DEFICIENCIES

Hereditary deficiencies in the innate immunity or complement system have highly variable clinical manifestations that are associated with the particular component of the immune system. Defects in regulatory complement proteins such as C1 inhibitor are associated with sudden onset of non-pruritic angioedema triggered by minor trauma or stress. In contrast, defects in regulatory proteins in the alternative pathway such as factors I or H can develop atypical hemolytic uremic syndrome. Individuals with defects in individual components of the classical or alternative complement cascade are susceptible to serious bacterial infections similar to patients with antibody deficiency. Complement deficiencies also carry an increased risk for development of autoimmune disease such as systemic lupus erythematosus, rheumatoid arthritis, and glomerulonephritis. Defects in the terminal components of the complement cascade will often develop chronic or recurrent infections by *Neisseria* (Table 28.1). Immune deficiency due to defects in toll-like receptor (TLR) signaling such as IRAK4 or Myd88 have recurrent serious bacterial infections in the absence of fever or signs of an inflammatory response.

OTHER DEFECTS IN INTRINSIC AND INNATE IMMUNITY

The presentation of these defects is highly variable because of their heterogeneous nature, depending on specific defects affecting either pattern-recognition receptors (PRRs) or the signaling pathways that should be activated by the PRRs. The patients may present with increased susceptibility to all types of infections but also with autoimmune manifestations.

LABORATORY ASSESSMENT OF IMMUNITY

The effective laboratory investigation of an immunodeficiency consists of a step-by-step assessment that correlates with the clinical manifestations of the immune disorder. In order to optimize the use of the clinical laboratory, testing should first focus on quantitative and qualitative screening evaluations followed by more targeted and specific testing to pinpoint the precise nature of the disorder and confirm the suspected.

Assessment of antibody-mediated immunity

MEASUREMENT OF SERUM IMMUNOGLOBULIN LEVELS

Immunoglobulin levels are most commonly measured using nephelometry that accurately measures IgG, IgA, IgM, and IgE in sera. All Ig levels should be interpreted in the context of the patient's age since infants and children have lower levels of IgG and IgA when compared to adolescents and adults, and therefore, normal values vary with age (Table 28.2).

Immunoglobulin assay is a fundamental element in the classification of immunodeficiencies (Table 28.3). A quantitative depression of one or more of the three major immunoglobulin isotypes is considered as compatible with a diagnosis of humoral immunodeficiency. If all immunoglobulin classes are depressed, the condition is designated as hypogammaglobulinemia. If the depression is very severe, and the combined levels of all three immunoglobulins are below 200 mg/dL, the patient is considered as having agammaglobulinemia.

IgG subclasses can also be quantified and the results of the assay may reveal subclass deficiencies. Patients with IgG subclass deficiency can have normal or slightly depressed total IgG. Low or absent IgG4 is common in healthy individuals, and its deficiency is not considered to be clinically significant.

Table 28.2 Normal values for human immunoglobulins[a]

	IgG	IgA	IgM
Newborn	636–1606	0	6–25
1–2 months	250–900	1–53	20–87
4–6 months	196–558	4–73	27–100
10–12 months	294–1069	16–84	41–150
1–2 years	345–1210	14–106	43–173
3–4 years	440–1135	21–159	47–200
5–18 years	630–1280	33–200	48–207
8–10 years	608–1572	45–236	52–242
Greater than 10 years	639–1349	70–312	57–352

[a] In mg/dL, as determined by immunonephelometry in the Department of Laboratory Medicine, Medical University of South Carolina.

Table 28.3 Immunoglobulin levels in immune deficiency[a]

Patient	IgG	IgA	IgM	Interpretation
A	850	2.8	128	IgA deficiency
B	1990	39.4	145	IgA deficiency
C	131	28.2	Traces	Severe hypogammaglobulinemia
D	690	16.0	264	IgA deficiency
E	154	60.0	840	Hyper IgM syndrome

[a] In mg/dL.

MEASUREMENT OF FUNCTIONAL ANTIBODY

In addition to determining total Ig levels, assessment of antibody deficiency should also include assessment of immune function, generally carried out by measuring antibody titers before and after a standard immunization. Pre- and postimmunization responses are classified based on whether the immunogen is T-dependent or T-independent antigens. Commonly used and validated T-dependent antigens include tetanus and diphtheria toxoids. Assays are performed prior to and 4–8 weeks following immunization. Reponses are optimally measured after the second immunization, following a priming initial vaccine. While a titer of >0.01 IU/mL is considered protective, most healthy individuals generate at titer >1.00 IU/mL or a greater than fourfold rise above the preimmunization titer. In contrast to T-independent antigens, infants and adults have similar postimmunization responses. Even preterm infants are able to mount antibody responses to T-dependent antigens.

Immunization with tetanus toxoid has also been used in the follow-up of the humoral immune response after a hematopoietic stem cell transplant to determine whether the immune function has reconstituted. As illustrated in Figure 28.2, this recovery may only be observed several months after the suspension of immunosuppressive therapy. It needs to be noted that the immunoglobulin levels may be normal while the patient shows a complete lack of response to immunization.

The antibody response to T-independent antigens is usually measured using the polyvalent (23 serotypes) pneumococcal polysaccharide vaccine. Healthy children under the age of 2 years cannot respond to T-independent antigens. It is recommended that young children and older adults with conditions that predispose for pneumococcal infections receive the 13-valent conjugated

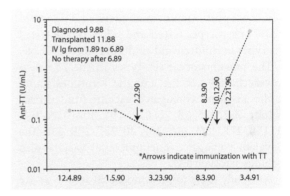

Figure 28.2 Longitudinal study of the serum levels of antitetanus toxoid (anti-TT) antibodies in a patient who received a bone marrow graft in December 1988. The patient received intravenous gammaglobulin from January to June 1989, as anti-infectious prophylaxis. The clinical evolution was excellent, and all therapy (immunosuppressive and immunoprophylactic) was discontinued in June 1989. The first assay of anti-TT antibody in December 1989 showed that the patient had low levels of antibody (0.15 U/mL). A first immunization with TT in February 1990 was followed by a paradoxical decrease of anti-TT antibody concentration. Only after three additional boosters given between August and February of 1991 was there a significant increase in anti-TT antibody concentration. At that time, the patient could be judged as immunologically recovered.

pneumococcal vaccines that are T-dependent antigens designed to include the most common invasive serotypes causing infection in the United States and Europe. In the case of older individuals with predisposing conditions (other than age), the administration of polyvalent (23 serotypes) vaccine a year after receiving the 13-valent conjugated pneumococcal vaccines has been recommended by some groups.

The response to the pure polysaccharide varies greatly among healthy individuals to the individual antigens within the vaccine and over time. In general, a titer ≥1.3 μg/mL is considered a normal titer following immunization. Healthy individuals generally mount at least a twofold rise above 1.3 μg/mL following immunizations and greater than fourfold rises are rare if the preimmunization titers are >4.4 μg/mL. Booster pneumococcal immunizations to test immune function are unnecessary and not recommended as repeated immunization may promote vaccine hyporesponsiveness. A normal response in children less than 5 years are postimmunization titers >1.3 μg/mL to >50% of serotypes tested and >70% of the tested serotypes in children and adults over 6 years of age.

The pneumococcal serotypes in the 23-valent polysaccharide vaccine and the serotypes found in the 13-valent conjugated vaccine (underlined) include, 2, 3, 4, 5, 6B, 7F, 8, 9N, 9V, 10A, 11A, 12F, 14, 15B, 17F, 18C, 19A, 19F, 20, 22F, 23B, 33F. The 13-valent conjugated pneumococcal vaccine also includes serotype 6A.

Antibody titers to pneumococcal serotypes are generally measured using enzyme immunoassay (EIA) or Luminex bead multiplexed assays. EIA techniques have been validated as a measure of immune function for many years. While a strength of this technique is little variation among assays, the lower limit of detection is only 1–1.3 μg/mL. Furthermore, most enzyme-linked immunosorbent assay (ELISA) commercial assays perform only 10–14 serotypes. In contrast, the Luminex assay can measure all 23 serotypes simultaneously with a lower limit of detection or 0.2–0.35 μg/mL ranges. However, the platforms for these assays have large variation among them, making it difficult to compare results among laboratories.

MEASUREMENTS OF PRIMARY IMMUNE RESPONSE

When patients are receiving immune globulin therapy, it is difficult to evaluate antibody production *in vivo* since the majority of circulating antibodies are passively acquired from the gammaglobulin coming from the donor pool. It is possible to measure responses to a primary or neoantigen in which the donor pool is unlikely to have been exposed, thus antibodies to these antigens will not be present in the donor pool. Generation of these antibodies would only have come from the immunized recipient. Rabies vaccine is an example of a vaccine that has been used

in that context, but measurement of rabies antibody has not been validated. An alternative has been bacteriophage φX-174, a highly immunogenic T cell–dependent neoantigen used *in vivo* to assess both primary and secondary antibody responses and designated by the World Health Organization Committee on Primary Immunodeficiency as a standard, potent, and safe antigen for assessment of immune response in humans (Figure 28.3). Antibodies to φX-174 produced by the immunized subject are used to neutralize the phage in a reverse lytic plaque assay. Phage immunization has been carried out by several groups in different countries and has been proven to be safe and effective.

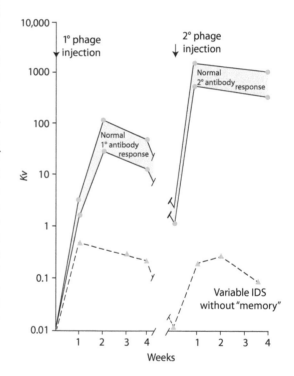

Figure 28.3 Primary and secondary antibody responses elicited by immunization with bacteriophage φX 174 in a patient with suspected humoral immunodeficiency. The shaded area between the solid lines indicates the range for normal responses. The patient's response, indicated by the interrupted line, showed a definite but diminished antibody response; the secondary response was not greater than the primary—no memory/amplification occurred. The immunoglobulin class of antibody in both primary and secondary responses was entirely IgM. (Reproduced with permission from Wedgewood et al. *Birth Defects: Original Article Series.* 11, 331, 1975.)

Basic screening tests for a patient with a suspected defect in antibody production include a complete blood count with differential, quantitative immunoglobulins by nephelometry, and testing of antibody immune function through the measurement of postimmunization vaccine titers. Other initial evaluations should include sweat chloride to evaluate for cystic fibrosis as well as total IgE and antigen-specific IgE to aeroallergens.

Confirmatory testing for antibody deficiency is based on the results of screening testing. For example, in patients who have selective IgA deficiency, measurement of IgG subclasses would be the next diagnostic test because the association between IgA deficiency and IgG2/IgG4 subclass deficiency has clinical relevance. Patients who have hypogammaglobulinemia should have B-cell enumeration using flow cytometry to differentiate between congenital agammaglobulinemia, where B cells are absent (Figure 28.4), from common variable immune deficiency in which patients have B cells but fail to produce antibody. If IgG and IgA are low but IgM is present, the patient may have hyper-IgM syndrome due to defects in either CD40 or its ligand, CD40L/CD154. Finally, severe forms of antibody deficiency should be confirmed using genetic analysis not only for the purpose of genetic counseling, but also to determine prognosis and associated risks for autoimmune disease and malignancy.

Laboratory assessment of cell-mediated immunity

Flow cytometry is the analysis of individual cells within a heterogeneous population using a fluidics system, lasers, and detectors interrogated to assess one cell at a time. Laser light deflected each cell passing though the fluidics system measures the cell's physical characteristics. Cell size is determined based on deflection of forward light scatter (FSC), and cellular internal complexity is assessed by side scatter light (SSC) deflection. Fluorochrome-conjugated monoclonal antibodies reacting with cell surface or internal protein complexes are preincubated with patient blood, tissue, or bone marrow. Multiple monoclonal antibodies, each tagged with a different fluorochrome, can be used to measure multiple cell protein complexes within a single sample. As cells traverse through the cytometer, they can be "gated" so that cells only with the size and internal complexity of the population of interest are analyzed. Since all lymphocytes, monocytes, and neutrophils are of hematopoietic origin, CD45, the leukocyte common antigen, is used to analyze all lymphocyte populations by gating on CD45 with the lymphocyte scatter gates.

Using flow cytometry, lymphocyte subpopulations can be accurately enumerated with very high precision and accuracy. All T cells express CD3,

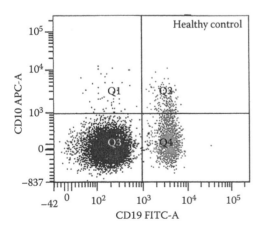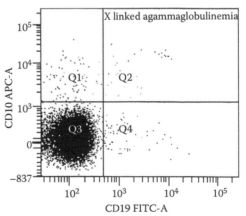

Figure 28.4 Flow cytometry assessment of patient with X-linked congenital agammaglobulinemia (XLA). (Right panel) Healthy control with normal populations of CD10+/CD19+ B cells. (Left panel) A patient with XLA where CD19 and CD10 B cells are absent.

Table 28.4 Distribution of the major human lymphocyte subpopulations in peripheral blood, as determined by flow cytometry

CD marker	Lymphocyte subpopulation	Normal range (%)	Normal range (absolute count)
CD19, CD20	B lymphocytes	4–20	96–421 cells/μL
CD3	T lymphocytes	62–85	700–2500 cells/μL
CD2	T lymphocytes; natural killer (NK) cells	70–88	840–2800 cells/μL
CD4	Helper T cells	34–59	430–1600 cells/μL
CD8	Cytotoxic T cells	16–38	280–1100 cells/μL

Source: Values obtained at the Flow Cytometry laboratory, Department of Pathology and Laboratory Medicine, Medical University of South Carolina.

part to the T-cell receptor complex, and either CD4 or CD8, which identify helper T cells or cytotoxic T cells, respectively. B cells are enumerated using either of two distinct B-cell markers, CD19 and CD20, while natural killer (NK) cells, which do not express CD3, are identified by coexpression of CD56 and CD16. Together the sum of these three populations makes up the lymphosome, consisting of 100% of the lymphocyte gate. Individual lymphocyte populations are quantified based on their percentage of the CD45-positive cells within the lymphocyte gate. These percentages are multiplied by the absolute lymphocyte count to report values both as a percentage of lymphocytes and absolute numbers in cells/microliter. These values are critical to the accurate interpretation of the results.

In healthy children and adults, CD3T cells make up 60%–70% of the total lymphocyte populations with children who have similar lymphocyte percentages but higher absolute T-cell counts when compared to adults. The normal ratio of CD4 to CD8T cells is greater than 1.0 and generally approaches 2:1. Inverted CD4/CD8 ratios that are abnormal most commonly reflect increased CD8 T cell activation and expansion or declines in CD4T cell numbers as seen in HIV-infected individuals. B cells make up less than 5%–10% and the lymphocyte populations with higher B-cell numbers and percentages in young infants. NK cells generally make up less than 5% of lymphocytes. Perturbations in numbers and percentages are caused in infections, immune suppression, autoimmune disease, and malignancy, and thus do not necessarily reflect primary immune deficiency. In addition to total CD3T cells, CD4, and CD8 expression T cells can be further subdivided in naïve (recent thymic emigrants) or memory T cells. Naïve T cells coexpress CD45RA, CD62L, CCR7, or CD31, while memory T cells express CD45RO. The normal distribution of lymphocyte subpopulations in a normal adult is shown in Table 28.4. Quantitative abnormalities may range from complete absence or pronounced deficiency of all or just a proportion of the given lymphocyte population.

NEWBORN SCREENING FOR CONGENITAL T-CELL DEFICIENCIES

Newborn screening (NBS) has proven to be highly effective in identifying and treating infants with genetic conditions. It is most effective when the incidence of the condition is high (at least 1:100,000 live births) and early diagnosis has a positive effect on long-term health or survival. Almost all U.S.-born infants are screened for more than 40 congenital diseases, and HIV screening is done on all pregnant women. There is variability of the screening panel among states, as each state department of health determines the conditions for which it screens. Any abnormal results require confirmatory testing prior to a definitive diagnosis. Screening for congenital T abnormalities fits into the paradigm for a condition where screening is effective at birth. Severe combined immune deficiency (SCID) has serious morbidity or mortality as almost all infants who go undiagnosed die before 2 years of age. Early diagnosis and treatment significantly improve prognosis, as nearly 90% of infants who receive hematopoietic stem cell transplantation before 3 months of life survive. SCID is not easily detected at birth by routine physical exam, as infants appear to be normal. There is a sensitive, specific, inexpensive test that utilizes existing NBS tools (Guthrie Card) to test dried blood spots obtained from heel sticks collected at birth. If the T-cell receptor excision circles (TREC) are below the threshold of normal lymphocyte counts, enumeration is performed using flow cytometry as the confirmatory test.

The method used for confirmation of SCID utilizes the TREC analysis to detect T-cell receptor recombination that takes place in the thymus. As shown in Figure 28.5, when TCR D-J and then V-DJ recombination occurs, the intervening circular DNA stays within the cell so that each naïve T cell leaving the thymus carries TREC. When T cells become activated and undergo clonal expansion, TRECs are diluted. Quantitative reverse transcription polymerase chain reaction (RTqPCR) can be used to identify any infants with SCID as well as other conditions that affect T-cell development, such as complete DiGeorge syndrome or SCID variants. Initial TREC numbers can be low in premature infants but normalize as they approach a term gestational age. Currently nearly all states perform NBS for SCID. Among the millions of newborns screened since Wisconsin implemented screening in 2008, the overall incidence of significant T-cell lymphopenia is 1:19,900. The incidence of SCID is approximately 1/60,000, and survival in these infants following hematopoietic transplant is 93%. The assays are highly specific as 0.08% of newborns required repeat testing and 0.016% required confirmatory flow cytometry testing. Conditions with low TREC numbers at birth include trisomy 21, ataxia-telangectasia, and the CHARGE syndrome, characterized by the presence of coloboma, heart defects, atresia choanae (also known as choanal atresia), growth retardation, genital abnormalities, and ear abnormalities. Secondary T-cell impairment leading to low TREC are thymectomy associated with surgery for congenital heart disease, chylothorax, and loss of lymphocytes due to gastrointestinal tract malformations.

IN VIVO TESTING OF DELAYED-TYPE HYPERSENSITIVITY

Delayed hypersensitivity responses are discussed in greater detail in Chapter 20. They are primarily mediated by activated T lymphocytes migrating to the dermis, where the antigen is associated to dermal dendritic cells. The result is a hyperstimulation of cell-mediated immunity in a localized area where the antigen was injected. Using controlled conditions, it is possible to challenge individuals with antigens known to cause this type of reaction as a way to explore their cell-mediated immunity. The two classical approaches to measure delayed-type hypersensitivity (DTH) responses in vivo are skin testing and induction of contact sensitivity.

Skin testing. First described by Koch in 1891, skin testing is based on eliciting a secondary response to an antigen to which the patient was previously sensitized. A small amount of soluble antigen is injected intradermally on the extensor surface of the forearm. The antigens used are usually microbial in origin (e.g., purified protein derivative [PPD] of tuberculin, tetanus toxoid, mumps antigens, and a variety of fungal extracts, including Candidin [from *Candida albicans*], coccidioidin [from *Coccidioides immitis*] and histoplasmin [from *Histoplasma capsulatum*]).

The area of the skin receiving the injection is observed for the appearance of erythema and induration, which are measured at 24 and 48 hours after the injection. A positive skin test is usually considered to be associated with an area of induration greater than 10 mm in diameter, but in patients with acquired immunodeficiency disease induration greater than 5 mm in diameter is considered positive. If no reaction is observed, the test may be repeated with a higher concentration of antigen.

If a patient has no reaction after being tested with a battery of antigens, it is assumed that a state of anergy exists. Anergy can be caused by immunological deficiencies, infections (such as measles or chronic disseminated tuberculosis), and can also be the result of errors in the technique of skin testing.

Although these tests have the theoretical advantage of testing the function of the T-cell system *in vivo,* they meet with a variety of problems. On

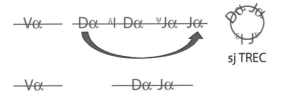

sj TREC

Figure 28.5 Use of T-cell receptor excision circles (TRECs) for the diagnosis of SCID. T-cell receptor recombination occurs within the thymus. The first step is the joining of the Dα to Jα gene segments with the intervening DNA, which forms the signal joining (SJ) TREC. This stable circular episomal DNA is amplified using quantitative reverse transcriptase polymerase chain reaction to determine the number of TREC copies within the dried blood spot obtained from all infants at the time of birth.

one hand, skin tests are difficult to reproduce, due to the difficulty in obtaining consistency among different sources and batches of antigens and to variations in the technique of inoculation among different investigators. On the other hand, the interpretation of negative tests has to be carefully weighed. Negative results after challenge with antigens to which there is no record of previous exposure can always be questioned, while a negative result with an antigen extracted from a microbial agent that has been documented as causing disease in the patient has a much stronger diagnostic significance, implying a functional defect in cell-mediated immunity.

IN VITRO ASSAYS OF T-CELL FUNCTION

There are limitations to the interpretation of numerical data, given the very loose correlation between membrane markers and biological function. However, numerical data are simpler and cheaper to obtain than functional data, which usually require cell isolation, performed in conditions that are anything but physiological (see Chapter 15). Human lymphocytes can be stimulated *in vitro* by specific antigens or by mitogenic substances.

Mitogenic stimulation assays. Cellular responses to mitogens are more quantitative and reproducible than delayed hypersensitivity responses elicited by skin testing. Mitogens nonspecifically activate large numbers of lymphocytes to induce cellular proliferation that can be measured by incorporation of tritiated thymidine (^{3}H-Tdr) in the *in vitro* culture system. The most commonly used T-lymphocyte mitogens are plant lectins such as phytohemagglutinin (PHA) and concanavalin A, which activate T cells only, and pokeweed mitogen, which activates both T and B lymphocytes. Cross-linking T-cell signaling pathways with immobilized monoclonal antibodies directed at CD3 and CD28 induce similar responses. Thymidine uptake by cells activated by the mitogen is compared to proliferation of lymphocytes incubated in media alone. Results are expressed as a stimulation index that divides the optimal (^{3}H-Tdr) uptake in the presence of the mitogen by the unstimulated control. In normal individuals, the mitogen stimulation index is 10- to 20-fold greater than the media control. Defects in T-cell signaling pathways result in mitogen responses many-fold lower than those of normal individuals. Lymphocyte proliferation responses to mitogens are very useful in the diagnosis of many of the T-cell immune disorders discussed in Chapter

29. An alternative methodology to measure cell stimulation by detecting intracellular ATP synthesis, which increases within the cells responding to the stimulant and thus correlates to cellular activation, has been recently introduced and has the advantage of not requiring the use of radiolabeled compounds (see Chapter 15).

Response to antigenic stimulation. The study antigen-specific T-cell response of lymphocytes *in vitro* may be more relevant, but the proportion of T cells responding to specific antigens is low, generally less than 1% of the cells in culture. As a result, proliferation response and (^{3}H-Tdr) uptake are lower, and a normal stimulation index to recall antigens is only three- to five-fold above the media control.

The probabilities of obtaining a measurable response can be increased if the lymphocytes are stimulated with antigens to which the lymphocyte donor has been previously exposed, and the cultures are incubated with the antigen for 5–7 days prior to addition of ^{3}H-Tdr.

Laboratory evaluation of phagocytic cell function

Phagocytic cell function tests were discussed in detail in Chapter 13. Testing for defects in phagocytic numbers and function involves three common tests for different types of phagocyte deficiency. A complete blood count with differential tests for congenital neutropenia as well secondary causes of neutropenia due to drug toxicity, infection, or malignancy. This confirmatory test for neutropenia requires bone marrow aspirate and biopsy. Leukocyte adhesion deficiency, types I, II, or III, can be made from cytometry. Loss of expression of CD11/18 markers on neutrophils and monocytes is used to diagnosis type I leukocyte adhesion deficiency, the most common subtype. In contrast to congenital neutropenia, these patients have persistently elevated white cell counts. Flow cytometry–based assays that measure the neutrophil oxidative burst by fluorescence changes in cells stimulated with phorbol myristate acetate (PMA) are widely used for the diagnosis of chronic granulomatous disease (CGD).

Diagnostic evaluation of complement function

The complement system can be activated by three different pathways, as discussed in Chapter 9.

All three pathways utilize C3 and the membrane attack complex (MAC), and the common effects of complement activation are opsonization, chemotaxis, and cell lysis.

Primary screening tests for complement deficiencies include the CH50 and AH50 assays. The total hemolytic complement assay (CH50) utilizes sheep erythrocytes coated with rabbit antisera. When complement is added and binds to the antibody coating of the sheep blood cells, the classical pathway is activated, the red cells are lysed, and hemoglobin is released into the supernatant, which can be measured using a spectrophotometer. A standard dilution of complement, used as reference, causes hemolysis of 50% of the red cells in the test. Since all complement components are necessary for the membrane attack complex, any absent factor in the classical or alternative pathway will prevent activation of the lytic sequence, and the result of the CH50 assay will be 0%. If any component is low, but not absent, such as in states of complement consumption or in heterozygous individuals with genetic complement deficiencies, the concentration of patient sera needed to achieve 50% lysis of red cells will be much higher than controls, and the calculated CH50 will be lower than normal. The alternative pathway hemolytic 50 (AH50) is based on the same principal except that red cell lysis is induced in the absence of antibody by rabbit erythrocytes, which are potent nonspecific activators of the alternative complement cascade. The results of the CH50 and AH50 assays can be used to identify which component of the complement cascade is deficient. Defects in C3 or the membrane attack complex, common to both pathways, will result in abnormal AH50 and CH50. A low CH50 with normal AH50 points to a defect in the initial components of the classical pathway. A low AH50 with normal CH50 points to an abnormality in the initial components of the alternative pathway. The next step is to use specific assays for different complement components and their fragments, to determine which complement component is deficient.

DIAGNOSTIC TESTING USING MOLECULAR GENETICS

Over 300 genes causing primary immune deficiency diseases have been identified, and with the application of whole exome sequencing, new genes are regularly identified. Confirming the genetic mutation is essential to the initiation of optimal treatments, determination of prognosis and future associated risks, identification of carriers, and implementation of effective family counseling. While some primary immune deficiencies, such as DiGeorge syndrome, can be diagnosed based on chromosomal cytogenetic studies (see Chapter 29), the majority of primary immune disorders are the result of single gene mutations, deletions, or duplications requiring careful sequencing of the genetic regions and cannot be detected by karyotyping or microarray alone. The advent of DNA- and RNA-based techniques now allows clinicians to accurately diagnose the majority of primary immune disorders. In most cases, the patient needs to be sufficiently characterized by laboratory-based assays described in this chapter to define the immune phenotype. Many patients lack a strong family history for the suspected underlying genetic mutation because as many as 40% of newly diagnosed patients with known primary immune disorders represent new mutations within the family or results of compound heterozygous mutations on the maternal and paternal alleles. If a genetic disorder is identified, all family members at risk should be screened because the penetrance of most primary immune deficiencies varies greatly among family members.

Two approaches to the diagnosis of primary immune deficiency are currently used clinically. The most common and straightforward is the application of a single gene of Sanger sequencing of genomic DNA from blood or buccal swab. For example, a single panel can probe the coding regions and splice junctions of the 26 different genes known to cause SCID. This method is accurate, inexpensive, and takes a few weeks to determine the results. Multiple commercial DNA sequencers are currently available, and the assays have been validated by the College of American Pathologists. However, if the initial genetic screen is not informative or the patient's clinical phenotype does not conform to a known primary immune deficiency, then whole exome massive parallel (or NextGen) sequencing can be performed using several available platforms. These assays involve paired-end reads and bidirectional sequencing. Reads are assembled and aligned to reference gene sequences and analyzed for sequence variants. In most cases, standard capillary sequencing is used to confirm pathogenic variants. NextGen sequencing should be done as a trio of the indexed patient and maternal and paternal samples to determine the alleles that carry the pathogenic variants. There are currently limitations to this technology. For example, in some cases, it cannot accurately identify deletions/duplications affecting these exons. It also cannot identify mutations in introns or epigenetic modification that affect gene expression. However, overall this is an emerging powerful technology for the diagnosis of primary immune deficiency as well as many other genetic disorders.

Besides the deficiency of genes directly related to the differentiation of the cells involved in immunological defenses, an increasing number of PID has been defined as secondary to deficiencies affecting intermediate but critical steps in cell activation and differentiation, described in detail in the 2015 classification from the International Union of Immunological Societies Expert Committee for Primary Immunodeficiency (e.g., MHC deficiencies, Zap-70 deficiency, JAK-3 deficiency, NF-κB and IκB deficiencies).

The ultimate goal of these studies is to determine whether by gene replacement, as it has been achieved for adenosine deaminase (ADA) deficiency and IL-2Rγ chain deficiency, as discussed in Chapter 29, or by the use of therapeutic agents able to correct metabolic deficiencies resulting from gene mutations, it will become possible to correct those disorders in a target-specific mode, a goal that is still distant but getting closer.

BIBLIOGRAPHY

Abraham RS, Aubert G. Flow cytometry, a versatile tool for diagnosis and monitoring of primary immunodeficiencies. *Clin Vaccine Immunol.* 2016;23:254–271.

Bousfiha A, Jeddane L, Picard C et al. The 2017 IUIS Phenotypic classification for primary immunodeficiencies. *J Clin Immunol.* 2018;38:129–143.

Conley ME, Notarangelo LD, Eizioni A. Diagnostic criteria for primary immunodeficiencies. *Clin Immunol.* 1999;93:190–197.

Fedson DS, Guppy MJ. Pneumococcal vaccination of older adults. Conjugate or polysaccharide? *Hum Vaccin Immunother.* 2013;9:1382–1384.

Gergen P, McQuillan GM, Kiely M et al. Serologic immunity to tetanus in the U.S. population: Implications for national vaccine programs. *New Engl J Med.* 1995;332:761–766.

Gunasekaran P, Noronha S, Pandey A, eds. *Current Developments in Biotechnology and Bioengineering. Functional Genomics and Metabolic Engineering.* New York, NY: Elsevier; 2017: 143–158.

Lim MS, Elenitoba-Johnson KSJ. The molecular pathology of primary immunodeficiencies. *J Mol Diagn.* 2004;6:59–83.

Locke BA, Dasu T, Verbsky JW. Laboratory diagnosis of primary immunodeficiencies. *Clin Rev Allergy Immunol.* 2014;46:154–168.

Lougaris V, Badoloato R, Ferrari S, Plebani, A. Hyper immunoglobulin M syndrome due to CD40 deficiency: Clinical, molecular, and immunological features. *Immunol Rev.* 2005;203:48–66.

Mahlaoui N, Warnatz K, Jones A et al. Advances in the care of primary immunodeficiencies (PIDS): From birth to adulthood. *J Clin Immunol.* 2017; 37:452–460.

Parker AR, Skold M, Ramsden DB et al. The clinical utility of measuring IgG subclass immunoglobulins during immunological investigation for suspected primary antibody deficiencies. *Lab Med.* 2017;48:314–325.

Picard C, Al-Herz W, Bousfiha A et al. Primary immunodeficiency diseases: An update on the classification from the International Union of Immunological Societies Expert Committee for Primary Immunodeficiency 2015. *J Clin Immunol.* 2015;35:696–726.

Smith LL, Buckley R, Lugar P. Diagnostic immunization with bacteriophage φx 174 in patients with common variable immunodeficiency/hypogammaglobulinemia. *Front Immunol.* 2014;5:410. doi: 10.3389/fimmu.2014.00410.

Wen L, Atkinson JP, Giclas PC. Clinical and laboratory evaluation of complement deficiency. *J Clin Immunol.* 2004;113:585–593.

29

Primary immunodeficiency diseases

JOHN W. SLEASMAN AND GABRIEL VIRELLA

INTRODUCTION

Primary immune deficiency diseases (PIDDs) are genetic defects with distinct clinical phenotypes resulting in a broad range of susceptibility to infection, malignancy, immune dysregulation with allergy, autoimmunity, and inflammation (Table 29.1). Based on Centers for Disease Control and Prevention (CDC) surveillance, there are over 250,000 individuals in the United States with primary immune deficiency (PID) and an estimated 500,000 individuals who are symptomatic but undiagnosed. These diseases result from over 300 separate inborn single- or multiple-gene errors. The International Union of Immunological Societies (IUIS) Expert Committee periodically updates this classification system based on the identification and characterization of new disorders. Each are cataloged based on common characteristics of their pathogenesis, genotype, and clinical phenotype. Proper classification requires in-depth assessment of the pattern of infections, associated autoimmune and malignant conditions, family history, and findings associated with known PID syndromes. Laboratory studies focused on particular aspects of the adaptive and innate immune response are required to pinpoint the arms of the immune system involved. The advent of next-generation sequencing has facilitated the discovery of new genes and gene combinations that make up the IUIS classification system. This chapter provides an overview of this classification of PID and cites specific examples of how genetic defects result in specific clinical phenotypes. Many of these disorders have provided great insight into the role of associated genes in normal human immune function.

IMMUNODEFICIENCIES AFFECTING CELLULAR AND HUMORAL IMMUNITY

Severe combined immunodeficiencies defined by CD3T cell lymphopenia

These heterogeneous disorders are subdivided on the basis of the relative impact on T-, B-, and natural killer (NK)-cell numbers and function. As the name implies, without treatment these conditions carry poor prognosis, with death due to infection or malignancy within the first few years of life. Subtype classification is based on the predominant arm of cellular immunity involved (T-, B+,

Table 29.1 International Union of Immunological Societies classification of primary immunodeficiencies

I. Combined T- and B-cell deficiencies
    a. SCID (based on T, B, NK phenotype)
    b. CID less profound than SCID
II. CID with syndromic features
III. Predominantly antibody deficiencies
    a. Hypogammaglobulinemia
    b. Other antibody deficiencies
IV. Diseases of immune dysregulation
    a. Hemophagocytic lymphohistiocytosis
    b. Syndromes with autoimmunity
V. Congenital defects in phagocytes
    a. Neutropenia
    b. Functional defects
VI. Defects in intrinsic and innate immunity
    a. Bacterial and parasitic
    b. MSMD and viral
VII. Auto-inflammatory disorders[a]
VIII. Complement deficiencies
IX. Phenocopies of PID

Source: Modified from 2017 International Union of Immunological Societies (IUIS) Bousfiha et al., *J. Clin. Immunol.*, 38, 129, 2018.
[a] This topic is discussed in Chapter 13.

NK+), (T−, B+, NK−), (T−, B−, NK+), (T−, B−, NK−). The advent of newborn screening using T-cell receptor excision circles (TRECs, see Chapter 28) has shown that overall incidence of SCID in the United States is 1:20,000 live births with variation in incidence and type of SCID among different ethnic groups.

T−, B+, NK+ SCID

Examples include IL-7Rα deficiency resulting in intrathymic arrest in T-cell development and FOXN1 deficiency that results in abnormal thymic epithelia. In both cases, T cells fail to develop, resulting in SCID phenotypes, but B cells and NK cells are spared.

T−, B+, NK− SCID

Most commonly this is the result of a mutation within the interleukin receptor common γ chain (γc). This X-linked condition impacts the function of the γc cell surface receptor responsible for signaling for multiple interleukin (IL) signaling pathways, including IL-2, IL-4, IL-7, IL-11 and IL-15.

Mutations in γc result in absent downstream cell surface signaling through the JAK/STAT transduction pathway, a critical component of interleukin-induced T-, B-, and NK-cell activation and differentiation. A form of SCID with an identical phenotype is JAK-3 deficiency because of its common link with γc IL signaling. Mutations in JAK-3 are inherited in an autosomal recessive pattern. Infants with these forms of SCID lack circulating T cells because of maturation arrest of T cell development within the thymus. B cells are present in normal or increased numbers but are deficient in function. NK cell numbers and function are also deficient.

T−, B−, NK+ SCID

This primarily results from deficient recombination of the T-cell and B-cell antigen receptors. Deficiencies in the recombinase-activating genes (RAG), Artemis (a DNA repair gene), and DNA Ligase IV all lead to this subtype of SCID because V(D)J recombination of the antigen receptors is critical to T-cell and B-cell development but not to the development of NK cells, which lack antigen receptors. Defects in DNA repair enzymes such as Artemis deficiency also carry the risk of radiosensitivity, leading to a high risk of malignancy and suppression of hematopoiesis.

T−, B−, NK− SCID

This is characteristic of adenosine deaminase (ADA) deficiency and reticular dysgenesis, in which all hematopoiesis is impacted. ADA catabolizes the deamination of adenosine and 2′-deoxyadenosine, converting them to inosine. Lack of ADA results in the intracellular accumulation of adenosine and 2′-deoxyadenosine, which are phosphorylated intracellularly, and the activity of the phosphorylating enzyme is greater than the activity of the dephosphorylating enzyme. Consequently, there is an accumulation of deoxyadenosine triphosphate (deoxyATP), which has a feedback inhibition effect on ribonucleotide reductase, an enzyme required for normal DNA synthesis. Overall, DNA synthesis is impaired, and no lymphocyte cellular proliferation is observed after stimulation. In addition, 2′-deoxyadenosine is a cellular toxin reported to cause chromosome breakage and ultimately severe lymphopenia impacting T cells, B cells, and NK cells because of their high mitotic turnover.

Combined immunodeficiencies generally less profound than SCID

Combined immunodeficiencies (CIDs) generally have a less profound clinical phenotype but still carry the hallmark of growth delay, susceptibility to opportunistic infections, autoimmunity (primarily in the form of autoimmune cytopenia), and malignancy. Similar to SCID defined by CD3 lymphopenia, different lymphocyte populations are impacted. For example, major histocompatibility complex (MHC) class-I or class-II deficiencies are associated with low levels of the CD8 or CD4 subsets. ZAP-70 deficiency results in a defective T-cell receptor signaling cascade either in the TCR/CD3 complex or downstream, resulting in deficient T-cell function as measured by poor proliferation to mitogens with normal numbers of CD3$^+$ and CD4$^+$ T cells but low numbers of CD8$^+$ T cells. Low B- and NK-cell numbers, lymphopenia, elevated IgE, low IgM, eosinophilia, severe atopic disease, and recurrent staphylococcal and viral infections characterize DOCK8 deficiency.

- **CD40 ligand/CD40 deficiency (hyper IgM syndrome)** results from the failure of the B cell to undergo T cell–induced immunoglobulin class switch resulting in low levels of IgG, IgA, and IgD in association with an elevation of IgM. This switch is triggered by the interaction of CD40 with its ligand (CD40L, CD154). Most cases are due to a mutation in CD40 ligand gene, located on Xq26-27, which is expressed on T cells, and due to the lack of expression of CD40L, the signal for class switch is not delivered to the B cells. In these patients, germinal centers do not differentiate in the peripheral lymphoid tissues and the impaired production of IgG antibodies leads to susceptibility to opportunistic infections such as those caused by *Pneumocystis jirovecii* and *Cryptosporidium*, autoimmunity, and carcinoma of the biliary system. Two other variants have similar phenotypes but are caused either by (1) defective activation-induced cytidine deaminase or uracil nucleoside glycosylase, enzymes involved in the processes of isotype switching and somatic hypermutation of immunoglobulin genes, or (2) absence of CD40 on B lymphocytes.
- **MHC-I deficiency (bare lymphocyte syndrome)** is a rare condition characterized by a deficient expression of HLA-A, B, and C markers and absence of β_2-microglobulin on lymphocyte membranes. The underlying genetic defects affect the genes coding for the transporters associated with antigen processing (TAP-1, TAP-2) or for a TAP-binding protein. Both TAP proteins and TAP-binding proteins are essential for proper intracellular assembly of the MHC-I molecules.

  Although some patients with this syndrome may be asymptomatic, most suffer from infections seen in cellular immune deficiencies including *Pneumocystis jirovecii* pneumonia and other fungal infections. Laboratory findings include lymphopenia, particularly low CD8 T cells, poor responses to mitogenic stimulation, low immunoglobulin levels, and lack of antibody responses to immunizations. B cells are usually detected, but plasma cells are absent. Molecular MHC DNA typing is normal because these germline genes are not affected.
- **MHC class-II deficiency** is also an autosomal recessive disease due to mutations in genes involved in the transcription of MHC-II genes; therefore, MHC-I genotyping is normal. Its clinical phenotypes are similar to severe forms of combined immunodeficiency, with absent cellular and humoral immune responses after immunization. These patients have a low number of CD4 T lymphocytes, which results in lack of differentiation of B lymphocytes into antibody-producing cells. Patients have increased susceptibility to fungal infections such as those caused by *Candida* or *Cryptosporidium*, the latter causing malabsorption and failure to thrive. Pulmonary infections are also frequent. The prognosis is very poor, and without hematopoietic stem cell transplantation, death occurs before the second decade of life. Laboratory findings include normal low numbers of CD4 T cells, inverted CD4/CD8 ratio, and low expression of MHC-II molecules (HLADR) on monocytes, B cells, and activated CD8 T cells.

Clinical presentation of SCID and combined immune deficiency

Essentially all forms of SCID begin with symptoms early in life, usually by 4 months of age. In most forms, survival beyond the first year of life is rare without aggressive therapy. Clinical presentations frequently include persistent infections of the lungs, often caused by opportunistic pathogens such as *Pneumocystis jirovecii,* systemic or extensive infections associated with *Candida* and herpes viruses, chronic infectious diarrhea, and failure to thrive. These manifestations are similar to those of AIDS, discussed in Chapter 30. Lymphoid tissues are generally underdeveloped, and approximately 20% of infants with SCID will develop graft-versus-host disease (GVHD), as a consequence of the transplacental transfer of maternal T lymphocytes late in gestation. The maternal T lymphocytes enter the fetal circulation but are not rejected, since the infants lack cell-mediated immunity. The maternal T cells, on the other hand, are activated by the infant's non-self MHC expressed in all cells and tissues and proliferate in the skin, gastrointestinal (GI) tract, and liver. Symptoms of GVHD include rash, jaundice, hepatitis, and chronic diarrhea. Children with SCID and other T-cell deficiencies can also develop GVHD following blood transfusions due to viable mononuclear cells transfused with the blood unit. To avoid this possibility, infants with suspected SCID should receive transfusions with irradiated blood. Children with SCID carry an increased risk of malignancy, particularly lymphomas driven by Epstein-Barr virus, and autoimmune cytopenia, most often thrombocytopenia.

Diagnosis

The general laboratory parameters seen in the various forms of SCID are outlined in Chapter 28. The hallmark is low to absent T cells with varying impact on B-cell and NK-cell numbers. Some forms of SCID have very low total lymphocyte counts.

Newborn screening using dried blood spots obtained from heel sticks at birth can be used to detect TREC and has become a highly effective means for mass screening for SCID with confirmation of the phenotype using flow cytometry (Figure 29.1). Functional cellular immunity, as measured by mitogen proliferation, is depressed (see Chapter 28). Immunoglobulins may be low or normal for age. The diagnosis of ADA deficiency is based on enzymatic analysis of red blood cells. In summary, SCID is a heterogeneous group of disorders with varying pathogenesis. Among the known causes, definitive diagnosis can be made through genetic sequencing to identify the mutated genes.

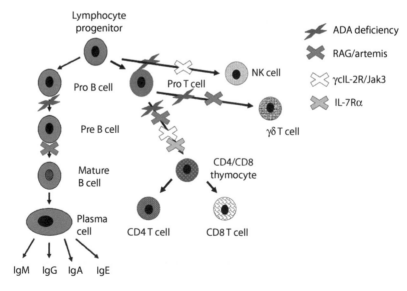

Figure 29.1 SCID subtypes detected though newborn screening (NBS). Different genes impacting T- and B-cell development impact the cellular phenotypes of SCID. All have low T-cell numbers and can be detected through NBS. Adenosine deaminase deficiency (ADA) affects T-cell, B-cell, and NK-cell development. RAG and Artemis deficiency result in absent T cells and B cells, but NK cell numbers are normal. Mutations in interleukin receptor common γ chain (γc IL-2R) and JAK 3 affect T- and NK-cell development, while B-cell numbers are normal, but they lack normal function. Mutations in IL-7α receptor cause T-cell maturation arrest in the thymus, but B-cell and NK-cell development is spared.

Therapy

Most cases of SCID lead to a fatal outcome due to infections or malignancy unless treated early in life. Initiating prophylaxis early in life can prevent *Pneumocystis jirovecii* pneumonia, as well as fungal and atypical mycobacterial infections. Immunoglobulin replacement therapy is needed as maternal IgG wanes. Pathogen exposure should be limited through reverse isolation, hence the term *bubble baby*. Children with suspected SCID and other defects of CID should not receive vaccines containing live, attenuated infectious agents. Therefore, rotavirus, measles, mumps, rubella, and chicken pox immunizations should not be given.

All forms of SCID can be effectively treated with hematopoietic stem cell (HSC) transplantation. Optimal survival occurs if the transplant occurs prior to the onset of infections in the first 3 months of life, from an HLA-matched related donor. If an HLA-matched related donor is not available, alternative strategies include the T-cell depleted haploidentical bone marrow cells from a parent, an HLA-matched unrelated bone marrow donor, or umbilical cord blood hematopoietic stem cells (HSC) from an unrelated donor, which provide a good chance for engraftment and cure. The risk for GVHD varies depending on the degree of HLA mismatch and the number of mature T cells within the transplanted cells. Preconditioning chemotherapy generally improves the chances of engraftment, but toxicity increases overall morbidity and mortality. A unique feature of HSC transplantation in SCID is that it can be successfully performed without conditioning to ablate pretransplant immunity. All HSC transplantation carries a GVHD risk, so immunosuppressive prophylaxis is often used.

Gene therapy has been applied to cure some forms of SCID. ADA deficiency was the first human disease successfully treated by gene therapy followed by IL-2Rγc deficiency. Gene therapy for single gene forms of PID involves harvesting HSC from the patient, transfecting a normal gene using a lentivirus vector, expanding the transfected cells *ex vivo*, and readministering them to the patient resulting in long-term immune reconstitution, recovery of immune function, and cure. Early trials of gene therapy using retroviral vectors for delivery resulted in lymphocytic leukemia in many of the recipients, apparently due to overexpression of the LMO-2 transcription factor, induced by the insertion of the retroviral vector near the 5' end of its coding domain leading to malignant transformation.

COMBINED IMMUNODEFICIENCY WITH ASSOCIATED OR SYNDROMIC FEATURES

These are disorders involving single or multiple genes that result in clearly recognizable clinical phenotypes. Most have several organ systems affected beyond immunity, and in many cases, immune dysfunction is a minor component of the syndrome. Following are specific examples that illustrate the broad range of these disorders.

Wiskott–Aldrich syndrome and X-linked thrombocytopenia

The triad of immunodeficiency, thrombocytopenia, and eczema characterizes Wiskott–Aldrich syndrome (WAS), an X-linked recessive disorder associated gene located in Xp11.23 encoding a protein known as Wiskott–Aldrich syndrome protein (WASP) expressed by hematopoietic cells to stabilize actin polymerization and cytoskeleton arrangement. Several different mutations have been identified resulting in either lack of synthesis or with synthesis of an abnormal WASP. As a result, cells of hematopoietic origin, particularly platelets and lymphocytes, have abnormal size, shape, and function. Platelets are small in size, aggregate poorly, and are sequestered and destroyed in the spleen. Hemorrhage due to thrombocytopenia is the major cause of morbidity and mortality. T cells are also small and show disorganization of the cytoskeleton and loss of microvilli associated with a predominant release of Th2 cytokines. Immunoglobulin levels are abnormal, IgA and IgE levels tend to be elevated, while IgM levels are low. Clinical manifestations include asthma, eczema, other allergic diseases, and autoimmunity diseases. Patients have increased susceptibility to viral infections and disseminated herpes simplex, Varicella-zoster, and *Molluscum contagiosum* infections are common. Antibody responses are poor leading to increased frequency of infections with encapsulated pyogenic bacteria, such as *Streptococcus pneumoniae*, *Neisseria meningitidis*, and *Haemophilus influenzae*. Diagnosis of affected individuals or female carriers of the trait can be confirmed by sequence analysis of the WASP gene.

Ataxia-telangiectasia

This autosomal recessive condition results from a deficiency of DNA repair enzymes leading to radiation sensitivity and high risk for lymphoreticular malignancies. The enzyme defects also impact tissue maturation that adversely impacts capillary beds in the cerebellum and causes progressive cerebellar ataxia with onset in early childhood. There is insidious development of telangiectasia starting with dilation of the conjunctival vessels. Laboratory findings include persistently elevated serum α-fetoprotein and carcinoembryonic antigen, selective IgA deficiency, and abnormal antibody production leading to recurrent sinopulmonary infections with bronchiectasis.

Most patients have thymic hypoplasia with low naïve T-cell counts and low total immunoglobulin levels. The prognosis is poor as there is no effective therapy. Correction of the immune deficiency through bone marrow transplant does not alter the course of the central nervous system deterioration. Death usually occurs before puberty, most frequently due to lymphoreticular malignancies or to the rupture of telangiectatic cerebral blood vessels.

DiGeorge syndrome

DiGeorge syndrome (DGS) is a result of the combination of thymic defects with additional congenital abnormalities. The thymus is hypoplastic resulting in varying degrees of T-cell deficiency. In addition, the patients have hypoparathyroidism, facial dysmorphism, and conotruncal cardiac defects. All those defects are believed to be the result of abnormal migration of neural crest cells forming the third and fourth pharyngeal arches during the fourth week of gestation. These embryonic structures form the development of the thymus, the parathyroid gland, the heart, and the face.

Approximately 90% of patients with DGS have an underlying microdeletion within chromosomal region 22q11.2. A number of critical genes in the region play a role in the clinical spectrum of the anomalies associated with the syndrome. Other genetic defects that result in a DiGeorge phenotype include deletions in chromosomes 10p13 and

17p13. Approximately 5% of DGS have no detectable genetic abnormality. While most deletions are sporadic, the presence of the deletion is inherited as an autosomal codominant condition, so half of the siblings will be at risk and 10% of affected children have an affected parent. Associated findings in DGS are listed in Table 29.2. Conotruncal cardiac defects, including truncus arteriosus, tetralogy of Fallot, interrupted aortic arch type b, or aberrant right subclavian artery are the most frequent cardiac features. Dysmorphic facial features include prominent nasal root with bulbous tip, protuberant ears, cup-shaped helices, and small, carp-like mouth. Cleft lip and palate and velopharyngeal insufficiency result in speech abnormalities. Hypoparathyroidism leads to hypocalcemia, often associated with neonatal tetany and seizures. Developmental and language delay, learning disabilities, and neuropsychiatric problems including schizophrenia are common.

Arrested T-cell development due to thymic aplasia or hypoplasia is a hallmark of the syndrome. In some cases, the thymus is absent or reduced in size, as can be noted on ante-posterior and lateral chest X-ray or by computed tomography scan. T cells can be absent (complete DiGeorge syndrome) or reduced in naïve T-cell numbers (partial DiGeorge syndrome). When CD3 counts are less than 500/μL, there can be a poor proliferation response

Table 29.2 **22q11.2 deletion syndrome: Phenotypic features**

Primary findings
Conotruncal heart defects
Cleft palate/abnormal facies
Thymic hypoplasia with low T-cell numbers
Hypoparathyroidism/hypocalcemia
Characteristic facial appearance

Associated findings
Developmental delays
Feeding difficulty
Motor/language delays
Autism/autistic spectrum
Chronic otitis media
Psychiatric disorders in childhood (schizophrenia, obsessive-compulsive disorder)
Increased risk of autoimmunity: Cytopenia, juvenile rheumatoid arthritis, thyroiditis
Renal anomalies (31%)

to T-cell mitogens such as phytohemagglutinin (PHA). Children with partial DGS most often have low T-cell numbers for age, elevated CD4 to CD8 T cell ratios, and low numbers of naïve T cells in the blood. The immune deficiency slowly corrects with age, but antibody abnormalities include poor response to immunizations, selective IgA deficiency, hypogammaglobulinemia, and autoimmunity, in the form of autoimmune cytopenias, can persist throughout life. While complete thymic aplasia occurs in only a small percentage of DGS, there are other genetic conditions associated with thymic aplasia. Examples include CHARGE syndrome, associated with mutations in chromodomain helicase DNA-binding protein-7 (CHD7) gene on chromosome 8q12 or with mutations in the semaphorin-3E gene (SEMA3E; 608166) on chromosome 7q21. Clinical and laboratory manifestations of CHARGE include coloboma of the eyes, heart anomalies, choanal atresia, CNS abnormalities and developmental delay, and genital and ear malformations. The T-cell numbers are absent or very low with deficient function.

Treatment for complete DGS is limited to thymus transplantation. Thymic tissues obtained during elective cardiac surgery can be implanted, and this has been successfully carried out without HLA matching or the risk of GVHD. Otherwise, treatment is focused on correction of the cardiac and parathyroid defects and prevention of opportunistic infections with prophylactic antibiotics.

Hyper-IgE syndrome (Job's syndrome)

This syndrome can be the result of at least two different genetic abnormalities. An autosomal dominant form is caused by STAT3 mutations, and a more clinically severe autosomal recessive form is caused by mutations of dedicator of cytokinesis 8 (DOCK8) that results in loss of signaling through STAT3. The DOCK8 mutations result in profound immune dysregulation with abnormal differentiation, survival, and function of B, T, and NK cells, including lack of differentiation of Th17 cells. As a consequence of those abnormalities, the patients have deficiencies and abnormalities in their immune cells. Immunoglobulin levels are variable, but most patients have very high levels of IgE. In contrast, their humoral responses are unusually short lived. Clinically, these patients are afflicted

with chronic atopic dermatitis, increased susceptibility to fungal infections by *Aspergillus* spp. and *Pneumocystis jirovecii*, disseminated *pyogenic contagiosum*, staphylococcal infections with abscesses in lymph nodes and skin, and pneumatoceles in the lungs. Ectodermal problems including retention of the primary teeth, hyperextensible joints, and early onset osteoporosis are also common, and patients have characteristic coarse facial features. A different mutation resulting in a STAT1 gain of function leads to a similar phenotype due to decreased impaired Th17 differentiation and reduced IL-17 production consequent to blocking of the RORγt signaling.

PREDOMINANTLY ANTIBODY DEFICIENCIES

Humoral immunodeficiencies are defects resulting from abnormal antibody production or function. As a group, they represent the most common clinically significant immune disorders. The clinical manifestations are summarized in Table 29.3. The predominant clinical signs of defective antibody production are recurrent sinopulmonary infections with encapsulated bacterial pathogens such as *Haemophilus influenzae* and *Streptococcus pneumoniae*. Other common clinical signs include polyarticular arthritis, recurrent otitis media, sinusitis, and bronchitis. Systemic bacterial infections such as pneumonia, empyema, meningitis, and septicemia are frequent and can be prevented with effective immune prophylaxis with human gammaglobulin. Recurrent pneumonia can lead to chronic obstructive lung disease and bronchiectasis. Chronic diarrhea and malabsorption caused by

Table 29.3 **Clinical features of defects in antibody production**

- Recurrent sinopulmonary infections with encapsulated bacteria
  (*Haemophilus influenzae, Streptococcus pneumoniae*)
- Chronic enteroviral gastroenteritis
- Chronic gastrointestinal giardiasis or cryptosporidiasis
- Bacterial sepsis, meningitis, osteomyelitis
- Chronic mycoplasma infection
- Chronic infectious arthritis

infection with *Giardia lamblia* are frequent, as is infectious arthritis of the large joints that develops in association with infection by pyogenic bacteria or *Ureaplasma urealyticum*. Patients are also at risk of developing chronic viral meningoencephalitis and other clinical manifestations of systemic infection by echovirus, particularly ECHO 11.

Hypogammaglobulinemia

Hypogammaglobulinemia can be subclassified depending on whether B cells are absent or present in low numbers, >1% of total blood lymphocytes.

X-LINKED AGAMMAGLOBULINEMIA

This condition is associated with absent B cells and results from a mutation in Bruton's tyrosine kinase (BTK) located on Xq21.2-22. Multiple mutations within these loci lead to the common phenotype of arrested B-cell development in the bone marrow. There are other rare forms of congenital agammaglobulinemia that appear in infancy but are inherited as autosomal recessive traits associated with deletions/mutations in genes encoding parts of either the Vλ region or of the Cμ heavy-chain region.

Infants with congenital agammaglobulinemia generally do not develop clinical symptoms until after the first year of life as maternally derived IgG wanes. The hallmark of agammaglobulinemia is absence of detectable B cells in blood, lymphoid tissues, and bone marrow leading to lack of any immunoglobulin isotype in the blood, although some patients may produce low amounts of IgM ("leaky phenotypes"). Histological examination of lymphoid tissues shows lack of germinal centers and secondary follicles in lymph nodes and peri-intestinal lymphoid tissues. Plasma cells are absent from both peripheral lymphoid tissues and bone marrow. Adenoids, tonsils, and peripheral lymph nodes are hypoplastic. The thymus has normal structure, and the T cell–dependent areas in peripheral lymphoid organs are normally populated. Unlike combined immune deficiencies, total peripheral blood lymphocyte counts, T-cell subsets, and T-cell function are normal.

COMMON VARIABLE IMMUNODEFICIENCY

The term common variable immunodeficiency (CVID) is applied to patients with hypogammaglobulinemia but with detectable B cells (>1% of normal). The designation CVID derives from the fact that this is the more common form of agammaglobulinemia and its pathogenesis is variable. This heterogeneous disorder is defined by the diagnostic criteria of low Ig levels (IgG and IgA, or IgM) for age, deficient antibody responses, as measured by the response to both polysaccharide and protein vaccines, variable age of onset, generally after 2 years of age, with a peak in early childhood and a second peak after age 20 years. Serum immunoglobulin levels are variably depressed (two standard deviations below the normal level for age or lower) for at least two of the major isotypes (IgG, IgA, or IgM). As a rule, patients produce some nonfunctional antibody of one of the major immunoglobulin isotypes. In contrast to congenital agammaglobulinemia, patients with CVID have low or normal numbers of B cells in peripheral blood but most have low numbers of class-switched and memory B cells.

Autoimmunity in the form of cytopenias, autoimmune thyroid disease, pernicious anemia, inflammatory arthritis, chronic enteropathy, polymyositis, and granulomatous disease that mimic sarcoidosis are common. In many cases, autoimmune thrombocytopenia is the first clinical manifestation. Lymphoproliferative disease with hyperplasia in the GI tract, tonsils, lymph nodes, and spleen is also a common manifestation, in contrast to congenital pathogen-driven malignancy such as Epstein–Barr virus (EBV)-associated non-Hodgkin's lymphoma and cancers of the GI system that are not increased in frequency in these patients.

About a third of CVID patients have defects in T-cell numbers and function, including inverted CD4/CD8 T cell ratios, increased expression of T-cell activation markers, and decreased response to mitogens. Most cases of CVID have no identified genetic cause. However, the advent of whole exome sequencing and other sophisticated genetic techniques have identified over 20 different genes and genetic loci associated with CVID. Identification of the precise genetic defect facilitates determining prognosis and associated morbidities within this heterogeneous patient population. Genetic defects associated with CVID often occur within signaling pathways that are key to normal B-cell differentiation such as the inducible costimulatory molecule (ICOS) and genes in the TNF receptor family such as the transmembrane activator and calcium-modulator and cyclophilin ligand inter-actor (TACI), which mediates Ig isotype switching. Other mutations that directly involve B cells are located in B-cell activation factor (BAFF), CD20, CD19, and other mutations that result in either loss of function or gain of function in the PIK3CD pathway.

OTHER ANTIBODY DEFICIENCIES

Added to each other, the disorders included in this group make up the most common antibody deficiencies. They have variable clinical manifesta-tions; from asymptomatic to recurrent infections requiring immunoglobulin replacement therapy.

Selective IgA deficiency with or without IgG subclass deficiency is most common, affecting a large proportion of the healthy population at a prevalence of 1/600–800 normal individuals. The pathogenesis of IgA deficiency is heterogeneous but is generally due to abnormal B-cell differentiation. In individuals with IgA deficiency and IgG subclass deficiency, IgG2 and IgG4 subclasses are low, but IgG1 and IgG3 are normal, as is B-cell function.

Anti-IgA antibodies reacting with isotypic or allotypic determinants of IgA can be detected in about one-third of the patients with selective IgA deficiency, suggesting that autoantibodies may play a role in the pathogenesis. When present in high titers, anti-IgA antibodies can trigger potentially fatal reactions when exposed to IgA-containing blood products, for example, through a blood or plasma transfusion.

While many patients with selective IgA defi-ciency are asymptomatic, recurrent bacterial upper respiratory infections, in particular, sinusitis, and GI infections with *Giardia lamblia* are common. Allergic diseases such as eczema, food allergies, and asthma are more frequent when compared to individuals with normal IgA levels. IgA deficiency can also be associated with GI disorders includ-ing celiac disease, nodular hepatitis, pernicious anemia, ulcerative colitis, and regional enteritis. Autoimmunity is more common than in the gen-eral population, particularly rheumatoid arthritis, idiopathic thrombocytopenia, and systemic lupus erythematosus. Similar to CVID, there is also an increased risk for GI malignancy, including GI lymphoma, adenocarcinoma of the stomach, and nodular lymphoid hyperplasia.

Blood IgA and IgG levels are developmen-tally regulated, and levels increase with age so the diagnosis of IgA or IgG subclass deficiency requires comparison to age-matched healthy con-trols. Newborn infants are completely deficient in IgA, and adult levels are not reached until puberty. Selective IgA deficiency is defined by IgA levels <10 mg/dL after age 4 years with normal for age levels of IgG and IgM. There is no effective replace-ment therapy for selective IgA deficiency, and Ig replacement therapy is not indicated as intra-venous IgG does not contain IgA. IgA-deficient patients who require blood transfusions should be given washed red blood cells, and alternatives for plasma infusions should be used. Patients should be educated about their increased risk of reactions to blood products.

Transient hypogammaglobulinemia of infancy is a disorder that is an accentuation of the normal physiologic decline in passively acquired maternal IgG. Normally, passively acquired mater-nal IgG is catabolized in a newborn infant with a half-life of approximately 1 month, but the infant's production is delayed, failing to maintain adequate IgG levels. As a result, IgG nadirs occur between 3 and 6 months of age. This process is more pro-nounced in preterm infants whose IgG levels are low at birth, as the transport of IgG across the placenta is greatest during the third trimester of gestation. If the infant's IgG nadir drops below two standard deviations for age, the criteria for transient hypo-gammaglobulinemia of infancy is fulfilled. Most of these patients most often are evaluated if they have increased frequency and/or severity of infections. Differentiation from more severe forms of humoral immunodeficiency is based on normal Ig function since these infants have normal response to immu-nization and normal B-cell enumeration.

GAMMAGLOBULIN REPLACEMENT THERAPY

For decades, Ig replacement therapy has been the mainstay for infection prophylaxis in patients with hypogammaglobulinemia. Even severe antibody deficiency diseases such as infantile agammaglob-ulinemia, CVID, and hyper-IgM syndrome can be effectively treated with regular repeated infusions of passive immunoglobulin. Most commonly, this is done using intravenous (IVIG) or subcutaneous (SCIG) Ig infused at regular weekly or monthly intervals. These immunoglobulin preparations are obtained from pooled human plasma from

3,000 to 60,000 healthy donors through the process of Cohn fractionation to isolate IgG (for the most part, serum IgA and IgM are removed in the fractionation process). Isolated IgG undergoes nanofiltration to remove potential pathogens and is reconstituted as a 5%, 10%, or 20% solutions that can be infused using an intravenous or subcutaneous pump with dosing tailored to achieve normal IgG levels. Donor screening for hepatitis C virus and other bloodborne pathogens is done prior to donation. Products are also treated with a detergent to inactivate pathogens and minimize the risks of blood-borne viruses. IVIG is administered monthly, while SCIG is divided into two or four equal aliquots for administration in the abdominal subcutaneous tissues using a small-gauge needle. This process minimizes some of the adverse reactions associated with IVIG and does not require intravenous access. The dosing of Ig is 500–800 mg/kg per month or the amount needed to maintain total IgG troughs at greater than 600 mg/dL. Adverse reactions to IVIg include aseptic (viral) meningitis that is associated with severe headaches. Because IgG crosses the blood-brain barrier poorly, viral infections in the central nervous system may require infusions with intraventricular Ig. Anaphylactoid reactions are rare but can be treated by slowing the infusion rate. In patients with IgA deficiency with recurring infections that do not respond to prophylactic antibiotic administration, administration of IVIg may be tried. Rarely this could be associated with an allergic reaction if the patient has anti-IgA antibodies and the purified IgG contains traces of IgA. Chronic infections of the GI tract sometimes require the use of human or bovine colostrum or oral Ig because IgG is not transported across the mucosa. It is important to note that replacement Ig can correct the antibody deficiency but does not correct all of the immune defects that can be associated with the immunodeficiency.

DISEASES OF IMMUNE DYSREGULATION

Hemophagocytic lymphohistiocytosis

Hemophagocytic lymphohistiocytosis (HLH) is a life-threatening disorder due to impaired lymphocyte cytotoxic activity due to defective formation of the immunologic cell-to-cell synapse that enables cytotoxic T cells and NK cells to kill an infected cellular target. The result is massive abnormal activation of T cells and macrophages, overproduction of γ-interferon, and infiltration of activated macrophages in the liver, bone marrow, spleen, and the central nervous system with massive hemophagocytosis. Clinical criteria include high fever with splenomegaly, autoimmune thrombocytopenia, neutropenia, and hemolytic anemia, and histologic evidence of hemophagocytosis in the tissues. Immune activation markers such as very high ferritin levels, hypofibrinogenemia, hyperlipidemia, and elevated plasma levels of soluble IL-2 receptor (sCD25) are usually found. Low NK numbers and activity are common. Familial forms can first appear in infancy or later in life and enable infection with human herpes viruses, particularly EBV. Mutations in Perforin, Syntaxin 11, and Munc 18 are the most common known genetic forms as all of these proteins play a critical role in tethering and formation of the immunologic synapse.

Hemophagocytic lymphohistiocytosis associated with hypopigmentation are a cluster of disorders resulting in defects in lysosomal trafficking modulators. These conditions include **Chediak-Higashi syndrome, Griscelli syndrome, and Hermansky Pudlak syndrome**. All are the result in abnormal assembly of cytoplasmic granules and fusion with phagosomes leading to abnormal NK, cytotoxic T cell, and granulocyte function due to failure to form the phagolysosome. Clinical manifestations include mucocutaneous albinism (Chediak-Higashi syndrome), abnormal hair structure and color (Griscelli syndrome), recurrent neutropenia, fever, hepatosplenomegaly and lymphadenopathy, and hemophagocytic lymphohistiocytosis following infections. Patients with Chediak-Higashi syndrome have morphological abnormalities in the PMN leukocytes (giant lysosomes), a finding that supports the diagnosis. Patients with Hermansky-Pudlak syndrome have partial albinism, nystagmus, and optic nerve abnormalities.

Immune dysregulation associated with autoimmunity

Diseases of immune dysregulation have clinical symptoms more often typical of autoimmune disease than recurrent infections. Genetic defects occur in key checkpoint signaling pathways that control transcriptional factors in cell cycle or the generation of T-helper cell subsets.

Autoimmune lymphoproliferative syndrome (ALPS) is a representative example of immune dysregulation due to defective T-cell apoptosis resulting in the accumulation of senescent T cells and autoimmunity. The condition is the result of mutation within the genes encoding the FAS/FAS ligand signaling pathways and of the caspase system including CD95, CD95L, caspases 10 and 8. Patients develop hepatosplenomegaly, generalized lymphadenopathy, and severe autoimmune hemolytic anemia and thrombocytopenia (Evan's syndrome). There is an accumulation of CD4$^-$/CD8$^-\alpha\beta$ CD3T cells in the blood and lymphoid tissues.

Immune dysregulation, polyendocrinopathy, enteropathy, X-linked (IPEX) is the result of mutation with the genes encoding FOXP3. Due to a defect in this transcriptional pathway, T-regulatory cells fail to develop, and there is an inability to generate peripheral immune tolerance. Clinical symptoms consist in development of type I diabetes in infancy, autoimmune thyroiditis, severe protein-losing enteropathy with villous atrophy, severe eczema, and autoimmune cytopenia. Even with hematopoietic bone marrow transplantation, death due to the enteropathy and autoimmune disease occurs in infancy. Diagnosis is based on the absence of intracellular expression FOXP3 on blood CD4T regulatory cells.

Autoimmune polyendocrinopathy with Candidiasis, and ectodermal dystrophy (APECED) is caused by a mutation in the **autoimmune regulator (AIRE)** gene that encodes a protein expressed in the thymus that contributes to self tolerance. Patients develop a variety of autoimmune disorders including hypoparathyroidism, adrenal and gonadal insufficiency, diabetes, and pernicious anemia, as well as mucocutaneous candidiasis, alopecia, dental enamel hypoplasia, and enteropathy.

CONGENITAL PHAGOCYTIC DEFECTS

Phagocytic disorders are classified based on whether they are associated with neutropenia or defective phagocyte function. Symptoms associated with phagocyte disorders include bacterial and fungal infections of soft tissues, cellulitis, and chronic recurrent lymphadenitis. Recurrent

Table 29.4 Clinical features of defects in phagocytic cells

- Poor wound healing
- Lymphadenitis/soft tissue abscesses and granulomas
- Gingivitis and periodontal disease
- Recurrent oral ulcers
- Chronic osteomyelitis
- Early onset inflammatory bowel disease
- Infection with catalase-positive organisms (*Staphylococcus aureus*, *Serratia* spp., *Escherichia coli*, *Candida* spp., *Aspergillus* spp.)

abscesses in organs such as lung, liver, and bone are also frequent and manifest as pneumonia, sepsis, meningitis, abscesses, and osteomyelitis. Common causes of infections are *Staphylococcus* species, *Pseudomonas* spp., *Candida*, and *Aspergillus* spp. Chronic or recurrent oral ulcers, poor wound healing (including delayed separation of the umbilical cord), and periodontal disease are also hallmark of deficiencies in phagocytic cell function or numbers (Table 29.4).

Neutropenia

Congenital neutropenias can occur due to a variety of genetic mutations, many of which involve other organ systems and have syndrome features. Neutropenia involves persistently low or cyclic declines in granulocytes to <100 cells/µL. Examples of syndromic-associated congenital neutropenia include autosomal recessive defects in SBDS (**Shwachman-Diamond syndrome**) and DNAJC21 with manifestations that include pancreatic insufficiency, pancytopenia, and chondrodysplasia. Mutation in 3-methylglutaconic acid (mutation in TAZ gene) is an X-linked disorder that results in congenital neutropenia, myopathy, cardiomyopathy, and growth retardation.

Nonsyndromic congenital neutropenias include **elastase deficiency** (SCN1 gene) resulting in cyclic neutropenia, susceptibility to myelodysplastic syndrome and leukemia, and in some cases, severe persistent neutropenia.

Mutations in HAX1 (**Kostmann disease**) result in severe neutropenia, cognitive deficiency, and susceptibility to myelodysplastic syndrome and leukemia.

Treatment of all congenital neutropenias involves aggressive antibiotic therapy for all febrile illnesses, the use of G-CSF, and in some cases hematopoietic bone marrow transplantation.

Functional defects of phagocytic cells

Leukocyte adhesion deficiency is the result of multiple autosomal recessive defects in neutrophil trafficking, the most common form is due to the lack of expression of the CD11/CD18 complex affecting both phagocytic cells and T lymphocytes. Clinical manifestations include a delayed separation of the umbilical cord, chronic, pyogenic infections, and with less frequency, fungal infections. Severe necrotizing gingivitis and periodontal disease are common. Patients have persistent leukocytosis (>25,000 cells/μL) due to the inability of leukocytes to normally marginate to vascular endothelial cells. Due to abnormal migration to infection sites, inflammation and pus are minimal. Specific infections include skin ulcers, delayed umbilical cord separation, and inflammation of the umbilical cord stump (omphalitis). Diagnosis is made using flow cytometry to enumerate expression of CD18 and CD11 subtypes on lymphocytes and granulocytes.

Chronic granulomatous disease (CGD) is the result of defects in the NAD/NADPH oxidase of the cytochrome B oxidase pathway. Lack of functional NADPH oxidase at the cell membrane level leads to failure to generate superoxide and H_2O_2, responsible for intracellular killing of bacteria and fungi within the phagosome. Both types of phagocytic cells (PMN leukocytes and monocytes) are affected. The killing defect leads to infections with catalase-positive organisms such as Staphylococci, *Serratia marscecens, Klebsiella* spp., *Aerobacter* spp., *Salmonella* spp., *Chromobacterium violaceum, Pseudomonas cepacia, Nocardia* spp., and *Aspergillus* spp. Catalase-negative organisms (such as *Streptococcus pneumoniae*) do not usually cause infections in these patients. The lack of involvement of catalase-negative organisms is due in part to generation of H_2O_2 by these organisms following ingestion that is not degraded by catalase. Progressive accumulation of H_2O_2 generated within the phagosome eventually reaches bactericidal levels.

The molecular basis of CGD is heterogeneous. The majority of cases are inherited as an X-linked trait, but autosomal-recessive inheritance is involved

in 25%–35% of the cases. The X-linked form is the result of a mutation in the α chain (91 Kd) phosphoprotein (gp91phox) of cytochrome b558. Molecular genetic studies have shown that in about half of the cases of X-linked CGD, there is a failure to express mRNA for the gp91phox protein and in the remainder of cases, mRNA is present but there is a failure to transport or properly insert the protein in the cytoplasmic membrane. The remaining cases of CGD are inherited as autosomal recessive traits, involving other proteins involved in the assembly of NADPH oxidase, such as neutrophil cytosolic factors 1 (p47phox) and 2 (p67phox), or the β chain (22 Kd) of cytochrome B (p22phox).

The clinical manifestations are dominated by recurrent bacterial and fungal infections. The most frequent infection sites are the lungs, lymph nodes, liver, skin, and soft tissues. The infections are characterized by the formation of microabscesses and noncaseating granulomas. Suppurative lymphadenitis, pyoderma, pneumonia with suppurative complications, liver abscesses, osteomyelitis, and severe periodontal disease are among the most frequently seen infections. Generalized lymphadenopathy and hepatosplenomegaly are frequently found on physical examination. Because the infectious agents are often sequestered within granulomas, obtaining a culture of the infecting organism is difficult unless a biopsy is obtained. It is common for blood cultures to be negative. Most patients have persistent immune activation with hypergammaglobulinemia and elevated C-reactive protein during times of infection. Diagnosis is usually confirmed by flow cytometry analysis of oxidative burst by neutrophils. These assays can also be used for the detection of female carriers. Treatment consists of prevention of fungal and bacterial infections with daily prophylaxis such as trimethoprim-sulfamethoxazole and antifungals such as itraconazole. The use of injections with γ-interferon may increase oxidative burst activity and has been shown to decrease infection frequency in some patients. Hematopoietic bone marrow transplantation requires conditioning for engraftment but is curative if successful.

DEFECTS IN INTRINSIC AND INNATE IMMUNITY

Two main types of defects in intrinsic and innate immunity can be identified: those due to genetic defects in pattern recognition molecules that trigger the immune response to pathogens and those due to deficiencies of the complement system.

Deficient pattern recognition

Clinical manifestations of deficient pattern recognition are based on the type of innate immune receptor or on the signaling pathway involved, leading to susceptibility to bacterial, parasitic and protozoal, mycobacterial, or viral infections. Predisposition to invasive bacterial infections is seen in IRAK4 and MYD88 deficiency critical to signaling through TLR 1, 2, 5, 6, 10, 4, and IL-1R. All of these receptors signal through MY88 and IRAK4 and deliver nuclear signals that enable the production of pro-inflammatory cytokines IL-1, IL-6, and TNFα. As a result, severe pyogenic infections occur without fever.

In contrast, STAT 1 gain of function mutations and IL17F deficiency result in chronic mucocutaneous candidiasis, ectodermal dysplasia, autoimmune endocrinopathy, and severe HSV infection.

CARD9 deficiency results in predisposition to invasive fungal infection and deep dermatophytoses. In contrast, increased susceptibility to mycobacterial disease is seen in complete interferon-γ receptor deficiency, manifest by disseminated mycobacterial infection in soft tissue, bone, lung, skin, and lymphoid tissues. Similar clinical phenotypes are seen with IL-12 deficiency and STAT 1 loss of function mutations. Susceptibility to viral infections, particularly human papillomaviruses is seen in WHIM syndrome (warts, hypogammaglobulinemia, infections, and myelokathexis) due to an autosomal-dominant gain of function mutation in CXCR4.

Mutations can lead to both autosomal-dominant and autosomal-recessive defects in TLR3 signaling defects and result in severe herpes simplex encephalitis early in life. In most of these conditions, standard laboratory immune testing is normal. Diagnosis depends on clinical presentation and direct assessment of the innate immune pathways.

Complement deficiencies

While there are known deficiencies in virtually all components of the complement cascade, clinical

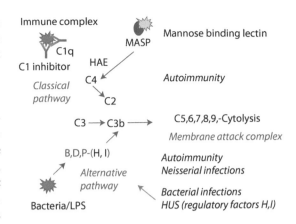

Figure 29.2 Complement cascade and clinical implications for defects in the complement system. The classical complement pathway is activated by C1q binding to immunoglobulin Fc. Activation is regulated by C1 inhibitor. Defects in C1 inhibitor production lead to hereditary angioedema (HAE). Defects in the classical pathway generally increase susceptibility to autoimmune disease. The alternative pathway is activated directly by bacteria or LPS. Defects in the alternative pathway increased susceptibility to bacterial infections. Defects in the alternative pathway regulatory proteins factors H and I increase susceptibility to atypical hemolytic uremic syndrome. Defects in the membrane attack complex increase susceptibility to chronic Neisseria infections and autoimmunity.

findings are highly variable and dependent on the pathway (classical or alternative) impacted by the defect. Symptoms range from an increased risk for the development of autoimmune disease, angioedema, to recurrent infections. Figure 29.2 shows the complement cascade and the location and phenotype of common deficiencies that are classified as based on high or low susceptibility to infections. Most complement deficiencies have autosomal-dominant inheritance except properdin deficiency, which is X-linked.

Defects in the early classical pathway (C1q, C2, and C4) result in SLE-like symptoms and increased susceptibility to infection with encapsulated bacteria. Deficiencies in late components of the membrane attack complex (C5, C6, C7, C8, and C9) place patients at risk for disseminated Neisseria infections, as does Properdin and factor D deficiencies in the alternative pathway. Deficiencies in the mannose binding lectin pathway include mannose binding lectin serine protease 2 (MASP2) deficiency and

Ficolin 3 deficiency. Both result in varying degrees of increased susceptibility to recurrent pyogenic infections. Abnormalities of factor H and factor I result in recurrent atypical hemolytic uremic syndrome. Deficiency in factor H and I results in a secondary fourfold increase in the catabolic rate of C3 complement component. Patients are prone to recurrent pyogenic infections, particularly with encapsulated bacteria such as *S. pneumoniae* and *N. meningitidis*. They are also prone to the development of immune complex disease. "Anaphylactoid" reactions secondary to the spontaneous generation of C3a are also frequently observed in these patients.

Diagnosis of complement deficiency is based on measurements of the function of the classical and alternative pathways using hemolytic assays to assess each pathway (see Chapter 28).

Hereditary angioedema (HAE) is due to a deficiency of C1 inhibitor that modulates the C1 binding in the classical pathway. Inability to produce protein (type 1) or production of a nonfunctional protein (type 2) results in the inability to downmodulate activation of the classical pathway leading to the production of complement split (C4a) productions and consumption of C4. C4a activates the Kallikrein pathway consisting of a group of serine proteases that activate bradykinins. This activation leads to uncontrolled nonpruritic angioedema of the lips, tongue, GI tract, and soft tissues and can result in life-threatening airway compromise. Activation is sporadic but is generally induced by mild trauma to the face or airways as can occur during routine dental and anesthesia procedures or simply by stress. Diagnosis is suspected on the basis of low C4 levels during attacks and confirmed based on measurements of serum levels and function of C1 inhibitor. Treatment options include treating attacks or giving regular prophylaxis by infusing purified C1 inhibitor isolated from human plasma administration of recombinant proteins that block the Kallikrein pathway.

PHENOCOPIES OF PRIMARY IMMUNE DEFICIENCY

These disorders are associated with somatic mutations or induced by autoantibodies to immune receptors that mimic genotypic PID. Somatic mutations can cause autoimmune lymphoproliferative syndrome, cryopyrinopathy mimicking Muckle–Wells syndrome (neonatal onset

multisystem inflammatory disease [NOMID]), and hypereosinophilic syndrome. Autoantibodies to the IL-17 can result in mucocutaneous candidiasis and polyendocrinopathy mimicking the symptoms of autoimmune polyendocrinopathy-candidiasis-ectodermal dystrophy (APECED). Autoantibodies to γ-interferon can increase susceptibility of mycobacterial infections. Autoantibodies to C1 inhibitor can lead to an acquired form of hereditary angioedema.

BIBLIOGRAPHY

Baker MW, Grossman WJ, Laessig RH et al. Development of a routine newborn screening protocol for severe combined immunodeficiency. *J Allergy Clin Immunol*. 2009;124:522–527.

Biggs CM, Keles S, Chatila TA. DOCK8 deficiency: Insights into pathophysiology, clinical features and management. *Clin Immunol*. 2017;181:75–82.

Bonilla FA, Geha RS. 12. Primary immunodeficiency diseases. *J Allergy Clin Immunol*. 2003;111(2 Suppl):S571–S581.

Bousfiha A, Jeddane L, Picard C et al. The 2017 IUIS phenotypic classification for primary immunodeficiencies. *J Clin Immunol*. 2018;38: 129–143.

Buckley RH. Molecular defects in human severe combined immunodeficiency and approaches to immune reconstitution. *Annu Rev Immunol*. 2004;22:625–655.

Cagdas DP, Cetinkaya G, Karaatmaca B et al. ADA deficiency: Evaluation of the clinical and laboratory features and the outcome. *J Clin Immunol*. 2018;38:484–493.

Casanova JL, Conley ME, Seligman SJ, Abel L, Notarangelo LD. Guidelines for genetic studies in single patients: Lessons from primary immunodeficiencies. *J Exp Med*. 2014;211: 2137–2149.

Castigli E, Geha RS. Molecular basis of common variable immunodeficiency. *J Allergy Clin Immunol*. 2006;117:740–746.

Chinen J, Cowan MJ. Advances and highlights in primary immunodeficiencies in 2017. *J Allergy Clin Immunol*. 2017;142:1041–1051.

Filipovich AH, Chandrakasan ß. Pathogenesis of hemophagocytic lymphohistiocytosis. *Hematol Oncol Clin North Am*. 2015;29:895–902.

Fischer A, Notarangelo LD, Neven B, Cavazzana M, Puck JM. Severe combined immunodeficiencies and related disorders. *Nat Rev Dis Primers*. 2015 Oct 29;1:15061.

Goldacke S, Warnatz K. Tackling the heterogeneity of CVID. *Curr Opin Allergy Clin Immunol*. 2005;5:504–509.

Hanson LA, Soderstrom R, Nilssen DE et al. IgG subclass deficiency with or without IgA deficiency. *Clin Immunol Immunopathol*. 1991;61(2 Pt 2):S70–S77.

Knight AK, Cunningham-Rundles C. Inflammatory and autoimmune complications of common variable immune deficiency. *Autoimmun Rev*. 2006;5:156–159.

Kohn DB, Hershfield MS, Puck JM et al. Consensus approach for the management of severe combined immune deficiency caused by adenosine deaminase deficiency. *J Allergy Clin Immunol*. 2019;143(3):852–863.

Leiding JW, Holland SM. Chronic granulomatous disease. In: Adam MP, Ardinger HH, Pagon RA et al. eds. *GeneReviews*, 1993–2018. Seattle, WA: University of Washington; August 9, 2012 [updated February 11, 2016]. Available from: https://www.ncbi.nlm.nih.gov/books/NBK99496/

Lougaris V, Badolato R, Ferrari S, Plebani A. Hyper immunoglobulin M syndrome due to CD40 deficiency: Clinical, molecular, and immunological features. *Immunol Rev*. 2005;203:48–66.

McDonald DR. Th17 deficiency in human disease. *J Allergy Clin Immunol*. 2012;129: 1429–1435.

Ochs HD. The Wiskott–Aldrich syndrome. *Semin Hematol*. 1998;3:332–345.

Panchal N, Booth C, Cannons JL, Schwartzberg PL. X-linked lymphoproliferative disease type 1: A clinical and molecular perspective. *Front Immunol*. 2018;9:666.

Routes J, Abinun M, Al-Herz W et al. ICON: The early diagnosis of congenital immunodeficiencies. *J Clin Immunol*. 2014;34:398–424.

Sleasman JW, Harville TO, White GB, George JF, Barrett DJ, Goodenow MM. Arrested rearrangement of TCR V ß genes in thymocytes from children with X-linked severe combined immunodeficiency disease. *J Immunol*. 1994; 153:442–448.

Tan QKG, Louie LR, Sleasman JW. IPEX syndrome. In: Adam MP, Ardinger HH, Pagon RA et al. eds. *GeneReviews*, 1993–2018. Seattle, WA: University of Washington; October 19, 2004 [updated July 19, 2018]. Available from: https://www.ncbi.nlm.nih.gov/books/NBK1118

Taubenheim N, von Hornung M, Durandy A et al. Defined blocks in terminal plasma cell differentiation of common variable immunodeficiency patients. *J Immunol*. 2005;175:5498–5503.

30

AIDS and other acquired immunodeficiencies

JOHN W. SLEASMAN AND GABRIEL VIRELLA

INTRODUCTION

Many factors influencing the function of the immune system can lead to variable degrees of immunoincompetence. Infections, exposure to toxic environmental factors, physical trauma, and therapeutic interventions can all be associated with immune dysfunction (see Table 30.1). In some cases, the primary disease that causes the immunodeficiency is very obvious, while in others a high degree of suspicion is necessary for its detection. The pathogenic mechanisms are very clear in some cases, and totally obscure in others. The following is a brief summary of some of the most common secondary immunodeficiencies, followed by a more detailed discussion of the acquired immunodeficiency syndrome (AIDS).

SECONDARY IMMUNODEFICIENCIES

Immunodeficiency associated with undernutrition

Immunodeficiency secondary to undernutrition has been reported in association with generalized malnutrition or in association with vitamin, mineral, and trace element deficiencies. Severe protein-calorie malnutrition is primarily associated with defects of both innate and adaptive immunity. Significant alterations of innate immunity include impairment of the epithelial barriers of the gut and skin, depressed granulocyte activity, and low complement levels. Defects of adaptive immunity include depression of cell-mediated immunity, low levels of secretory IgA, low numbers of circulating T and B cells, and lymphoid organ atrophy. Different groups have reported anergy, depressed lymphocyte reactivity to phytohemagglutinin (PHA), and depressed Th1 cytokine release in undernourished populations. In kwashiorkor, which is due to a combination of protein-calorie malnutrition and deficiency in trace elements and vitamins, the degree of immunodeficiency seems to be more profound.

Several causes for the immune deficiency associated with undernutrition have been suggested, including general metabolic depression, thymic atrophy with low levels of thymic factors, depressed numbers of helper T lymphocytes (which could account for the variable compromise of humoral immunity), and impaired cytokine release. A practical consideration to bear in mind is that malnourished children should not be vaccinated with live, attenuated vaccines, which are generally contraindicated in immunodeficient patients. It is also believed that undernutrition is a contributing factor to the high incidence of recurrent tuberculosis

Table 30.1 Causes of secondary immunodeficiency

- Malnutrition
- Systemic disorders
  - Immunoglobulin hypercatabolism
  - Excessive loss of immunoglobulins
  - Renal insufficiency
  - Extensive burns
- Drug induced
  - Cytotoxic drugs
  - Glucocorticoids
  - Antimalarial agents
  - Captopril
  - Carbamazepine
  - Fenclonefac
  - Gold salts
  - Phenytoin
  - Sulfasalazine
  - Alcohol, cannabinoids, opiates
- Surgery
- Malignancies
  - B-cell and plasma cell malignancies
  - Immunodeficiency with thymoma
  - Non-Hodgkin's lymphoma
- Infectious diseases
  - HIV
  - Congenital rubella
  - Congenital cytomegalovirus infection
  - Congenital toxoplasmosis
  - Epstein–Barr virus

in adults and of the high mortality among HIV-infected patients in Austral Africa.

Several vitamin deficiencies are associated with and may play a role in inducing abnormalities of the immune response, particularly when associated with protein-calorie undernutrition. The molecular mechanisms underlying these deficiencies have not been defined. Deficiencies of pyridoxine, folic acid, and vitamin A are usually associated with cellular immunodeficiency. Vitamin D3 deficiency negatively affects both innate and adaptive immune responses against *Mycobacterium tuberculosis*. Also, vitamin D3 deficiency is associated with enhanced inflammation, which in the case of tuberculosis contributes significantly to its pathogenesis.

There is also evidence that children born from undernourished mothers may undergo epigenetic modifications that negatively affect the development of the immune system.

In spite of all of these factors, malnourished children respond to vaccination, although the duration of vaccine-induced protection may be shorter than in normal children, Attenuated vaccines need to be considered carefully because of the possible risk of developing the disease against which the vaccine is supposedly protecting.

Immunodeficiency associated with zinc deficiency

The significance of zinc deficiency for the normal functioning of the immune system is underlined by observations performed in patients with acrodermatitis enteropathica, a rare congenital disease in which diarrhea and malabsorption (affecting zinc, among other nutrients) play a key pathogenic role. Affected patients often present with epidermolysis bullosa and generalized candidiasis, associated with combined immunodeficiency that can be corrected with zinc supplementation.

Secondary zinc deficiency is considerably more frequent and can develop as a consequence of low meat consumption, a high-fiber diet, chronic diarrhea, chronic kidney insufficiency, anorexia nervosa and bulimia, alcoholism, diabetes, psoriasis, hemodialysis, parenteral alimentation, etc. The depletion caused by these conditions, however, does not seem to be severe enough to cause symptomatic immunodeficiency but may be one of several factors adversely affecting the immune system.

The basis for the depression of cell-mediated immunity in zinc deficiency is not fully known, but it has been proposed that zinc may be essential for the normal activity of cellular protein kinases involved in signal transduction during lymphocyte activation.

Immune deficiency associated with renal failure

Patients with renal failure have depressed cell-mediated immunity, as reflected in cutaneous anergy, delayed skin graft rejection, lymphopenia, and poor T-lymphocyte responses to mitogenic stimulation. Humoral immunity can also be affected, particularly in patients with the nephrotic syndrome, who may lose significant amounts of IgG in their urine.

The impairment of cell-mediated immunity is apparently secondary to the retention of low molecular weight metabolites in uremic patients, including homocystein, methylguanidine, "middle molecules" (molecular weight 1200), phenylacetic acid, and others. These metabolites inhibit lymphocyte activation, induce lymphocyte apoptosis, and induce the oxidative burst in phagocytic cells.

Chronic oxidative stress will contribute to the oxidation of a variety of proteins, including low-density lipoprotein (LDL), thus enhancing the inflammatory response and increase the levels of pro-atherogenic LDL, adding to the many other factors that contribute to the acceleration of atherosclerosis.

Uremia is also associated to intestinal bacterial overgrowth that has pathogenic consequences. The production of uremic toxins is increased and the production of immunoregulatory short-chain fatty acids decreased. The uremic toxins, as well as proinflammatory products released by pathogens (e.g., lipopolysaccharide [LPS]) enter the systemic circulation, particularly in patients with uremia-associated hypervolemia, which increases the permeability of the intestinal barrier. LPS and other proinflammatory compounds will activate innate immune systems, but they have a paradoxical immunosuppressive effect on the adaptive immune response.

Burn-associated immunodeficiency

Bacterial infections are frequent and severe complications in burn patients, often leading to death. There are several factors that may contribute to the incidence of infections in burned patients, including the presence of open and infected wounds, a general metabolic disequilibrium, and a wide spectrum of immunological abnormalities.

Depressed neutrophil function is a major factor contributing to the lowered resistance to infection. Defective chemotaxis and reduced respiratory burst are the most prominent abnormalities. Several factors may contribute to this depression:

- Exaggerated complement activation (mostly by proteases released in injured tissues) causes the release of large concentrations of C5a that may disturb proper chemotactic responses and cause massive activation of granulocytes. When the already activated granulocytes reach the infected tissues they may no longer be responsive to additional stimulation.

- Bacterial endotoxin, prostaglandins, and β-endorphins have been suggested as additional factors that adversely affect neutrophil functions. The involvement of prostaglandins has been supported by studies in experimental animals, in which administration of cyclooxygenase blockers normalizes phagocytic cell functions.

- Another contributing factor seems to be the low opsonizing power of the burn blister fluid, which has very low levels of both complement and immunoglobulins.

Macrophage activation. Macrophages harvested from patients with burn injury appear to be in a state of activation, releasing increased amounts of interleukin (IL)-1, tumor necrosis factor (TNF), IL-6, transforming growth factor (TGF-β), and prostaglandin 2 (PGE2). These same cytokines are measured in increased levels in the circulation of patients with severe burns. Of these cytokines, IL-6 has been shown to be the one that is consistently elevated after thermal injury. It has been proposed that this state of activation increases the response of macrophages to other stimuli, such as endotoxin, therefore increasing the susceptibility of burn patients to sepsis.

Depressed cell-mediated immunity. Impairment of cell-mediated immunity is suggested by a prolongation of skin homograft survival and depressed delayed hypersensitivity responses. Laboratory studies have documented low responses to mitogenic stimuli and depressed mixed lymphocyte culture reactions. A major functional abnormality of T lymphocytes isolated from burned patients is their depressed release of IL-2 after mitogenic stimulation. This depression may be secondary to the release of immunosuppressive factors by the burned tissues, including a 10 Kd glycopeptide, a 1000 Kd lipid-protein complex, and PGE2. PGE2 is released by overactive monocytes and causes an increase of intracellular cAMP in T cells, inhibiting their proliferation. In addition, the circulating levels of TGF-β are elevated 6–8 days postinjury. Given the immunosuppressive effects of TGF-β on both T cells and B cells, it is not surprising that some investigators have suggested that TGF-β plays a significant role in causing immunosuppression in patients with severe burns.

Iatrogenically induced immune deficiencies

A wide range of therapeutic interventions has been shown to cause functional depression of the immune system. On top of the list is the administration of cytotoxic/immunosuppressive drugs, but many other medical procedures have unexpected effects on the immune system.

Neutropenia. The reduction of the total number of neutrophils is the most frequent cause of infection due to defective phagocytosis. Although there are rare congenital forms of neutropenia of variable severity, most frequently neutropenia is secondary to a variety of causes (see Table 30.2). Administration of cytotoxic drugs is almost inevitable followed by neutropenia (see Chapter 24), but

Table 30.2 **Causes of neutropenia**

I. Congenital
II. Secondary (acquired)
   A. Depressed bone marrow granulocytosis
      1. Drug induced
      2. Tumor invasion
      3. Nutritional deficiency
      4. Unknown cause (idiopathic)
   B. Peripheral destruction of neutrophils
      1. Autoimmune (Felty's syndrome)[a]
      2. Drug induced

[a] An association of rheumatoid arthritis, splenomegaly, and neutropenia.

a variety of drugs of other groups may cause idiosyncratic neutropenia with variable frequency.

Postsurgery immunodeficiency. Both surgery and general anesthesia are associated with transient depression of immune functions, affecting the mitogenic responses of PBL, cutaneous hypersensitivity, and antibody synthesis. Multiple factors seem to contribute to the depression of the immune system (Figure 30.1), such as transient severe lymphopenia that can occur in the immediate postoperative period; the exaggerated release of PGE2, due to the posttraumatic activation of inflammatory cells, which depresses T-lymphocyte and accessory cell functions; blood loss, which can be associated with a reduction of IL-2 release by activated T lymphocytes and of MHC-II expression by accessory cells with reduced B-lymphocyte responses to antigenic stimulation; transfusions have a poorly understood immunosuppressive effect; and anesthesia and administration of opiates (as painkillers) can lead to a depression of phagocytic cell functions and to a reduced activity of NK cells.

Complete normalization of the immune function may take 10 days (for mitogenic responses) to a month (for delayed hypersensitivity reactions and the humoral immune response).

It also needs to be kept in mind that postsurgical infection is facilitated by a variety of factors associated with surgery, which even in its simplest form is traumatic to the patient. For example, the surgical incision disrupts the integrity of the skin, a very important barrier against infection. Special types

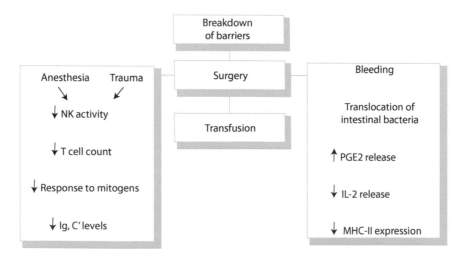

Figure 30.1 **Different factors contributing to the immune suppression associated with surgery.**

of surgery, such as intestinal surgery, promote the spreading of bacteria from a highly contaminated organ into surrounding tissues. The introduction of intravenous lines and catheters, often associated with surgical procedures, opens new routes for the penetration of opportunistic agents into the skin. Severe blood loss during surgery can cause massive entrance of intestinal bacteria into the portal circulation, and subsequently, into the systemic circulation (phenomenon known as *bacterial translocation*). If one adds a depressed immune system to these factors, it is easy to understand the clinical significance of postsurgical infection.

Splenectomy deserves special reference as a cause of immune depression. The removal of the spleen represents the loss of an important filtration organ, very important for the removal of circulating bacteria. In addition, the spleen plays a significant role in recruiting immunocytes in the initial phases of the immune responses. Splenectomized patients are weakly responsive to polysaccharides, and if we add this fact to the inability to remove bacteria, particularly those with polysaccharide capsules, from circulation it is easy to understand why splenectomized patients are prone to severe septicemia. The most commonly offending organisms include *Streptococcus pneumoniae* (50% of the cases), *Haemophilus influenzae*, and *Neisseria meningitidis*—all of them pyogenic bacteria with antiphagocytic polysaccharide capsules. Other organisms involved as frequent causes of infection in splenectomized patients include *Staphylococcus aureus* and group A *Streptococcus*. It has also been demonstrated that about one-third of the cases of human infection by *Babesia*, an intracellular sporozoan, occur in splenectomized patients.

Similar defects are noticed in patients with **sickle cell anemia**, who develop splenic atrophy as a consequence of repeated infections and fibrosis (autosplenectomy). Noteworthy is the fact that patients with sickle cell anemia are particularly prone to develop salmonella bacteremia involving strains of *Salmonella enteritidis*, which do not disseminate in the bloodstream of normal individuals. This allows *S. enteritidis* to spread to organs other than the intestine, namely, the bones. (*S. enteritidis* is the most frequent cause of osteomyelitis in patients with sickle cell anemia.)

Thymectomy is frequently done in neonates with congenital heart disease, to ensure proper surgical access. It is generally believed that thymectomy after birth has few (if any) effects on the development of the immune system of humans, and there is no conclusive evidence suggesting otherwise.

Immunosuppression associated with drug abuse

There is considerable interest in defining the effects of drug abuse on the immune system. Unfortunately, most data concerning the immunological effects of drugs of abuse are based on *in vitro* experiments or on studies carried out with laboratory animals, which may or may not reflect the *in vivo* effects of these compounds in humans.

Alcohol. Chronic alcoholism is associated with a depression of both cell-mediated and humoral immunity, but it could be argued that factors other than ethanol consumption, such as undernutrition and vitamin deficiencies, could be the major determinants of the impairment of the immune system. A direct effect of ethanol is supported by animal experiments, in which both T-lymphocyte functions and B-lymphocyte responses to T-dependent antigens are compromised after 8 days of ethanol administration.

Cannabinoids. There is little concrete evidence for an immunosuppressive effect of cannabinoids in humans, except for depressed results in *in vitro* T-lymphocyte function tests and for an increased incidence of *Herpes genitalis* among young adults who use cannabinoids. In laboratory animals, cannabinoid administration predominantly affects T- and B-lymphocyte functions, increases the sensitivity to endotoxin, and increases the frequency of infections by intracellular agents, such as *Listeria monocytogenes*. However, the conditions of administration of these compounds to laboratory animals are rather different than the conditions surrounding their use as recreational drugs.

Opiates. *Cocaine* has been shown to have direct effects over human T lymphocytes *in vitro*, but the required concentrations greatly exceed the plasma levels measured in addicts. The results of studies carried out in addicts have been contradictory.

Intravenous heroin use is associated with a high frequency of infections. In many instances, the infection (thrombophlebitis, soft tissue abscesses, osteomyelitis, septic arthritis, hepatitis B and D, and HIV infection) seems clearly related to the use of infected needles, but in other cases (bacterial pneumonia, tuberculosis), the infection could result from a depression of the immune system. However, to date, no conclusive evidence supporting a depressive effect of heroin over the immune system has been published.

Immunosuppression associated with infections

A wide variety of infectious agents have acquired the ability to thwart the immune system in a variety of ways, and in doing so, ensure their ability to survive in the host for at least the time necessary for their replication.

Bacterial infections. Disseminated mycobacterial infections are often associated with a state of anergy. The patients fail to respond to the intradermal inoculation of tuberculin and other antigens, and their *in vitro* lymphocyte responses to PHA and to mycobacterial antigens are depressed. The mechanisms leading to anergy are poorly understood and probably involve more than a single factor:

- An increased production of IL-10 and IL-4 could reduce the activity of Th1 helper lymphocytes, thus depressing cell-mediated immunity.
- Mycobacteria infect phagocytic monocytes, and intracellular infection is associated with a depression of both the antigen-presentation capacities and the ability to deliver costimulatory signals to T lymphocytes (e.g., the expression of the CD80/86 molecules is depressed). In addition, infected monocytes/macrophages may release nitric oxide, which inactivates lymphocytes in the proximity of the infected cells.

The release of soluble immunosuppressor compounds has been demonstrated for several bacteria. Several different substances, including enzymes (ribonuclease and asparaginase), exotoxins (such as staphylococcal enterotoxins), and other proteins, have been shown to have immunosuppressive properties, although probably their effects are limited to reducing the specific anti-infectious immune response. The staphylococcal enterotoxins are part of a group of bacterial proteins known as superantigens (see Chapter 14). *In vitro*, most superantigens have stimulatory properties, but when administered *in vivo*, induce generalized immunosuppression (perhaps as a consequence of indiscriminate nonspecific T-cell activation).

Parasitic infections. Parasitic infections due to protozoa seem to be often associated with suppression of the immune response to the parasite itself. In some cases, however, there is evidence of the induction of a more generalized state of immunosuppression. For example, acute infections with *Trypanosoma cruzi* are associated with cell mediated immunity depression that can be easily reproduced in laboratory animals. Both in humans and experimental animals, there is a reduced expression of IL-2 receptors, which can be interpreted as resulting from a downregulation of Th1 cells, either by cytokines or by suppressor compounds released by the parasite. Similar mechanisms seem to account for the generalized immunosuppression observed in experimental animals infected with *Toxoplasma, Schistosoma, Leishmania*, and *Plasmodia*.

Viral infections. The AIDS epidemic has certainly focused our attention in the interplay between viruses and immunity. However, HIV is certainly not the only virus able to interfere with the immune system. A classical example is the temporary immunosuppression associated with viral influenza, which facilitates secondary bacterial infections, particularly in the lungs, and the development of a transitory state of anergy during the acute stage of measles, which was first reported by Von Pirquet in 1908.

The mechanisms responsible for the transitory state of anergy associated with measles were revisited in modern times. We now know that during the 3–4 weeks following the acute phase of measles, patients show lymphopenia, and the residual population of peripheral blood lymphocytes shows poor responses to mitogens and antigens such as PHA and *Candida albicans*. The function of antigen-presenting cells, including dendritic cells, is also impaired, with reduced release of IL-12. This state of anergy seems to be caused by the release of viral proteins by infected cells that have immunosuppressive properties. A viral nucleoprotein interacts with the FcγR on dendritic cells, and viral envelope glycoproteins interact with the viral hemagglutinin receptor, CD46. Other targets of viral proteins are CD150, TLR2, and FcγRII.

Other viruses, such as cytomegalovirus (CMV) and the rubella virus, can cause immunosuppression. CMV mainly depresses the specific response to the virus, while the rubella virus induces a generalized immunosuppression, similar to that caused by the measles virus. Viruses can also release suppressor factors (*Herpes simplex* virus secretes a protein similar to IL-10, which can downregulate cytokine release by activated T lymphocytes) and interfere with antigen presentation (adenovirus infection is associated with a depressed expression of MHC-I molecules). However, patients infected with these viruses do not develop generalized immunosuppression, so it seems likely that the significance of these mechanisms is mostly related to promoting conditions favorable for the persistence of the infection.

HIV INFECTION AND AIDS

HIV infection, the cause of AIDS, was first recognized as a distinct clinical entity in the early 1980s as an association of severe immune deficiency with increased incidence of severe infection with *Pneumocystis jirovecii* pneumonia and Kaposi's sarcoma among men who have sex with men in the United States and Europe. A human retrovirus as the cause of AIDS was established in 1983 by Drs. Françoise Barre-Sinoussi and J.C. Chermann, at the Pasteur Institute in Paris, France. It was given the designation of HIV, a member of the *Lentiviridae* family of retrovirus. Two major variants of the virus have been identified. HIV-1, the first to be isolated, exhibits a high degree of genetic

diversity but can be classified into distinct groups or clades that vary in their geographic distribution, tropism, and phylogenetic makeup (Figure 30.2). In contrast, HIV-2, prevalent in West Africa, was isolated a few years later. It is less virulent and is more restricted geographically. Both viruses are derived from simian immune deficiency virus (SIV), and there is now strong genetic evidence to support that HIV is derived from the chimpanzee form of SIV.

Epidemiology of HIV/AIDS

According to UNAIDS, as of 2018 there were estimated to be about 37 million people living with HIV/AIDS worldwide with approximately 1.8 million new infections per year, representing a nearly 35% decline since 2009 due largely to worldwide efforts to contain the epidemic. The highest numbers of infected people live in Sub-Saharan Africa (25 millions), followed by South and Southeast Asia (7.1 million), Latin American (1.7 million), Eastern Europe and Central Asia (1.4 million), and North America (1 million). The highest infection rates occur in Sub-Saharan Africa (7.5%) and the Caribbean (2.3%). Each year approximately 1 million people die worldwide as a consequence of HIV infection. HIV is primarily a sexually transmitted disease with highest risk among populations with high prevalence, such as men who have sex with

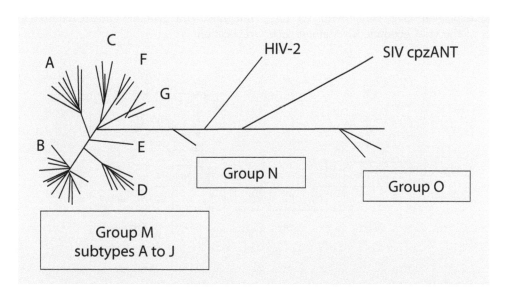

Figure 30.2 Phylogenetic relationships among worldwide HIV-1 strains relative to groups, M, N, and O and within subtypes of M (A–J). Relative phylogenetic distance to HIV-1 and SIV chimpanzee is shown.

men in Europe and North America, and through heterosexual transmission in countries of high prevalence. Other routes of transmission include sharing needles among IV drug users and mother-to-child transmission that can occur *in utero* during late pregnancy, at the time of delivery, and through breastfeeding. In the absence of antiretroviral therapy (ART) to prevent transmission, about a third of HIV-exposed infants become infected.

Characteristics of HIV and viral life cycle

Structurally, HIV-1 and HIV-2 are constituted by two identical strands of (+)RNA associated with matrix proteins, a double protein capsid, and a lipid envelope with inserted glycoproteins. The integrated form of HIV-1 (provirus) is approximately 9.8 kilobases in length. Both ends of the provirus are flanked by a repeated sequence known as the long terminal repeats (LTRs) which play a key role in the viral life cycle.

The genetic organization of HIV-1 contains three major genes, *gag, pol,* and *env* common to all retroviruses, bounded by the LTR and accessory genes *vif, vpr tat, rev,* and *nef* interspersed between *pol* and *env* (Figure 30.3). The *gag* gene gives rise to a 55-kilodalton (kD) Gag precursor protein (p55). During translation, the *N*-terminus of p55 is myristylated, triggering its association with the cytoplasmic aspect of cell membranes. The membrane-associated Gag polyprotein recruits two copies of the viral genomic RNA along with

other viral and cellular proteins that trigger the budding of the viral particle from the surface of an infected cell. After budding, p55 is cleaved by the virally encoded aspartic protease (see later) during the process of viral maturation into four smaller proteins designated MA (matrix [p17]), CA (capsid [p24]), NC (nucleocapsid [p9]), and p6. The *pol* gene encodes a protein that in its native form functions as a reverse transcriptase, but after cleavage can function as a ribonuclease and an endonuclease involved in integration into the host chromosome. The *env* gene encodes the envelope glycoproteins. The translated product of *env* is gp160, which is cleaved by a cellular protease into gp120 and gp41. The gp41 moiety contains the transmembrane domain of env, while gp120 is located on the surface of the infected cell and of the virion through noncovalent interactions with gp41. gp120 mediates the viral attachment between HIV and the CD4 molecule and one of two possible coreceptors CCR5 and CXCR4. Genetic variability is not uniform across gp120 that has five highly variable loops, V1 to V5, which play a key role in viral attachment and immune escape. gp41 contains an *N*-terminal fusogenic domain mediating fusion of the viral and cellular membranes, thereby allowing entry of the virion into the cytoplasm. The regulatory proteins encoded by noncontiguous segments of the genome, in some cases read in alternative frames, have as their main function to promote the transcription and transport to the cytoplasm of integrated viral genomes and are required for viral replication.

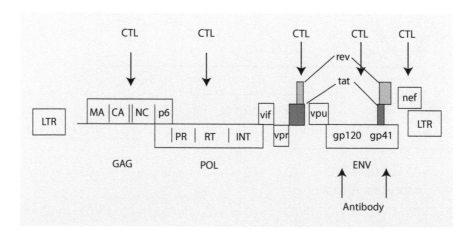

Figure 30.3 Structure and organization of the HIV genome with primary cytotoxic T-cell epitopes and antibody epitopes shown with arrows.

Viral life cycle. The primary HIV cellular targets are memory CD4T cells expressing CCR5 and CD45R0 as well as macrophages. However, CD4T cells are the primary source of replicating virus. The initial interaction of HIV and CD4 cells involves specific regions of gp120 binding at the CD4 binding domain between V4 and V5 followed by binding of the V3 loop to one of the chemokine coreceptors on the cell membrane. CCR5 and CXCR4 are G-protein coupled, 7-transmembrane β-chemokine receptors (see Chapter 11) with CCR-5 predominantly on memory T cells and macrophages, and CXCR-4 expressed on naïve T lymphocytes. The interaction between the CD120 and the coreceptor molecules results in exposure of the fusogenic domain of gp41 that can then interact with the cell membrane. This, in turn, results in the fusion of the membrane and the viral envelope, and penetration of the nucleocapsid into the cytoplasm. Once HIV enters a cell, its RNA is reverse transcribed into proviral DNA and transported to the nucleus to integrate into the host genome using the viral-encoded enzyme integrase. Virus can remain within latently infected cells for months to years depending on the degree of cellular activation. The next phase of the viral life cycle is viral expression that depends on cellular activation. Viral replication begins with initiation of transcription of viral genomic proviral DNA to RNA and translation of viral proteins. Viral polypeptides are cleaved by both cellular and viral proteases as the virus is assembled and buds from an infected cell and forms a viable virion. The steps of the viral life cycle are shown in Figure 30.4.

HIV pathogenesis

HIV-1 enters via mucosal surfaces in the rectal or genital track where it binds to dendritic cells by gp-120 binding to DC SIGN, a peptide expressed on DC and other antigen-presenting cells (DC). These cells migrate to the regional lymph nodes where they interact with CD4 T cells to induce initial viremia, generally within 3 days of initial exposure. The presence of genital ulcers induced by other infections increases the risk of infection. Initial viremia disseminates virus to T cells throughout the body, particularly CD4 CD45RO memory T cells in the Peyer's patches, inguinal, and mesenteric lymph nodes of the gastrointestinal tract. By 21 days postinfection, up to 60% of the memory CD4T cells with the gut-associated lymphoid tissue (GALT) have become infected and undergone apoptosis and cell death and are never totally replaced, even with effective therapy. This massive loss of T cells in the GALT is not reflected in the peripheral blood.

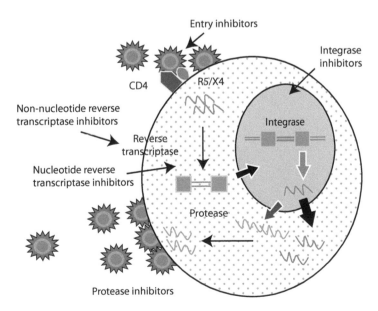

Figure 30.4 HIV life cycle and the points of action of antiretroviral agents. Entry inhibitors block viral attachment CD4 and CCR5 or CXCR4. Sites of action of nonnucleotide reverse transcriptase inhibitors, nucleotide reverse transcriptase inhibitors, integrase inhibitors, and protease inhibitors are indicated in the diagram.

The paradigm of HIV immune pathogenesis is characterized by *tap* and *drain* T-cell dynamics in which susceptible memory CD4 T cells become infected by virus and express viral proteins, making them susceptible to HIV-specific cytotoxic CD8 T cells (CTL) (Figure 30.5). If these infected cells are not cleared by cytotoxic T cells, they produce new infectious virus prior to cell death by apoptosis (the drain). The half-life of an infected T cell is about 2 days and 6–12 hours for a free virion. The *tap* is the capacity of the immune system to regenerate CD4 T cells in the thymus or lymph nodes. Approximately 95% of blood free virus comes from acutely infected CD4 T cells. A small percentage of CD4 T cells do not die but develop into latently infected long-term memory T cells in which virus infection can persist for years in spite of effective ART. Dendritic cells and macrophages can also harbor virus.

Microbial translocation and chronic macrophage activation. During the initial phases of viremia and infection of memory CD4 T cells within the GALT, the massive T-cell loss results in increased intestinal permeability to gastrointestinal microbes. The subsequent microbial translocation of bacterial cell wall products, particularly lipopolysaccharide (LPS), binds to toll-like receptor 4 (TLR4) on macrophages throughout the body. Global macrophage activation is evident by elevated plasma levels of soluble CD14 and high levels of macrophage-derived pro-inflammatory cytokines such as TNF. Microbial translocation creates a chronic state of macrophage-derived inflammation that is not reversed by control of viral replication by ART.

HIV-specific immune response. The initial control of HIV replication is primarily by HIV-specific cytotoxic T lymphocytes (CTL) emerging by the third week of infection to control the initial phase of viremia. During acute infection, viral levels peak at $>10^6$ viral copies/mL, and with activation of CTL, viral load falls to achieve a lower, steady-state set point determined by the effectiveness of host MHC-I restricted CTL responses. Certain HLA haplotypes, for example HLA-B*5701, are more effective than other HLA types, such as HLA-B51 or B35 in controlling viremia. Viral set point correlates directly with disease progression to AIDS. Over 60% of untreated patients with set points >100,000 copies/mL will develop AIDS within 5 years, while <10% of patients with viral

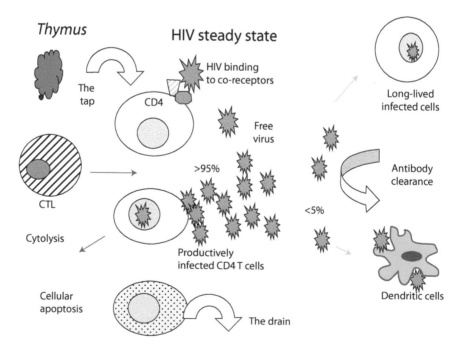

Figure 30.5 Pathogenesis of HIV infection *in vivo*. Steady-state free virus comes primarily (>95%) from infected CD4 T cells producing virus prior to CTL killing or apoptosis. Latently infected long-lived CD4 T cells and dendritic cells serve as the primary viral reservoirs. Antibody clearance plays a minor role once infection is established.

set points <1000 will develop AIDS over the same time frame. The primary CTL epitopes are peptides derived from *gag, env, tat, nef,* and *pol* (Figure 30.3).

During acute infection, HIV-specific antibodies can also be detected, but antibody response is not as effective as CTL in controlling viral replication due to rapid viral immune escape. However, broadly neutralizing antibodies directed against epitopes of gp120 and gp41 have been identified against conserved regions of these envelope proteins, particularly the CD4 binding site located between V4 and V5 and the membrane proximal region of gp41. Antibody inhibits HIV replication through direct neutralization and through ADCC-promoting antibodies. The rate of disease progression is considerably higher in individuals lacking neutralizing antibodies. The inability of an infected individual to mount a durable effective adaptive immune response to HIV antigens has been a major challenge in creating an effective HIV vaccine.

HIV escape mechanisms. Most HIV-infected patients develop disease progression in spite of evidence of a strong antiviral antibody and CTL responses. Loss of immunologic recognition or *immune escape* results in increased viral replication and is the best predictor of progression to AIDS within the first 5 years of infection. Multiple factors contribute to HIV escape from the immune response; the most predominant is the HIV mutation rate that is many-folds faster than what is observed in most other viruses. The error rate of HIV reverse transcriptase is about 1 in 10^4 base pairs or approximately one new nucleotide per new virion. This high mutation rate coupled with the 10^9 new virions produced each day results in a high degree of genetic variability within the replicating pool of viruses. Viruses that have mutations in CTL and antibody epitopes have a selective advantage for ongoing replication. As HIV replicates, it alters its coreceptor use allowing it to expand its coreceptor use. In many patients with advanced disease, the predominant replicating virus utilizes CXCR4 and replicates most effectively in T cells.

HIV causes downregulation of HLA-A and HLA-B expression without affecting the expression of HLA-C and HLA-E. allowing infected cells to evade detection by CTL. This mechanism does not impact NK cells. Humoral immune responses are relatively inefficient in eliminating viral-infected cells. The highly glycosylated variable regions in gp120V1 and V2 *shield* the most effective immunodominant antibody epitopes directed at the CD4 binding domains.

CD4 T cell depletion and viral persistence. Ongoing viral replication leads to progressive decline in the numbers and percentages of CD4T cells (Figure 30.6). The principal T-cell population lost is memory CD4 CD45RO$^+$ T cells. Total T-cell depletion is directly correlated with the degree of immunosuppression and risk for AIDS-associated opportunistic infections in infected patients. Several factors account for the depletion of CD4$^+$ T cells. The primary mechanisms are direct cytotoxicity caused by virus replication and cross-linking of CD4 by gp120 that primes T lymphocytes for apoptosis. In spite of the relatively short life of an HIV-infected T cell, persistent replication of

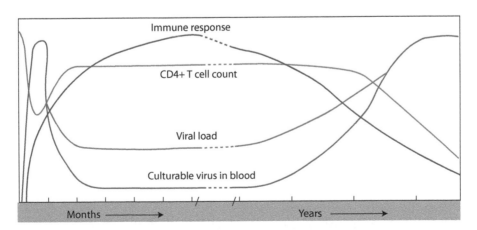

Figure 30.6 Longitudinal evolution of laboratory parameters during the course of an untreated HIV infection. (Adapted from Saag, M.S. et al., *Nat. Med.*, 2, 625, 1996.)

competent provirus within latent memory T cells is a major determinant factor in the failure of effective ART to eradicate latent reservoirs in lymphoid tissues and the central nervous system (CNS). Virus can persist because HIV peptides are not expressed on resting cells; thus, they are not CTL or antibody targets. However, even with optimal suppression, latently infected cells are able to produce new virus when activated. Latently infected memory T cells persist for decades, which is why in spite of millions of HIV infections worldwide, cure has been elusive.

Other factors contributing to AIDS-associated immune suppression. Several other factors beyond the depletion of CD4T cells seem to contribute to the state of marked immune dysregulation evident prior to development of AlDS. HIV infection also adversely impacts immune regulation through the depletion of regulatory T cells and Th17T cells that constitutively express CD4. HIV also has a direct effect on B-cell function leading to chronic B-cell activation, loss of memory B cells, hypergammaglobulinemia, and dysgammaglobulinemia resulting in increased susceptibility to bacterial infections.

Clinical history of HIV infection

As early as 5–10 days after infection, viral mRNA can be detected in the plasma, peaking at 10–20 days after infection. Seroconversion, when enzyme-linked immunosorbent assay (ELISA) or Western blot can detect HIV antibodies, does not occur until 4–6 weeks postinfection, resulting in a window of time in which an infected individual will test negative but be highly infectious due to high viral loads. CTL activation is evident by elevated CD8 T cell numbers resulting in an inverted CD4/CD8 T-cell ratio. As antibody and CTL responses control viral replication, a steady-state viral set point is reached. Without ART, most HIV-infected patients will develop AlDS. The following is a summary of clinical stages of HIV infection:

- **Acute retroviral infection**: In most cases, patients experience a mononucleosis-like illness with fever and adenopathy, viral RNA is detectable in the blood using PCR-based assays. HIV ELISA and Western blot are initially negative.
- **Asymptomatic infection**: Minimal symptoms with the exception of the presence of

lymphadenopathy, viral load has dropped to set point levels, ELISA and Western blot are positive. Blood CD4 T-cell counts are generally in the normal range (Centers for Disease Control and Prevention [CDC] stage A).
- **Symptomatic infection**: Increasingly symptomatic; chronic non-life-threatening infections; CD4 T cells decline, early signs of pathogen-driven malignancies (CDC stage B).
- **Advanced infection**: High risk for opportunistic infections, wasting syndrome, AIDS (CDC stage C).

ACUTE ILLNESS ASSOCIATED WITH SEROCONVERSION (ACUTE RETROVIRAL SYNDROME)

The period of acute viral infection can result in *acute retroviral syndrome* during the first 2–6 weeks between exposure and onset of symptoms. Clinical symptoms can include fever, malaise, myalgia, and headache as commonly seen in acute infectious mononucleosis or influenza infection. Other symptoms include fever, sore throat, myalgia, swollen lymph nodes, enlarged spleen, and a maculopapular rash as the most predominant symptoms. Although these symptoms occur often, almost 30% of patients have not reported symptoms at all. Most newly infected individuals do not seek medical care. Less frequently presenting symptoms include acute hepatitis or aseptic meningitis. Most patients recover completely from the acute infection, although adenopathy may persist.

ASYMPTOMATIC INFECTION

Following acute infection, the majority of HIV-infected patients enter a period of clinical latency with relatively few symptoms. Lasting in some cases for decades, even in untreated patients, the duration of this period is directly associated with viral load and CD4 T-cell counts. However, virus is actively replicating and patients are infectious to others. The CDC classifies this time as category A, based on minimal symptoms; CD4 counts can vary, but almost all patients have an inverted CD4/CD8 T-cell ratio.

EARLY SYMPTOMATIC HIV INFECTION

Eventually the CD4 T-cell count declines and symptomatic disease emerges. During the early symptomatic phase, CDC category B, constitutional symptoms including fevers, night sweats, fatigue, chronic diarrhea, and headache are common. Clinical symptoms of oral candidiasis, herpes zoster (shingles), thrombocytopenia, pelvic and rectal abscesses, and peripheral neuropathy are among the conditions seen during this disease stage. CD4 counts are generally in the 200–500 cells/µL range. During asymptomatic HIV infection coinfections such as syphilis, hepatitis B, and tuberculosis can accelerate HIV progression. Similarly, HIV infection often results in reactivation of latent tuberculosis. Coinfection with human papillomaviruses (HPVs) and increased risk for the development of cervical and anal carcinoma is common.

Late-stage symptomatic infection/AIDS

The late stages of HIV disease are characterized by severe life-threatening opportunistic infections and CD4 T cells below 200 cells/µL. Disseminated infections and malignancies such as Kaposi's sarcoma, lymphoma, and HPV-associated carcinoma can occur. With the progressive decline of CD4 T-cell counts, the risk for development of opportunistic infections increases. The onset of opportunistic infections is considered as the clinical hallmark for diagnosis of AIDS. The designation of AIDS is applied when an HIV-infected individual develops clinical advanced symptoms or has CD4 T-cell counts <200 cells/µL.

Opportunistic infections are defined as infections that generally do not cause life-threatening disease in an immune-competent host but can be severe or fatal in an immune-compromised host. A list of the most common opportunistic infections associated with AIDS is shown in Table 30.3. Many of these infections such as *Pneumocystis jirovecii* pneumonia and *Mycobacterium avium-intracellulare* can be prevented if chemoprophylaxis is given when CD4 T-cell counts fall below 200/µl. Opportunistic infections with fungal and parasitic pathogens such as invasive candidiasis, cryptosporidiosis, toxoplasmosis, and invasive aspergillosis are AIDS-defining illnesses.

In addition to opportunistic infections, AIDS patients have a higher morbidity and mortality when infected by pathogens not considered as opportunistic, such as recurrent bacterial pneumonia or pulmonary tuberculosis. Recurrent bacterial infections are the most common infectious presentation of HIV-infected infants and children. Specific neoplastic diseases, such as Kaposi's sarcoma, AIDS-related lymphoma, and HPV-associated invasive cervical and anal carcinoma are also hallmarks of AIDS.

AIDS-related lymphoma is a consequence of combined long-term stimulation and proliferation of B cells caused by HIV itself in combination with reactivation of Epstein–Barr virus (EBV) infection as T-immunity wanes. Translocations involving chromosomes 8 and 14, as well as overexpression of

Table 30.3 Opportunistic infections characteristically associated with AIDS

- *Pneumocystis carinii* (*jirovecii*) pneumonia
- Chronic cryptosporidiosis or isosporiasis causing untractable diarrhea
- Toxoplasmosis
- Extraintestinal strongyloidosis
- Candidiasis (oral candidiasis is common as a prodromal manifestation and is considered as a marker of progression toward AIDS; esophageal, bronchial, and pulmonary candidiasis are pathognomonic)
- Cryptococcosis
- Histoplasmosis
- Infections caused by atypical Mycobacteria, such as *M. avium intracellulare*
- Pulmonary and extrapulmonary tuberculosis (often resistant to therapy)
- Disseminated cytomegalovirus infection (may affect the retina and cause blindness)
- Disseminated herpes simplex infection
- Multidermatomal herpes zoster
- Recurrent *Salmonella* bacteremia
- Progressive multifocal leukoencephalopathy
- Invasive nocardiosis

EBV's LMP-1 are often detected in these lymphomas. The prognosis in patients with AIDS-related lymphoma is related to absolute CD4 T-cell counts, with the lowest counts ($<100/\mu L$) having the worst prognosis. Kaposi's sarcoma is caused by a virus of the herpes family (human herpes virus 8, HHV-8). Infections with this virus in HIV-positive patients seem to be associated with exaggerated release of IL-6, IL-1, TNF, and oncostatin M by activated macrophages, which would act synergistically in promoting the development of the vascular proliferative lesions typical of the tumor. The frequency of Kaposi's sarcoma has decreased after introduction of effective therapeutic modalities.

HIV is a neurotropic virus, and neurocognitive disorders such as encephalopathy (dementia) and progressive multifocal leukoencephalopathy (due to reactivation of an infection with the JC virus) are AIDS-defining illnesses. HIV-infected individuals are also susceptible to invasive CNS infections such as cryptococcal meningitis, HSV encephalitis, CNS toxoplasmosis, and bacterial meningitis.

Other HIV-related conditions are not directly related to coinfections. These include cardiomyopathy, nephropathy (which may progress to renal failure), bone marrow suppression, and peripheral neuropathy. Chronic hepatitis B or C in HIV-infected patients has faster rates of progression to hepatic failure and cirrhosis and poorer response to therapy.

As a direct result of microbial translocation and macrophage activation though TLR4, HIV infection becomes a chronic inflammatory state. Clinical manifestations include higher rates of cardiovascular disease such as myocardial infarction and stroke (three- to fivefold higher rates than in HIV-uninfected individuals with similar risk factors). Other clinical manifestations of chronic macrophage activation include HIV-associated osteopenia and associated higher bone fracture risk, metabolic syndrome manifest by type II diabetes, and neurocognitive decline due to macrophage activation that persists even when viral replication is optimally controlled by ART.

Long-term nonprogression and HIV cure. In spite of millions of individuals infected and multiple treatments to delay disease progression, an HIV cure has been elusive. There are many factors known to delay disease progression, even without treatment. The genetics of CTL responses against viral epitopes have a major influence on disease progression. Population genetics show that the HLA B region plays the dominant role in determining which patients develop AIDS in less than a year and which do not progress for decades. Genetic changes in HIV receptors may play a major role in determining both susceptibility to initial infection and disease progression. Individuals with a homozygous CCR5Δ32 mutation are less likely to become infected, even with repeated exposure. Individuals with heterozygous CCR5Δ32 mutations that become infected tend to be slow progressors. The only patient with a presumed HIV cure has been a patient in Berlin, Germany, who received a bone marrow transplant for a malignancy from a homozygous CCR5Δ32 mutation donor. This patient has been off ART for many years and has not shown signs of viral replication of disease progression. Patients who are on effective ART who have undetectable replicating virus in the plasma still harbor virus in latent reservoirs. Virus rebounds when ART is interrupted, but the timing of rebound varies, and some patients have not shown evidence of viral replication up to a year after stopping therapy. The major source of latently infected cells is in resting, nondividing, memory CD4 T cells and dendritic within the lymphoid tissues, with the CNS as another source of latent virus.

Pediatric HIV infection

The most common route of HIV infection in children is through maternal-to-child transmission, although prior to the screening of blood products, many children, like adults, became infected through blood transfusions and HIV-contaminated blood products such as Factor VIII in the case of patients with hemophilia. Mother-to-child transmission can occur *in utero*, intrapartum, or through breastfeeding. In the absence of ART to prevent infection, intrapartum transmission is most common. Mothers with high viral load due to advanced disease or during acute infection are most likely to transmit HIV to their infants. Prior to ART prophylaxis, breastfeeding accounted for 5%–12% of cases, but with implementation of ART this has become less prevalent. Even in the absence of ART, only about a third of infants born to HIV-infected mothers become infected.

Due to transplacental transfer of IgG, virtually all infants born to HIV-infected mothers will test positive based on ELISA and Western blot. In uninfected infants, these antibodies will wane by 12 months of age, and the child will be antibody negative. Detection of infected infants requires the use of antigen-based detection methods such as the quantitative PCR to detect viral RNA or PCR-based methods to detect proviral DNA in peripheral blood. Similar to adults, the rate of disease progression varies in children based on HLA types and coinfections. Children infected *in utero* tend to have more rapid disease infection. Children also show more severe CNS involvement and have more severe morbidity with common bacterial infections such as pneumococcal disease when compared to HIV-infected adults.

Laboratory diagnosis and monitoring of HIV infection

The best rapid test for initial screening is the application of assays to detect HIV antibodies. There are several rapid and standardized enzyme-linked immunoassay tests that have high sensitivity and specificity for infection. These screening tests are used effectively to screen blood donors and are cost effective, so they can be applied to screen large at-risk populations. Confirmatory testing using the more specific Western blot (immunoblot) detects antibodies to specific HIV proteins. A Western blot is considered positive if antibodies to structural proteins (e.g., p24), enzymes (gp41), and envelope glycoproteins (gp41 or gp120) are simultaneously detected. The sensitivity and specificity of the combined ELISA and Western blot assays is over 99.5%.

Direct detection of HIV-1 is performed quantitatively by PCR to detect viral RNA in plasma. These assays can detect as low as 20 viral copies/μL. Patients on effective ART have viral copies below the level of detection (<40 copies/μL) but remain infected and capable of transmitting virus to others. HIV proviral DNA or cell-associated virus can be detected using a nonquantitative PCR assay that detects viral DNA. These assays are used to monitor viral levels in patients being treated with ART, to detect virus acute infection, prior to seroconversion, and to detect infected infants who test positive by ELISA due to passive maternal antibody. Monitoring disease progression also involves periodic assessment of CD4 T-cell counts using flow cytometry for both their number and percentage in the blood.

Treatment of HIV

ART agents are used in combination to impair multiple steps in the viral life cycle (Figure 30.4). This treatment strategy is similar to using multiple agents to treat malignancy or tuberculosis. The current treatment of HIV infection involves a combination of agents classified according to their viral primary targets and steps in the viral replication. Drugs vary in their potency, half-life, and side effects.

Reverse transcriptase inhibitors are subclassified into different categories based on their mechanism of action. **Nucleoside analogs**, such as zidovudine (azidodideoxythymidine, ZDV), zalcitabine (2', 3'-dideoxycytidine, ddC), didanosine (2', 3'-dideoxyinosine, ddI), stavudine (2'3'-didehydro-3'deoxythymidine, d4T), lamivudine (2'-deoxy-3'-thiacytidine, 3TC), emtricitabine (FTC), and abacavir are phosphorylated by cellular thymidine kinases and taken up preferentially by the HIV reverse transcriptase. **Nucleotide analogs**, such as tenofovir disoproxil and tenofovir alafenamide, are similar to nucleoside analogs in that both agents terminate DNA elongation upon incorporation into nascent DNA chains. Tenofovir and FTC have long half-lives and can be administered once daily. These agents are equally effective against HIV-1 and HIV-2. **Nonnucleoside reverse transcriptase inhibitors (NNRTIs)**, such as nevirapine, delavirdine, and efavirenz, bind to a hydrophobic pocket of the reverse transcriptase at a site different from active site to block the enzymatic activity by steric hindrance. These agents are highly effective in inhibiting HIV replication and viral load falls within hours after initial administration. Because of the different binding sites, strains of HIV resistant to nucleoside reverse transcriptase inhibitors are not cross-resistant to NNRTIs. However, mutations within reverse transcriptase changing a single amino acid can confer resistance to the entire class of NNRTIs.

Entry inhibitors block viral binding to CCR5 or impair penetration mediated by gp41. Enfurtivide is a synthetic peptide that blocks the interaction of gp41 with the plasma membrane. Its use is constrained because it requires drug delivery by injection. Maraviroc is a negative allosteric modulator of the CCR5 that binds to this coreceptor blocking the binding of HIV gp120.

Protease inhibitors are nonhydrolyzable synthetic peptides that compete as substrates for the HIV protease. HIV-infected cells exposed to these compounds accumulate gag polyprotein precursors that remain uncleaved due to the inhibition of the protease activity, resulting in noninfectious virions. Currently approved protease inhibitors include amprenavir, atazanavir, darunavir, fosamprenavir, indinavir, lopinavir, nelfinavir, ritonavir, saquinavir, and tipranavir, all of which vary in their half-lives and side effects. Most protease inhibitors cause hyperlipidemia, glucose intolerance, and lipodystrophy. However, these agents are also highly effective in inhibiting viral replication, and unlike NNRTIs, multiple amino acid substitutions are required for the development of drug resistance.

Integrase inhibitors or integrase strand inhibitors (INSTIs) are the newest class of ART, targeting the integrase enzyme that incorporates the proviral DNA into the T-cell genome. Currently approved INSTIs include dolutegravir, elvitegravir, and raltegravir, with long-acting (>1 month) injectable agents in development. These agents have better toxicity profiles than many other antivirals and are less prone to the development of drug resistance.

Combination therapy (cART). Most first-line HIV treatment protocols involve combinations of NRTI or NNRIT plus one highly active agent such as an NNRTI, PI, or integrase inhibitor. The rationale for the association is to combine nucleoside analogs that require different HIV mutations for drug resistance to develop. The probability of emergence of a double mutant polymerase retaining functional activity is relatively low. cART lowers viral load very rapidly with a 2–3 log10 reduction with 1–2 days of initiating treatment and a phase II decline to undetectable (<40 copies/μL) by 4–6 weeks of treatment. With good adherence to therapy, most patients can achieve and sustain control of viral replication between 12 and 24 weeks. Current treatment calls for all patients to start cART at the time of diagnosis. Waiting to initiate treatment results in higher viral levels and lower CD4 T-cell counts, increasing the risk for treatment failure. More importantly, low viral levels reduce the likelihood of transmission to an uninfected individual. Since viral replication is necessary for the generation of new mutations, effective viral suppression does not lead to the emergence of drug resistance.

Immune reconstitution of CD4 T cells coincides with reduction in viral load. This is a biphasic process with initial increases in CD4 CD45RO memory T cells followed by a slow increase in naïve CD4 CD45RA T cells. As expected, naïve T-cell reconstitution is greater in children than adults. In patients with advanced disease and coinfections with CMV or tuberculosis, an acute severe immune reconstitution inflammatory syndrome (IRIS) often develops during the early phase of immune reconstitution. These coinfections can be prevented by optimal treatment prior to starting cART. cART results in improved immune function as treated patients have better responses to vaccines and higher T-cell mitogenic response. However. cART does not result in reversal of macrophage activation, as levels of sCD14 and plasma LPS levels remain elevated even after years of effective cART. While cART reduces the viral load to undetectable levels, HIV-specific CD4 and CD8 responses remain depressed. Periodic interruptions of antiretroviral therapy were initially performed to allow for a burst of HIV replication to induce specific immunity, but larger-scale clinical trials show that this strategy resulted in increased morbidity and mortality.

Combination antiretroviral therapy has had a dramatic impact on the HIV epidemic changing HIV from a lethal disease to a chronic condition requiring life-long treatment but with a relatively normal quality of life and life expectancy. The establishment of the President's Emergency Plan for AIDS Relief (PEPFAR) and the Global Fund to Fight AIDS have brought resources to sub-Saharan Africa and other regions of the world hit hardest by the epidemic. As a result, the goal to have 90% of infected individuals know their HIV status, 90% on therapy, and 90% have undetectable viral levels is feasible in the next 10 years if funding continues.

HIV prevention

In the absence of a cure, prevention of infection offers the best hope to stop the HIV epidemic. ART has been shown to be highly effective in preventing mother-to-child transmission. Although not all antivirals are appropriate for infants or pregnant women, certain cART combinations reduce transmission risk from >30% to <1% when cART is administered during pregnancy, during labor, and after delivery. It is not practical to administer cART to infants, so transmission through breastfeeding still results in nearly 100,000 newly infected infant infections per year worldwide. Based on the success of ART to protect the fetus and newborn from infection, preexposure prophylaxis (PrEP) is also effective in protecting uninfected individuals from HIV acquisition when their sexual partner is infected. Postexposure prophylaxis is effective in preventing HIV acquisition after sexual exposure and accidental needle sticks in the health-care setting.

Recently, broadly neutralizing monoclonal antibodies with prolonged half-lives have been developed which target conserved regions of HIV such as the membrane proximal region of gp41 and the CD4 binding site for gp120. These monoclonals share unique characteristics of long CDR3 lengths and have high hydrophobicity. They are administered as injectable agents to individuals at high risk for acquisition such as HIV discordant couples and breastfeeding infants of HIV-infected mothers.

Nonpharmacologic means of preventing HIV infection are simple and cost effective. Public campaigns to raise awareness of HIV infection to promote the use of male and female condoms are highly effective when appropriately targeted. Male circumcision reduces the risk of heterosexual transmission significantly. Delivering newborns by elective C-section in high-risk untreated mothers reduces the risk of transmission to the newborn.

HIV vaccines

The development of an effective HIV vaccine has been elusive since the epidemic was first recognized. HIV evolution to evade immunity is a major barrier to development of an infective vaccine. Therapeutic vaccines have been tested in humans and nonhuman primates to enhance the cellular and humoral responses within infected patients. The focus has been to identify conserved CTL targets to better control or eradicate infected cells. So far, this strategy had been ineffective in restoring or enhancing cellular immune responses in patients who have undergone treatment interruption.

Vaccines to prevent acquisition have been an even greater challenge. Recombinant viral particles made by inserting HIV glycoprotein genes in vaccinia virus or canary poxvirus genomes, for example, have been shown to induce neutralizing antibodies in both human and nonhuman primates. A vaccine trial testing a strategy to prime with a canary pox vector and three genetically engineered HIV genes (env, gag, and pol) termed ALVAC HIV (vCP1521), followed by a boost with an engineered gp120 protein (AIDSVAX B/E) has shown promise for providing protection to humans. Correlates of protection mapped to antibodies to variable regions 1 (V1) and 2 (V2). These studies provide promising evidence that an effective vaccine could be developed.

BIBLIOGRAPHY

Andiman WA. Transmission of HIV-1 from mother to infant. *Curr Opin Pediatr.* 2002;14:78–85.

Bourke CD, Berkley JA, Prendergast AJ. Immune dysfunction as a cause and consequence of malnutrition. *Trends Immunol.* 2016;37:386–398.

Brand J-M, Kirchner H, Poppe C, Schmucker P. The effects of general anesthesia on human peripheral immune cell distribution and cytokine production. *Clin Immun Immunopath.* 1997; 83:190–194.

Chandrasekaran P, Saravanan N, Bethunaickan R, Tripathy S. Malnutrition: Modulator of immune responses in tuberculosis. *Front Immunol.* 2017 Oct 18;8:1316. doi: 10.3389/fimmu.2017.01316.

Cunningham-Rundles S, McNeeley DF, Moon A. Mechanisms of nutrient modulation of the immune response. *J Allergy Clin Immunol.* 2005;115:1119–1128.

Dahabieh MS, Battivelli E, Verdin E. Understanding HIV latency: The road to an HIV cure. *Annu Rev Med.* 2015;66:407–421.

Department of Health and Human Services (DHHS) Panel on Antiretroviral Guidelines for Adults and Adolescents. *Guidelines for the Use of Antiretroviral Agents in HIV-1-Infected Adults and Adolescents.* Department of Health and Human Services; 2017. Available from: http://aidsinfo.nih.gov/ContentFiles/Adultand AdolescentGL.pdf

Fauci AS. HIV reservoirs as obstacles and opportunities for an HIV cure. *Nat Immunol.* 2015;16: 584–589.

Field CJ, Johnson IR, Schley PD. Nutrients and their role in host resistance to infection. *J Leukoc Biol.* 2002;71:16–32.

Friedman H, Eisenstein TK. Neurological basis of drug dependence and its effects on the immune system. *J Neuroimmunol.* 2004;147:106–108.

Harris BH, Gelfand JA. The immune response to trauma. *Semin Pediatr Surg*. 1995;4:77–82.

Kerdiles YM, Sellin CI, Druelle J, Horvat B. Immunosuppression caused by measles virus: Role of viral proteins. *Rev Med Virol*. 2006;16: 49–63.

Kurts C, Panzer U, Anders HJ, Rees AJ. The immune system and kidney disease: Basic concepts and clinical implications. *Nat Rev Immunol*. 2013; 13:738–775.

Lafeuillade A. Eliminating the HIV reservoir. *Curr HIV/AIDS Rep*. 2012;9:121–131.

Migueles SA, Sabbaghian MS, Shupert WL et al. HLA B*5701 is highly associated with restriction of virus replication in a subgroup of HIV-infected long term nonprogressors. *Proc Nat Acad Sci USA*. 2000;97:2709–2714.

O'Connell R J, Kim JH, Excler JL. The HIV-1 gp120V1V2 loop: Structure, function and importance for vaccine development. *Expert Rev Vaccines*. 2014;13:1489–1500.

Pavia CS, La Mothe M, Kavanagh M. Influence of alcohol on antimicrobial immunity. *Biomed Pharmacother*. 2004;58:84–89.

Schwacha MG. Macrophages and post-burn immune dysfunction. *Burns* 2003;29:1–14.

Sleasman JW, Goodenow MG. HIV. *J Allergy Clin Immunol*. 2003;111:S582–S592.

Stenvinkel P, Ketteler M, Johnson RJ et al. IL-10, IL-6, and TNF-α: Central factors in the altered cytokine network of uremia—The good, the bad, and the ugly. *Kidney Int*. 2005;67:1216–1233.

Walker B, McMichael A. The T-cell response to HIV. *Cold Spring Harb Perspect Med*. 2012;2(11). doi: 10.1101/cshperspect.a007054. www.cdc.gov/hiv/statistics/surveillance/terms.html; Terms, Definitions, and Calculations Used in CDC HIV Surveillance Publications, 2018.

Index

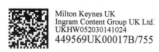

9 781032 087771